Food Safety, Security, Sustainability and Nutrition as Priority Objectives of the Food Sector

Food Safety, Security, Sustainability and Nutrition as Priority Objectives of the Food Sector

Editors

António Raposo
Fernando Ramos
Dele Raheem
Ariana Saraiva
Conrado Javier Carrascosa Iruzubieta

MDPI • Basel • Beijing • Wuhan • Barcelona • Belgrade • Manchester • Tokyo • Cluj • Tianjin

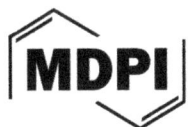

Editors

António Raposo
CBIOS Research Center for
Biosciences and Health
Technologies
Universidade Lusófona de
Humanidades e Tecnologias
Lisboa
Portugal

Fernando Ramos
Pharmacy Faculty
University of Coimbra
Coimbra
Portugal

Dele Raheem
Northern Institute for
Environmental and Minority
Law (NIEM), Arctic Centre
University of Lapland
Rovaniemi
Finland

Ariana Saraiva
Department of Animal
Pathology and Production,
Bromatology and Food
Technology
Universidad de Las Palmas
de Gran Canaria
Arucas
Spain

Conrado Javier Carrascosa
Iruzubieta
Department of Animal
Pathology and Production,
Bromatology and Food
Technology
Universidad de Las Palmas
de Gran Canaria
Arucas
Spain

Editorial Office
MDPI
St. Alban-Anlage 66
4052 Basel, Switzerland

This is a reprint of articles from the Special Issue published online in the open access journal *International Journal of Environmental Research and Public Health* (ISSN 1660-4601) (available at: www.mdpi.com/journal/ijerph/special_issues/priority_food).

For citation purposes, cite each article independently as indicated on the article page online and as indicated below:

LastName, A.A.; LastName, B.B.; LastName, C.C. Article Title. *Journal Name* **Year**, *Volume Number*, Page Range.

ISBN 978-3-0365-2290-6 (Hbk)
ISBN 978-3-0365-2289-0 (PDF)

© 2021 by the authors. Articles in this book are Open Access and distributed under the Creative Commons Attribution (CC BY) license, which allows users to download, copy and build upon published articles, as long as the author and publisher are properly credited, which ensures maximum dissemination and a wider impact of our publications.

The book as a whole is distributed by MDPI under the terms and conditions of the Creative Commons license CC BY-NC-ND.

Contents

About the Editors ix

Preface to "Food Safety, Security, Sustainability and Nutrition as Priority Objectives of the Food Sector" xi

António Raposo, Fernando Ramos, Dele Raheem, Ariana Saraiva and Conrado Carrascosa
Food Safety, Security, Sustainability and Nutrition as Priority Objectives of the Food Sector
Reprinted from: *Int. J. Environ. Res. Public Health* **2021**, *18*, 8073, doi:10.3390/ijerph18158073 . . . 1

Ariana Saraiva, Conrado Carrascosa, Dele Raheem, Fernando Ramos and António Raposo
Maltitol: Analytical Determination Methods, Applications in the Food Industry, Metabolism and Health Impacts
Reprinted from: *Int. J. Environ. Res. Public Health* **2020**, *17*, 5227, doi:10.3390/ijerph17145227 . . . 5

Ariana Saraiva, Conrado Carrascosa, Dele Raheem, Fernando Ramos and António Raposo
Natural Sweeteners: The Relevance of Food Naturalness for Consumers, Food Security Aspects, Sustainability and Health Impacts
Reprinted from: *Int. J. Environ. Res. Public Health* **2020**, *17*, 6285, doi:10.3390/ijerph17176285 . . . 33

Conrado Carrascosa, Dele Raheem, Fernando Ramos, Ariana Saraiva and António Raposo
Microbial Biofilms in the Food Industry—A Comprehensive Review
Reprinted from: *Int. J. Environ. Res. Public Health* **2021**, *18*, 2014, doi:10.3390/ijerph18042014 . . . 55

Dele Raheem, Conrado Carrascosa, Fernando Ramos, Ariana Saraiva and António Raposo
Texture-Modified Food for Dysphagic Patients: A Comprehensive Review
Reprinted from: *Int. J. Environ. Res. Public Health* **2021**, *18*, 5125, doi:10.3390/ijerph18105125 . . . 87

Jianming Wang, Ninh Nguyen and Xiangzhi Bu
Exploring the Roles of Green Food Consumption and Social Trust in the Relationship between Perceived Consumer Effectiveness and Psychological Wellbeing
Reprinted from: *Int. J. Environ. Res. Public Health* **2020**, *17*, 4676, doi:10.3390/ijerph17134676 . . . 111

Elena Bogdanova, Sergei Andronov, Ildiko Asztalos Morell, Kamrul Hossain, Dele Raheem, Praskovia Filant and Andrey Lobanov
Food Sovereignty of the Indigenous Peoples in the Arctic Zone of Western Siberia: Response to COVID-19 Pandemic
Reprinted from: *Int. J. Environ. Res. Public Health* **2020**, *17*, 7570, doi:10.3390/ijerph17207570 . . . 125

Longji Hu, Rongjin Liu, Wei Zhang and Tian Zhang
The Effects of Epistemic Trust and Social Trust on Public Acceptance of Genetically Modified Food: An Empirical Study from China
Reprinted from: *Int. J. Environ. Res. Public Health* **2020**, *17*, 7700, doi:10.3390/ijerph17207700 . . . 143

Rachel A. Cassinat, Meg Bruening, Noe C. Crespo, Mónica Gutiérrez, Adrian Chavez, Frank Ray and Sonia Vega-López
Effects of a Community-Based Pilot Intervention on Home Food Availability among U.S. Households
Reprinted from: *Int. J. Environ. Res. Public Health* **2020**, *17*, 8327, doi:10.3390/ijerph17228327 . . . 163

Laura Piombo, Gianluca Nicolella, Giulia Barbarossa, Claudio Tubili, Mayme Mary Pandolfo, Miriam Castaldo, Gianfranco Costanzo, Concetta Mirisola and Andrea Cavani
Outcomes of Culturally Tailored Dietary Intervention in the North African and Bangladeshi Diabetic Patients in Italy
Reprinted from: *Int. J. Environ. Res. Public Health* **2020**, *17*, 8932, doi:10.3390/ijerph17238932 . . . **175**

Yen-Cheng Chen and Hsiang-Chun Lin
Exploring Effective Sensory Experience in the Environmental Design of Sustainable Cafés
Reprinted from: *Int. J. Environ. Res. Public Health* **2020**, *17*, 8957, doi:10.3390/ijerph17238957 . . . **187**

Chunshan Zhou, Rongrong Zhang, Xiaoju Ning and Zhicheng Zheng
Spatial-Temporal Characteristics in Grain Production and Its Influencing Factors in the Huang-Huai-Hai Plain from 1995 to 2018
Reprinted from: *Int. J. Environ. Res. Public Health* **2020**, *17*, 9193, doi:10.3390/ijerph17249193 . . . **203**

Sónia Pedreiro, Sandrine da Ressurreição, Maria Lopes, Maria Teresa Cruz, Teresa Batista, Artur Figueirinha and Fernando Ramos
Crepis vesicaria L. subsp. *taraxacifolia* Leaves: Nutritional Profile, Phenolic Composition and Biological Properties
Reprinted from: *Int. J. Environ. Res. Public Health* **2020**, *18*, 151, doi:10.3390/ijerph18010151 . . . **223**

Ingrid C. Fideles, Rita de Cassia Coelho de Almeida Akutsu, Rosemary da Rocha Fonseca Barroso, Jamacy Costa-Souza, Renata Puppin Zandonadi, António Raposo and Raquel Braz Assunção Botelho
Food Insecurity among Low-Income Food Handlers: A Nationwide Study in Brazilian Community Restaurants
Reprinted from: *Int. J. Environ. Res. Public Health* **2021**, *18*, 1160, doi:10.3390/ijerph18031160 . . . **239**

Mackenzie J. Ferrante, Juliana Goldsmith, Sara Tauriello, Leonard H. Epstein, Lucia A. Leone and Stephanie Anzman-Frasca
Food Acquisition and Daily Life for U.S. Families with 4- to 8-Year-Old Children during COVID-19: Findings from a Nationally Representative Survey
Reprinted from: *Int. J. Environ. Res. Public Health* **2021**, *18*, 1734, doi:10.3390/ijerph18041734 . . . **255**

Zabihollah Nemati, Zahra Moradi, Kazem Alirezalu, Maghsoud Besharati and António Raposo
Impact of Ginger Root Powder Dietary Supplement on Productive Performance, Egg Quality, Antioxidant Status and Blood Parameters in Laying Japanese Quails
Reprinted from: *Int. J. Environ. Res. Public Health* **2021**, *18*, 2995, doi:10.3390/ijerph18062995 . . . **269**

Heesup Han, Linda Heejung Lho, António Raposo, Aleksandar Radic and Abdul Hafaz Ngah
Halal Food Performance and Its Influence on Patron Retention Process at Tourism Destination
Reprinted from: *Int. J. Environ. Res. Public Health* **2021**, *18*, 3034, doi:10.3390/ijerph18063034 . . . **283**

Adele Evans, Anthony J. Slate, I. Devine Akhidime, Joanna Verran, Peter J. Kelly and Kathryn A. Whitehead
The Removal of Meat Exudate and *Escherichia coli* from Stainless Steel and Titanium Surfaces with Irregular and Regular Linear Topographies
Reprinted from: *Int. J. Environ. Res. Public Health* **2021**, *18*, 3198, doi:10.3390/ijerph18063198 . . . **297**

Carmen Rubio-Armendáriz, Soraya Paz, Ángel J. Gutiérrez, Verena Gomes Furtado, Dailos González-Weller, Consuelo Revert and Arturo Hardisson
Toxic Metals in Cereals in Cape Verde: Risk Assessment Evaluation
Reprinted from: *Int. J. Environ. Res. Public Health* **2021**, *18*, 3833, doi:10.3390/ijerph18073833 . . . **313**

Ashleigh Domingo, Kerry-Ann Charles, Michael Jacobs, Deborah Brooker and Rhona M. Hanning
Indigenous Community Perspectives of Food Security, Sustainable Food Systems and Strategies to Enhance Access to Local and Traditional Healthy Food for Partnering Williams Treaties First Nations (Ontario, Canada)
Reprinted from: *Int. J. Environ. Res. Public Health* **2021**, *18*, 4404, doi:10.3390/ijerph18094404 . . . **325**

Hongyu Wang, Xiaolei Wang, Apurbo Sarkar and Fuhong Zhang
How Capital Endowment and Ecological Cognition Affect Environment-Friendly Technology Adoption: A Case of Apple Farmers of Shandong Province, China
Reprinted from: *Int. J. Environ. Res. Public Health* **2021**, *18*, 7571, doi:10.3390/ijerph18147571 . . . **341**

Lluís Serra-Majem, Laura Tomaino, Sandro Dernini, Elliot M. Berry, Denis Lairon, Joy Ngo de la Cruz, Anna Bach-Faig, Lorenzo M. Donini, Francesc-Xavier Medina, Rekia Belahsen, Suzanne Piscopo, Roberto Capone, Javier Aranceta-Bartrina, Carlo La Vecchia and Antonia Trichopoulou
Updating the Mediterranean Diet Pyramid towards Sustainability: Focus on Environmental Concerns
Reprinted from: *Int. J. Environ. Res. Public Health* **2020**, *17*, 8758, doi:10.3390/ijerph17238758 . . . **357**

Walter Willett
Mediterranean Dietary Pyramid
Reprinted from: *Int. J. Environ. Res. Public Health* **2021**, *18*, 4568, doi:10.3390/ijerph18094568 . . . **377**

Maria Luz Fernandez, Dele Raheem, Fernando Ramos, Conrado Carrascosa, Ariana Saraiva and António Raposo
Highlights of Current Dietary Guidelines in Five Continents
Reprinted from: *Int. J. Environ. Res. Public Health* **2021**, *18*, 2814, doi:10.3390/ijerph18062814 . . . **379**

About the Editors

António Raposo

António Raposo is Assistant Professor at Lusófona University and he is an Integrated Member of CBIOS.

He graduated in Nutritional Sciences from Egas Moniz Higher Institute of Health Science, Portugal, in 2009, and obtained his Ph.D. with European Mention in Animal Health and Food Safety from the University of Las Palmas de Gran Canaria, Spain, 2013.

His main research interests are Studies on the utilization of *Catostylus tagi* jellyfish in health sciences, particularly as a food ingredient, food habits, food safety evaluation, food innovation, natural food products, food security, and sustainability.

He is a member of the editorial board of relevant international peer-reviewed journals in his research field. He has published more than 55 papers in indexed JCR journals, as well as scientific book chapters, a patent model, and co-authored a book in English with a special focus on Nutrition, Food Security, and Food Safety Sciences. He has been acting as Guest Editor of several Special Issues published in high-impact JCR journals. He has collaborated as a Visiting Professor at Portuguese, Spanish, Chilean, and Vietnamese Universities.

Fernando Ramos

Fernando Ramos is an Associate Professor with tenure and Dean of the Faculty of Pharmacy of the University of Coimbra. He is Senior Research of REQUIMTE/LAQV. He collaborates with EFSA, being a member of the Scientific Panel on Additives and Products or Substances used in Animal Feed (FEEDAP). He is the Vice-Chair of the Scientific Committee of the Portuguese Food and Economic Safety Authority (ASAE). He has published more than 150 papers in indexed JCR journals, namely in developing analytical methodologies for determining drug residues in food and in feed. He has written 22 book chapters and edited four books, two in Portugal and two in the USA. In addition, he is on the Roster of JECFA (Joint FAO/WHO Expert Committee on Food Additives) related to the safety of drug residues in foods.

Dele Raheem

Dele Raheem is Associate Professor (Docent) in Food Microbiology, University of Helsinki, Finland. He holds a Doctor of Food Sciences from the University of Helsinki, Finland; he is also an Adjunct Professor of Food Microbiology. Dele's research interest is in food bioprocessing, preservation, and crosscutting issues related to food security. He has gained extensive research and industrial experience in the past three decades. He also obtained a Master's degree in education from the University of Greenwich, London, UK. He has co-authored and published one book, eight book chapters, and 30 articles in peer-reviewed journals. He is a reviewer and member of the editorial board for many international journals. He is a professional member of the Finnish Association of Academic Agronomists and the Food Climate Research Network based in Oxford, UK. Currently, he is affiliated with the Northern Institute for Environmental and Minority Law, Arctic Centre at the University of Lapland as a Senior researcher.

Ariana Saraiva

Ariana Saraiva is a Ph.D. student at the University Institute of Animal Health and Food Safety, University of Las Palmas de Gran Canaria.

She graduated in Nutritional Sciences from Instituto Superior de Ciências da Saúde Egas Moniz, Portugal, and obtained her Master's degree in Food Safety from the University of Coimbra, Portugal.

Her main research interests are food safety evaluation, food innovation, and natural food products.

She has published more than 15 papers in indexed JCR journals and co-authored a book with Professor António Raposo in English. She has been acting as Guest Editor of Special Issues published in the International Journal of Environmental Research and Public Health.

Conrado Javier Carrascosa Iruzubieta

Conrado Carrascosa Iruzubieta is an Associate Professor with tenure of the Faculty of Veterinary Faculty of the Las Palmas University, Spain. He is a Veterinary graduate (Las Palmas University) and Food Science Technology graduate (Universidad Politécnica de Valencia). He has worked for 17 years as a technician at Proquimia Company (Cleaning and disinfection products). His field of expertise is at Pseudomonas fluorescens in foods, cleaning and disinfection in the food industry, and biofilm. He has published more than 42 papers in indexed JCR journals. He has written four book chapters. In addition, he has realized his stay in the Microbiology at Interfaces Laboratory in the Faculty of Science and Engineering, Manchester Metropolitan University, Manchester Metropolitan University, UK.

Preface to "Food Safety, Security, Sustainability and Nutrition as Priority Objectives of the Food Sector"

Food systems are at the center of global environmental, social, and economic challenges such as resource scarcity, ecosystem degradation, and climate change. The current food systems are generating negative outcomes, such as land, water, and ecosystem degradation, biodiversity loss, excessive greenhouse gas emissions, persistent malnutrition and hunger, and are failing to eradicate poverty, particularly in rural populations in the global South. The future food systems will have to provide food and nutrition security while facing unprecedented sustainability challenges: this underlines the need for a transition to more sustainable food systems. Taking into account these premises and considering the complexity of food systems, this book presents 24 papers published by researchers from 24 different countries all over the world, including Australia, Brazil, Canada, Cape Verde, China, Croatia, Finland, France, Greece, Iran, Italy, Israel, Korea, Malaysia, Malta, Morocco, Portugal, Russia, Spain, Sweden, Taiwan, the UK, the USA, and Vietnam.

The editors are very grateful to their families and friends for all of the support they provided. We would also like to extend a very special thanks for the commitment and dedication of all researchers who published their works herein and the entire MDPI team. Only in this way was it possible to carry out this successful project.

António Raposo, Fernando Ramos, Dele Raheem, Ariana Saraiva, Conrado Javier Carrascosa Iruzubieta
Editors

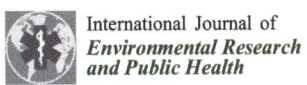

Editorial

Food Safety, Security, Sustainability and Nutrition as Priority Objectives of the Food Sector

António Raposo [1,*], Fernando Ramos [2,3], Dele Raheem [4], Ariana Saraiva [5] and Conrado Carrascosa [5]

1 CBIOS (Research Center for Biosciences and Health Technologies), Universidade Lusófona de Humanidades e Tecnologias, Campo Grande 376, 1749-024 Lisboa, Portugal
2 Pharmacy Faculty, University of Coimbra, Azinhaga de Santa Comba, 3000-548 Coimbra, Portugal; framos@ff.uc.pt
3 REQUIMTE/LAQV, R. D. Manuel II, Apartado, 55142 Oporto, Portugal
4 Northern Institute for Environmental and Minority Law (NIEM), Arctic Centre, University of Lapland, 96101 Rovaniemi, Finland; braheem@ulapland.fi
5 Department of Animal Pathology and Production, Bromatology and Food Technology, Faculty of Veterinary, Universidad de Las Palmas de Gran Canaria, Trasmontaña s/n, 35413 Arucas, Spain; ariana_23@outlook.pt (A.S.); conrado.carrascosa@ulpgc.es (C.C.)
* Correspondence: antonio.raposo@ulusofona.pt

Keywords: environmental health; food safety; food security; nutrition; sustainability

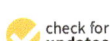

Citation: Raposo, A.; Ramos, F.; Raheem, D.; Saraiva, A.; Carrascosa, C. Food Safety, Security, Sustainability and Nutrition as Priority Objectives of the Food Sector. *Int. J. Environ. Res. Public Health* **2021**, *18*, 8073. https://doi.org/10.3390/ijerph18158073

Received: 22 July 2021
Accepted: 26 July 2021
Published: 30 July 2021

Publisher's Note: MDPI stays neutral with regard to jurisdictional claims in published maps and institutional affiliations.

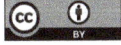

Copyright: © 2021 by the authors. Licensee MDPI, Basel, Switzerland. This article is an open access article distributed under the terms and conditions of the Creative Commons Attribution (CC BY) license (https://creativecommons.org/licenses/by/4.0/).

Food systems are at the center of global environmental, social, and economic challenges such as resource scarcity, ecosystem degradation, and climate change [1]. The current food systems are generating negative outcomes, such as land, water, and ecosystem degradation, biodiversity loss, excessive greenhouse gas emissions, persistent malnutrition and hunger, and are failing to eradicate poverty, particularly of rural populations in the global South [2]. The future food systems will have to provide food and nutrition security while facing unprecedented sustainability challenges: this underlines the need for a transition to more sustainable food systems. Taking into account these premises and considering the complexity of food systems, this Special Issue presents 23 papers published by researchers from 24 different countries all over the world, including Australia, Brazil, Canada, Cape Verde, China, Croatia, Finland, France, Greece, Iran, Italy, Israel, Korea, Malaysia, Malta, Morocco, Portugal, Russia, Spain, Sweden, Taiwan, the UK, the USA, and Vietnam.

Regarding the review articles included in this Special Issue, it is possible to find four works that address the following themes: the bulk sweetener maltitol, where the analytical determination methods, applications in the food industry, metabolism, and health impacts are discussed in depth [3]; the relevance of food naturalness for consumers, food security aspects, sustainability, and health impacts, focused on natural sweeteners [4]; biofilm concerns from many angles, including biofilm-forming pathogens in the food industry, biofilm disinfectant resistance, and biofilm identification methods [5]; how texture and rheology might be evaluated in the food industry with specific attention on dysphagia [6].

In terms of research articles, we can mention 17 relevant works that focus on different areas common to the objectives of this Special Issue, namely: the study of green food intake and social trust as mediators in the relationship between perceived consumer effectiveness and psychological wellbeing [7]; the investigations by Bogdanova et al. [8] focused on integrating many components of the reindeer food value chain in a multidisciplinary manner to promote indigenous peoples' food sovereignty in Western Siberia's Arctic zone, as well as reflections on the key issues of the COVID-19 pandemic; an empirical study from China analyzing the effects of epistemic and social trust on public acceptance of genetically modified food [9]. This research adds to our understanding of how trust influences the acceptance of emerging technologies, and it is crucial for risk-management practices. The quasi-experimental pilot study assessed the effects of a pilot community-based behavioral intervention on the home food environment in U.S. [10]. In Italy, the results of a culturally tailored dietary intervention in diabetic patients from North Africa and Bangladesh were investigated by Piombo et al. [11]. Chen and Lin [12] have investigated and constructed the important and appropriate factors for designing a green café ambiance and empirically analyzed indicators with high operability that are suitable for green café ambience design. Another study from China used exploratory spatial data analysis, a gravity center model, a spatial panel data model, and a geographically weighted regression model to examine the spatial–temporal characteristics in grain production and their influencing factors using climate and socioeconomic data from 1995 to 2018 [13]. The nutritional profile, phenolic composition, and biological properties of *Crepis vesicaria* L. subsp. *taraxacifolia* leaves were analyzed in a research conducted by Pedreiro et al. [14]. The study by Fideles et al. [15] looked at food insecurity among Brazilian Community restaurant food handlers and the factors that contribute to it. In the U.S., Ferrante et al. [16] designed a survey to look at how COVID-19 affects parents' lifestyles (e.g., work, child care, grocery shopping), as well as current family food acquisition and food habits (e.g., cooking, restaurant use); Nemati et al. [17] conducted a study to evaluate the effects of using different levels of ginger powder on the productive performance, eggs quality, and blood parameters in laying Japanese quails; Professor Heesup Han and colleagues have investigated the impact of halal food performance, which includes criteria such as availability, health/nutrition, accreditation, and cleanness/safety/hygiene, on Muslim traveler retention in a non-Islamic destination [18]. Evans et al. [19] investigated how surface characteristics (chemistry and topography) and cleaning direction affected the removal of bacteria and meat exuded from surfaces. The amounts of Al, Cd, Cr, Ni, Pb, and Sr in frequently consumed cereals and cereal-based products were determined in a study conducted in the Cape Verde Islands, and the risk associated with them was analyzed [20]. The study about the Indigenous community perspectives of food security, sustainable food systems, and strategies to enhance access to local and traditional healthy food for partnering Williams Treaties First Nations (Ontario, Canada) can be used to develop Indigenous community-based projects and initiatives aimed at improving food security, establishing more sustainable food systems, and achieving food sovereignty [21]; Wang et al. [22] investigated the effects of ecological compensation, capital endowment, and ecological cognition on the adoption of environmentally friendly technology by farmers.

On 25 November 2020, Professor Lluís Serra-Majem and his co-workers published an important Update of the Pyramid of the Mediterranean Diet, considering sustainability and focusing on environmental concerns [23]. This work has more strongly emphasized the lower consumption of red meat and bovine dairy products, and the higher consumption of vegetables and locally grown eco-friendly plant foods as much as possible. This paper is already an Editor's Choice article and promoted the publication of two pertinent commentary papers: a work carried out by Professor Maria Luz Fernandez and collaborators on highlights of current dietary guidelines around the world [24], and also a text produced by the well-known Professor Walter Willett, mentioning that "all countries can benefit by considering this updated Mediterranean Dietary Pyramid when developing their dietary guidelines and food systems" [25].

There is a need for a 'food systems thinking' that takes cognizance of the link between the safety of food, food security, nutrition, and health at both individual and planetary levels. Our food system needs to be sustainable, as alluded to by some of the authors in this Special Issue. The food sector will need to make necessary changes and respond to sustainability challenges in our current food system; these include the negative outcomes mentioned earlier [1,2], population growth, climate change, and pandemics. This transformation of the food system, whose goal is to help stakeholders better understand and manage the complex choices that affect the future of food systems and to accelerate progress toward the Sustainable Development Goals, has already been discussed in several fora on a global level and will culminate at the UN SDG Food System summit in New

York, the USA, by September 2021 [26]. The topics addressed in this Special Issue are thought-provoking and worth considering by researchers, academics, policymakers, food processors, indigenous peoples, and other stakeholders.

Last but not the least, the editors believe that this Special Issue gives an important contribution in the form of essential ingredients of 'food for thought', when safety, sustainability, and nutrition are considered as priority objectives in the food sector.

Author Contributions: This Special Issue was edited jointly by A.R., F.R., D.R., A.S. and C.C. This editorial was written jointly by the editors. All authors have read and agreed to the published version of the manuscript.

Funding: This research received no external funding.

Institutional Review Board Statement: Not applicable.

Informed Consent Statement: Not applicable.

Data Availability Statement: Not applicable.

Acknowledgments: The authors are very grateful to their families and friends for all of the support they provided. We also would like to extend a very special thanks for the commitment and dedication of all researchers who published their works in this Special Issue and the entire MDPI team. Only in this way was it possible to carry out this successful project.

Conflicts of Interest: The authors declare no conflict of interest.

References

1. Horton, P.; Banwart, S.A.; Brockington, D.; Brown, G.W.; Bruce, R.; Cameron, D.; Holdsworth, M.; Koh, S.C.L.; Ton, J.; Jackson, P. An agenda for integrated system-wide interdisciplinary agri-food research. *Food Sec.* **2017**, *9*, 195–210. [CrossRef]
2. El Bilali, H.; Callenius, C.; Strassner, C.; Probst, L. Food and nutrition security and sustainability transitions in food systems. *Food Energy Secur.* **2019**, *8*, e00154. [CrossRef]
3. Saraiva, A.; Carrascosa, C.; Raheem, D.; Ramos, F.; Raposo, A. Maltitol: Analytical Determination Methods, Applications in the Food Industry, Metabolism and Health Impacts. *Int. J. Environ. Res. Public Health* **2020**, *17*, 5227. [CrossRef] [PubMed]
4. Saraiva, A.; Carrascosa, C.; Raheem, D.; Ramos, F.; Raposo, A. Natural Sweeteners: The Relevance of Food Naturalness for Consumers, Food Security Aspects, Sustainability and Health Impacts. *Int. J. Environ. Res. Public Health* **2020**, *17*, 6285. [CrossRef]
5. Carrascosa, C.; Raheem, D.; Ramos, F.; Saraiva, A.; Raposo, A. Microbial Biofilms in the Food Industry—A Comprehensive Review. *Int. J. Environ. Res. Public Health* **2021**, *18*, 2014. [CrossRef] [PubMed]
6. Raheem, D.; Carrascosa, C.; Ramos, F.; Saraiva, A.; Raposo, A. Texture-Modified Food for Dysphagic Patients: A Comprehensive Review. *Int. J. Environ. Res. Public Health* **2021**, *18*, 5125. [CrossRef] [PubMed]
7. Wang, J.; Nguyen, N.; Bu, X. Exploring the Roles of Green Food Consumption and Social Trust in the Relationship between Perceived Consumer Effectiveness and Psychological Wellbeing. *Int. J. Environ. Res. Public Health* **2020**, *17*, 4676. [CrossRef]
8. Bogdanova, E.; Andronov, S.; Asztalos Morell, I.; Hossain, K.; Raheem, D.; Filant, P.; Lobanov, A. Food Sovereignty of the Indigenous Peoples in the Arctic Zone of Western Siberia: Response to COVID-19 Pandemic. *Int. J. Environ. Res. Public Health* **2020**, *17*, 7570. [CrossRef]
9. Hu, L.; Liu, R.; Zhang, W.; Zhang, T. The Effects of Epistemic Trust and Social Trust on Public Acceptance of Genetically Modified Food: An Empirical Study from China. *Int. J. Environ. Res. Public Health* **2020**, *17*, 7700. [CrossRef] [PubMed]
10. Cassinat, R.A.; Bruening, M.; Crespo, N.C.; Gutiérrez, M.; Chavez, A.; Ray, F.; Vega-López, S. Effects of a Community-Based Pilot Intervention on Home Food Availability among U.S. Households. *Int. J. Environ. Res. Public Health* **2020**, *17*, 8327. [CrossRef] [PubMed]
11. Piombo, L.; Nicolella, G.; Barbarossa, G.; Tubili, C.; Pandolfo, M.M.; Castaldo, M.; Costanzo, G.; Mirisola, C.; Cavani, A. Outcomes of Culturally Tailored Dietary Intervention in the North African and Bangladeshi Diabetic Patients in Italy. *Int. J. Environ. Res. Public Health* **2020**, *17*, 8932. [CrossRef]
12. Chen, Y.-C.; Lin, H.-C. Exploring Effective Sensory Experience in the Environmental Design of Sustainable Cafés. *Int. J. Environ. Res. Public Health* **2020**, *17*, 8957. [CrossRef]
13. Zhou, C.; Zhang, R.; Ning, X.; Zheng, Z. Spatial-Temporal Characteristics in Grain Production and Its Influencing Factors in the Huang-Huai-Hai Plain from 1995 to 2018. *Int. J. Environ. Res. Public Health* **2020**, *17*, 9793. [CrossRef]
14. Pedreiro, S.; da Ressurreição, S.; Lopes, M.; Cruz, M.T.; Batista, T.; Figueirinha, A.; Ramos, F. *Crepis vesicaria* L. subsp. *taraxacifolia* Leaves: Nutritional Profile, Phenolic Composition and Biological Properties. *Int. J. Environ. Res. Public Health* **2021**, *18*, 151. [CrossRef] [PubMed]

15. Fideles, I.C.; de Cassia Coelho de Almeida Akutsu, R.; da Rocha Fonseca Barroso, R.; Costa-Souza, J.; Zandonadi, R.P.; Raposo, A.; Botelho, R.B.A. Food Insecurity among Low-Income Food Handlers: A Nationwide Study in Brazilian Community Restaurants. *Int. J. Environ. Res. Public Health* **2021**, *18*, 1160. [CrossRef]
16. Ferrante, M.J.; Goldsmith, J.; Tauriello, S.; Epstein, L.H.; Leone, L.A.; Anzman-Frasca, S. Food Acquisition and Daily Life for U.S. Families with 4- to 8-Year-Old Children during COVID-19: Findings from a Nationally Representative Survey. *Int. J. Environ. Res. Public Health* **2021**, *18*, 1734. [CrossRef] [PubMed]
17. Nemati, Z.; Moradi, Z.; Alirezalu, K.; Besharati, M.; Raposo, A. Impact of Ginger Root Powder Dietary Supplement on Productive Performance, Egg Quality, Antioxidant Status and Blood Parameters in Laying Japanese Quails. *Int. J. Environ. Res. Public Health* **2021**, *18*, 2995. [CrossRef] [PubMed]
18. Han, H.; Lho, L.H.; Raposo, A.; Radic, A.; Ngah, A.H. Halal Food Performance and Its Influence on Patron Retention Process at Tourism Destination. *Int. J. Environ. Res. Public Health* **2021**, *18*, 3034. [CrossRef]
19. Evans, A.; Slate, A.J.; Akhidime, I.D.; Verran, J.; Kelly, P.J.; Whitehead, K.A. The Removal of Meat Exudate and *Escherichia coli* from Stainless Steel and Titanium Surfaces with Irregular and Regular Linear Topographies. *Int. J. Environ. Res. Public Health* **2021**, *18*, 3198. [CrossRef]
20. Rubio-Armendáriz, C.; Paz, S.; Gutiérrez, Á.J.; Gomes Furtado, V.; González-Weller, D.; Revert, C.; Hardisson, A. Toxic Metals in Cereals in Cape Verde: Risk Assessment Evaluation. *Int. J. Environ. Res. Public Health* **2021**, *18*, 3833. [CrossRef]
21. Domingo, A.; Charles, K.-A.; Jacobs, M.; Brooker, D.; Hanning, R.M. Indigenous Community Perspectives of Food Security, Sustainable Food Systems and Strategies to Enhance Access to Local and Traditional Healthy Food for Partnering Williams Treaties First Nations (Ontario, Canada). *Int. J. Environ. Res. Public Health* **2021**, *18*, 4404. [CrossRef] [PubMed]
22. Wang, H.; Wang, X.; Sarkar, A.; Zhang, F. How Capital Endowment and Ecological Cognition Affect Environment-Friendly Technology Adoption: A Case of Apple Farmers of Shandong Province, China. *Int. J. Environ. Res. Public Health* **2021**, *18*, 7571. [CrossRef]
23. Serra-Majem, L.; Tomaino, L.; Dernini, S.; Berry, E.M.; Lairon, D.; Ngo de la Cruz, J.; Bach-Faig, A.; Donini, L.M.; Medina, F.-X.; Belahsen, R.; et al. Updating the Mediterranean Diet Pyramid towards Sustainability: Focus on Environmental Concerns. *Int. J. Environ. Res. Public Health* **2020**, *17*, 8758. [CrossRef]
24. Fernandez, M.L.; Raheem, D.; Ramos, F.; Carrascosa, C.; Saraiva, A.; Raposo, A. Highlights of Current Dietary Guidelines in Five Continents. *Int. J. Environ. Res. Public Health* **2021**, *18*, 2814. [CrossRef] [PubMed]
25. Willett, W. Mediterranean Dietary Pyramid. *Int. J. Environ. Res. Public Health* **2021**, *18*, 4568. [CrossRef] [PubMed]
26. United Nations Food Systems Summit. The United Nations Food System Summit, New York. 2021. Available online: https://www.un.org/en/food-systems-summit/about (accessed on 21 July 2021).

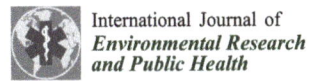

Review

Maltitol: Analytical Determination Methods, Applications in the Food Industry, Metabolism and Health Impacts

Ariana Saraiva [1], Conrado Carrascosa [1], Dele Raheem [2], Fernando Ramos [3,4] and António Raposo [5,6,*]

1. Department of Animal Pathology and Production, Bromatology and Food Technology, Faculty of Veterinary, Universidad de Las Palmas de Gran Canaria, Trasmontaña s/n, 35413 Arucas, Spain
2. Northern Institute for Environmental and Minority Law (NIEM), Arctic Centre, University of Lapland, 96101 Rovaniemi, Lapland, Finland
3. Pharmacy Faculty, University of Coimbra, Azinhaga de Santa Comba, 3000-548 Coimbra, Portugal
4. REQUIMTE/LAQV, University of Oporto, 4051-401 Porto, Portugal
5. Department for Management of Science and Technology Development, Ton Duc Thang University, Ho Chi Minh City, Vietnam
6. Faculty of Environment and Labour Safety, Ton Duc Thang University, Ho Chi Minh City, Vietnam
* Correspondence: antonio.raposo@tdtu.edu.vn

Received: 22 May 2020; Accepted: 14 July 2020; Published: 20 July 2020

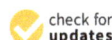

Abstract: Bulk sweetener maltitol belongs to the polyols family and there have been several dietary applications in the past few years, during which the food industry has used it in many food products: bakery and dairy products, chocolate, sweets. This review paper addresses and discusses in detail the most relevant aspects concerning the analytical methods employed to determine maltitol's food safety and industry applications, its metabolism and its impacts on human health. According to our main research outcome, we can assume that maltitol at lower doses poses little risk to humans and is a good alternative to using sucrose. However, it causes diarrhoea and foetus complications at high doses. Regarding its determination, high-performance liquid chromatography proved the primary method in various food matrices. The future role of maltitol in the food industry is likely to become more relevant as processors seek alternative sweeteners in product formulation without compromising health.

Keywords: food additives; food industry; food safety; health impacts; maltitol; metabolism; sweeteners

---

1. Introduction

Maltitol ($C_{12}H_{24}O_{11}$; 4-O-α-glucopyranosyl-D-sorbitol) is a hygroscopic non-reducing sugar and disaccharide polyol that is listed as an alternative sweetener to sugar because, except for browning, it possesses roughly 75–90% of sucrose's sweetness and has similar properties [1]. Of all polyols, maltitol has the closest solubility curve to that of sucrose and is freely soluble in water: 220 g of sucrose is soluble in 100 mL of water at 37 °C, whereas 200 g of maltitol is soluble in 100 mL of water at 37 °C. Once dissolved, the viscosities of sugar solutions and maltitol are equivalents, with viscosities of 18 millipascal seconds (mPa.s; 50% solution in water at 20 °C) and 23 mPa.s, respectively. Comparable solubility helps maltitol to dissolve in the mouth in almost exactly the same way as sucrose, leaving the mouth able to feel the expected sweetened taste of a given food product [2].

Given its high crystalline purity and chemical composition, in its natural crystalline form maltitol is less hygroscopic than sugar. At about 40 °C, maltitol absorbs ambient moisture even at a relative humidity of 82% and higher, as opposed to 80% for sucrose. This would mean improved shelf stability of those goods made with maltitol rather than sucrose when processed under given atmospheric/climate conditions. When employed as a covering on confectionery and chewing gum, maltitol's low hygroscopicity leads to long-lasting crunchiness. Reduction in the carbonyl group enhances maltitol's thermo-chemical stability during the conversion from maltose into maltitol. It does not react with amino acids when heated, which avoids Maillard reactions and, thus, lowers excessive browning potential [2].

Maltitol occurs naturally in different fruits and vegetables. Small amounts of maltitol naturally exist in roasted malt and chicory leaves. Maltitol is commercially produced from the starch of cereals such as corn, wheat and potatoes. Manufacturers resort to D-maltose catalytic hydrogenation to create hydrogenated disaccharide composed of a glucose molecule and a sorbitol molecule that are bonded together [2,3].

As with other sugar alcohols, maltitol is poorly absorbed in the small intestine, and has lower insulinaemic (35 vs. 45) and glycaemic indices (35 vs. 68), and a lower caloric value (2.4 vs. 4 kcal/g) and sweetening power (approx. 90%) than sucrose [4,5]. The metabolism of maltitol follows a known pathway [6–8]. This compound is partly absorbed only in the proximal intestine and enters the lower intestine and colon. As a result, digestive tolerance to maltitol has been previously examined in chocolate in healthy adult volunteers [9–11]. Adults can eat as much as 40 g of maltitol/day with no significant symptoms, while children can consume 15 g [9–12]. So maltitol is used primarily as a sugar substitute in food products as it has a bulking effect compared to intense sweeteners [3]. Maltitol is also employed in pharmaceuticals or oral care products (toothpaste) [13,14]. Apart from its technological and nutritional qualities, maltitol also possesses similar organoleptic properties to glucose [15] and provides good digestive tolerance. This permits its widespread use for both children and adults in various dietary applications, mostly in the sweet food categories such as cakes, pastries, sugar confectionery, chocolate, chewing gum and snack bars as well as its use as a tabletop sweetener [10,12,16]. Maltitol exhibits certain prebiotic effects in rats or humans [17,18]. As nine hydroxyl groups exist in the molecule, it is reasonable to believe that maltitol is able to act as an additive to avoid moisture loss and to further delay stalling in foods like bread [1].

As very little work on maltitol can be found in the literature, this paper aims to review analytical methods for its determination, its chief food industry and safety applications, and its metabolism and impacts on human health that stem from its utilisation.

2. Analytical Methods for Maltitol Determination

Assessing maltitol in food and beverages with low/no sugar content is relevant in both nutritional and quality control terms. The analytical procedures followed in sugar alcohol analyses are similar to those employed for other sugars. Nonetheless, sugar alcohols are characterised by high chemico-thermal stability (up to 180 °C). High-performance liquid chromatography (HPLC) methods are the most widespread choice thanks to their robustness, high sensitivity and easy sample preparation [19]. However, maltitol entails several analytical problems, as we discuss below.

Food products are complex matrices given major differences in their composition, which comprises several types of thickeners, preservatives, macromolecules, and colour additives. As many food matrix components have similar polarities to maltitol, this compound is not easy to isolate. Moreover, the maltitol levels encountered in some food products entail adjusting the sample concentration to the analytical method's linear range by dilution [19].

An analytical method for determining a target compound in a given matrix usually goes through three main stages: (1) sampling; (2) sample preparation; and (3) determination of the analyte. In the first stage, it is essential to ensure that the samples are representative, taken without contamination and transported swiftly and properly to the laboratory. When samples are not analysed immediately, storage conditions must be established to avoid changes in the sample quality. The second stage, sample preparation, comprises the process of isolating the compound of interest from interferents in the matrix prior to analysis, with the most suitable instrumental tools. This step is critical for the determination of the analyte, in this case maltitol, and is usually the most time-consuming process to conduct and optimise [19,20]. The sample preparation method depends on the complexity of the matrix, but in general homogenisation, extraction, clean-up and pre-concentration may be required, depending on sample complexity, to remove chemical interferences and determine whether or not a sample contains maltitol and at what concentration [21,22].

Preparing liquid samples is normally simple, but this is limited to dilution and filtration. In already filtered samples, injection is frequently performed directly. Carbonated drinks need to be degassed in an ultrasonic bath, either under vacuum or by sparging with nitrogen [19,23]. Some sample solutions may need to be treated with clarifying agents, such as Carrez solutions, which are suitable for the elimination of suspended solid material, proteins and lipids. Organic solvents, such as ethanol and acetonitrile, are used to selectively precipitate thickeners and polysaccharides. Besides, during sample preparation, acids such as acetic, metaphosphoric and formic acid can also be employed to precipitate food matrix components or to adjust the pH of the sample [20,22]. Whatever the procedure, filtration is always mandatory before the final analysis [21]. A single filtration step with a membrane filter is often enough to achieve the desired characteristics, but sometimes preliminary filtration using filter paper or centrifuge may be necessary [24]. All samples must be subjected to replicated analysis.

Grembecka et al. performed analysis of four sugars and five sugar alcohols, including maltitol, in fruit juices, fruit drinks, nectars and syrups [25]. The sample pretreatment applied was the slightest; it consisted of a first filtration through filter paper to remove particulate matter, followed by a dilution with 75% acetonitrile, and finally a second filtration with 0.45 µm membrane filters [25]. This minimal sample preparation procedure is suitable for many simpler samples and has the advantage of being economical, simple and speedy.

The addition of an extraction step is the most widely used sample preparation technique. For this purpose, the most commonly employed organic solvents are methanol, acetonitrile and chloroform [20]. Liquid-liquid extraction (LLE) can be employed because it is inexpensive but is not easy to automate and normally requires large quantities of solvents. More complex solid matrices may require more elaborate extraction and purification techniques such as solid phase extraction (SPE) or ultrasound-assisted extraction (UAE) with different solvents, even though extraction with water suffices in some cases [19,23].

Andersen et al. analysed four sugars and six sugar alcohols, including maltitol, in several types of matrices, namely desserts, cakes, candies, liquorice, wine, gums, chocolate and pastilles [26]. The samples were ground and the extraction was carried out with water at 60 °C for 4 h at room temperature, followed by centrifugation and filtration through a folded filter (S&S, 592.5, diameter = 125 mm), dilution and a second filtration through a Minisart 0.2 µm [26]. As can be seen from this case, heat is sometimes applied to aid in the extraction process. Overall, the adopted sample preparation protocol was relatively simple.

A quite different approach was used by Nojiri et al., which reported the analysis of five sugar alcohols, including maltitol, in confectionery products [27]. In this case, sample preparation consisted of extraction with 30% ethanol, followed by centrifugation, evaporation, and derivatisation with a 10% solution of p-nitro-benzoyl chloride. The reagent excess was eliminated and the sample was evaporated. Finally, the residue was dissolved in chloroform and purified in an SPE (solid phase extraction) cartridge (Sep-Pak C18) [27]. The use of ethanol is advantageous in relation to water, as it inhibits metabolic enzymes, thus contributing to the preservation of the sugar composition [23]. SPE is a well-established tool for the pre-concentration and clean-up of target compounds from aqueous samples and extracts. The bases of this technique are identical to those of conventional liquid-solid chromatography (LSC) and HPLC [22]. The most highly employed SPE cartridges for the extraction of sweeteners from foods are those with columns packed with octadecylsilyl silica (ODS-C18) [21,24]. Briefly, the SPE protocol consists in conditioning the cartridge, followed by the loading of the extract, and finally the washing of the cartridge. Ultimately, the elution of the compounds of interest is carried out with a suitable solvent. It is crucial that interfering compounds are not trapped and elute almost immediately, or that they have a high affinity for the stationary phase in order to be strongly adsorbed. It is worth mentioning that the sensitivity of the final analysis can be increased through a pre-concentration strategy, that is, by evaporation of the eluate until dryness and re-dissolving it in a small volume of solvent suitable for the subsequent analysis [20,21,24]. The solubility of maltitol in the processing solvent is naturally of major relevance.

In general, SPE sample preparation procedures are a good option for samples of a more complex nature ("dirty samples"), as they are undemanding, reasonably inexpensive and swift [21,24]. Moreover, owing to the lower column sizes and volumes, they require the use of less mobile phase volume, which leads to both less waste and less exposure of laboratory technicians to organic solvents, as well as leading to additional cost savings. The sample capacity and eluant volume are usually suitable also for direct injection into HPLC equipment without the need for additional sample preparation processes, thereby reducing both the risk of sample loss and contamination [22]. Furthermore, SPE exhibit greater potential for selective isolation, i.e., sample fractionation into different compounds or classes of compounds [28]. Finally, SPE systems have been increasingly improved in terms of throughput, precision and accuracy, and are compatible with the most commonly used analytical instrumentation [21].

In another study, Joshi et al. developed a method for the quantification of maltitol in flavoured milk, burfi and yoghurts [29]. Sample extraction was carried out with water under sonication for 20 min at 40 °C. A treatment with Carrez reagents was applied to remove proteins, followed by filtration through filter paper and a 0.22 μm syringe filter [29].

UAE is an efficient, economical and green technique for sample preparation. When compared to the classic extraction procedures, it allows the reduction of the amount of solvent and glassware used, as well as of the extraction time, wherefore it has been increasingly used. This technique explores the cavitation process that is observed when an extractive solvent in contact with a solid matrix is exposed to ultrasound energy. The mechanical effect generated induces a greater solvent penetration into the solid, and causes its mechanical erosion, which results in a superior mass transfer, with a consequent increase in the efficiency of the sample's extraction and a good recovery of the analyte [30].

After the sample extraction process, certain components of the food matrix may still be contained in the extract and act as a source of interference in the final determination. These undesirable compounds can be co-extracted with maltitol owing to their similar solubility profile. The occurrence of chemical interferents in the extract may bring about accuracy problems in the method, wherefore additional clean-up steps may be essential to obtain proper separation, detection and quantification [21]. As seen in the examples above, precipitation is a commonly applied technique, usually with Carrez solutions, sodium hydroxide/zinc sulphate and similar agents, followed by filtration or centrifugation. Other common clean-up methods include SPE, as earlier discussed, LLE and dialysis. An adequate extraction/clean-up process improves the recovery of maltitol and is indispensable to avoid problems such as clogging of the HPLC columns [21].

To summarise, proper sample preparation/clean-up can shorten analysis time, improve method sensitivity and selectivity, and optimise maltitol identification/quantification. The addition of a pre-concentration step can be interesting, as it can lower the detection limits during the analysis. On the other hand, a filtration step before the final analysis, usually with 0.45 μm filters, is essential for all samples, in order to remove particulate matter that can cause damage to the equipment and interfere with the results [20]. It is recommended also that a guard column filled with the same material as the main column be used, in order to act as a filter, prolong the lifetime of the analytical column and improve its performance [31]. Besides, ultrapure solvents should preferably be used in sample preparation, as this provides greater purity, stability and durability of the analytical instruments [20]. Lastly, the sample preparation procedure chosen to determine maltitol depends on the nature of the matrix and the analytical system to be used in quantification and can be more or less costly and demanding. As general rule, it should be kept as simple as possible to reduce error.

As a final remark, it should be noted that, even though the traditional sample pretreatment methods are still widely used, there is a growing trend in this field to minimise the use of organic solvents and sample sizes, and adopt extraction procedures that allow the analysis of compounds of different classes simultaneously, ideally likely to be automated [20].

That said, and once the correct sample preparation is complete, the foodstuff is ready for analysis. Research papers have reported different approaches to determine maltitol in food products, as discussed below. Table 1 summarises details of practical applications.

Table 1. Analytical procedures used in the determination of maltitol in food samples.

Analyte	Matrix	Technique	Sample Preparation	Mobile Phase/ Electrolyte	Column/ Capillary	Analytical Parameters	Ref.
Xylitol Meso-erythritol D-glucitol D-mannitol Maltitol Parachinit	Confectionery products	HPLC-UV (260 nm)	Extraction with 30% ethanol, followed by centrifugation, evaporation, and derivatisation with a 10% solution of p-nitro-benzoyl chloride. Excess reagent was destroyed and the sample was evaporated. The residue was dissolved in chloroform and purified in an SPE cartridge.	Acetonitrile–water (67:33)	GL Sciences stainless-steel column (250 × 4.5 mm) packed with Inertsil Ph-3	LOD 0.1% LOQ n.a. Recovery 73.2–109.0% RSD ≤ 9.0%	[27]
Maltitol	Milk Burfi Yoghurts	HPLC-RI	Extraction with water under sonication for 20 min at 40 °C. Treatment with Carrez reagents to remove proteins was applied, followed by filtration (filter paper and 0.22 μm syringe filter).	Acetonitrile–water (75:25)	Waters Spherisorb Amino column (5 μm, 250 × 4.6 mm) with a guard column Waters μBondpack (10 μm NH$_2$)	LOD 10 μg/mL LOQ 25 μg/mL Recovery 97.81–98.54% RSD ≤ 1.93%	[29]
Lactose Sucrose Fructose Glucose Xylitol Isomalt Sorbitol Erythritol Maltitol	Desserts	HPLC-RI	Extraction with distilled water (50 °C) in a water bath 60 °C for 15 min, precipitation with sodium hydroxide and zinc sulphate, and filtration (0.45 μm membrane filters).	Distilled water	Shodex Sugars SP0810 column (300 × 8.0 mm) with lead (II) ions and a guard column Shodex SP-G (5 μm, 50 × 6 mm)	LOD 0.01–0.17 mg/mL LOQ 0.03–0.56 mg/mL Recovery 91–109% RSD ≤ 8%	[32]
Fructose Sucrose Glucose Lactose Maltose Erythritol Sorbitol Xylitol Inositol Mannitol Lactitol Isomalt Maltitol	Sweets Jellies Gums Chocolalte Processed chocolate products Snacks	UPLC-ELSD	Extraction with water at 80 °C for 30 min (gums and sweets) or 50% alcohols at 80 °C for 30 min after fat removal (chocolate and processed chocolate products), centrifugation, and filtration (0.22 μm PVDF syringe filter).	Acetonitrile (eluent A) and water (eluent B) both containing 0.05% (v/v) ethanolamine and triethylamine as modifiers	Acquity BEH Amide column (1.7 μm, 150 × 2.1 mm)	LOD 0.006–0.018% LOQ 0.020–0.059% Recovery 89.13–105.32% RSD ≤ 1.55%	[33]

Table 1. Cont.

Analyte	Matrix	Technique	Sample Preparation	Mobile Phase/Electrolyte	Column/Capillary	Analytical Parameters	Ref.
Maltose Sucrose Fructose Glucose Xylitol Sorbitol Erythritol Mannitol Maltitol	Fruit juices Fruit beverages Nectars Dietary supplements (syrups)	HPLC-CAD	Filtration (through filter paper to remove solid particles), dilution with 75% acetonitrile, and second filtration (0.45 μm membrane filters).	Water (eluent A) and acetonitrile (eluent B)	Shodex Asahipak NH2P-50 4E column (5 μm, 250 × 4.6 mm)	LOD 0.12–0.44 μg/mL LOQ 0.40–1.47 μg/mL Recovery 95.6–105% RSD ≤ 4.97%	[25]
Cl$^-$ K$^+$ Br$^-$ SO$_4^{2-}$ NO$_3^-$ Erythrose Arabinose Fructose Galactose Glucose Lactose Isomaltulose Maltose Lyxose Maltotriose Mannose Rhamnose Raffinose Ribose Sucrose Xylose Sorbose Erythritol Inositol Lactitol Mannitol Maltitol Xylitol Sorbitol Acarbose	Energy drinks Beer Soft drinks Wine Coffee Milk Smoothies Tea Fruit juices Ketchup Yoghurts Honey	HILIC-CAD	Dilution in 60% acetonitrile and centrifugation. Samples with gas were degassed in an ultrasonic bath prior to dilution.	85% acetonitrile (eluent A) and 60% acetonitrile (eluent B), both with 10 mM of ammonium acetate adjusted to pH 8.25 with ammonium hydroxide	WATERS Acquity UPLC BEH Amide column (1.7 μm, 150 × 2.1 mm) and an Acquity UPLC BEH Amide VanGuard precolumn	LOD 0.032–2.675 mg/L LOQ 0.107–8.918 mg/L Recovery n.a. RSD ≤ 4.94%	[34]

Table 1. Cont.

Analyte	Matrix	Technique	Sample Preparation	Mobile Phase/ Electrolyte	Column/ Capillary	Analytical Parameters	Ref.
Glucose Xylose Fructose Sucrose Lactose Sorbitol Lactitol Isomaltitol Maltitol	Biscuits Cakes Creams Toffees Chocolate Roasted malt Chicory	HPAEC-PAD	Extraction with water under sonication, centrifuged and filtered. Treatment with Carrez reagents to remove proteins and fats was applied to some products, followed by dilution and filtration (0.2 μm nylon membranes).	40 mM of sodium hydroxide + 1 mM of barium acetate	Dionex CarboPac PA100 column (250 × 4 mm) and a guard column CarboPac PA100 column (50 × 4 mm) A gold working electrode and a silver/silver chloride reference electrode were employed. The optimal detection potential was +0.10 V.	LOD 10–20 pmol LOQ n.a. Recovery n.a. RSD ≤ 2%	[35]
Glucose Lactose Sucrose Maltose Xylitol Sorbitol Mannitol Lactitol Isomaltitol Maltitol	Desserts Cakes Sweets Liquorice Wine Gums Chocolate Pastilles	HPAEC-PAD	Extraction with water (60 °C) for 4 h at room temperature, centrifugation, filtration (through a folded filter S&S, 592.5, diameter = 125 mm), dilution and second filtration (0.2 μm Minisart).	100% 1M of NaOH (eluent A) and 100% water (eluent B)	Dionex CarboPac MA1 column (250 × 4 mm) and a guard column Dionex CarboPac MA1 (50 × 4 mm)	LOD 0.3–1.1 mg/l LOQ 1–4 mg/L Recovery 85.8–107% RSD ≤ 5.2%	[26]
Cyclamate Saccharin Sucralose Dulcin Aspartame Neoheperidine Dihydrochalcone Acesulfame potassium Alitame Neotame Rebaudioside A Stevioside Erythritol Xylitol Maltitol	Carbonated and non-carbonated beverages Hard sweets Yoghurts	UHPLC-MS/MS	Beverages were simply diluted with water, except those containing gas, which were first sonicated to remove it. Hard sweets were dissolved in water, vortexed and diluted. Yoghurts were processed using solid phase extraction (SPE). All samples were filtered (0.20 μm membrane filters) prior to injection.	10 mM of ammonium acetate in water/methanol (98/2, v/v) (eluent A) and 10 mM of ammonium acetate in water/methanol (1/99, v/v) (eluent B)	Waters Acquity UPLC BEH C18 column (1.7 μm, 100 × 2.1 mm) with a Vanguard pre-column (1.7 μm, 5 × 2.1 mm)	LOD 0.1–1.8 ng/mL (drinks) and 0.1–2.5 ng/g (sweets and yoghurts) LOQ n.a. Recovery 70–114% RSD ≤ 15%	[36]

Table 1. Cont.

Analyte	Matrix	Technique	Sample Preparation	Mobile Phase/ Electrolyte	Column/ Capillary	Analytical Parameters	Ref.
Erythritol Xylitol Sorbitol Maltitol	Chocolate	CE-C⁴D	Extraction with water and ultrasound, followed by filtration (0.22 μm membrane filters) and dilution.	25 mM of sodium borate, pH adjusted to 8.5 with boric acid	Fused silica capillary column (70 cm × 50 μm) C⁴D parameters were 2 V (peak to peak), 628 kHz	LOD 2.7–4.8 μg/g LOQ 9–15.9 μg/g Recovery 70–116% RSD ≤ 19%	[37]

LOD—Limit of detection; LOQ—Limit of quantification; RSD—Relative standard deviation; n.a.—Not available.

Assessing maltitol by ultraviolet (UV) detectors is challenging because its structure lacks chromophore groups. However, UV detectors are not expensive and this obstacle can be overcome by the derivatisation technique using a chromophoric reagent. Nojiri et al. developed a method to analyse six sugar alcohols, including maltitol, in several confectionery products by HPLC after nitro-benzoylation [27]. Using p-nitro-benzoyl chloride permitted maltitol to be converted into a strong UV absorbing derivative [27]. Despite these good results, having to apply derivatisation is a disadvantage that should be considered for routine analyses. This technique increases sensitivity and selectivity, but is lengthy, and the presence of reagents in samples can negatively impact on analysis results. Many foods contain UV active compounds and can cause interference [36].

Another detector that has been described for maltitol determination is the refractive index (RI). The RI detector allows simple and fast analysis of compounds that change the refractive index of the solvent, which are virtually all analytes [34]. Joshi et al. successfully established a procedure for maltitol analysis in dairy products, which was based on the use of an amino column containing a silica-based aminopropyl bonded stationary phase linked with an RI detector [29]. An isolation method based on enzymatic treatment with β-galactosidase was applied for the lactose hydrolysis, which allowed the removal of the lactose peak that had a retention time coincident with maltitol [29]. Hadjikinova et al. also developed and validated an HPLC-RI method for the simultaneous determination of four sugars and five sugar alcohols including maltitol in desserts [32]. Briefly, the sample preparation consisted of extraction with distilled water (50 °C) in a water bath at 60 °C for 15 min, precipitation with sodium hydroxide and zinc sulphate, and filtration (0.45 μm membrane filters). In this case, a column specially designed for the separation of sugars and sugar alcohols (Shodex Sugars SP0810) was employed [32].

The main problem of RI detection is its limitation to isocratic methods. An RI detector is very sensitive to changes in temperature and flow rate [23,34]. Ultraviolet–visible (UV/VIS) detection with a diode array detector (DAD) presents similar limits of detection (LODs) to those of the HPLC-RI procedure, but implies pre- or post-column derivatisation. Hence a gradient elution can be employed, but sample preparation is more time-consuming [34]. Another option is HPLC coupled with fluorescence detectors (FDs), which yields higher selectivity and sensitivity than those of HPLC-DAD, but FDs are costly and require derivatisation [34].

Evaporative light scattering detectors (ELSD) also have been employed. The mobile phase in ELSD is nebulised by air or nitrogen to produce particles, and the light scattered by the resulting particles is measured [23]. Koh et al. developed a method with both an amide-based column and ELS detection [33]. Sample extraction was performed with water at 80 °C for 30 min for gums and candies, and with 50% alcohols at 80 °C for 30 min, after fat removal, for chocolate and processed chocolate products, followed by centrifugation and filtration (0.22 μm PVDF syringe filter) [33]. Unlike amino-based columns, amide-based columns are able to retain analytes over a wide pH range in the mobile phase [38]. These authors tested columns of various lengths (50, 100, 150 mm) and recommended employing the longest column because shorter lengths negatively impact resolution [33]. Nonetheless, the response peaks achieved in the longer columns are often wider, which means less sensitivity given increased diffusion [38]. This method resulted in separation of eight sugar alcohols and five sugars within 15 min without derivatisation, which is a noteworthy outcome. Ethanolamine and triethylamine were added to eluents to modify the stationary phase. The developed analytical system was applied to commercial samples of gums, chocolate, sweets, processed snacks and chocolate products at 0.21–46.41% of sugars and sugar alcohols. Maltitol appeared in gums and sweets [33].

Compared to the RI, ELSD offers much a higher sensitivity and stability of the chromatographic baseline, even in the gradient eluent mode. The required sample pretreatment is normally minimal [23]. Having said that, the pulsed amperometric detector (PAD) and the Corona charged aerosol detector (CAD) are considered superior to ELSD and RI detectors in sensitivity, selectivity and reproducibility terms [25,31].

CAD has the following characteristics regardless of the chemical properties of the compound of interest: high sensitivity to mass, gradient compatibility, wide dynamic range, high precision, and consistent response [23]. CAD works on the principle of the eluent's nebulisation with nitrogen to produce analyte particles. This is followed by drying to eliminate the mobile phase. Particles are then charged with a high-voltage corona wire. The quantity of charge measured by an electrometer is proportional to the quantity of the analyte of interest in the sample [23,34].

CAD mobile phases must be volatile as they are for ELSD [23]. Grembecka et al. successfully and simultaneously determined by the HPLC-CAD method five sugar alcohols and four sugars, including maltitol, in drinks and dietary supplements, with no extraction step [25]. After analysing commercial samples, maltitol was found only in syrup (dietary supplement) [25].

The hydrophilic interaction liquid chromatography (HILIC) mode is an alternative to HPLC for separating polar compounds like maltitol. The principle of separation is in accordance with the differential distribution of the compounds between a relative hydrophobic eluent and a water rich layer immobilised in a hydrophilic stationary phase [39]. More recently, Pitsch et al. set up a HILIC-CAD method that allows for the simultaneous determination of 30 compounds. It comprises five ions, 17 sugars and seven sugar alcohols, including maltitol, in 24 food and beverage samples [34]. The applied pretreatment was a minimal dilution in 60% acetonitrile with centrifugation. Samples with gas were degassed in an ultrasonic bath prior to dilution. Analyte separation was done in an amide-based column. The use of 60% acetonitrile led to some matrix interference in complex beer samples without affecting the quantification results. It has been suggested that matrix interferences could be further decreased by employing SPE or increasing the acetonitrile concentration in the sample diluent. Separating maltitol from sugars and other sugar alcohols is quite challenging owing to chemical similarities and implies that high-efficiency separation columns and long runs are normally necessary. The above-cited authors took a quantification approach based on peak height instead of peak area, which was successful. They obtained results during a shorter period and did not compromise reliability. The method was generally a sound tool for routine analyses [34].

Sugar alcohols, including maltitol (pKa 12.84), possess weak acid properties, with ionising under high pH conditions, at least partially, so they can be separated by ion-exchange mechanisms. So another possible maltitol analysis method is high-performance anion-exchange chromatography (HPAEC), which is usually coupled with PAD, and allows the quantification of non-derivatised sugars and sugar alcohols at low concentrations in the order of pmol. This method is characterised by its high sensitivity, and it neither entails complex sample pretreatments nor uses organic solvents [23].

PAD can be interesting to determine maltitol as it directly detects it (with no pre- or post-column derivatisation) and offers high sensitivity and selectivity with complex commercial samples. PAD only detects analytes with functional groups that are oxidisable at the specific voltage applied to detection which makes the required sample preparation simple. Sodium hydroxide gradients can be used, as detection is not affected by salt concentration changes [23]. Cataldi et al. set up an HPAEC-PAD method for separating and quantifying four sugar alcohols and five sugars, including maltitol, in cakes, biscuits, toffees, creams, chocolate, chicory and roasted malt [35]. The extraction was performed with water under sonication, followed by centrifugation and filtration. A treatment with Carrez reagents to remove proteins and fats was applied in some products, followed by dilution and filtration (0.2 μm nylon membranes) prior to injection. A pellicular column with a relatively low ion-exchange capacity was successfully employed. It is well-known that data reproducibility in HPAEC is strongly affected by the interference of carbonate ions, which tend to occupy the column's active sites, and thus reduces the retention of both sugar and sugar alcohol molecules. Regardless of taking all the precautions when preparing the alkaline eluent, this divalent ion still remains. The authors have shown that the presence of barium ions in the alkaline mobile phase increases both selectivity and reproducibility, but cuts analysis times, because it enables the precipitation of carbonate ions. This means that either taking precautions while preparing the alkaline eluent or regenerating the column between runs is no longer necessary. The method was applied to commercial samples. Maltitol was found in all the matrices, except for sponge cakes and creams. The levels detected in chicory and roasted malt were very low [35]. Andersen et al. also proposed a HPAEC-PAD method for quantifying six sugar alcohols and four sugars, including maltitol [26], but the kit performed poorly when separating maltitol and fructose [26].

Despite the merits of the different aforementioned detectors, mass spectrometry (MS) is still widely employed in both qualitative and quantitative analyses of sugars/sugar alcohols as it is able to identify compounds with high levels of sensitivity and specificity. MS allows maltitol to be directly detected without derivatisation. In this context, electrospray ionization (ESI) is normally coupled with HPLC-MS and MS/MS systems [19]. Shah et al. developed a method to simultaneously determine 14 non-nutritive sweeteners, including maltitol, in food and beverages by ESI with UHPLC (ultra-high-performance liquid chromatography) MS/MS in the negative ion mode [36]. The method required minimal sample preparation/clean-up. The beverages were simply diluted with water, except those containing gas, which were first sonicated to remove it. Hard candies were dissolved in water, vortexed and diluted. Yoghurts were processed using SPE. All samples were filtered (0.20 µm membrane filters) prior to injection. The authors tested different kinds of reversed-phase columns, including C8 and C30. The C18 column performed best, i.e., with easier and faster separation. The method enabled the quantification and monitoring of all the analytes by multiple reactions with three isotopically labelled internal standards. Obtaining two structurally significant MS product ions for both analytes and internal standards led to more selectivity and confirmation, which implies a major advantage [36].

Coupling MS with chromatography offers a powerful technique to selectively determine sugars and sugar alcohols in a single run. However, this detection method requires costly analytical instruments and specialised technicians [38]. High-purity organic solvents are also necessary for liquid chromatography [40]. An alternative analytical technique is capillary electrophoresis (CE), which offers good separation efficiency with low operating costs and minimal waste and has, therefore, been increasingly used to study several types of analytes in relatively complex matrices. The separation principles of sugar alcohols in CE systems are similar to those which apply to HPAEC [40].

The usability of CE in analysing maltitol has been recently proven by Coelho et al., who proposed using a method with CE and capacitively coupled contactless conductivity detection (C^4D) [37]. The target analytes were four sugar alcohols, which included maltitol. Chocolate was the studied matrix. Extraction was performed using water and ultrasound, followed by filtration (0.22 µm membrane filters) and dilution. The strong alkaline background electrolyte was 25 mM of sodium borate (pH 8.5), which allowed negatively charged borate esters to form, produced by the borate ions-sugar alcohol interaction. The separation of all analytes was achieved in an impressive time: less than 6 min. This method was applied to commercial chocolate samples and revealed that most contained maltitol as the main sweetener [41].

By way of conclusion, the method of choice for maltitol determination in different food matrices is HPLC because it is compatible with its physico-chemical characteristics, it is able to meet multi-analyte detection needs, and demonstrates simplicity, high sensitivity and robustness. CE is an interesting alternative that often incurs lower running costs. However, it would appear that its robustness is limited [19]. Repeatability and reproducibility issues have been pointed out by several authors, which are mainly caused by inconsistent injection amount and unstable electroosmotic flow rate in the capillaries [42]. Some quantitative studies have directly compared the performance of CE and HPLC. In research conducted by Prado et al. CE provided a swifter analysis, whilst RP-HPLC displayed both superior repeatability (relative standard deviation (RSD) 0.98% vs. RSD 1.62%) and sensitivity (three times less LOD (limit of detection)) [43]. Similarly, Velikinac et al. reported higher selectivity for CE method, but the HPLC method was more sensitive (LOD 2.5 times less) and delivered superior precision (RSD < 2% vs. RSD < 4.5%) [44]. Gas chromatography is not a popular option given the need for derivatisation [34]. As UHPLC-MS/MS systems become increasingly common in laboratories, more methods using this technique will be developed and will enable foodstuffs to be analysed at high-throughput levels. Multi-analyte methods are most advantageous [19]. For the time being, the development of robust reliable methods to determine maltitol and other sweeteners in complex food matrices is an omnipresent challenge. Sound analytical methods are crucial for fulfilling growing needs in the food quality and safety fields.

3. Applications in the Food Industry and Safety

Huge efforts have been made to cut sugar intake in many food products for health reasons, particularly related to cardiovascular diseases and diabetes. This worrying phenomenon has attracted a 'sugar tax' that is imposed on food and drink industries in many countries. As confectioneries are more frequently consumed in the Western world, replacing sucrose is an ongoing challenge for food product developers to focus on alternatives that match aromas, sweetness, mouthfeel and texture. Maltitol forms part of the polyol group used for replacing sugar in the food industry. Polyols are generally relevant to the food industry for combatting weight control, diabetes and tooth decay.

Maltitol is a sugar alcohol that comes from maltose, a disaccharide with a similar sweetness to that of sucrose. Maltitol has many applications in food products like bakery and dairy products, chocolate and sweets. It is commercially available as maltitol syrup (E965ii) and crystalline maltitol (E965i) and is already included in a wide range of foods like chewing gum, chocolate, tableted mints, and other related products such as hard and chewy sweets.

Maltitol is a promising alternative to sugar as a bulk sweetener because its sweetness is almost 85–95% of that of sucrose. Its hygroscopicity is low, and it possesses excellent flow properties and a crystalline structure that results in end products with a very good taste and mouthfeel. Maltitol has a low glycaemic response of 29 and a calorie value of 2.4 kcal per gram in both Europe and the USA, which are lower figures than for traditional bulk sweeteners like sucrose [2]. The glycaemic index (GI) of crystalline maltitol is 36 and the GI for syrup is 52 with a higher hydrogenated oligosaccharides content [45]. Table 2 compares some unique properties of maltitol are compared to those of sucrose.

Table 2. A comparison of some physico-chemical properties for sucrose and maltitol.

Physico-Chemical Properties	Sucrose	Maltitol
Molecular weight	342	344
Sweetness	1.0	0.9
Solubility at 22 °C	67%	65%
Melting point (°C)	168–170	144–152
Heat of solution (cal/g)	4.3	−5.5
* ERH for water uptake (20 °C)	84%	89%
Calories (kcal/g)	4.0	2.4 (EU)
Glycaemic index (GI)	68	35
Molecular formula	$C_{12}H_{22}O_{11}$	$C_{12}H_{24}O_{11}$
Chemical structure		

* ERH—Equilibrium relative humidity. Adapted from Grembecka [41].

Given its many physico-chemical properties, the replacement of sugar with maltitol and its application in foods makes it extremely versatile. The main considerations for the food industries include cooling effect, solubility, hygroscopicity in response to relative humidity, sweetness and taste [46]. Maltitol can act as a bulking agent, humectant, emulsifier, sweetener stabilizer, or thickener in food and drink applications [41].

Awareness about eating low-calorie sweeteners, not only in patients with diabetes but also in the general population, has increased because sweeteners are employed as ingredients in many low-calorie foods: e.g., powdered drink mixes, soft drinks, dairy products, desserts, baked goods, chocolates, sweets, puddings, canned foods, jams and jellies, confectionery and chewing gum. Low-calorie sweeteners can be employed as table-top sweeteners at home, in restaurants and in cafeterias [47].

This section discusses how these properties offer advantages for developing food products, with further details in the following sections on metabolism and health impacts.

Maltitol's sweetness is pleasant and clean and accounts for up to 90% of that attributed to sucrose, but its calorie value is 2.1–2.4 kcal/g (Table 2). Maltitol is also a non-cariogenic agent. Given its slow absorption, the insulin response associated with its ingestion significantly reduces. When applied simultaneously with short-chain fructo-oligosaccharides in sugar-free food product formulations, it lowers postprandial glycaemic responses [41]. As its hygroscopicity is low and it remains stable at high temperature, it is used in many baked products, and also as a variety of low-fat, reduced calorie and sugar-free food. Given its similarities to sucrose, maltitol can replace it in many formulations on a weight-for-weight basis. This allows many healthy snacks to be produced, including "sugar-free" or those with "no added sugar."

A summary of common food products in which sucrose is replaced with maltitol is shown in Table 3.

Table 3. A summary of common food products where sucrose is replaced with maltitol.

Food Product	Impact of the Replacement on Quality Attributes
Reduced sugar baked goods	improved taste and reduced staling
Chocolate powder	improved textural and sensory properties
Milk powder	improved rheological properties
Frozen dairy foods and ice cream	improved creaminess, lower glycaemic index
Drinkable yoghurts and flavoured milk	reduced calorific content, better texture and sweetness profile
Candies and hard sweets	visual appearance is maintained during thermal processing
Pectin jellies	lower energy value, better physicochemical properties
Marshmallow	fine granulometry maltitol powder and increased stability

Common maltitol applications include reduced-sugar baked goods, in which it can act as a 1:1 replacement for sucrose. Its sweetening and bulking properties are equivalent to those of sucrose. For instance, addition of maltitol significantly impacts the quality of dough and bread by affecting water mobility, thermal properties and retrogradation, which denote structure-function relations. Maltitol can lower dough fermentation rates and specific bread volumes to a certain extent. One study has shown that the presence of maltitol can rise the gelatinisation temperature of wheat starch and reduce its enthalpy.

Hardness and chewiness of bread tend to become lower when maltitol is applied, which suggests that maltitol can improve bread tasting properties. Low Field-Nuclear Magnetic Resonance data reveal a weaker interaction between water and starch chains or the gluten network when maltitol is present [1]. This study demonstrated that maltitol performed a binding potential with water and retarded the staling of bread. These phenomena are attributable to hydrophilicity and the hydroxyl number in maltitol, and to its further restriction in water mobility. The crust lightness of maltitol biscuits decreased by 25% because Maillard reactions did not occur, and biscuit texture was significantly softer with significantly better overall acceptance [1]. This study showed that maltitol can be a potential food additive to improve taste and to hinder the staling of bread. Nonetheless, more accurate comprehensive research into the interactions among maltitol, starch and the gluten network, and more rheological experiments, are needed.

Maltitol's low hygroscopicity makes it a polyol of choice for chocolate applications because it contributes to high stability during conching and storage. Maltitol's low hygroscopic character allows chocolate to be refined under the same conditions as sucrose and for conching at temperatures up to 80 °C. Addition of sweeteners to chocolate helps to cut cocoa bitterness, and its impact on rheological properties is also important for chocolate in end-product quality terms. Sucrose composition in chocolate is about 40–50%, depending on the type, which confers many functional properties to chocolate like sweetness, mouthfeel, texture, or particle size distribution (PSD) [48]. Employing maltitol as an alternative sweetener in chocolate improves its textural and sensory characteristics and enhances its storage stability due to anti-blooming effects [49].

The influence of maltitol and xylitol as bulking agents on the rheological properties of compound milk chocolate with a simplex-lattice mixture design has been investigated. The results showed that using maltitol and xylitol instead of sucrose can provide low-calorie compound milk chocolate with no undesirable rheological effects on samples. The results demonstrated that chocolate combinations containing 87.8% maltitol and 12.2% xylitol are optimum concentrations that produce the most acceptable rheological properties [50].

Drinkable yoghurts and flavoured milks have become increasingly popular in recent years as an alternative to high-sugar beverages, and also as delivery systems for prebiotics. High-potency sweeteners and hydrocolloid stabilisers are used to lower these products' energy content. This approach gives a product with a distorted texture and an unpleasant mouthfeel. A more practical approach is to add maltitol or maltitol syrup to replace sugar solids because maltitol significantly contributes to these products' overall sweetness and texture [51]. It is important to ensure that the polyol content of food products remains below 20 g per serving to avoid possible laxative effects. With maltitol, developed end products not only have a better texture because of more equivalent solids but also a more rounded sweetness profile.

Maltitol and maltitol syrups can be suitably applied to bakery products, chocolate and hard sweet production as they neither participate in Maillard reactions nor alter the product's attractive appearance during thermal processing [51].

Maltitol is a useful fat substitute and sugar replacement in frozen dairy food and ice cream as it makes products creamy, sweet and sticky, and extends their shelf life. This makes the freezing point and sweetness of no-added-sugar ice cream similar to that of full-sugar ice cream for the same molecular weight, and sucrose results in a low-glycaemic-index ice cream without its texture being compromised. Taste and sweetness can, thus, be adjusted for sensory optimisation with a combination of sugars, including maltitol and sucralose supplementation to boost sweetness whenever necessary [52]. Dairy flavour and desire for sweetness strongly correlate with vanilla flavour perception that is lacking in alternative formulations. From the studied product formulations, a combination of tagatose (6%), polydextrose (6%) and maltitol (3%) or maltitol (15%) and trehalose (2.5%) in a formulation with milk cream and milk protein concentrate proves to be a potential formulation to meet both sensory and physico-chemical requirements [52].

Hard sweets are essentially constituted of sugar syrup (sucrose and glucose syrup in traditional products) that has been heated to reduce the moisture content to a very low level, insofar as the product's glassy state remains upon cooling [53]. Aerated confectionery, such as marshmallow formulated with maltitol syrup and maltitol powder to replace glucose syrup and sucrose, has been successfully developed. Maltitol syrups containing 55–65% maltitol make good products, in which maltitol forms the major component of these formulations up to 70% of dry solids. For dusting powder applied to outer surfaces, a fine granulometry maltitol powder provides stable products, and its use is preferred to other polyols [53]. It can be used as a sweetener for sugar-free soft sweets and prevents other polyols in the formulation being obtained from crystallising. Sweets made with maltitol have better chewing and are not as sticky.

Maltitol syrup is an excellent polyol for pectin jellies. While producing pectin jellies, their final moisture content can slightly increase (0.3 ± 0.5%) to obtain a similar texture and shelf life to traditional glucose sucrose jellies, and a small amount of carrageenan (0.4 ± 0.5%) can be added to increase the firmness of products stored at high temperature and humidity [46]. These authors also recommended a higher maltitol content of almost 75% to help to prevent pectin from setting too quickly, and they advise depositing at temperatures above 90 °C [46].

In a recent study into reduced sugar jellies formulation from *Physalis peruviana* L. fruit, otherwise known as Cape gooseberry, Inca berry, Peruvian groundcherry, or goldenberry, the authors showed that the physicochemical and textural properties of jellies made their use promising in different foods with a sweet taste, and offer further opportunities for future research into product development [54]. These authors suggested that maltitol and maltitol syrup sweetener are the most functional sugar substitutes in the composition of jellies from physalis juice, as jelly with maltitol and maltitol syrup had a 90% lower total sugar content than that of the jelly made with sucrose and 83% of that produced with fructose.

In addition, the jelly obtained with maltitol and maltitol syrup had the lowest energy value compared to jellies obtained with sugar and fructose. Henceforth according to the terms of EU Regulation No. 1924/2006, jellies with physalis juice and maltitol/maltitol syrup can be classified with nutrition claims such as "food with no added sugars" and "energy-reduced food" [54].

Maltitol is generally recognised as 'halal' as it is permitted by Islamic law and it is kosher pareve as it meets all "kashruth" requirements. It is regarded as vegan-friendly and is GMO-free because raw material starch comes from non-GMO plants [45]. Depending on the overall formulation, products containing maltitol can display a number of label claims, including "no sugar added", "sugar-free" and "low-calorie".

According to the evaluation of the European Food Safety Authority (EFSA) and the Codex Alimentarius Commission, maltitol and other low-calorie sweeteners are safe for human consumption and will not cause cancer or other health-related problems as long as they are consumed at acceptable daily intakes (ADI) [47]. Similarly, extensive toxicological testing by the Joint FAO/WHO Expert Committee of Food Additives (JECFA) has shown that maltitol syrups are safe for human consumption and were given an ADI status. The EFSA is currently reviewing the technico-toxicological data on maltitol and other sweeteners that are authorised as food additives in the EU. This on-going re-evaluation is expected to be completed by the end of 2020 [55].

As maltitol is fermented in the colon, its digestion rate is slow and it is not completely digested, which means a slower rise in blood sugar and insulin levels compared to glucose and sucrose [2] in a study that evaluated the impact of confectionary sweeteners on the composition of gut microbiota. An optimal dose of 34.2 g for maltitol plus polydextrose significantly increased the numbers of faecal bifidobacteria, lactobacilli, and short-chain fatty acids after maltitol ingestion compared to sucrose intake [17]. To date, however, not enough data are available to determine the specific effects of maltitol on gut microbiota, so more studies are necessary [47].

Compared to the reactions that occur after consuming standard sucrose-containing chocolate, the occasional or regular consumption of increasing doses of maltitol is not associated with significant digestive symptoms but does result in increased diarrhoea [10]. Generally speaking, most polyols, including maltitol, have a few side effects when overeaten, such as laxative, gastrointestinal symptoms, bloating, diarrhoea and abdominal pain. Therefore, if any food product contains more than 10% added maltitol or other polyols, it must include the statement "excessive consumption may have laxative effects" [56].

4. Metabolism

Maltitol has substituted for sucrose in many food applications on a weight-for-weight basis due to its slow unfinished absorption through the small intestine and fermentative degradation by intestinal microbiota [4]. The laxative effect of polyols is frequently cited as the main cause of their lack of market penetration (other than their cost vs. sugars). Luckily however, maltitol is one of the best tolerated polyols.

The main features of the metabolism of polyols xylitol, sorbitol, erythritol, mannitol, isomalt, lactitol, maltitol and hydrogenated starch hydrolysates have been described by many authors [57–59]. They include their metabolism, absorption and glycaemic effects, energy utilisation, gastrointestinal tolerance and dental properties. Although structural similarities exist between these polyols, data reveal that the metabolic characteristics of each polyol, especially their calorific values, have to be individually considered [4]. Moreover, we should consider each person's specific condition. Basically, studies on maltitol metabolism have focused on its degradation in the intestines and its effects on the adaptation of dental plaque to metabolise maltitol. Thus, we focus on these two topics.

Maltitol is added to many foods as a sweetener and sugar substitute in relation to its possible interaction with different ingredients. Some studies have reported that the concentration of a sweetener and the characteristics of foodstuff remain stable throughout their shelf life and do not significantly vary when looking at normal food products: yoghurt, burfi, flavoured milk [29], and chocolate [49].

Regarding the oral metabolism of maltitol, it is noteworthy that the oral cavity is a complex ecosystem with the most diverse microbial populations and the second largest diverse microbiota after the gut, with over 700 species of bacteria [60]. In the oral cavity, most habitats are dominated by *Streptococcus*, and other species are located in different areas, followed by *Haemophilus* in buccal mucosa, *Actinomyces* in supragingival plaque, and *Prevotella* in the immediately adjacent (but low-oxygen) subgingival plaque [61,62].

A very important element of pH regulation is saliva (pH 6.5–7), with buffer capacity in the oral cavity. Thus, saliva pH lowers more after consuming snacks containing maltitol. After 10, 15, 20 and 30 min, significant changes take place in saliva pH compared to the initial pH (the zero minute) [63]. Some research has found [63,64] that patients at high caries risk have a significantly lower saliva pH than patients at low caries risk. The type of sweetener in snacks also affects saliva pH, as shown by a reduction after patients have eaten snacks containing sucrose compared to those who ate snacks containing maltitol. This may be because *Streptococcus mutans* cannot change maltitol into acid because essential enzymes are lacking, even though maltitol can penetrate into the membrane of the bacteria cell, which reduces the activity of glucosyltransferase [65] Sucrose can easily be fermented into lactic acid and piruvic acid and, thus, enhance the enzymatic activity of glucosyltransferase [66].

For other polyols, it has been demonstrated both in vivo and in vitro that xylitol and sorbitol inhibit the growth of a number of cariogenic bacteria, including *Streptococcus mutans* and *Streptococcus sobrinus* [67–71]. The mechanism is assumed to be due to the accumulation of sugar alcohol in the cell upon uptake, which results in the formation of a toxic sugar phosphate [71,72]. The effect of maltitol on dental plaque has been studied by Keijser et al. [57], and knowledge about its microbiota is a key element in studying the degradation of polyols. Upper buccal plaque microbiota is dominated by members of the phylum Proteobacteria (30.9%), Firmicutes (26.4%), Actinobacteria, (19.2%) Bacteroidetes (14.0%) and Fusobacteria (9.0%). Lower-lingual plaque is dominated by Fusobacteria (28.2%), Bacteroides (20.6%), Proteobacteria (19.8%), Firmicutes (18%) and Actinobacteria (12.0%). The dominant genera in upper-buccal plaque samples are *Haemophilus, Streptococcus, Corynebacterium* and *Neisseria*. Lower-lingual plaque samples are dominated by *Leptotrichia, Fusobacterium, Prevotella, Veillonella* and *Capnocytophaga*. The effects of polyol-sweetened gums on healthy oral microbiota have not yet been established [57].

Another study indicates that dental plaque adjustment in order to metabolise sucrose and sorbitol occurs with frequent exposure to these sweeteners, while frequent exposure to maltitol and xylitol does not result in plaque adjustment to metabolise these sweeteners [65].

Regarding the intestinal metabolism of maltitol, it is relevant to consider that low-digestible carbohydrates are consumed incompletely, or not, in the small intestine, but are at least partially fermented throughout the large intestine by bacteria [73]. Maltitol belongs to this group (glucose plus sorbitol) as it is included in polyols. Carbohydrates of at least two units usually need to be reduced enzymatically into monosaccharides before they can be absorbed in the small intestine and enter circulation.

During a clinical trial, the consumption of maltitol-polydextrose chocolate contributed to intestinal prebiotic effects, but these findings cannot be clearly extrapolated due to the mixture of putative functional ingredients in the experimental diet [17]. Tolerance to slowly absorbed bulking sweeteners like sugar alcohols is often assessed by fasting healthy volunteers eating large or increasing quantities of the test substance, either on its own or diluted in water [10]. Stool excretion after ingesting sugar alcohols is negligible, which implies that sugar alcohols reach the large intestine when they are almost completely digested by colonic flora [74]. Yet this malabsorption has certain side effects, such as the fermentation of unabsorbed sugar leading to flatulence. As polyol molecules are osmotically active, diarrhoea may occur when the ability of colonic flora to ferment these low-molecular-weight carbohydrates is surpassed and osmotic stress arises in the intestinal lumen [75]. Regular maltitol consumption did not lead to increased rectal gases and in breath H_2 production did not lower compared to occasional maltitol consumption. This means that regular maltitol consumption did not result in colonic flora adaptation and was variable with different unabsorbable sugars [76]. These results demonstrate that a larger part of ingested maltitol is fermented by intestinal microbes than is hydrolysed by digestive enzymes. Although maltitol is catabolised to carbon dioxide via intestinal microbes, there is much less available energy than that of digestible sugars like sucrose [8].

Several carbohydrates, such as isomalt, sorbitol and lactitol, were worse tolerated than similar amounts of maltitol [9]. We only found one study that has compared the effects of maltitol to those of polyglycitol [74], but with different amounts of both. It can y be inferred that certain sugar alcohols are just as well tolerated at the respective intakes (no diarrhoea or other side effects).

According to research into rats and humans, Hosoya [77] concluded that maltitol would not be hydrolysed, but only slightly absorbed from the small intestine before being quickly excreted again. Other investigators, however, stated different degrees of absorption. The detailed study of Rennhard and Bianchine [69] concluded that maltitol is partially hydrolysed in the stomach, partially absorbed intact from the small intestine, and partially degraded by gut flora to volatile fatty acids, which are easily absorbed and utilised by the microbiota.

According to research into rats and humans, Hosoya [77] concluded that maltitol would not be hydrolysed, but absorbed only slightly from the small intestine before being quickly excreted again. Other investigators, however, stated different degrees of absorption. The detailed study of Rennhard and Bianchine [78] concluded that maltitol is partially hydrolysed in the stomach, partially absorbed intact from the small intestine, and partially degraded by gut flora into volatile fatty acids, which are easily absorbed and utilised by the microbiota.

Another benefit of several sweeteners is the relation with H_2 production in the small intestine, which can reduce hepatic oxidative stress, diminish the severity of neurological disorders [79,80], lead to lower concentrations of inflammatory cytokines [81], and has been employed as a drug for the suppression of postprandial hyperglycaemia by inhibiting the digestion of disaccharides. It can also suppress the risk of myocardial infarction in patients with type 2 diabetes [82].

Hydrogen breath studies have indirectly tested malabsorption by measuring hydrogen expiration, a result of colonic fermentation. The major source of exogenous H_2 is the intestinal microbiome which produces it from indigestible components whose source can be dietary fibre (non-digestible carbohydrates and lignin), including functional fibre (isolated non-digestible carbohydrates shown to have beneficial physiologic effects on humans) [83], and can be responsible for inducing H_2 production. Matsumoto et al. [84] concluded that a combination of the different chemical structures of indigestible components, such as H_2-producing milk containing sugar alcohol (maltitol), may be important and effective for H_2 production by various intestinal microbiomes (Rikenellaceae, Clostridiales Incertae, Clostridiales, Ruminococcaceae and *Alistipes*).

Table 4 summarises several benefits of the regular consumption of maltitol versus other sweeteners.

Table 4. Several benefits of the regular consumption maltitol versus other sweeteners.

Maltitol Consumption Benefits	Reference(s)
Does not reduce the saliva pH	[65]
Excellent relation with different ingredient of foodstuff	[29]
It is not fermented in the oral cavity	[66]
The oral cave micro-organisms cannot produce an adjustment to metabolise the maltitol	[65]
Possible probiotic effects	[17]
Produces less energy in small intestine	[17]
Partially hydrolysed in the stomach	[78]
Partially absorbed in the small intestine	[78]
Easily absorbed and utilised by the microbiota	[78]
Improvement of the H_2 production by intestinal microbiomes	[84]

5. Impacts on Health

Thorough toxicological studies have proven that maltitol is safe for use. The Joint FAO/WHO Expert Committee of Food Additives (JECFA) has assigned it as an acceptable "not specified" daily intake [85–87]. It is authorised in most countries for food use, although some countries (EU, USA) have their own particular legal standards and purity specifications for this substance, while others do not and instead follow the Codex Alimentarius specification for maltitol. Polyols are known as food additives in the EU, and their use in food is regulated by Sweeteners in Food Regulations. Maltitol (and maltitol syrups) have been assigned E number E965 and are approved for use in food at quantum satis for a variety of food items specified in the regulations, usually bakery goods, confectionery, ice cream, desserts and fruit preparations. Polyols are not usually permitted in drinks (except erythritol) due to over-consumption laxation issues. Maltitol (and other polyols) cannot be used in foods in association with sugars in the EU unless the polyol is employed, as a result of the mixture, for a technical purpose other than sweetness or towards a 30% reduction in calories that results from the combination. Prohibitions on using polyols in conjunction with sugars do not exist in the USA, and the Food and Drug Administration (FDA) finds polyols to be a food additive or 'Generally Recognized as Safe' (GRAS). Maltitol has a self-affirmed GRAS status [4,88]. Of all sugar alcohols, maltitol most resembles sugar flavour. It is not cariogenic and is safe for diabetics [89,90].

Its usage does not facilitate tooth decay [6,88,91] because it cannot be fermented by oral bacteria [7,92]. Daily use of gum containing maltitol induces the inhibition of some bacteria present in supragingival plaque microbiota, many of which are known as first dental surface colonisers [57]. Several in vitro and animal experiments [93,94] have identified the oral health impact of maltitol, as have clinical trials [95,96]. Yet maltitol's health advantage is not restricted to dental care. Evidence from previous research works indicates that maltitol can have major anti-hyperglycaemic potential [3,6,97,98]. This is because a single oral administration of 50 g of maltitol to healthy individuals resulted in substantially lower glycaemic and insulin responses compared to administering the same volume of glucose or sucrose [99,100]. It has also been documented that the intake of 30 or 50 g of maltitol as a single oral dose leads to a lower glucose and insulin response compared to diabetic subjects' ingestion of an equal volume of maltose or glucose [101,102]. Overweight participants fed low-fat, low-calorie and high-amylose cornstarch-sweetened maltitol muffins displayed lower glucose, insulin and lipidaemic responses, but improved satiety versus those fed traditional sugar-sweetened muffins [98]. Two prior reports recorded a single oral maltitol administration, namely sorbitol mixture (60:7) [100] or 50 g of maltitol [103], which significantly reduced blood insulin and glucose responses in relation to administering the same volume of glucose in both normal and diabetic participants.

A study by Kang et al. [104] documented in vitro alpha glucosidase, alpha amylase and sucrase inhibitory maltitol activity, which indicates that maltitol can be useful for regulating carbohydrate digestion and postprandial hyper-glycaemia. Contrarily to this, Matsuo [97] stated that maltitol did not inhibit intestinal glucosidase, sucrase or maltase operations with a single oral dose of a maltitol and sucrose mixture (25:25 g) or of sucrose (50 g) or maltitol (50 g) given to healthy individuals. Based on the findings of the above-mentioned studies, it can be argued that maltitol may show a hypoglycaemic reaction by other mechanisms, such as inhibiting the absorption of intestinal glucose and/or increasing muscle glucose uptake, rather than inhibiting intestinal carbohydrate digesting enzyme activities [105]. Thabuis et al. [3] also noted that, in accordance with FAO recommendations, the maltitol glycaemic response (GR) was significantly lower than the glucose GR up to 90 min after its administration. The insulin-emic response (IR) to maltitol was substantially lower than the glucose IR up to 2 h after administration, according to FAO recommendations. Maltitol showed few glycaemic and insulinaemic responses. Both substances were well tolerated by all the volunteers who participated in the study up to a single intake of 50 g.

Chukwuma et al. [105] observed that maltitol prevents the synthesis of intestinal glucose and improves the accumulation of insulin-mediated muscle glucose ex vivo, but not in normal and type 2 diabetic rats when co-ingested with glucose. Dietary glucose is consumed quickly from the small intestine. However, experiments in vitro have indicated that the proximal [106] or mid-small intestine (part of the duodenum and jejunum) [107] shows the highest glucose absorption. Hence the jejunal rat intestine portion was used in the ex vivo procedure to study glucose absorption. It is also recognised that osmotic pressure can affect the absorption of intestinal water and glucose. Previous in vitro research has indicated that lowering osmolality in isolated rat duodenums enhanced the uptake of luminal water and glucose [108].

The peak value of 5.20 ± 0.72 mg/cm jejunum of glucose absorption was found in the ex vivo absorption research by Chukwuma et al. [105], which lowered to 3.00 ± 0.35 mg/cm jejunum in the presence of 2.5% maltitol. Maltitol's inhibitory effect on jejunal glucose absorption was concentration-dependent, with the lowest value of 1.20 ± 0.20 mg/cm jejunum at 20% maltitol. These results indicate a concentration-dependent inhibitory influence of maltitol on ex vivo jejunal glucose absorption, which may be attributed partly to a growing osmolarity (388.48–896.68 mOs m/L) influence of increasing maltitol concentrations (2.5–10%). Unlike the major ex vivo inhibitory effect of maltitol on jejunal glucose absorption, however, a single oral maltitol administration that was co-ingested with glucose did not significantly affect or lower the glucose absorption index in intestinal segments. This effect similarly translates into the observed marginal effect in normal glycaemic and diabetic animals on postprandial blood glucose levels. As seen in several previous studies [78,109,110], this finding under in vivo conditions may be related to maltitol hydrolysis by disaccharidases of small intestinal mucosa. The recent findings of Chukwuma et al. [105] tend to further clarify the apparent inconsistency between the documented effects of maltitol on alpha glucosidase and alpha amylase, which ranged from in vitro [104] to in vivo experimental conditions [97].

Gastric emptying and digesta gastrointestinal tract transit levels primarily affect nutrient absorption in the small intestine. Previous research has shown that delayed gastric emptying and rapid digestive transit can lead to less intestinal absorption of nutrients and food intake [111,112], which is believed to be a mode of action of acarbose in regulating postprandial blood glucose production in diabetic patients [113]. A single oral dose of maltitol has recently been shown to have no major impact on gastric emptying in normal or diabetic animals, which could be partly responsible for the negligible effect of maltitol on small intestinal glucose absorption [105]. Nevertheless, maltitol accelerated the digestive transit in the caecum of diabetic rats, but not other parts, which did not affect overall intestinal glucose absorption because most glucose absorption occurs in the first quarter to the mid-small intestine [106,107].

Circulating glucose uptake by cells is a significant mechanism for the body to preserve glucose homeostasis, as blood glucose rises owing to glycogen degradation, dietary glucose absorption and gluconeogenesis [114] for either storage or energy metabolism. Insulin is the main controlling hormone in activating the clearance of circulating glucose through insulin-mediated glucose absorption in cells [114]. Some previous studies have stated that hyperosmolarity improves muscle glucose absorption by AMP-Kinase (adenosine monophosphate-Kinase) regulation and/or glucose transporter type 4 endocytosis inhibition [115], but recent ex vivo research has revealed that while maltitol demonstrates insulin-mediated glucose uptake (GU50 = 7.31 ± 2.08%), it does not have any substantial insulin-free glucose uptake effect on isolated rat psoas muscle (GU50 = 111.12 ± 19.36%) [105]. This result may indicate that maltitol can potentiate insulin-mediated glucose absorption in muscles, at least in ex vivo environments, when increased osmolarity (388.48–896.68 mOsm/L) due to higher maltitol concentrations cannot be an influential factor in this regard.

Regarding maltitol's possible genotoxicity and teratogenicity, a few decades ago Takizawa and Hachiya [116] stated that maltitol was not mutagenic in *Escherichia coli* and *Salmonella typhimurium* strains and did not induce the frequency of micronucleus in mice bone marrow cells. Canimoglu and Rencuzogullari [117] also stated that maltitol did not induce the mean of sister chromatid exchanges and the percentage of chromosome aberrations at all concentrations and for all treatment periods in human lymphocytes but did induce the micronucleus frequency with no dose dependency.

In a study by Canimoglu and Rencuzogullari [118], conducted to reveal the genotoxicity and cytotoxicity of maltitol, rats were intraperitoneally administered with up to 10 g/kg body weight (bw) maltitol concentrations; that is, a very high dose. Despite this dose, maltitol was neither genotoxic nor cytotoxic. It ought not to be believed that 10 g/kg bw of maltitol should be given to humans in one day. Hence the maximal employed maltitol dose cannot be surpassed, and it can be inferred that maltitol has no genotoxic impact on the in vivo test system.

Maltitol was not proven cytotoxic in rat bone marrow cells because it did not lower the mitotic index. Maltitol was not cytotoxic in human lymphocytes [117], but for other sweeteners there are reports that some were cytotoxic [119–121] and some were not [122]. Maltitol was not shown to be teratogenic, but an embryotoxic influence was demonstrated by reducing the weight of foetuses and inducing growth retardation at a very high concentration (4 g/kg bw) [112].

Therefore, at lower doses, it can be inferred that maltitol poses a low risk for humans but may induce diarrhoea when taken at high doses [112]. Additionally, maltitol may induce hyper-glycaemia and lower embryo weight during pregnancy when used at high doses over long periods, particularly during the first trimester of pregnancy [112]. Accordingly, caution must be taken in utilising it at higher concentrations in food and beverages for the health of our generation and future generations. Table 5 summarises the main attributes of consumed maltitol and its relations to health impacts.

Table 5. The main attributes of maltitol for its consumption, taking into account impacts on health.

Attribute	Reference(s)
Not cariogenic	[89,90]
Prevents tooth decay	[6,88,91,95,96]
Antihyperglycaemic	[3,6,97,98,104,105]
Insulin-mediated glucose uptake	[105]
Not genotoxic	[118]
Not cytotoxic	[118]
Not teratogenic	[118]
Decreases foetus weight	[118]
Causes growth retardation at high doses (4 g/kg body weight)	[118]

6. Conclusions

Maltitol remains innocuous and helps to improve consumers' health quality due to benefits such as exerting prebiotic effects, lowering calorie consumption due to sucrose, and promoting dental health. Due to the similarity of the physicochemical features of maltitol and sucrose, the latter can be easily substituted for maltitol in several foodstuffs; we therefore considered several analytical methods in the determination of maltitol in food samples and its identification can be executed by HPLC methods, which are the most widely used analytical methods of choice. When considering the pros and cons of different analytical methods, HPLC is easier and widely used to detect maltitol in foods.

Based on our literature review, in order to gain a better understanding of the metabolism of maltitol and its impacts on human health, more studies need to be conducted to determine the effects of larger maltitol doses over longer periods of time on gastrointestinal tolerance, gut microbiota in both the small and large intestines, and oral cavity. Since a high consumption of maltitol has some adverse effects such as flatulence and laxative effects, adequate information has to be provided to consumers. Labelling foodstuffs containing sweeteners (>10%) that "excessive consumption may have laxative effects" is an important way to provide information on such effects.

Author Contributions: A.S., C.C., F.R., D.R. and A.R. equally contributed to review the literature, and worked on summarising the results, conceptualization, and discussion, and also wrote the manuscript. They read the manuscript and approved this submission. All authors have read and agreed to the published version of the manuscript.

Funding: This research received no external funding.

Acknowledgments: The authors are very grateful to their families and friends for all the support they provided.

Conflicts of Interest: The authors declare no conflict of interest.

References

1. Ding, S.; Peng, B.; Li, Y.; Yang, J. Evaluation of specific volume, texture, thermal features, water mobility, and inhibitory effect of staling in wheat bread affected by maltitol. *Food Chem.* **2019**, *283*, 123–130. [CrossRef]
2. Rozzi, N.L. Sweet Facts about Maltitol. *Food Prod. Des.* **2007**, *17*, 10.
3. Thabuis, C.; Rodriguez, B.; Gala, T.; Salvi, A.; Parashuraman, M.; Wils, D.; Guerin-Deremaux, L. Evaluation of glycemic and insulinemic responses of maltitol in Indian healthy volunteers. *Int. J. Diabetes Dev. Ctries.* **2015**, *35*, 482–487. [CrossRef]
4. Kearsley, M.W.; Deis, R.C. Maltitol powder. In *Sweeteners and Sugar Alternatives in Food Technology*, 2nd ed.; O'Donnell, K., Kearsley, M.W., Eds.; John Wiley & Sons, Ltd.: Chichester, UK, 2012; pp. 295–308.
5. Livesey, G. Glycaemic responses and toleration. In *Sweeteners and Sugar Alternatives in Food Technology*, 2nd ed.; O'Donnell, K., Kearsley, M.W., Eds.; John Wiley & Sons, Ltd.: Chichester, UK, 2012; pp. 3–26.
6. Livesey, G. Health potential of polyols as sugar replacers, with emphasis on low glycaemic properties. *Nutr. Res. Rev.* **2003**, *16*, 163–191. [CrossRef] [PubMed]
7. Matsuo, T. Lactic acid production from sugar alcohol, maltitol and lactitol, in human whole saliva. *Shigaku* **1973**, *60*, 760.
8. Oku, T.; Akiba, M.; Lee, M.H.; Moon, S.J.; Hosoya, N. Metabolic fate of ingested [14C]-maltitol in man. *J. Nutr. Sci. Vitaminol.* **1991**, *37*, 529–544. [CrossRef]
9. Koutsou, G.A.; Storey, D.M.; Lee, A.; Zumbe, A.; Flourie, B.; LeBot, Y.; Olivier, P. Dose-related gastrointestinal response to the ingestion of either isomalt, lactitol or maltitol in milk chocolate. *Eur. J. Clin. Nutr.* **1996**, *50*, 17.
10. Ruskone-Fourmestraux, A.; Attar, A.; Chassard, D.; Coffin, B.; Bornet, F.; Bouhnik, Y. A digestive tolerance study of maltitol after occasional and regular consumption in healthy humans. *Eur. J. Clin. Nutr.* **2003**, *57*, 26–30. [CrossRef] [PubMed]
11. Storey, D.M.; Koutsou, G.A.; Lee, A.; Zumbe, A.; Olivier, P.; Le Bot, Y.; Flourie, B. Tolerance and breath hydrogen excretion following ingestion of maltitol incorporated at two levels into milk chocolate consumed by healthy young adults with and without fasting. *J. Nutr.* **1998**, *128*, 587–592. [CrossRef]
12. Thabuis, C.; Cazaubiel, M.; Pichelin, M.; Wils, D.; Guerin-Deremaux, L. Short-term digestive tolerance of chocolate formulated with maltitol in children. *Int. J. Food Sci. Nutr.* **2010**, *61*, 728–738. [CrossRef]
13. Imfeld, T.N. Clinical caries studies with polyalcohols. A literature review. *Schweiz. Monatsschr. Zahnmed.* **1994**, *104*, 941–945. [PubMed]
14. Ito, I.; Ito, A.; Unezaki, S. Preparation and evaluation of gelling granules to improve oral administration. *Drug Discov. Ther.* **2015**, *9*, 213–220. [CrossRef] [PubMed]

15. Portmann, M.O.; Kilcast, D. Psychophysical characterization of new sweeteners of commercial importance for the EC food industry. *Food Chem.* **1996**, *56*, 291–302. [CrossRef]
16. Lee, A.; Wils, D.; Zumbe, A.; Storey, D.M. The comparative gastrointestinal responses of children and adults following consumption of sweets formulated with sucrose, isomalt and lycasin HBC. *Eur. J. Clin. Nutr.* **2002**, *56*, 755–764. [CrossRef]
17. Beards, E.; Tuohy, K.; Gibson, G. A human volunteer study to assess the impact of confectionery sweeteners on the gut microbiota composition. *Br. J. Nutr.* **2010**, *104*, 701–708. [CrossRef]
18. Thabuis, C.; Herbomez, A.C.; Desailly, F.; Ringard, F.; Wils, D.; Guérin-Deremaux, L. Prebiotic-like effects of SweetPearl® Maltitol through changes in caecal and fecal parameters. *Food Nutr. Sci.* **2012**, *3*, 1375. [CrossRef]
19. Shah, R.; de Jager, L.S. Recent analytical methods for the analysis of sweeteners in food: A regulatory perspective. *Food Drug Adm. Papers.* **2017**, *5*, 13–32.
20. Kokotou, M.G.; Asimakopoulos, A.G.; Thomaidis, N.S. Sweeteners. In *Food Analysis by HPLC*; Nollet, L.M.L., Toldrá, F., Eds.; CRC Press: Boca Raton, FL, USA, 2012; pp. 493–513.
21. Nikoleli, G.-P.; Nikolelis, D.P. Low Calorie Nonnutritive Sweeteners. In *Sweeteners: Nutritional Aspects, Applications, and Production Technology*; Varzakas, T., Labropoulos, A., Anestis, S., Eds.; CRC Press: Boca Raton, FL, USA, 2012; pp. 80–117.
22. Kokotou, M.G.; Asimakopoulos, A.G.; Thomaidis, N.S. Intense Sweeteners. In *Handbook of Food Analysis*; Nollest, L.M.L., Toldrá, F., Eds.; CRC Press: Boca Raton, FL, USA, 2016; pp. 219–232.
23. Grembecka, M. Sugar Alcohols. In *Encyclopedia of Analytical Science*, 3rd ed.; Worsfold, P., Poole, C., Townshend, A., Miró, M., Eds.; Elsevier: Amsterdam, The Netherlands, 2019; pp. 290–299.
24. Zygler, A.; Wasik, A.; Namieśnik, J. Analytical methodologies for determination of artificial sweeteners in foodstuffs. *TrAC-Trends Anal. Chem.* **2009**, *28*, 1082–1102. [CrossRef]
25. Grembecka, M.; Lebiedzińska, A.; Szefer, P. Simultaneous separation and determination of erythritol, xylitol, sorbitol, mannitol, maltitol, fructose, glucose, sucrose and maltose in food products by high performance liquid chromatography coupled to charged aerosol detector. *Microchem. J.* **2014**, *117*, 77–82. [CrossRef]
26. Andersen, R.; Sørensen, A. Separation and determination of alditols and sugars by high-pH anion-exchange chromatography with pulsed amperometric detection. *J. Chromatogr. A* **2000**, *897*, 195–204. [CrossRef]
27. Nojiri, S.; Taguchi, N.; Oishi, M.; Suzuki, S. Determination of sugar alcohols in confectioneries by high-performance liquid chromatography after nitrobenzoylation. *J. Chromatogr. A* **2000**, *893*, 195–200. [CrossRef]
28. Otles, S.; Ozyurt, V.H. Sampling and Sample Preparation. In *Handbook of Food Chemistry*; Cheung, P.C.K., Mehta, B.M., Eds.; Springer: Berlin, Germany, 2015; pp. 151–164.
29. Joshi, K.; Kumari, A.; Arora, S.; Singh, A.K. Development of an analytical protocol for the estimation of maltitol from yoghurt, burfi and flavoured milk. *LWT-Food Sci. Technol.* **2016**, *70*, 41–45. [CrossRef]
30. Albero, B.; Sánchez-Brunete, C.; García-Valcárcel, A.I.; Pérez, R.A.; Tadeo, J.L. Ultrasound-assisted extraction of emerging contaminants from environmental samples. *TrAC-Trends Anal. Chem.* **2015**, *71*, 110–118. [CrossRef]
31. Martínez Montero, C.; Rodríguez Dodero, M.C.; Guillén Sánchez, D.A.; Barroso, C.G. Analysis of low molecular weight carbohydrates in food and beverages: A review. *Chromatographia* **2004**, *59*, 15–30.
32. Hadjikinova, R.; Petkova, N.; Hadjikinov, D.; Denev, P.; Hrusavov, D. Development and validation of HPLC-RID method for determination of sugars and polyols. *J. Pharm. Sci. Res.* **2017**, *9*, 1263–1269.
33. Koh, D.-W.; Park, J.-W.; Lim, J.-H.; Yea, M.-J.; Bang, D.-Y. A rapid method for simultaneous quantification of 13 sugars and sugar alcohols in food products by UPLC-ELSD. *Food Chem.* **2018**, *240*, 694–700. [CrossRef] [PubMed]
34. Pitsch, J.; Weghuber, J. Hydrophilic interaction chromatography coupled with charged aerosol detection for simultaneous quantitation of carbohydrates, polyols and ions in food and beverages. *Molecules* **2019**, *24*, 4333. [CrossRef]
35. Cataldi, T.R.; Campa, C.; Casella, I.G.; Bufo, S.A. Determination of maltitol, isomaltitol, and lactitol by high-pH anion-exchange chromatography with pulsed amperometric detection. *J. Agric. Food Chem.* **1999**, *47*, 157–163. [CrossRef]

36. Shah, R.; Farris, S.; De Jager, L.S.; Begley, T.H. A novel method for the simultaneous determination of 14 sweeteners of regulatory interest using UHPLC-MS/MS. *Food Addit. Contam. Part A* **2015**, *32*, 141–151. [CrossRef]
37. Coelho, A.G.; DeJesus, D.P. A simple method for determination of erythritol, maltitol, xylitol, and sorbitol in sugar free chocolates by capillary electrophoresis with capacitively coupled contactless conductivity detection. *Electrophoresis* **2016**, *37*, 2986–2991. [CrossRef]
38. Cortés-Herrera, C.; Artavia, G.; Leiva, A.; Granados-Chinchilla, F. Liquid chromatography analysis of common nutritional components, in feed and food. *Foods* **2019**, *8*, 1. [CrossRef] [PubMed]
39. Sanz, M.L.; Martínez-Castro, I. Recent developments in sample preparation for chromatographic analysis of carbohydrates. *J. Chromatogr. A* **2007**, *1153*, 74–89. [CrossRef]
40. Pokrzywnicka, M.; Koncki, R. Disaccharides determination: A review of analytical methods. *Crit. Rev. Anal. Chem.* **2018**, *48*, 186–213. [CrossRef] [PubMed]
41. Grembecka, M. Sugar alcohols—their role in the modern world of sweeteners: A review. *Eur. Food Res. Technol.* **2015**, *241*, 1–14. [CrossRef]
42. Nowak, P.M.; Woźniakiewicz, M.; Gładysz, M.; Janus, M.; Kościelniak, P. Improving repeatability of capillary electrophoresis—A critical comparison of ten different capillary inner surfaces and three criteria of peak identification. *Anal. Bioanal. Chem.* **2017**, *409*, 4383–4393. [CrossRef] [PubMed]
43. Prado, M.S.A.; Steppe, M.; Tavares, M.F.M.; Kedor-Hackmann, E.R.M.; Santoro, M.I.R.M. Comparison of capillary electrophoresis and reversed-phase liquid chromatography methodologies for determination of diazepam in pharmaceutical tablets. *J. Pharm. Biomed. Anal.* **2005**, *37*, 273–279. [CrossRef] [PubMed]
44. Velikinac, I.; Čudina, O.; Janković, I.; Agbaba, D.; Vladimirov, S. Comparison of capillary zone electrophoresis and high performance liquid chromatography methods for quantitative determination of ketoconazole in drug formulations. *Farmaco* **2004**, *59*, 419–424. [CrossRef]
45. Food Additives. What is Maltitol (E965) in Food? Uses, Health benefits, Safety, Side Effects. Available online: https://foodadditives.net/sugar-alcohols/maltitol/ (accessed on 1 May 2020).
46. Zumbe, A.; Lee, A.; Storey, D. Polyols in confectionery: The route to sugar-free, reduced sugar and reduced calorie confectionery. *Br. J. Nutr.* **2001**, *85*, S31–S45. [CrossRef]
47. Ruiz-Ojeda, F.J.; Plaza-Díaz, J.; Sáez-Lara, M.J.; Gil, A. Effects of sweeteners on the gut microbiota: A review of experimental studies and clinical trials. *Adv. Nutr.* **2019**, *10* (Suppl. 1), S31–S48. [CrossRef]
48. Aidoo, R.P.; Depypere, F.; Afoakwa, E.O.; Dewettinck, K. Industrial manufacture of sugar-free chocolates–Applicability of alternative sweeteners and carbohydrate polymers as raw materials in product development. *Trends Food Sci. Technol.* **2013**, *32*, 84–96. [CrossRef]
49. Son, Y.J.; Choi, S.Y.; Yoo, K.M.; Lee, K.W.; Lee, S.M.; Hwang, I.K.; Kim, S. Anti-blooming effect of maltitol and tagatose as sugar substitutes for chocolate making. *LWT-Food Sci. Technol.* **2018**, *88*, 87–94. [CrossRef]
50. Pirouzian, H.R.; Peighambardoust, S.H.; Azadmard-Damirchi, S. Rheological properties of sugarfree milk chocolate: Comparative study and optimisation. *Czech J. Food Sci.* **2017**, *35*, 440–448.
51. Dobreva, V.; Hadjikinova, M.; Slavov, A.; Hadjikinov, D.; Dobrev, G.; Zhekova, B. Functional properties of maltitol. *Agric. Sci. Technol.* **2013**, *5*, 168–172.
52. Whelan, A.P.; Vega, C.; Kerry, J.P.; Goff, H.D. Physicochemical and sensory optimisation of a low glycemic index ice cream formulation. *Int. J. Food Sci. Technol.* **2008**, *43*, 1520–1527. [CrossRef]
53. Flambeau, M.; Respondek, F.; Wagner, A. Maltitol syrups. In *Sweeteners and Sugar Alternatives in Food Technology*, 2nd ed.; O'Donnell, K., Kearsley, M.W., Eds.; John Wiley & Sons, Ltd.: Chichester, UK, 2012; pp. 309–330.
54. Hadjikinova, R.; Stankov, S.; Popova, V.; Ivanova, T.; Stoyanova, A.; Mazova, N.; Marudova, M.; Damyanova, S. Physicochemical and textural properties of reduced sugar jellies from *Physalis peruviana* L. fruit. *Ukr. Food J.* **2019**, *8*, 560–570. [CrossRef]
55. EFSA. Call for Technical and Toxicological Data on Sweeteners Authorised as Food Additives in the EU. June 2017. Available online: https://www.efsa.europa.eu/sites/default/files/engage/170621.pdf (accessed on 1 May 2020).
56. Petković, M. Alternatives for Sugar Replacement in Food Technology: Formulating and Processing Key Aspects. In *Food Engineering*, 1st ed.; Coldea, T.E., Ed.; IntechOpen, Ltd.: London, UK, 2019. [CrossRef]

57. Keijser, B.J.; van den Broek, T.J.; Slot, D.E.; van Twillert, L.; Kool, J.; Thabuis, C.; Ossendrijver, M.; van der Weijden, F.A.; Montijn, R.C. The impact of maltitol-sweetened chewing gum on the dental plaque biofilm microbiota composition. *Front. Microbiol.* **2018**, *9*, 381. [CrossRef]
58. Mooradian, A.D.; Smith, M.; Tokuda, M. The role of artificial and natural sweeteners in reducing the consumption of table sugar: A narrative review. *Clin. Nutr. ESPEN* **2017**, *18*, 1–8. [CrossRef]
59. Theka, T.; Rodgers, A. Glycaemia and phosphatemia after oral glucose and maltitol ingestion in subjects from two different race groups: Preliminary evidence of inter-race differences in metabolism and possible implications for urinary stone disease. *Int. Urol. Nephrol.* **2017**, *49*, 1369–1374. [CrossRef]
60. Deo, P.N.; Deshmukh, R. Oral microbiome: Unveiling the fundamentals. *J. Oral Maxillofac. Pathol.* **2019**, *23*, 122.
61. Huttenhower, C.; Gevers, D.; Knight, R.; Abubucker, S.; Badger, J.H.; Chinwalla, A.T.; Creasy, H.H.; Earl, A.M.; FitzGerald, M.G.; Fulton, R.S.; et al. Structure, function and diversity of the healthy human microbiome. *Nature* **2012**, *486*, 207.
62. Segata, N.; Waldron, L.; Ballarini, A.; Narasimhan, V.; Jousson, O.; Huttenhower, C. Metagenomic microbial community profiling using unique clade-specific marker genes. *Nat. Methods* **2012**, *9*, 811. [CrossRef]
63. Widowati, W.; Akbar, S.H.; Tin, M.H. Saliva pH Changes in Patients with High and Low Caries Risk After Consuming Organic (Sucrose) and Non-Organic (Maltitol) Sugar. *Int. Med. J. Malays.* **2013**, *12*.
64. Sardana, V.; Balappanavar, A.Y.; Patil, G.B.; Kulkarni, N.; Sagari, S.G.; Gupta, K.D. Impact of a modified carbonated beverage on human dental plaque and salivary pH: An in vivo study. *J. Indian Soc. Pedod. Prev. Dent.* **2012**, *30*, 7. [PubMed]
65. Maguire, A.; Rugg-Gunn, J.; Wright, G. Adaptation of dental plaque to metabolise maltitol compared with other sweeteners. *J. Dent.* **2000**, *28*, 51–59. [CrossRef]
66. Wolff, M.S.; Larson, C. The cariogenic dental biofilm: Good, bad or just something to control? *Braz. Oral Res.* **2009**, *23*, 31–38. [CrossRef] [PubMed]
67. Thabuis, C.; Cheng, C.Y.; Wang, X.; Pochat, M.; Han, A.; Miller, L.; Wils, D.; Guerin-Deremaux, L. Effects of maltitol and xylitol chewing-gums on parameters involved in dental caries development. *Eur. J. Paediatr. Dent.* **2013**, *14*, 303–308.
68. Söderling, E.; Hirvonen, A.; Karjalainen, S.; Fontana, M.; Catt, D.; Seppä, L. The effect of xylitol on the composition of the oral flora: A pilot study. *Eur. J. Dent.* **2011**, *5*, 24–31. [CrossRef]
69. Haghgoo, R.; Afshari, E.; Ghanaat, T.; Aghazadeh, S. Comparing the efficacy of xylitol-containing and conventional chewing gums in reducing salivary counts of Streptococcus mutans: An in vivo study. *J. Int. Soc. Prev. Community Dent.* **2015**, *5* (Suppl. 2), S112.
70. Mäkinen, K.K. Gastrointestinal disturbances associated with the consumption of sugar alcohols with special consideration of Xylitol: Scientific review and instructions for dentists and other health-care professionals. *Int. J. Dent.* **2016**, *2016*, 5967907. [CrossRef]
71. Trahan, L.; Bourgeau, G.; Breton, R. Emergence of multiple xylitol-resistant (fructose PTS-) mutants from human isolates of mutans streptococci during growth on dietary sugars in the presence of xylitol. *J. Dent. Res.* **1996**, *75*, 1892–1900. [CrossRef]
72. Miyasawa-Hori, H.; Aizawa, S.; Takahashi, N. Difference in the xylitol sensitivity of acid production among Streptococcus mutans strains and the biochemical mechanism. *Oral Microbiol. Immunol.* **2006**, *21*, 201–205. [CrossRef] [PubMed]
73. Grabitske, H.A.; Slavin, J.L. Gastrointestinal effects of low-digestible carbohydrates. *Crit. Rev. Food Sci. Nutr.* **2009**, *49*, 327–360. [CrossRef] [PubMed]
74. Beaugerie, L.; Flourié, B.; Marteau, P.; Pellier, P.; Franchisseur, C.; Rambaud, J.C. Digestion and absorption in the human intestine of three sugar alcohols. *Gastroenterology* **1990**, *99*, 717–723. [CrossRef]
75. Hammer, H.F.; Santa Ana, C.A.; Schiller, L.R.; Fordtran, J.S. Studies of osmotic diarrhea induced in normal subjects by ingestion of polyethylene glycol and lactulose. *J. Clin. Investig.* **1989**, *84*, 1056–1062. [CrossRef] [PubMed]
76. Stone-Dorshow, T.; Levitt, M.D. Gaseous response to ingestion of a poorly absorbed fructo-oligosaccharide sweetener. *Am. J. Clin. Nutr.* **1987**, *46*, 61–65. [CrossRef]
77. Hosoya, N. Effect of sugar alcohols on the intestine. In *Chàvez, Bourges, Basta, Nutrition. Proc. 9th Int. Congr. Nutr., Mexico 1972*; Vol. 1: Review of basic knowledge; Karger: Basel, Switzerland, 1975; pp. 164–168.

78. Rennhard, H.H.; Bianchine, J.R. Metabolism and caloric utilization of orally administered carbon-14-labeled maltitol in rat, dog, and man. *J. Agric. Food Chem.* **1976**, *24*, 287–291. [CrossRef]
79. Nishimura, N.; Tanabe, H.; Sasaki, Y.; Makita, Y.; Ohata, M.; Yokoyama, S.; Asano, M.; Yamamoto, T.; Kiriyama, S. Pectin and high-amylose maize starch increase caecal hydrogen production and relieve hepatic ischaemia–reperfusion injury in rats. *Br. J. Nutr.* **2012**, *107*, 485–492. [CrossRef]
80. Tanabe, H.; Sasaki, Y.; Yamamoto, T.; Kiriyama, S.; Nishimura, N. Suppressive effect of high hydrogen generating high amylose cornstarch on subacute hepatic ischemia-reperfusion injury in rats. *Biosci. Microbiota Food Health* **2012**, *31*, 103–108. [CrossRef]
81. Nishimura, N.; Tanabe, H.; Adachi, M.; Yamamoto, T.; Fukushima, M. Colonic hydrogen generated from fructan diffuses into the abdominal cavity and reduces adipose mRNA abundance of cytokines in rats. *J. Nutr.* **2013**, *143*, 1943–1949. [CrossRef]
82. Hanefeld, M.; Cagatay, M.; Petrowitsch, T.; Neuser, D.; Petzinna, D.; Rupp, M. Acarbose reduces the risk for myocardial infarction in type 2 diabetic patients: Meta-analysis of seven long-term studies. *Eur. Heart J.* **2004**, *25*, 10–16. [CrossRef]
83. Lupton, J.R.; Brooks, J.A.; Butte, N.F.; Caballero, B.; Flatt, J.P.; Fried, S.K. *Dietary Reference Intakes for Energy, Carbohydrate, Fiber, Fat, Fatty Acids, Cholesterol, Protein, and Amino Acids*; National Academy Press: Washington, DC, USA, 2002; pp. 589–768.
84. Matsumoto, M.; Fujita, A.; Yamashita, A.; Kameoka, S.; Shimomura, Y.; Kitada, Y.; Tamada, H.; Nakamura, S.; Tsubota, K. Effects of functional milk containing galactooligosaccharide, maltitol, and glucomannan on the production of hydrogen gas in the human intestine. *J. Funct. Foods* **2017**, *35*, 13–23. [CrossRef]
85. Joint, F.A.O. WHO Expert Committee on Food Additives, & World Health Organization (JECFA). In *Evaluation of Certain Food Additives: Twenty-Fourth Report of the Joint FAO*; World Health Organization: Geneva, Switzerland, 1980.
86. Joint, F.A.O. WHO Expert Committee on Food Additives, & World Health Organization (JECFA). In Proceedings of the Toxicological evaluation of certain food additives and contaminants/prepared by the 29th meeting of the Joint FAO/WHO Expert Committee on Food Additives, Geneva, Switzerland, 3–12 June 1985.
87. Joint, F.A.O. WHO Expert Committee on Food Additives, & World Health Organization (JECFA). In *Evaluation of Certain Food Additives Food Additives, Forty-Ninth Report of the Joint fao/WHO Expert Committee on Food Additives*; WHO Technical Report Series; World Health Organization: Geneva, Switzerland, 1999; p. 884.
88. Awuchi, C.G.; Echeta, K.C. Current Developments in Sugar Alcohols: Chemistry. Nutrition, and Health Concerns of Sorbitol, Xylitol, Glycerol, Arabitol, Inositol, Maltitol, and Lactitol. *Int. J. Adv. Acad. Res.* **2019**, *5*, 1–33.
89. Carocho, M.; Morales, P.; Ferreira, I.C. Sweeteners as food additives in the XXI century: A review of what is known, and what is to come. *Food Chem. Toxicol.* **2017**, *107*, 302–317. [CrossRef] [PubMed]
90. Washburn, C.; Christensen, N. *Sugar Substitutes: Artificial Sweeteners and Sugar Alcohols*; Cooperative extension of Utah State University: Logan, UT, USA, 2012.
91. Lee, E.J.; Jin, B.H.; Paik, D.I.; Hwang, I.K. Preventive effect of sugar-free chewing gum containing maltitol on dental caries in situ. *Food Sci. Biotechnol.* **2009**, *18*, 432–435.
92. Van Loveren, C. Sugar alcohols: What is the evidence for caries-preventive and caries-therapeutic effects? *Caries Res.* **2004**, *38*, 286–293. [CrossRef]
93. Izumitani, A.; Fujiwara, T.; Minami, T.; Suzuki, S.; Ooshima, T.; Sobue, S. Non-cariogenicity of maltitol in vitro and animal experiments. *Shoni Shikagaku Zasshi* **1989**, *27*, 1018–1024.
94. Ooshima, T.; Izumitani, A.; Minami, T.; Yoshida, T.; Sobue, S.; Fujiwara, T.; Hamada, S. Noncariogenicity of maltitol in specific pathogen-free rats infected with mutans streptococci. *Caries Res.* **1992**, *26*, 33–37. [CrossRef]
95. Li, X.J.; Zhong, B.; Xu, H.X.; Yi, M.; Wang, X.P. Comparative effects of the maltitol chewing gums on reducing plaque. *Huaxi Kouqiang Yixue Zazhi* **2010**, *28*, 502–504.
96. Keukenmeester, R.S.; Slot, D.E.; Rosema, N.A.M.; Van Loveren, C.; Van der Weijden, G.A. Effects of sugar-free chewing gum sweetened with xylitol or maltitol on the development of gingivitis and plaque: A randomized clinical trial. *Int. J. Dent. Hyg.* **2014**, *12*, 238–244. [CrossRef]
97. Matsuo, T. Estimation of glycemic response to maltitol and mixture of maltitol and sucrose in healthy young subjects. *Tech. Bull. Fac. Kagawa Univ.* **2003**, *55*, 57–61.

98. Quílez, J.; Bullo, M.; Salas-Salvadó, J. Improved postprandial response and feeling of satiety after consumption of low-calorie muffins with maltitol and high-amylose corn starch. *J. Food Sci.* **2007**, *72*, S407–S411. [CrossRef] [PubMed]
99. Secchi, A.; Pontiroli, A.E.; Cammelli, L.; Bizzi, A.; Cini, M.; Pozza, G. Effects of oral administration of maltitol on plasma glucose, plasma sorbitol, and serum insulin levels in man. *Klin. Wochenschr.* **1986**, *64*, 265–269. [CrossRef] [PubMed]
100. Wheeler, M.L.; Fineberg, S.E.; Gibson, R.; Fineberg, N. Metabolic response to oral challenge of hydrogenated starch hydrolysate versus glucose in diabetes. *Diabetes Care* **1990**, *13*, 733–740. [CrossRef] [PubMed]
101. Mimura, G.; Koga, T.; Oshikawa, K.; Kido, S.; Sadanaga, T.; Jinnouchi, T.; Kawaguchi, K.; Mori, N. Maltitol tests with diabetics. *Jpn. J. Nutr. Diet.* **1972**, *30*, 145–152. [CrossRef]
102. Vessby, B.; Karlstrom, B.; Skarfors, E. Comparison of the effects of maltitol with those of sucrose, fructose and sorbitol on blood glucose and serum insulin concentrations in healthy and non-insulin dependent diabetic subjects: Studies after an oral load and after addition to a standard breakfast meal. *Diabetes Nutr. Metab. Clin. Exp.* **1990**, *3*, 231–237.
103. Moon, S.; Lee, M.; Huh, K.; Lee, K. Effects of maltitol on blood glucose and insulin responses in normal and diabetic subjects. *Korean J. Nutr.* **1990**, *23*, 270–278.
104. Kang, Y.R.; Jo, S.H.; Yoo, J.I.; Cho, J.B.; Kim, E.J.; Apostolidis, E.; Kwon, Y.I. Anti-hyperglycemic effect of selected sugar alcohols (829.32). *FASEB J.* **2014**, *28* (Suppl. 1), 829–832.
105. Chukwuma, C.I.; Ibrahim, M.A.; Islam, M.S. Maltitol inhibits small intestinal glucose absorption and increases insulin mediated muscle glucose uptake ex vivo but not in normal and type 2 diabetic rats. *Int. J. Food Sci. Nutr.* **2017**, *68*, 73–81. [CrossRef]
106. Rider, A.K.; Schedl, H.P.; Nokes, G.; Shining, S. Small intestinal glucose transport: Proximal-distal kinetic gradients. *J. Gen. Physiol.* **1967**, *50*, 1173–1182. [CrossRef]
107. Levin, R. Digestion and absorption of carbohydrate from embryo to adult. In *Digestion in the Fowl*, 1st ed.; Boorman, R.N., Freeman, B.M., Eds.; British Poultry Science Ltd.: Edinburgh, UK, 1976; pp. 63–116.
108. Cohen, M.I.; Mcnamara, H.; Finberg, L. Intestinal osmolality and carbohydrate absorption in rats treated with polymerized glucose. *Pediatr. Res.* **1978**, *12*, 24–26. [CrossRef]
109. Kamoi, M. Study on metabolism of maltitol Part 1: Fundamental experiment. *J. Jpn. Diab. Soc.* **1975**, *18*, 243–249.
110. Lian-Loh, R.; Birch, G.G.; Coates, M.E. The metabolism of maltitol in the rat. *Br. J. Nutr.* **1982**, *48*, 477–481. [CrossRef] [PubMed]
111. Salminen, E.; Salminen, S.; Porkka, L.; Koivistoinen, P. The effects of xylitol on gastric emptying and secretion of gastric inhibitory polypeptide in the rat. *J. Nutr.* **1984**, *114*, 2201–2203. [CrossRef] [PubMed]
112. Shafer, R.B.; Levine, A.S.; Marlette, J.M.; Morley, J.E. Effects of xylitol on gastric emptying and food intake. *Am. J. Clin. Nutr.* **1987**, *45*, 744–747. [CrossRef]
113. Ranganath, L.; Norris, F.; Morgan, L.; Wright, J.; Marks, V. Delayed gastric emptying occurs following acarbose administration and is a further mechanism for its anti-hyperglycaemic effect. *Diabetic Med.* **1998**, *15*, 120–124. [CrossRef]
114. Aronoff, S.L.; Berkowitz, K.; Shreiner, B.; Want, L. Glucose metabolism and regulation: Beyond insulin and glucagon. *Diabetes Spectr.* **2004**, *17*, 183–190. [CrossRef]
115. Gual, P.; Le Marchand-Brustel, Y.; Tanti, J.F. Positive and negative regulation of glucose uptake by hyperosmotic stress. *Diabetes Metab.* **2003**, *29*, 566–575. [CrossRef]
116. Takizawa, Y.; Hachiya, N. Bacterial reversion assay and micronucleus test carried out on hydrogenated glucose syrups 'Malti-Towa'(powder) and maltitol crystal. *Mutat. Res./Genet. Toxicol.* **1984**, *137*, 133–137. [CrossRef]
117. Canimoglu, S.; Rencuzogullari, E. The cytogenetic effects of food sweetener maltitol in human peripheral lymphocytes. *Drug Chem. Toxicol.* **2006**, *29*, 269–278. [CrossRef]
118. Canimoglu, S.; Rencuzogullari, E. The genotoxic and teratogenic effects of maltitol in rats. *Toxicol. Ind. Health* **2013**, *29*, 935–943. [CrossRef]
119. Lorenzi, M.; Cagliero, E.; Toledo, S. Glucose toxicity for human endothelial cells in culture: Delayed replication, disturbed cell cycle, and accelerated death. *Diabetes* **1985**, *34*, 621–627. [CrossRef] [PubMed]
120. Rencuzogullari, E.; Tüylü, B.A.; Topaktaş, M.; Ila, H.B.; Kayraldız, A.; Arslan, M.; Diler, S.B. Genotoxicity of aspartame. *Drug Chem. Toxicol.* **2004**, *27*, 257–268. [CrossRef] [PubMed]

121. Tucker, J.D.; Christensen, M.L. Effects of anticoagulants upon sister-chromatid exchanges, cell-cycle kinetics, and mitotic index in human peripheral lymphocytes. *Mutat. Res. Lett.* **1987**, *190*, 225–228. [CrossRef]
122. Damasceno, D.C.; Gonçalves, M.A.; Durante, L.C.; Castro, N.C.; Moura, C.H.; Oliveira, C.B. Effects of a saccharin and cyclamate mixture on rat embryos. *Vet. Hum. Toxicol.* **2003**, *45*, 157–159. [PubMed]

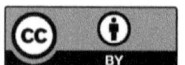

© 2020 by the authors. Licensee MDPI, Basel, Switzerland. This article is an open access article distributed under the terms and conditions of the Creative Commons Attribution (CC BY) license (http://creativecommons.org/licenses/by/4.0/).

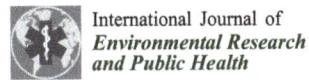

Review

Natural Sweeteners: The Relevance of Food Naturalness for Consumers, Food Security Aspects, Sustainability and Health Impacts

Ariana Saraiva [1], Conrado Carrascosa [1], Dele Raheem [2], Fernando Ramos [3,4] and António Raposo [5,6,*]

1. Department of Animal Pathology and Production, Bromatology and Food Technology, Faculty of Veterinary, Universidad de Las Palmas de Gran Canaria, Trasmontaña s/n, 35413 Arucas, Spain
2. Northern Institute for Environmental and Minority Law (NIEM), Arctic Centre, University of Lapland, 96101 Rovaniemi, Lapland, Finland
3. Pharmacy Faculty, University of Coimbra, Azinhaga de Santa Comba, 3000-548 Coimbra, Portugal
4. REQUIMTE/LAQV, R. D. Manuel II, 55142 Apartado, Oporto, Portugal
5. Department for Management of Science and Technology Development, Ton Duc Thang University, Ho Chi Minh City, Vietnam
6. Faculty of Environment and Labour Safety, Ton Duc Thang University, Ho Chi Minh City, Vietnam
* Correspondence: antonio.raposo@tdtu.edu.vn

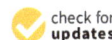

Received: 28 July 2020; Accepted: 27 August 2020; Published: 28 August 2020

Abstract: At a moment when the population is increasingly aware and involved in what it eats, both consumers and the food sector are showing more interest in natural foods. This review work discusses, addresses and provides details of the most important aspects of consumer's perceptions of and attitudes to natural foods and in-depth research into natural sweeteners. It also includes issues about their use and development as regards health impacts, food security and sustainability. In line with our main research outcome, we can assume that consumers are very keen on choosing foods with clean labelling, natural ingredients, preferably with other functional properties, without the loss of taste. In response to such a phenomenon, the food industry offers consumers alternative natural sweeteners with the advantage of added health benefits. It is noteworthy that Nature is a superb source of desirable substances, and many have a sweet taste, and many still need to be studied. Finally, we must stress that being natural does not necessarily guarantee market success.

Keywords: consumer's perceptions and attitudes; food industry; food security; health impacts; natural food products; natural sweeteners; sustainability

1. Introduction

In the 20th century, developed countries resolved the lack of food security with a major contribution from agri-food industrialisation [1–3]. Food processing has played a vital role in prolonging food products' shelf life, mitigating food losses and reducing waste and in enhancing the production of nutrients and their availability [4,5]. Yet day-to-day consumer perceptions rely on other factors apart from these achievements. In modern societies, more globalised markets and more manufacturing efforts made in the food chain have led to knowledge gaps and a perceived separation between local manufacturers and citizens (e.g., how foods are produced, where they are produced, etc.) [6,7]. Consumers are gradually becoming more aware to natural ingredients, while the growing importance of naturalness among consumers has meant key implications for the food industry [8]. This could well have implications for not only developing and selling food, but also for the increase in emerging food technologies. It is possible that those food products not perceived as natural are not accepted by lots of consumers in the majority of countries.

The demand for zero-calorie and naturally derived sweeteners has dramatically grown in the last decade because consumers are more mindful of their health [9]. For decades sweeteners have been used to make food more flavourful and to attract consumers. They were first adopted because of high-calorie sugar-to-diet ratio, and this favoured obesity in the general population, which became widespread in infants and children [10]. Thus, a low-calorie sweetener, saccharine, became available in the 1980s. As this sweetener was so popular, others followed, including cyclamates, aspartame and acesulfame K, which are the most widespread. Sweeteners have long-since been the object of controversies and conflicts over the years, which have included allegations of liver and bladder toxicity, carcinogenicity, foetus malformations, along with other dangers [11]. Whereas all these allegations have been investigated, sweeteners were considered safe [12], although some loss of consumer trust remains as some are not permitted in the USA, while others are allowed in the EU (e.g., cyclamate and cyclamic acid), but are not permitted in the USA (under E 952). Hence the need for natural substitutes is crucial [13]. Natural sweeteners and synthetic sweeteners have the same purpose: to act as a sweet flavour while fewer or no calories at all to diet. Natural sweeteners can be classified as two categories: high-potency sweeteners and bulk sweeteners. The former's potency is greater than the sweetness of one sucrose molecule. The latter's potency is the equivalent to one sucrose molecule, or less, with sucrose being the international standard for sweetness.

The main aims of this review were to provide details of and understand consumers perceptions and attitudes to natural food products, and to study in-depth natural sweeteners, mostly aspects related to their use and production in health impacts, food security and sustainability terms. Special attention was given to sweeteners, which are unanimously considered in the literature to have a good taste, high solubility and high stability, be safe with an acceptable cost-on-use, namely, erythritol glycyrrhizin, tagatose, steviol glycosides and thaumatin.

2. Consumer Perceptions of and Attitudes to Natural Food Products

Humans are inherently connected to natural objects [14], so it should come as no surprise that most humans have clearly preferred natural foods in the last few decades [8,15]. The findings of the Nielsen Global Health and Wellness Survey [16], which was conducted in 60 countries and involved 30,000 consumers, revealed that the most essential food characteristics are naturalness, freshness and minimal processing. The findings of the Kampffmeyer Food Innovation Study [17], conducted with over 4000 consumers from eight European countries, indicate that food naturalness is a "decisive buying incentive," and that approximately three quarters of respondents perceived a close "natural" + "health" link. The market research outcomes generally suggest that many consumers in developed countries usually eat natural foods. From the natural science point of view, naturalness definitely does not imply that a food product is healthier, less dangerous or tastier, although this is not how most people perceive naturalness [18,19].

Consumers perceive naturalness as a beneficial characteristic of food items. However, the relative importance of food naturalness varies across lands, cultures and throughout history [20]. Human beings have conventionally sought to monitor and reduce environmental threats. The arrival of increasingly processed foods in developed countries in the 1950s provided longer food shelf life, and better food and nutrition security [4,5]. It was at that time when consumers started showing a strong preference for processed foods. Conversely, consumers' everyday experience depends on other things apart from these accomplishments. Today, highly globalised markets and intensified food chain production in industrialized economies have added to a knowledge gap and perceived distance between food manufacturers and consumers [6,7].

Globalisation and industrialisation go hand in hand with a more man-made and higher risk that enhance citizens' perception of modernity risks [21]. In the last few decades, food safety incidents have impacted Europe, such as dioxin and bovine spongiform encephalopathy [22,23]. Consumers are concerned about excess pesticide use by traditional industrial agricultural methods [24], the employment of artificial ingredients, colourants or additives like E133 [25], and questionable food innovations, like genetically modified organisms [26], being introduced. This has made consumers suspicious or sceptical about the negative health consequences that this food system entails [3]. Growing public concern about what the food system does to climate change and its general negative impact on sustainability [27] mean that consumers now question the social and environmental consequences of food production [28,29].

Consumers generally prefer food to be nutrient-fed and satiated, while price and taste are other important factors [30,31]. However, it is often suggested that food consumption in industrialized societies is presently affected by three particular major trends: convenience, health concerns, sustainability [32]. Health concerns are driven by consumers' affluence, but are also explained by not only the rising number of food- and lifestyle-related diseases (i.e., obesity, diabetes, etc.) [7,33], but also increasing intolerances and allergies to certain components and specific food products like gluten. These aspects also motivate consumers to pay more attention to healthy food items that promote healthier lifestyles at older ages and that lower the incidence of some diseases. Sustainability concerns come over according to increasing knowledge of emissions released by traditional agricultural activities [1]. This has led to an ever-growing expansion of organic farming and markets, and can also explain why some consumers seek products, such as 'local food' products (food miles) and why they are willing to pay more for water-saving products [34]. Convenience food refers to the number of meals not eaten at home or home-delivered meals as opposed to homemade meals. This figure has significantly risen in past decades [35], which suggests that consumers are involved in additional capabilities of food items to save time (e.g., frozen foods, ready meals, microwavable food, etc.).

By analysing the factors that impact individual differences in the perceived importance of naturalness, although high mean values of the importance of naturalness in foods (INF) were found in most studies, individual differences appeared in how important naturalness was perceived [8]. For psychological factors, several works have indicated the importance of consumers' values for explaining INF. Idealism [36], tradition and universalism [37] were positively associated with INF, whereas hedonism and power correlated negatively with INF [37]. Interest shown in health correlated positively with INF [38,39], and attitudes to novel technologies, chemicals and functional foods correlated negatively [38,40–45]. Some experiments revealed a certain conceptual similarity between predictors and how INF was calculated. Attitudes to traditional and organic food, along with food involvement and neophobia were positively related to INF in a number of research works [46–51]. The research by Olbrich et al. [47], which included over 10,000 German consumers, revealed that attitudes to organic food were related to INF. Similar findings are reported in Taiwan by Hsu et al. [48]. These two experiments indicated that no difference appeared between INF and items assessing organic food preferences. Very few experiments examined the relation linking INF with personality characteristics. Steptoe et al. [39] reported a positive association for INF and the control locus, while Huotilainen et al. [52] found that the perceived INF value was not related to consumer willingness to accept food innovations.

As for consumer attitudes to food naturalness affecting their behaviour and intentions, some studies report INF measurement items overlapping measuring intentions or behaviours in relation to eating organic food [49,51,53,54]. INF influences intention to eat in a more enviro-friendly way [55] with fresh [56], local/traditional [52,57] natural [58] and low-calorie food items [59]. The results cross-country analysis obtained by Hemmerling et al. [57] were inconclusive; INF had a strong impact on local/traditional foods in Italy and Germany, but was negligible in The Netherlands, Poland, France and Switzerland. Only two experiments have investigated how INF affects consumer decisions about eating functional food, but the results were inconclusive. Kraus [60] reported substantial effects in Poland, but the research by Urala and Lähteenmäki in Finland [61] proved unsubstantial. Lähteenmäki et al. [62] also reported that INF adversely affected purchase intention to buy genetically modified cheese in Finland, Denmark, Sweden and Norway. In their works, Lusk et al. [63] saw that INF increased the probability of selecting non-clone or non-hormone milk as opposed to the clone or hormone variety. Many research works undertaken in different countries have revealed that INF significantly affects eating healthy [64–68], organic [69] and traditional foods [46,70], and eating unhealthy [66,67] and convenience foods [71]. Roininen and Tuorila [72] and Zandstra et al. [73] found that INF did not affect unhealthy or healthy eating. Small sample sizes ($n = 144$ and $n = 132$) could potentially explain such insignificant results. With their survey of 197 Spanish consumers, Carrillo et al. [74] found that perceived naturalness of functional foods increased their sales.

Regarding natural food ingredients, which have attracted far more attention from public and food manufacturers, for a few decades now it has been worth emphasising that consumers mainly choose food without additives but, if they are not available, the same consumer chooses food containing natural additives rather than synthetic ones [11,13]. Consumer research has revealed that consumers have increasingly become more knowledgeable of food additives and more frequently prefer natural additives to their artificial analogues [40,75,76]. Unlike artificial sweeteners, which are all capable of structural modification in the hope that better tasting analogues will be discovered, natural sweeteners must be used 'as are' simply because any structural change made to a natural sweetener to improve its taste profile will automatically destroy the 'natural' proposition and position. So, although the consumer interest level is high, identifying a natural sweetener with the requisite sensory quality is no trivial undertaking [77].

3. Natural Sweeteners

Preference for sweet taste is not only innate, but universal [78]. Food products related to a sweet taste characteristically contain simple carbohydrates in the forms of fructose, glucose and sucrose, which are metabolised to produce energy rapidly, as wee as complex carbohydrates in the form of starch for long sustained energy and storage. However, the sweet taste can be induced by the presence of peptides, D-amino acids, glycosides, proteins, coumarins, ureas, substituted aromatic compounds, dihydrochalcones and other nitrogenous substances [79]. Yet all sweet-tasting compounds interact and activate a single receptor, which is expressed on the surface of taste buds, the TAS1R2-TAS1R3 heterodimer, and contains multiple binding sites to explain the range of compounds that induce perceived sweetness [80].

Honey used to be the main sweetener in human diet. However, in the 18th century, the process of extracting sucrose from sugar beet and sugar cane grew exponentially and clearly assumed preponderance. Nowadays, sucrose, or common table sugar, remains the most traditionally used sweetener, and is available in a variety of refined forms [81]. In 2018 and 2019, global sucrose consumption came to 174 million metric tons [82]. In the last few years, sugar overconsumption has become pandemic, with serious consequences in public health terms. There is clear evidence for an association between eating too much sugar and being at higher risk for dental caries, type II diabetes obesity and cardiovascular diseases, among other non-communicable diseases [83]. Given this scenario, sweeteners in food products have spread, and this product is major a target of much interest for the industrial and scientific communities.

Many synthetic sweeteners have been developed, but today demand undoubtedly lies in natural sweeteners, preferably the high-intensity kind; i.e., with low-calorie contributions. This trend stems from not only growing consumer concern about the harmful effects of a diet that includes too much sugar, but also the problems that arise from employing artificial food additives. Although many low-calorie sweeteners are readily available, only a few can be used by the food industry, mainly because of safety concerns and technological problems [81]. It is worth noting that, apart from sweetening, these compounds can influence a product's colour, flavour, texture and shelf life [84].

The most important aspects when selecting a sweetener have to do with its physico-chemical properties, such as thermal stability and solubility in water, but also production cost and safety [85,86]. Its sweetness potency is extremely relevant; that is to say, sweeteners can be classified in line with their intrinsic characteristics (nutritive value, sweetening power) and origin (synthetic, semisynthetic and natural) [87]. Depending on their sweetness level in relation to sucrose, considered an international reference (sweetness potency = 1), sweeteners are grouped into two classes: bulk and intense. Bulk sweeteners have a similar or less sweetening potency vs. sucrose, and are used to typically confer low-calorie food products preservative action, bulk and texture [88]. They can be employed in baked food products, breakfast cereals, preserved foods, desserts, cakes, jams, ice cream and sauces [89]. To the sweeteners in this category we indicate sugar alcohols like maltitol, sorbitol, lactitol, xylitol, erythritol, mannitol, isomalt, hydrogenated starch hydrolysates and hydrogenated glucose syrups [86]. Trehalose and tagatose are two new compounds with a similar suitability to sugar alcohols [86,89]. Bulk sweeteners are frequently utilised in the food industry for the benefits they offer over sucrose in both functional aspects (e.g., lowering the freezing point of a frozen desert or of the Maillard reaction) and nutritional terms (e.g., slower assimilation). However, these sweeteners do not substantially lower the calorie value of a food [89].

The sweetness that intense sweeteners provide is much more than sucrose and in different potencies [88]. Given their high sweetness potency, very small amounts are required to accomplish the desired sweetening effect. Hence their contribution to a product's energy value is minimum, which is most advantageous [87]. Despite them often being called "artificial sweeteners", such compounds can be synthetic (e.g., saccharin, aspartame, sucralose, acesulfame-potassium, cyclamate, alitame, neotame, dulcin), semisynthetic (e.g., neohesperidine dihydrochalcone) or natural (e.g., rebaudioside and stevioside) [88]. Intense sweeteners are of widespread use in processed foods, especially carbonated and non-carbonated drinks, canned food, baked food, sweets, jellies and puddings [89].

Although an origin-based sweetener classification is not considered by authorities like the European Food Safety Authority (EFSA) or the US Food and Drug Administration (FDA), we adopt this classification because, given their growing popularity, we pay attention to natural sweeteners.

Natural sweeteners encompass wide-ranging compounds like sugars, sugar alcohols, amino acids, proteins, terpenoid glycosides and some polyphenols [84,85]. Having said that, only those that possess relevant characteristics, e.g., safety, good taste, high stability, good solubility and reasonable cost, are found on the market as widely used sweeteners [11,90]. The present review focuses on the natural sweeteners that comply with these principles.

3.1. Sugars

The relative sweetness potency of carbohydrates is consistently lower than that of sucrose (a reference compound), except for fructose, which is the sweetest natural sugar (relative sweetness = 1.43) which is abundance in fruit, agave nectar, honey and some vegetables [85]. Fructose and glucose and are the two most widely adopted monosaccharides as natural sweeteners by the food industry [85]. Fructose replaces sucrose in a range of food products thanks to its lower glycaemic index, sweetening strength and low cost, and its ability to improve overall end product quality characteristics; flavour, colour texture, and shelf-life stability [84]. High fructose syrups are widely employed, mostly those produced with corn starch by an elaborate technological process, and given their interesting texturising ability, flavour profile [85]. When ingested as large amounts, malabsorption and consequent gastrointestinal disturbances may occur, and excessive intake may lead to metabolic changes; e.g., insulin resistance, high plasma triglycerides, etc. [84,91].

In this context it is worth highlighting two new compounds: trehalose and tagatose. They have been relatively recently approved as novel food ingredients or novel foods and appear on the market as sucrose alternatives [86]. The trehalose disaccharide comprises two glucose units linked by an α-1,1-glucosidic bond and occurs naturally in plants, fungi, insects, algae bacteria and yeasts [86]. The commercial product is acquired from starch by following an enzymatic process [92] and it has a relative sweetness power of 0.43 [85]. Trehalose is well appeciated because it induces a low glycaemic response and helps to maintain dehydrated and frozen food products fresh via the stabilisation of colour, texture and flavour [86]. It reduces starch retrodegradation and does not participate in Maillard reactions. It is an ingredient frequently found in sports drinks and health bars [93]. Tagatose is a fructose isomer found naturally-occurring in certain fruit and dairy products [90]. It is considered a prebiotic and a flavour enhancer [11]. In industrial terms, it is produced from lactose following a multistep enzymatic process, plus fractionation and purification [14]. Its sweetness potency comes close to that of sucrose, 0.92, with the advantage of being differently metabolised by contributing to fewer calories, evoking a weaker glycaemic response [86,87,90] and does not favour dental caries. As it is only partly digested, tagatose can bring about diarrhoea, abdominal discomfort and flatulence when ingested as high doses [86]. Tagatose is used to prepare energy bars, breakfast cereals, chocolate gums, caramel, ice cream, soft drinks and yogurt [11,90].

3.2. Sugar Alcohols

Sugar alcohols, or polyols, are low-digestible carbohydrates that occur naturally in fruit, vegetables, mushrooms and algae [94], and have been employed as an alternative type of sweetener in recent years. The sugar alcohols allowed by the food industry to be used as nutritive or bulk sweeteners include maltitol, mannitol, sorbitol, xylitol, erythritol, isomalt and lactitol. Some other relevant compounds that enter this category are arabitol and hydrogenated starch hydrolysates, despite not being permitted in the EU [87]. They are obtained generally by catalytic hydrogenation from the corresponding aldose sugars [84]. For certain sugar alcohols, like erythritol, methods based on fermentation or enzymatic conversion with osmophilic yeasts or fungi have been followed [11]. By the way, mannitol, sorbitol and maltitol are easily extracted from brown algae (i.e., *Laminaria* species) [95]. Sugar alcohols are frequently employed for food product reformulation purposes where, other than sweetness, texture and the bulk of sugar play a key role in sugar-free cookies, cakes, sweets, chocolate and gums [86,96]. They are applied to pharmaceutical products like throat lozenges [86]. Polyols offer two major advantages over sugar as food ingredients: (1) do not favour tooth decay because they are not fermentable by oral bacteria; (2) lower calorie content and glycaemic index, which are most interesting for diabetics [86]. Sugar alcohols also present prebiotic properties and, like fibres, contribute to healthy intestinal microbiota [97]. Sugar alcohols are universally considered safe and have no established acceptable daily intake (ADI), but should be used in line with good manufacturing practices (GMP) [84,94].

Sugar alcohols are frequently used together with intense sweeteners to mask off-flavours of the latter, while conferring the bulkiness that low-calorie sweeteners cannot [84,98]. Unlike sugars, they are not subject to Maillard reactions and leave a cooling effect in the mouth, which could be desirable for certain products, but particularly in many others (e.g., baked goods) [94]. Overall, of all the allowed sugar alcohols, the properties of xylitol, erythritol and maltitol come the closest to those of sucrose, with a relative sweetness of 0.63, 0.87 and 0.97, respectively. This is why they are the most widely used [85,99]. Unlike sucrose and glucose, sugar alcohols are not totally digested, which is why excess ingestion can lead to gastrointestinal symptoms even in healthy people, like laxative side effects, so consumers with inflammatory bowel disease should be very careful with them [97]. Notwithstanding, frequent intake seems to result in better tolerance [99]. Besides the above-cited side effect, they display no other health-related problems in association with high-potency artificial sweeteners [10]. As with all sweeteners, the safety of sugar alcohols is currently being reassessed by EFSA and new data are expected to become available at the end of 2020 [100].

3.3. Terpenoid Glycosides

Steviol glycosides are a group of sweet compounds which are extracted from the leaves of a plant native to South America called *Stevia rebaudiana* Bertoni (Asteraceae), which is currently grown in some countries in Europe and Asia. Typically, the above-mentioned glycosides represent up to 15% of the dry matter in plant leaves. Ten main ent-kaurane diterpenoid glycosides exist, and they all have the same steviol core structure. Stevioside, followed by rebaudioside A, are the two most abundant and commercially relevant ones [90]. They leave a very sweet taste in the mouth that is hundreds of times superior to sucrose, which makes them very interesting sweeteners [85]. Rebaudioside A, whose relative sweetness is 250–450, is the most appealing steviol glycoside, and offers a taste like sucrose with no off-tastes, while stevioside has a slight bitter side effect [85,101]. Seeing as the leaves of the plant cannot be utilised directly in the USA and EU, steviol glycosides are extracted with water before being redissolved and recrystallixed from a hydro-alcoholic solution [87]. Steviol glycosides are hydrolysed to steviol by colonic microbiota. Most steviol is absorbed by the intestine before reaching the liver, where it goes through a process of conjugation with glucuronic acid to produce steviol glucoronides, which are finally excreted mostly in urine [102]. Consuming steviol glycosides is safe provided it lies within the 4 mg/kg of body weight/day limit [103]. Both their calorie contribution is non-significant, so they are suitable for diabetic patients. They have also been attributed anti-inflammatory and immunomodulatory diuretic and anti-hypertensive properties [104]. As for their physico-chemical characteristics, they remain moderately stable at high temperature and may be used within a pH range from 2 to 10 [87]. Steviol glycosides have been widely used to produce confectionery, chocolates, baked goods, yoghurts, ice cream, gums, sauces, jam dairy products and drinks [11,105].

Another interesting sweetening compound is glycyrrhizin, or glycyrrhizic acid, which is isolated from *Glycyrrhiza glabra* L. roots (Fabaceae), which is a liquorice plant [90]. This molecule offers a relative sweetness of 90 [85]. Its use as a sweetener is permitted in Japan and other countries, but not in the USA and EU [85], where glycyrrhizin is approved only as a surfactant and flavouring agent, and also in the form of ammoniated glycyrrhizin, which is considered Generally Recognised as Safe (GRAS) [106]. Glycyrrhizin intake should never exceed 100 mg/day, considering all its sources in the diet, given the risk of toxic effects: hypertension and hypokalaemia-induced secondary disorders [107,108]. Some authors indicate that glycyrrhizin could have beneficial effects on intestinal microbiota [97]. The applications of glycyrrhizin as foaming agent and flavour enhancer include baked goods, ice cream, confectionery, gums and beverages [99].

3.4. Proteins

Sweet-tasting proteins are naturally-occurring in some exotic plants, and their sweetness is hundreds to thousands of times superior to sucrose [85]. Thaumatin comprises a mixture of six closely interrelated proteins, thaumatin I, II, III, a, b and c, extracted from *Thaumatococcus daniellii* Benth fruit (Marantaceae), which is native to western Africa. Thaumatin I and II are the main forms, despite all isoforms being sweet-tasting [90]. No unanimous value for its sweetening potency exists, but it is estimated to be about 1600–3000-fold higher than sucrose [11,85]. Extraction is performed by water and mechanical methods [87]. Current thaumatin production does not meet demand, and alternative methods to produce it through microorganisms and transgenic plants are growing [109]. Thaumatin is permitted in both the EU and the USA, where it is GRAS [97]. Owing to lack of toxicity, its ADI is still to be established [110]. There is, however, a risk of allergic reactions [111]. The metabolism of thaumatin is similar to that of any other protein in human diet. Its energy input is 4 kcal/g, which is negligible as minor amounts are used in practice [101]. The main problems with its use are late onset of action and a slight liquorice off-taste, which may interfere with consumer acceptance. Hence its use in large amounts is not recommended. Nevertheless, it works extremely well when employed in conjunction with other sweeteners to diminish bitterness and confer foods an umami flavour [90]. As regards physico-chemical properties, it is highly soluble in water, and well resists high temperature and acidic pH [87]. Thaumatin is frequently employed in processed vegetables, sauces, soups, poultry, products deriving from egg, gums and fruit juice [87].

Several other sweet proteins are known, with the most promising ones being brazzein, mabinlin, monelin, miraculin, pentadine, curculin (neoculin) and lysozyme, but more studies are necessary to ensure their safety and applicability [90].

4. Production of Safe Enviro-Friendly Natural Sweeteners

Natural sweetener production must remain safe with no adverse environmental consequences. It is presently necessary to guarantee that our food system does not pose health problems to consumers and our planet, as reflected in the recent 'EU green deal' [112]. This section summarises the production of the following sweeteners, which are highlighted in preceding sections given their relevance for industrial food processing.

4.1. Erythritol

Industrial erythritol production has gained prominence with the rapid development of the electrochemical process. During this process, erythrose and erythritol are produced by the electrolytic decarboxylation of arabinoic or ribonic acid. The substrates for the reaction are obtained by the decarboxylation of C-6 sugars [113]. However, a more natural method involves the biotechnological process, which results in higher yields from fermenting a sugar source. Erythritol derives from fermentation processes, conducted mostly by fungi or synthesized by lactic acid bacteria. In order to produce erythritol, the common pathways among east-like fungi genera include: *Trigonopsis, Candida, Pichia, Moniliella, Yarrowia, Pseudozyma, Trichosporonoides, Aureobasidium, Trichoderma* [114]. For industrial production purposes, *Yarrowia lipolytica*, *Moniliella pollinis* and *Trichosporonoides megachiliensis* are reported as effective [113]. One main part of the production process involves separation and purification steps because they are crucial when erythritol is taken as a food additive. A patent describes that to recover erythritol from the culture medium, separation from fermenting microorganisms is required, followed by ion exchange chromatography and crystallization. Moreover, a chromatographic separation step was subject to activated-carbon treatment in order to recover the erythritol fraction [115].

4.2. Tagatose

As a natural sweetener, biotechnological tagatose production by enzymatic isomerisation is a preferred alternative to chemical processes. For biological D-tagatose manufacturing, several biocatalyst sources can be resorted to; e.g., L-arabinose isomerase (l-AI) EC 5.3.1.4, which can catalyse the conversion of D-galactose into D-tagatose, and also for converting L-arabinose into L-ribulose, due to the similar configurations of substrates [116,117] yet biological D-tagatose production is limited given the less bioconversion efficiency of l-AI, a metal ion requirement, and the poor thermostability and low affinity of the enzyme for D-galactose. It has, thus, been suggested that applying protein engineering and genomic tools may enhance the bioconversion efficiency for D-tagatose production by amending the functional properties of l-AI [118]. Applying high-throughput screening or a selection method helps to evaluate individual protein variants and, hence, increase the possibility of screening specific mutants with greater catalytic activity. During D-tagatose production, the safety problem caused by enzyme or cells of not GRAS hosts can be overcome by transferring the gene of L-arabinose isomerase to GRAS hosts like *C. Glutamicum*, *Corynebacterium ammonagenes* and *Bacillus megaterium* [119]. Ultimately, more research needs to be conducted to explore new sources of biocatalysts from GRAS microorganisms, apart from enzyme secretion and expression in a food-grade microbial host.

4.3. Steviol Glycosides

The raw materials employed in the manufacturing process of Steviol glycosides preparations are crushed leaves from the perennial shrub *Stevia rebaudiana* (Bertoni) Bertoni of the family Asteraceae (Compositae). The literature indicates several alcohols and ion exchange resins used during the manufacturing process [120]. Extracting glycosides from stevia leaves involves thermal extraction and maceration. Both the quality and yield of the extracted products can increase by following techniques like supercritical fluids, ultrasonic waves and microwaving [121]. Besides, a multistage membrane process, which has been developed to concentrate glycoside sweeteners, is also highlighted in the report, with bitter-tasting components from the sweetener concentrate being washed out during the nanofiltration process.

The conventional extraction processes described in the literature often follow a similar methodology, whereby stevia leaves are extracted with hot water or alcohols. In certain cases, leaves are pre-treated with non-polar solvents (e.g., hexane or chloroform hexane) to eliminate lipids, essential oils, chlorophyll and other non-polar substances. With this pre-treatment, extracts are clarified by precipitation with either salt or alkaline solutions, and then finally concentrated and redissolved in methanol for the crystallisation of glycosides [122]. Other extraction procedure steps involved are described in [123], where stevia leaves were soaked in warm water to dissolve glycosides before the precipitation and filtration of the resultant solution, followed by concentration by evaporation, ion exchange purification, spray drying and crystallisation to produce a white powder and crystals. Rao et al. [124] applied ultra- and nano-filtration membranes to develop a simple eco-friendly and low-cost process to isolate steviol glycosides, which resulted in the final product's improved taste profile.

4.4. Glycyrrhizin

The methods followed to prepare glycyrrhizic acid (GA) from liquorice roots have been investigated by several researchers. The literature reports a number of procedures as regards solvent extraction by various organic solvents, purification by ion exchange and polymeric resins, chromatographic separation, adsorption, foam separation, supercritical fluid extraction, microwave-assisted extraction (MAE) and multistage counter-current extraction (MCE) to extract GA [125]. Most existing processes to extract and purify the sweet ingredients from liquorice roots involve several steps and large quantities of solvents and chemicals. Extracting GA from roots includes extraction with hot water at ambient pressure in the presence of a number of additives, such as alkalis, as well as mineral acids, ethyl alcohol like aqueous ammonia, methanol and ethanol, which are the most well-accepted technologies. The primary aqueous extract from liquorice roots contains GA and many other water-soluble substances, which are then subjected to further process more purified products. Pure GA is also prepared from liquorice roots using alcohol as the extraction solvent in an ultrasonic device, followed by purification [126]. The conventional solvent extraction technique followed to extract GA from liquorice offers several disadvantages, namely considerable solvent requirements, longer extraction time, lower yields and higher extraction temperature. All this requires developing an effective economical extraction method [126]. The purification procedure involves the acidification of the extract by adding acids like H_2SO_4 or HCl acids to form the solid product of GA salt (at pH 1–2). Ultrasound assisted extraction has shown that the extraction rate rises due to cavitation because the developed cavity grows in size and then abruptly collapses with the release of energy at an enormous rate, which thus increases the local temperature and pressure [127]. Therefore, greater solvent penetration in cellular materials takes place, which improves the cell content release in the bulk medium [127].

4.5. Thaumatin

The thaumatin production process can be strongly affected depending on the quality and availability of source materials [128]. In order to achieve stabler protein production that meets its demand, a series of studies were conducted, which involved thaumatin production with genetically engineered microorganisms and transgenic plants (see the studies by [129,130]).

Although using a plant system offers some advantages over microbial systems in terms of its scalability, safety and economy, they still lack some benefits that can be obtained from microbial hosts, such as the possibility of controling growth conditions and product consistencies from batch to batch [128]. Biochemical production methods have been considered because the natural production of these proteins is normally too expensive. Recombinant DNA technology is applied to produce sweet proteins in a host organism. The most promising host known is the methylotrophic yeast *Pichia pastoris*. This yeast has a tight regulated methanol-induced promoter that well controls recombinant protein production [128]. Despite thaumatin having been studied by several researchers in the last 30 years, there is still much to be done to improve its production by biochemical routes. As the literature evidences, biological products are emerging as a promising applicant in the food industry, hence the huge potential for future research to centre on using advanced computational techniques to optimise thaumatin bioproduction.

Other natural sweeteners with enviro-friendly production methods that are becoming popular food ingredients for health-conscious consumers are briefly described below:

(1) Raw Honey: one of the oldest natural sweeteners. Honey is sweeter than sugar, and is the only sweetener obtained from an animal source (insect bees, minilivestock). Honey is a sugar secretion that is deposited on honeycombs by bees *Apis mellifera*, *Apis indica* (Indian Bee), *Apis dorsata* (Rock Bee), among other Apis species of the family Apidae [131].

(2) Blackstrap Molasses: the by product from raw sugar refinery or a sugarcane factory; it is the thick dark, viscous liquid that is left after the final sugar crystallisation stage from which no more sugar can be crystallised economically by usual methods [132].

(3) Real Maple Syrup: it is made from the sap exuded from stems of the genus *Acer*, usually in spring. Sap primarily contains water and sucrose, with varying amounts of amino and organic acids and phenolic substances, which is concentrated by heating to produce a wide range of flavour compounds [133].

(4) Coconut Sugar: it is locally produced from the phloem sap of coconut palm tree (*Cocos nucifera* L.) blossom. Juice collectors climb palm trees and cut off unopened inflorescences with sickles. The escaping sap is collected in bamboo or plastic containers for 8–12 h. Lime is sometimes added to prevent sap from fermenting [132].

(5) Other combinations: they involve production that blends several natural product sweeteners, such as a low concentration of steviol glycosides (<0.5 percent per dry leaf weight) with a small amount of raw organic sugar cane. Similarly, a combination of sweetening solutions, e.g., Erysweet+, a stevia erythritol blend, and KetoseSweet+, an allulose, stevia and monk fruit blends are becoming popular beverages [134].

Consumers are eager to purchase products with natural ingredients and clean labels, preferably with further functional properties, but which do not compromise taste. In order to achieve this trend, food industries are now willing to reformulate their food products to include alternative natural sweeteners to sugar.

5. Health Impacts

For natural sweeteners are deemed suitable to be extensively used and marketed, they must be safe, offer good flavour with a high degree of solubility and a good level of stability, and offer reasonable cost-effective applications [135]. This paper only investigates the natural sweeteners that meet all these criteria [11] in relation to their health impacts.

The two major compounds of bulk sweeteners are erythritol and tagatose. Erythritol is allowed in both the USA and the EU, but there are restrictions on use in drinks with the latter. As a bulk sweetener, it has approximately 65% of sucrose sweetness, but it does not lead to tooth decay and is neither toxic nor carcinogenic for the amounts added to food. The main products for which erythritol is employed are baked goods, frostings, coatings, chocolate, fermented milk, low-calorie beverages, chewing gums, sweets, among others [129,135]. In 2014, a scientific panel, mandated by EFSA, ruled out its laxative properties and declared it safe for use without defining its acceptable daily intake (ADI) [136]. Based on acute toxicity investigations, and following oral administration, erythritol is graded as being essentially non-toxic. Subchronic research further enhances erythritol's safety. Chronic research (up to 2 years) has demonstrated that erythritol has no effect on either survival or carcinogenicity [137,138]. At high doses (up to 16 g/kg body weight), erythritol affects neither the reproductive capacity nor fertility of parental rats. No adverse effects have been observed on developing foetuses [137–140]. Erythritol has no mutagenic potential, as observed in the Ames and chromosomal aberration tests [137,138,141,142]. Animal toxicity tests and human clinical trials have reliably shown that erythritol is safe. Erythritol has never been predicted to have adverse effects when applied for its intended use in food [137,138].

Erythritol has been found to reduce the risk of caries in several trials [143–147]. As erythritol does not affect insulin levels or glucose, it is an appropriate sugar substitute in diabetes patients, and also for individuals who wish or need to regulate their blood sugar levels because of prediabetes or compromised carbohydrate metabolism [148,149]. Diabetes patients can benefit from the vascular effects of erythritol, as mentioned above. It is assumed that endothelium is not compromised by erythritol in non-diabetic subjects, but in diabetic subjects where endothelium is under diabetic stress, erythritol can transfer a range of damage and dysfunction parameters to a safer side, as *in vitro, ex vivo* and *in vivo* studies report [148,150,151]. Erythritol can also be regarded as a substance with a beneficial impact on the endothelium under high-glucose conditions by contributing to avoid or delay the onset of diabetic complications [152]. The erythritol attribute has minor effects on several targets and can also prove beneficial. A compound with a strong biological effect is not as appropriate for chronic supplementation as required in diabetes. The option would be to use a substance like erythritol with moderate protective effects. Erythritol is not only valuable, but should be considered a recommended sugar replacement for the rapidly increasing numbers of people with diabetes or prediabetes to reduce their chances of developing diabetic complications [152,153].

Tagatose comes in very small amounts in fruit and heat-treated dairy products. Its potency vs. sucrose is 92%, which means that it comes close in taste, but only adds 1.5 kcal/g, which makes it safe for diabetics to use without harming teeth. Tagatose is approved in the US as a GRAS compound, is permitted in the EU as a food ingredient and in many other countries with practically no toxicity associated with its use. Tagatose uses in the food industry include yoghurts, frostings, cereals, beverages, chewing gum, fudge, caramel, fondant, chocolate and ice cream [129,135,154].

Tagatose's safety and toxicity dimensions have been explored in animal and human subjects [118]. As tagatose intake increases above 10%, adverse reactions (increased liver weight and hypertrophy) have been reported in rats [155]. Consequently, the 5% tagatose level is a known safe dose that has no side effects. at reproductive performance is not impaired, even when tagatose intake is as high as 20 g/kg body weight/day [156]. Human clinical experiments to study D-tagatose use have been based mainly on its gastrointestinal and urecaemic consequences. High plasma uric acid levels are associated with purine metabolism disorder and gout development. A significant rise in the plasma uric acid concentration occurs in both the healthy and non-insulin-dependent diabetes mellitus populations after a single oral 75 g dose of D-tagatose [157]. A lower D-tagatose dose (45 g/day; 15 g, 3 times/day [TID]) is considered safe for healthy human subjects because it has no adverse effects on glycogen levels, plasma uric acid, and liver function [158]. An intake of 45 g D-tagatose/day (15 g TID) for 1 year does not induce any adverse effects on plasma uric acid levels in patients with non-insulin-dependent diabetes mellitus [159]. The above D-tagatose dose also tends to reduce postprandial plasma glucose levels. However, very few records suggest any gastrointestinal problems (nauseas, mild to severe flatulence and diarrhoea) following the intake of 30 g of D-tagatose as a single dose [160]. Given the above considerations, the "No Observed Adverse Effect Level" (NOAEL) for tagatose is set at 45 g/day or 0.75 g/kg body weight/day [161].

Regarding high-potency sweeteners, steviol glycosides (E 960) [162] are a good example of natural compounds disseminated widely worldwide. Steviosides have been used in large quantities in Japan for more than 20 years and have no documented side effects. Stevia safety is also responsible mostly for the low-absorption steviol glycosides in both humans and rats in stomach and upper intestine [121].

The use and safety of steviol glycosides has been reviewed and evaluated worldwide by a range of scientific bodies and regulatory organisation. High-purity extracts of stevia leaves have been approved for use in food and beverages by over 150 countries and regions [163]. During its 69th meeting, the Joint FAO/WHO Expert Committee on Food Additives (JECFA) set an ADI of 4 mg/kg bw/day for steviol glycosides in 2008, expressed as steviol equivalents. JECFA reaffirmed this ADI during its 82nd meeting in 2016 [164]. The Food Standards Australia New Zealand [165] and EFSA [166] have defined an ADI of 4 mg/kg bw/day for steviol glycosides (expressed as steviol equivalents). Stevia mutagenicity has been studied in many trials, although they gave contradictory results. For example, two studies concluded that, in certain assays, stevia demonstrated a dose-dependent mutagenic effect, but the same studies also concluded that stevioside is non-mutagenic [167,168]. Several other findings indicate that the plant lacks mutagenic effects [169,170]. Despite reports not being harmonious, the FDA continues to monitor this herb as a sugar replacement, while other findings reveal that steviol and stevioside do not interfere with DNA and have no genotoxicity [171]. Mizushina et al. [172] suggested that stevioside is not involved in bladder carcinogenesis. Up to 2500 mg/kg body weight/day has been safely used in rats and enabled their normal growth and reproduction [173]. After 14 consecutive days of administering steviosides as part of acute toxicity trials, no histopathologicity, no lethality and no morphological modifications were recorded in rodents [174]. In another study, the oral administration of an aqueous extract taken from stevia leaves (up to 10%) revealed no adverse effects on female rat fertility and no teratogenic effects [175]. It has also been shown that both stevia and stevioside are safe when used as sweeteners. This is appropriate for diabetic and phenylketonuric patients, and also for obese individuals who wish to lose weight and to remove sucrose from their diet. After intake, no allergic reactions or toxicity were reported [176]. In the long term, randomised, double-blind, placebo-controlled trials indicate using steviol glycosides as a sweetener with no toxic effects for humans [177]. Stevia's safety has also been confirmed by recent studies, which demonstrated that steviol glycosides are not mutagenic, carcinogenic or teratogenic, they and do not cause toxicity [178,179]. Recently, following oral administration, a toxicological stevia leaf ethanolic extract evaluation revealed no harmful effects on subchronic oral toxicity and genotoxicity. The authors proposed that stevia leaves have the potential to be considered functional food and a nutritional supplement, rather than sweetener [180].

Another high-potency sweetener is glycyrrhizin (E 958) [181]. This compound, which is also known as glycyrrhizic acid, can act as a sweetener with a potency 50-fold sweeter than sucrose, but is also employed as a foaming agent and a flavour enhancer. This substance is legally used in both the US and EU as mono-ammonium glycyrrhizinate and ammoniated glycyrrhizin. Glycyrrhizin has antiviral, anticancer antioxidant, anti-inflammatory and hepatoprotective effects [97], but also has potential hypertensive effects and an intense aftertaste [182]. In the gut, glycyrrhizin is de-glycosylated to glycyrrhetic acid (a major product) by *Eubacterium* spp. *Bacteroides* J-37 and to 18β glycyrrhetic acid 3-*O*-monoglucuronide (the minor product) by *Bacteroides* J-37 and *Streptococcus* LJ-22. *Eubacterium* spp. can be used to convert 18β-glycyrrhetic acid 3-*O*-monoglucuronide into glycyrrhetic acid [182–184]. These glycyrrhizin metabolites (particularly 18β-glycyrrhetinic acid) are significant anti-tumour cytotoxic agents with potent inhibitory effects on anti-platelet aggregation activity and rotavirus infection [185]. Some results indicate that the glycyrrhizin/intestinal microbiota interaction has beneficial effects on hosts [183,184,186].

Thaumatin (E 957), a mixture of five proteins (thaumatin I, I, III, a, b), is also employed as a sweetener in many countries. If we consider its health effects, thaumatin does not induce tooth decay and is suitable for diabetics, as opposed to artificial sweeteners [187]. The metabolism of this sweetener is the equivalent to other dietary proteins. The research work by Hsu et al. [188] demonstrates that thaumatin is digested more quickly than egg albumin. Moreover, several studies addressing thaumatin safety aspects indicate that this sweetener induces neither toxicity nor allergenicity [128]. Some studies have evaluated thaumatin toxicity; e.g., the Joint FAO/WHO Expert Committee on Food Additives, Food and Agriculture Organization of the United Nations and World Health Organization [189] study reveals that protein is void of toxic, genotoxic or teratogenic effects. Several studies offer compelling evidence that thaumatin is not an allergen to either oral mucosa or other treatment-associated allergic effects [128]. Higginbotham et al. [190] also state that thaumatin has no harmful impact when employed as a flavour additive or a partial sweetener at a particular intake level. This protein's safety has been evaluated by the Scientific Committee for Food of the European Commission (SCF) and JECFA, which concluded that it should be listed as an acceptable ingredient [110]. This sweet protein has been approved in the European Union since 1984 (E957) according to Annex II of Regulation (EC) No. 1333/2008 [110] and maintains its GRAS status in the USA. It was licensed for use in pharmaceuticals and food in the UK in 1983, except for baby food. It is an approved high-intensity sweetener and flavour enhancer in most other countries [191]. The Panel on Additives and Products or Substances used in Animal Feed (FEEDAP) [192] also indicates the safety of this protein in animals and its use is permitted as an additive from 1 to 5 mg/kg. Thaumatin is also employed as a sweetener in some foodstuffs like ice cream and sweets at the permitted 50 mg/kg dose. In dairy products and soft drinks, it is primarily utilised as a flavour enhancer within the range from 0.5 mg/L and 5 mg/kg [89].

There are a few other natural sweeteners that can be used in the future, but are not actually found in foodstuffs. Some examples of these substances are brazzein and monatin, which is attributable to their rarity and low yield when isolated from plant matrices.

Table 1 lists the main attributes of natural sweeteners for their use by taking into account health impacts.

Table 1. The main attributes of natural sweeteners for their use by taking into account health impacts.

Natural Sweetener	Attribute(s) and Reference(s)
Erythritol	Non-carcinogenic [137,138]; Non-mutagenic [137,138,141,142]; does not affect glucose or insulin levels [148,149]; beneficially impacts the endothelium [152]
Tagatose	Lowers postprandial plasma glucose levels [160]
Steviol glycosides	Non-genotoxic [171]; non-carcinogenic [172,178,179]; non-allergic [176]; non-teratogenic and non-mutagenic [178,179]
Glycyrrhizin	Anticancer, antiviral, antioxidant, anti-inflammatory, and hepatoprotective [97,185]
Thaumatin	Does not induce tooth decay [187]; not toxic and non-allergic [128]

6. Conclusions

Society is becoming increasingly aware of the utmost importance of eating a balanced diet to maintain and promote health. Excess sugar consumption is now a cross-cutting concern, but this habit is not an easy one to break, so sugar-free or low-sugar foods and drinks are in great demand and the sweetening agents that make them feasible are high-value ingredients. Today the food industry applies bulk and intense sweeteners, which are mainly synthetic in origin, to substitute sugar (sucrose). Consumers are all the more eager to eat products with natural ingredients and clean labels, preferably with other functional properties, and that do not compromise taste. To achieve this trend, the food industry now has alternative natural sweeteners at its disposal, like high-fructose corn syrup, sugar alcohols (polyols) and, quite recently, steviol glycosides tagatose and thaumatin, which offer consumers the advantage of additional health benefits. Nature is an incredible source of valuable compounds, including those with a sweet taste, of which many have not yet been explored. Nevertheless, it must be emphasised that being natural does not ensure their success on the market. It should also be noted that a long traditional use in some restricted societies and areas around the globe, and this despite providing some reassurance, cannot rule out the need to conduct detailed scientific studies to prove the safety of the natural compounds to be used as food additives and, for example, as sweeteners. The food industry needs to face the challenge of developing new products with natural functional sweeteners to continue innovating and satisfying consumers. Finally, although compounds like glycyrrhizin, an approved flavour enhancer, are not used as a sweetener, can play a relevant role in improving product characteristics, such as flavour, and need to be considered by industry.

Author Contributions: Conceptualization, A.S., C.C., D.R., F.R. and A.R.; methodology, A.S., C.C., D.R., F.R. and A.R.; software, A.S., C.C., D.R., F.R. and A.R.; validation, A.S., C.C., D.R., F.R. and A.R.; formal analysis, A.S., C.C., D.R., F.R. and A.R.; investigation, A.S., C.C., D.R., F.R. and A.R.; resources, A.S., C.C., D.R., F.R. and A.R.; data curation, A.S., C.C., D.R., F.R. and A.R.; writing—original draft preparation, A.S., C.C., D.R., F.R. and A.R.; writing—review and editing, A.S., C.C., D.R., F.R. and A.R.; visualization, A.S., C.C., D.R., F.R. and A.R.; supervision, A.S., C.C., D.R., F.R. and A.R.; project administration, A.S., C.C., D.R., F.R. and A.R.; funding acquisition, A.S., C.C., D.R., F.R. and A.R. All authors have read and agreed to the published version of the manuscript.

Funding: This research received no external funding.

Acknowledgments: The authors are very grateful to their families and friends for all the support they provided.

Conflicts of Interest: The authors declare no conflict of interest.

References

1. Asioli, D.; Aschemann-Witzel, J.; Caputo, V.; Vecchio, R.; Annunziata, A.; Næs, T.; Varela, P. Making sense of the "clean label" trends: A review of consumer food choice behavior and discussion of industry implications. *Food Res. Int.* **2017**, *99*, 58–71. [CrossRef] [PubMed]
2. Lusk, J.L. *Unnaturally Delicious: How Science and Technology Are Serving up Super Foods to Save the World*, 1st ed.; St. Martin's Press: New York, NY, USA, 2016; pp. 189–213.
3. Meneses, Y.; Cannon, K.J.; Flores, R.A. Keys to understanding and addressing consumer perceptions and concerns about processed foods. *Cereal Foods World.* **2014**, *59*, 141–146. [CrossRef]
4. Augustin, M.A.; Riley, M.; Stockmann, R.; Bennett, L.; Kahl, A.; Lockett, T.; Osmond, M.; Sanguansri, P.; Stonehouse, W.; Zajac, I.; et al. Role of food processing in food and nutrition security. *Trends Food Sci. Technol.* **2016**, *56*, 115–125. [CrossRef]
5. Weaver, C.M.; Dwyer, J.; Fulgoni, V.L., III; King, J.C.; Leveille, G.A.; MacDonald, R.S.; Ordovas, J.; Schnakenberg, D. Processed foods: Contributions to nutrition. *Am. J. Clin. Nutr.* **2014**, *99*, 1525–1542. [CrossRef]
6. Princen, T. The shading and distancing of commerce: When internalization is not enough. *Ecol Econ* **1997**, *20*, 235–253. [CrossRef]
7. Weis, T. *The Global Food Economy: The Battle for the Future of Farming*, 1st ed.; Fernowood Publishing: Black Point, NS, Canada, 2007; pp. 11–47.
8. Román, S.; Sánchez-Siles, L.M.; Siegrist, M. The importance of food naturalness for consumers: Results of a systematic review. *Trends Food Sci. Technol.* **2017**, *67*, 44–57. [CrossRef]
9. Philippe, R.N.; De Mey, M.; Anderson, J.; Ajikumar, P.K. Biotechnological production of natural zero-calorie sweeteners. *Curr. Opin. Biotechnol.* **2014**, *26*, 155–161. [CrossRef]
10. Mooradian, A.D.; Smith, M.; Tokuda, M. The role of artificial and natural sweeteners in reducing the consumption of table sugar: A narrative review. *Clin. Nutr. Espen* **2017**, *18*, 1–8. [CrossRef]
11. Carocho, M.; Morales, P.; Ferreira, I.C. Natural food additives: Quo vadis? *Trends Food Sci. Technol.* **2015**, *45*, 284–295. [CrossRef]
12. Serra-Majem, L.; Raposo, A.; Aranceta-Bartrina, J.; Varela-Moreiras, G.; Logue, C.; Laviada, H.; Socolovsky, S.; Pérez-Rodrigo, C.; Aldrete-Velasco, J.A.; Meneses Sierra, E.; et al. Ibero–American consensus on low-and no-calorie sweeteners: Safety, nutritional aspects and benefits in food and beverages. *Nutrients* **2018**, *10*, 818. [CrossRef]
13. Carocho, M.; Barreiro, M.F.; Morales, P.; Ferreira, I.C. Adding molecules to food, pros and cons: A review on synthetic and natural food additives. *Compr. Rev. Food Sci. Food Saf.* **2014**, *13*, 377–399. [CrossRef]
14. Wilson, E.O. *Biophilia*, 1st ed.; Harvard University Press: Cambridge, MA, USA, 1984; pp. 1–23.
15. Rozin, P.; Fischler, C.; Shields-Argelès, C. European and American perspectives on the meaning of natural. *Appetite* **2012**, *59*, 448–455. [CrossRef] [PubMed]
16. Nielsen. *We Are What We Eat, Healthy Eating Trends around the World.* January 2015. Available online: https://www.nielsen.com/wp-content/uploads/sites/3/2019/04/january-2015-global-health-and-wellness-report.pdf (accessed on 27 July 2020).
17. GoodMills Innovation. *Kampffmeyer Food Innovation Study.* November 2012. Available online: http://goodmillsinnovation.com/sites/kfi.kampffmeyer.faktor3server.de/files/attachments/1_pi_kfi_cleanlabelstudy_english_final.pdf (accessed on 27 July 2020).
18. Rozin, P. The meaning of "natural" process more important than content. *Psychol. Sci.* **2005**, *16*, 652–658. [CrossRef]
19. Rozin, P. Naturalness judgments by lay Americans: Process dominates content in judgments of food or water acceptability and naturalness. *Judgm. Decis. Mak.* **2006**, *1*, 91–97.
20. Rozin, P.; Spranca, M.; Krieger, Z.; Neuhaus, R.; Surillo, D.; Swerdlin, A.; Wood, K. Preference for natural: Instrumental and ideational/moral motivations, and the contrast between foods and medicines. *Appetite* **2004**, *43*, 147–154. [CrossRef] [PubMed]
21. Beck, U. *Risk Society: Towards a New Modernity*, 1st ed.; Sage Publications Ltd.: London, UK, 1992; pp. 19–91.

22. Bánáti, D. Consumer response to food scandals and scares. *Trends Food Sci. Technol.* **2011**, *22*, 56–60. [CrossRef]
23. Knowles, T.; Moody, R.; McEachern, M.G. European food scares and their impact on EU food policy. *Br. Food J.* **2007**, *109*, 43–67. [CrossRef]
24. Aktar, W.; Sengupta, D.; Chowdhury, A. Impact of pesticides use in agriculture: Their benefits and hazards. *Interdiscip. Toxicol.* **2009**, *2*, 1–12. [CrossRef]
25. Lucová, M.; Hojerová, J.; Pažoureková, S.; Klimová, Z. Absorption of triphenylmethane dyes Brilliant Blue and Patent Blue through intact skin, shaven skin and lingual mucosa from daily life products. *Food Chem. Toxicol.* **2013**, *52*, 19–27. [CrossRef]
26. Grunert, K.G.; Bredahl, L.; Scholderer, J. Four questions on European consumers' attitudes toward the use of genetic modification in food production. *Innov. Food Sci. Emerg. Technol.* **2003**, *4*, 435–445. [CrossRef]
27. Godfray, H.C.J.; Beddington, J.R.; Crute, I.R.; Haddad, L.; Lawrence, D.; Muir, J.F.; Pretty, J.; Robinson, S.; Thomas, S.M.; Toulmin, C. Food security: The challenge of feeding 9 billion people. *Science* **2010**, *327*, 812–818. [CrossRef] [PubMed]
28. Asioli, D.; Canavari, M.; Pignatti, E.; Obermowe, T.; Sidali, K.L.; Vogt, C.; Spiller, A. Sensory experiences and expectations of Italian and German organic consumers. *J. Int. Food Agribus. Mark.* **2014**, *26*, 13–27. [CrossRef]
29. Caputo, V.; Nayga, R.M., Jr.; Scarpa, R. Food miles or carbon emissions? Exploring labelling preference for food transport footprint with a stated choice study. *Aust. J. Agric. Econ.* **2013**, *57*, 465–482. [CrossRef]
30. Frewer, L.J.; van Trijp, H. *Understanding Consumers of Food Products*, 1st ed.; Woodhead Publishing Limited: Cambridge, UK, 2007; pp. 21–24.
31. MacFie, H. Preference mapping and food product development. In *Consumer-Led Food Product Development*, 1st ed.; MacFie, H., Ed.; Woodhead Publishing Limited: Cambridge, UK, 2007; pp. 551–593.
32. Grunert, K.G. Trends in food choice and nutrition. In *Consumer Attitudes to Food Quality Products: Emphasis on Southern Europe*, 1st ed.; Klopčič, M., Kuipers, A., Hocquette, J.-F., Eds.; Wageningen Academic Publishers: Wageningen, The Netherlands, 2013; pp. 23–30.
33. Kearney, J. Food consumption trends and drivers. *Philos. Trans. R. Soc. B* **2010**, *365*, 2793–2807. [CrossRef] [PubMed]
34. Krovetz, H. The effect of water-use labeling and information on consumer valuation for water sustainable food choices in California. In Proceedings of the Environmental Sciences Senior Thesis Symposium, University of California at Berkeley, Berkeley, CA, USA, 23 April 2016.
35. Lachat, C.; Nago, E.; Verstraeten, R.; Roberfroid, D.; Van Camp, J.; Kolsteren, P. Eating out of home and its association with dietary intake: A systematic review of the evidence. *Obes. Rev.* **2012**, *13*, 329–346. [CrossRef]
36. Chrysochou, P.; Askegaard, S.; Grunert, K.G.; Kristensen, D.B. Social discourses of healthy eating. A market segmentation approach. *Appetite* **2010**, *55*, 288–297. [CrossRef] [PubMed]
37. Pohjanheimo, T.; Paasovaara, R.; Luomala, H.; Sandell, M. Food choice motives and bread liking of consumers embracing hedonistic and traditional values. *Appetite* **2010**, *54*, 170–180. [CrossRef]
38. Mai, R.; Hoffmann, S. How to combat the unhealthy = tasty intuition: The influencing role of health consciousness. *J. Public Policy Mark.* **2015**, *34*, 63–83. [CrossRef]
39. Steptoe, A.; Pollard, T.M.; Wardle, J. Development of a measure of the motives underlying the selection of food: The food choice questionnaire. *Appetite* **1995**, *25*, 267–284. [CrossRef]
40. Bearth, A.; Cousin, M.E.; Siegrist, M. The consumer's perception of artificial food additives: Influences on acceptance, risk and benefit perceptions. *Food Qual. Prefer.* **2014**, *38*, 14–23. [CrossRef]
41. Chen, M.F. The gender gap in food choice motives as determinants of consumers' attitudes toward GM foods in Taiwan. *Br. Food J.* **2011**, *113*, 697–709. [CrossRef]
42. Chen, M.F. Consumers' health and taste attitude in Taiwan: The impacts of modern tainted food worries and gender difference. *Br. Food J.* **2013**, *115*, 526–540. [CrossRef]
43. Dickson-Spillmann, M.; Siegrist, M.; Keller, C. Attitudes toward chemicals are associated with preference for natural food. *Food Qual. Prefer.* **2011**, *22*, 149–156. [CrossRef]
44. Huotilainen, A.; Tuorila, H. Social representation of new foods has a stable structure based on suspicion and trust. *Food Qual. Prefer.* **2005**, *16*, 565–572. [CrossRef]
45. Siegrist, M.; Stampfli, N.; Kastenholz, H.; Keller, C. Perceived risks and perceived benefits of different nanotechnology foods and nanotechnology food packaging. *Appetite* **2008**, *51*, 283–290. [CrossRef] [PubMed]

46. Pieniak, Z.; Verbeke, W.; Vanhonacker, F.; Guerrero, L.; Hersleth, M. Association between traditional food consumption and motives for food choice in six European countries. *Appetite* **2009**, *53*, 101–108. [CrossRef]
47. Olbrich, R.; Hundt, M.; Grewe, G. Willingness to pay in food retailing—An empirical study of consumer behaviour in the context of the proliferation of organic products. In *European Retail Research*, 1st ed.; Foscht, T., Morschett, D., Rudolph, T., Schnedlitz, P., Schramm-Klein, H., Swoboda, B., Eds.; Springer Gabler: Wiesbaden, Germany, 2015; pp. 67–101.
48. Hsu, S.Y.; Chang, C.C.; Lin, T.T. An analysis of purchase intentions toward organic food on health consciousness and food safety with/under structural equation modeling. *Br. Food J.* **2016**, *118*, 200–216. [CrossRef]
49. Bäckström, A.; Pirttilä-Backman, A.M.; Tuorila, H. Willingness to try new foods as predicted by social representations and attitude and trait scales. *Appetite* **2004**, *43*, 75–83. [CrossRef] [PubMed]
50. Eertmans, A.; Victoir, A.; Vansant, G.; Van den Bergh, O. Food-related personality traits, food choice motives and food intake: Mediator and moderator relationships. *Food Qual. Prefer.* **2005**, *16*, 714–726. [CrossRef]
51. Onwezen, M.C.; Bartels, J. Development and cross-cultural validation of a shortened social representations scale of new foods. *Food Qual. Prefer.* **2013**, *28*, 226–234. [CrossRef]
52. Huotilainen, A.; Pirttilä-Backman, A.M.; Tuorila, H. How innovativeness relates to social representation of new foods and to the willingness to try and use such foods. *Food Qual. Prefer.* **2006**, *17*, 353–361. [CrossRef]
53. Urala, N.; Lähteenmäki, L. Consumers' changing attitudes towards functional foods. *Food Qual. Prefer.* **2007**, *18*, 1–12. [CrossRef]
54. Mouta, J.S.; de Sá, N.C.; Menezes, E.; Melo, L. Effect of institutional sensory test location and consumer attitudes on acceptance of foods and beverages having different levels of processing. *Food Qual. Prefer.* **2016**, *48 Pt A*, 262–267. [CrossRef]
55. Tobler, C.; Visschers, V.H.; Siegrist, M. Eating green. Consumers' willingness to adopt ecological food consumption behaviors. *Appetite* **2011**, *57*, 674–682. [CrossRef] [PubMed]
56. Gomez, P.; Schneid, N.; Delaere, F. How often should I eat it? Product correlates and accuracy of estimation of appropriate food consumption frequency. *Food Qual. Prefer.* **2015**, *40*, 1–7. [CrossRef]
57. Hemmerling, S.; Canavari, M.; Spiller, A. Preference for naturalness of european organic Consumers: First evidence of an attitude-liking-gap. *Br. Food J.* **2016**, *118*, 2287–2307. [CrossRef]
58. Oellingrath, I.M.; Hersleth, M.; Svendsen, M.V. Association between parental motives for food choice and eating patterns of 12-to 13-year-old Norwegian children. *Public Health Nutr.* **2013**, *16*, 2023–2031. [CrossRef]
59. Phan, U.T.; Chambers, E. Motivations for choosing various food groups based on individual foods. *Appetite* **2016**, *105*, 204–211. [CrossRef]
60. Kraus, A. Factors influencing the decisions to buy and consume functional food. *Br. Food J.* **2015**, *117*, 1622–1636. [CrossRef]
61. Urala, N.; Lähteenmäki, L. Attitudes behind consumers' willingness to use functional foods. *Food Qual. Prefer.* **2004**, *15*, 793–803. [CrossRef]
62. Lähteenmäki, L.; Grunert, K.; Ueland, Ø.; Åström, A.; Arvola, A.; Bech-Larsen, T. Acceptability of genetically modified cheese presented as real product alternative. *Food Qual. Prefer.* **2002**, *13*, 523–533. [CrossRef]
63. Lusk, J.L.; Crespi, J.M.; Cherry, J.B.C.; Mcfadden, B.R.; Martin, L.E.; Bruce, A.S. An fMRI investigation of consumer choice regarding controversial food technologies. *Food Qual. Prefer.* **2015**, *40*, 209–220. [CrossRef]
64. Grubor, A.; Djokic, N.; Djokic, I.; Kovac-Znidersic, R. Application of health and Taste attitude scales in Serbia. *Br. Food J.* **2015**, *117*, 840–860. [CrossRef]
65. Pollard, J.; Greenwood, D.; Kirk, S.; Cade, J. Motivations for fruit and vegetable consumption in the UK Women's Cohort Study. *Public Health Nutr.* **2002**, *5*, 479–486. [CrossRef]
66. Pollard, T.M.; Steptoe, A.; Wardle, J. Motives underlying healthy eating: Using the Food Choice Questionnaire to explain variation in dietary intake. *J. Biosoc. Sci.* **1998**, *30*, 165–179. [CrossRef]
67. Steptoe, A.; Wardle, J. Motivational factors as mediators of socioeconomic variations in dietary intake patterns. *Psychol Health* **1999**, *14*, 391–402. [CrossRef]
68. Thong, N.T.; Solgaard, H.S. Consumer's food motives and seafood consumption. *Food Qual. Prefer.* **2017**, *56*, 181–188. [CrossRef]
69. Lockie, S.; Lyons, K.; Lawrence, G.; Mummery, K. Eating "Green": Motivations behind organic food consumption in Australia. *Sociol. Rural.* **2002**, *42*, 23–40. [CrossRef]

70. Pieniak, Z.; Perez-Cueto, F.; Verbeke, W. Nutritional status, self identification as a traditional food consumer and motives for food choice in six european countries. *Br. Food J.* **2013**, *115*, 1297–1312. [CrossRef]
71. Brunner, T.A.; Van der Horst, K.; Siegrist, M. Convenience food products. Drivers for consumption. *Appetite* **2010**, *55*, 498–506. [CrossRef]
72. Roininen, K.; Tuorila, H. Health and taste attitudes in the prediction of use frequency and choice between less healthy and more healthy snacks. *Food Qual. Prefer.* **1999**, *10*, 357–365. [CrossRef]
73. Zandstra, E.H.; De Graaf, C.; Van Staveren, W.A. Influence of health and taste attitudes on consumption of low-and high-fat foods. *Food Qual. Prefer.* **2001**, *12*, 75–82. [CrossRef]
74. Carrillo, E.; Prado-Gascó, V.; Fiszman, S.; Varela, P. Why buying functional foods? Understanding spending behaviour through structural equation modelling. *Food Res. Int.* **2013**, *50*, 361–368. [CrossRef]
75. Devcich, D.A.; Pedersen, I.K.; Petrie, K.J. You eat what you are: Modern health worries and the acceptance of natural and synthetic additives in functional foods. *Appetite* **2007**, *48*, 333–337. [CrossRef]
76. Pokorný, J. Natural antioxidants for food use. *Trends Food Sci. Technol.* **1991**, *2*, 223–227. [CrossRef]
77. Lindley, M.G. Natural High-Potency Sweeteners. In *Sweeteners and Sugar Alternatives in Food Technology*, 2nd ed.; O'Donnell, K., Kearsley, M.W., Eds.; John Wiley & Sons, Ltd.: Chichester West Sussex, UK, 2012; pp. 185–212.
78. Drewnowski, A.; Mennella, J.A.; Johnson, S.L.; Bellisle, F. Sweetness and food preference. *J. Nutr.* **2012**, *142*, 1142–1148. [CrossRef]
79. Marcus, J.B. A taste primer. In *Aging, Nutrition and Taste: Nutrition, Foods Science and Culinary Perspectives for Aging Tastefully*; Academic Press: New York, NY, USA, 2019; p. 114.
80. Belloir, C.; Neiers, F.; Briand, L. Sweeteners and sweetness enhancers. *Curr. Opin. Clin. Nutr. Metab. Care* **2017**, *20*, 279–285. [CrossRef]
81. Laffitte, A.; Neiers, F.; Briand, L. Characterization of taste compounds: Chemical structures and sensory properties. In *Flavour: From Food to Perception*; Guichard, E., Salles, C., Morzel, M., Le Bon, A.-M., Eds.; Wiley-Blackwell: Oxford, UK, 2017; pp. 154–191.
82. Statista. Sugar Consumption Worldwide 2009/10–2019/20. Available online: https://www.statista.com/statistics/249681/total-consumption-of-sugar-worldwide/ (accessed on 12 May 2020).
83. World Health Organization (WHO). Guideline: Sugars Intake for Adults and Children. Available online: http://www.who.int/nutrition/publications/guidelines/sugars_intake/en/ (accessed on 12 May 2020).
84. Grembecka, M. Natural sweeteners in a human diet. *Rocz. Państwowego Zakładu Hig.* **2015**, *66*, 195–202.
85. Chéron, J.-B.; Marchal, A.; Fiorucci, S. Natural sweeteners. In *Encyclopedia of Food Chemistry*; Varelis, P., Melton, L., Shahidi, F., Eds.; Elsevier: Amesterdam, The Netherlands, 2019; Volume 1, pp. 189–195.
86. Kroger, M.; Meister, K.; Kava, R. Low-calorie sweeteners and other sugar substitutes: A review of the safety issues. *Compr. Rev. Food Sci. Food Saf.* **2006**, *5*, 35–47. [CrossRef]
87. Carocho, M.; Morales, P.; Ferreira, I.C.F.R. Sweeteners as food additives in the XXI century: A review of what is known, and what is to come. *Food Chem. Toxicol.* **2017**, *107*, 302–317. [CrossRef]
88. Shah, R.; Jager, L.S. Recent analytical methods for the analysis of sweeteners in food: A regulatory perspective. *Food Drug Adm. Pap.* **2017**, *5*, 13–32.
89. Mortensen, A. Sweeteners permitted in the European Union: Safety aspects. *Scand. J. Food Nutr.* **2006**, *50*, 104–116. [CrossRef]
90. Fry, J.C. Natural low-calorie sweeteners. In *Natural Food Additives, Ingredients and Flavourings*; Baines, D., Seal, R., Eds.; Woodhead Publishing: Cambridge, UK, 2012; pp. 41–75.
91. Tappy, L.; Le, K.A. Metabolic effects of fructose and the worldwide increase in obesity. *Physiol. Rev.* **2010**, *90*, 23–46. [CrossRef]
92. The Commission of the European Communities. Commission decision of 25 September 2001 authorising the placing on the market of trehalose as a novel food or novel food ingredient under Regulation (EC) No 258/97 of the European Parliament and of the Council. *Off. J. Eur. Communities* **2001**, *L269*, 17.
93. BeMiller, J.N. Oligosaccharides. In *Carbohydrate Chemistry for Food Scientists*; Elsevier: Amesterdam, The Netherlands, 2019; pp. 49–74.
94. Grembecka, M. Sugar alcohols—their role in the modern world of sweeteners: A review. *Eur. Food Res. Technol.* **2015**, *241*, 1–14. [CrossRef]
95. Chades, T.; Scully, S.M.; Ingvadottir, E.M.; Orlygsson, J. Fermentation of mannitol extracts from brown macro algae by *Thermophilic Clostridia*. *Front. Microbiol.* **2018**, *9*, 1931. [CrossRef]

96. Andersen, R.; Sørensen, A. Separation and determination of alditols and sugars by high-pH anion-exchange chromatography with pulsed amperometric detection. *J. Chromatogr. A* **2000**, *897*, 195–204. [CrossRef]
97. Ruiz-Ojeda, F.J.; Plaza-Díaz, J.; Sáez-Lara, M.J.; Gil, A. Effects of sweeteners on the gut microbiota: A review of experimental studies and clinical trials. *Adv. Nutr.* **2019**, *10*, 31–48. [CrossRef]
98. Saraiva, A.; Carrascosa, C.; Raheem, D.; Ramos, F.; Raposo, A. Maltitol: Analytical Determination Methods, Applications in the Food Industry, Metabolism and Health Impacts. *Int. J. Environ. Res. Public Health* **2020**, *17*, 5227. [CrossRef]
99. *Alternative Sweeteners*, 4th ed.; O'Brien-Nabors, L. (Ed.) CRC Press: Boca Raton, FL, USA, 2016.
100. European Food Safety Authority (EFSA). Call for Technical Data on Sweeteners Authorised as Food Additives in the EU. Available online: https://www.efsa.europa.eu/en/consultations/call/call-technical-data-sweeteners-authorised-food-additives-eu (accessed on 12 May 2020).
101. Swiader, K.; Wegner, K.; Piotrowska, A.; Tan, F.-J.; Sadowska, A. Plants as a source of natural high-intensity sweeteners: A review. *J. Appl. Bot. Food Qual.* **2019**, *92*, 160–171.
102. Gu, W.; Rebsdorf, A.; Anker, C.; Gregersen, S.; Hermansen, K.; Geuns, J.M.C.; Jeppesen, P.B. Steviol glucuronide, a metabolite of steviol glycosides, potently stimulates insulin secretion from isolated mouse islets: Studies in vitro. *Endocrinol. Diabetes Metab.* **2019**, *2*, 1–9. [CrossRef] [PubMed]
103. European Food Safety Authority Panel on Food Additives and Flavourings (EFSA-FAF Panel). Safety of a proposed amendment of the specifications for steviol glycosides (E 960) as a food additive: To expand the list of steviol glycosides to all those identified in the leaves of *Stevia rebaudiana* Bertoni. *EFSA J.* **2020**, *18*, 6106.
104. Chatsudthipong, V.; Muanprasat, C. Stevioside and related compounds: Therapeutic benefits beyond sweetness. *Pharmacol. Ther.* **2009**, *121*, 41–54. [CrossRef] [PubMed]
105. Pielak, M.; Czarniecka-Skubina, E.; Trafiałek, J.; Głuchowski, A. Contemporary trends and habits in the consumption of sugar and sweeteners—A questionnaire survey among poles. *Int. J. Environ. Res. Public Health* **2019**, *16*, 1164. [CrossRef]
106. U.S. Food and Drug Administration (FDA). Food Additive Status List. Available online: https://www.fda.gov/food/food-additives-petitions/food-additive-status-list (accessed on 12 May 2020).
107. Nazari, S.; Rameshrad, M.; Hosseinzadeh, H. Toxicological effects of *Glycyrrhiza glabra* (licorice): A review. *Phyther. Res.* **2017**, *31*, 1635–1650. [CrossRef]
108. European Commission's Scientific Committee on Food (EC-SCF). Opinion of the Scientific Committee on Food on Glycyrrhizinic Acid and Its Ammonium Salt. Available online: https://ec.europa.eu/food/sites/food/files/safety/docs/sci-com_scf_out186_en.pdf (accessed on 12 May 2020).
109. Masuda, T. Sweet-tasting protein thaumatin: Physical and chemical properties. In *Sweeteners: Pharmacology, Biotechnology, and Applications*; Merillon, J.-M., Ramawat, K.G., Eds.; Springer: Berlin, Germany, 2017; pp. 493–523.
110. European Food Safety Authority Panel on Food Additives and Nutrient Sources added to Food (EFSA-ANS Panel). Scientific Opinion on the safety of the extension of use of thaumatin (E 957). *EFSA J.* **2015**, *13*, 4290.
111. Tschannen, M.P.; Glück, U.; Bircher, A.J.; Heijnen, I.; Pletscher, C. Thaumatin and gum arabic allergy in chewing gum factory workers. *Am. J. Ind. Med.* **2017**, *60*, 1–6. [CrossRef]
112. European Commission. From Farm to Fork. May 2020. Available online: https://ec.europa.eu/info/strategy/priorities-2019--2024/european-green-deal/actions-being-taken-eu/farm-fork_en (accessed on 26 May 2020).
113. Rzechonek, D.A.; Dobrowolski, A.; Rymowicz, W.; Mirończuk, A.M. Recent advances in biological production of erythritol. *Crit. Rev. Biotechnol.* **2018**, *38*, 620–633. [CrossRef]
114. Moon, H.J.; Jeya, M.; Kim, I.W.; Lee, J.K. Biotechnological production of erythritol and its applications. *Appl. Microbiol. Biotechnol.* **2010**, *86*, 1017–1025. [CrossRef]
115. Horikita, H.; Hattori, N.; Takagi, Y.; Kawaguchi, G.; Maeda, T. Process for Producing Erythritol. U.S. Patent 4,923,812, 8 May 1990.
116. Cheetham, P.S.J.; Wootton, A.N. Bioconversion of d-galactose into d-tagatose. *Enzym. Microb. Technol.* **1993**, *15*, 105–108. [CrossRef]
117. Roh, H.J.; Kim, P.; Park, Y.C.; Choi, J.H. Bioconversion of d-galactose into d-tagatose by expression of l-arabinose isomerase. *Biotechnol. Appl. Biochem.* **2000**, *31*, 1–4. [CrossRef] [PubMed]
118. Roy, S.; Chikkerur, J.; Roy, S.C.; Dhali, A.; Kolte, A.P.; Sridhar, M.; Samanta, A.K. Tagatose as a potential nutraceutical: Production, properties, biological roles, and applications. *J. Food Sci.* **2018**, *83*, 2699–2709. [CrossRef] [PubMed]

119. Oh, D.K. Tagatose: Properties, applications, and biotechnological processes. *Appl. Microbiol. Biotechnol.* **2007**, *76*, 1–8. [CrossRef]
120. Food and Agriculture Organization. Steviol Glycosides, Chemical and Technical Assessment Prepared by Harriet Wallin. June 2004. Available online: http://www.fao.org/fileadmin/templates/agns/pdf/jecfa/cta/63/Steviol.pdf (accessed on 20 May 2020).
121. Mathur, S.; Bulchandani, N.; Parihar, S.; Shekhawat, G.S. Critical Review on Steviol Glycosides: Pharmacological, Toxicological and Therapeutic Aspects of High Potency Zero Caloric Sweetener. *Int. J. Pharm.* **2017**, *13*, 916–928.
122. Pasquel, A.; Meireles, M.A.A.; Marques, M.O.M.; Petenate, A.J. Extraction of stevia glycosides with CO_2+ water, CO_2+ ethanol, and CO_2+ water+ ethanol. *Braz. J. Chem. Eng.* **2000**, *17*, 271–282. [CrossRef]
123. Singh, B.; Singh, J.; Kaur, A. Agro-production, processing and utilization of *Stevia rebaudiana* as natural sweetener. *J. Agric. Eng. Food Technol.* **2014**, *1*, 28–31.
124. Rao, A.B.; Reddy, G.R.; Ernala, P.; Sridhar, S.; Ravikumar, Y.V.L. An improvised process of isolation, purification of steviosides from *Stevia rebaudiana* Bertoni leaves and its biological activity. *Int. J. Food Sci. Technol.* **2012**, *47*, 2554–2560. [CrossRef]
125. Mukhopadhyay, M.; Panja, P. A novel process for extraction of natural sweetener from licorice (*Glycyrrhiza glabra*) roots. *Sep. Purif. Technol.* **2008**, *63*, 539–545. [CrossRef]
126. Liao, J.; Qu, B.; Zheng, N. Extraction of Glycyrrhizic Acid from *Glycyrrhiza uralensis* Using Ultrasound and Its Process Extraction Model. *Appl. Sci.* **2016**, *6*, 319. [CrossRef]
127. Charpe, T.W.; Rathod, V.K. Extraction of glycyrrhizic acid from licorice root using ultrasound: Process intensification studies. *Chem. Eng. Process.* **2012**, *54*, 37–41. [CrossRef]
128. Joseph, J.A.; Akkermans, S.; Nimmegeers, P.; Van Impe, J.F. Bioproduction of the recombinant sweet protein thaumatin: Current state of the art and perspectives. *Front. Microbiol.* **2019**, *10*, 695. [CrossRef] [PubMed]
129. Nabors, L.O.; Gelardi, R. *Alternative Sweeteners*, 3rd ed.; Marcel Dekker: New York, NY, USA, 2001; pp. 1–12.
130. Jain, T.; Grover, K. Sweeteners in human nutrition. *Int. J. Health Sci. Res.* **2015**, *5*, 439–451.
131. Priya, K.; Gupta, V.R.M.; Srikanth, K. Natural sweeteners: A complete review. *J. Pharm. Res.* **2011**, *4*, 2034–2039.
132. Chen, J.C.; Chou, C.C. *Cane Sugar Handbook: A Manual for Cane Sugar Manufacturers and Their Chemists*, 12th ed.; John Wiley & Sons: New York, NY, USA, 1993; pp. 375–435.
133. Perkins, T.D.; van den Berg, A.K. Maple syrup—Production, composition, chemistry, and sensory characteristics. *Adv. Food Nutr. Res.* **2009**, *56*, 101–143.
134. Beverage Industry. Natural Sweeteners Resonate with Consumers. September 2018. Available online: https://www.bevindustry.com/articles/91414-natural-sweeteners-resonate-with-consumers?oly_enc_id=3136G3707801F0X (accessed on 20 May 2020).
135. Baines, D.; Seal, R. *Natural Food Additives, Ingredients and Flavourings*, 1st ed.; Woodhead Publishing: Cambridge, UK, 2012; pp. 23–26.
136. EFSA. Scientific opinion on the safety of the proposed extension of use of erythritol (E968) as a food additive. *EFSA J.* **2015**, *13*, 4033. [CrossRef]
137. Bernt, W.O.; Borzelleca, J.F.; Flamm, G.; Munro, I.C. Erythritol: A review of biological and toxicological studies. *Regul. Toxicol. Pharm.* **1996**, *24*, S191–S197. [CrossRef]
138. Munro, I.C.; Berndt, W.O.; Borzelleca, J.F.; Flamm, G.; Lynch, B.S.; Kennepohl, E.; Bär, E.A.; Modderman, J. Erythritol: An interpretive summary of biochemical, metabolic, toxicological and clinical data. *Food Chem. Toxicol.* **1998**, *36*, 1139–1174. [CrossRef]
139. Waalkens-Berendsen, D.H.; Smits-van Prooije, A.E.; Wijnands, M.V.; Bär, A. Two-generation reproduction study of erythritol in rats. *Regul. Toxicol. Pharm.* **1996**, *24*, S237–S246. [CrossRef]
140. Shimizu, M.; Katoh, M.; Imamura, M.; Modderman, J. Teratology study of erythritol in rabbits. *Regul. Toxicol. Pharm.* **1996**, *24*, S247–S253. [CrossRef]
141. Kawamura, Y.; Saito, Y.; Imamura, M.; Modderman, J.P. Mutagenicity studies on erythritol in bacterial reversion assay systems and in Chinese hamster fibroblast cells. *Regul. Toxicol. Pharm.* **1996**, *24*, S261–S263. [CrossRef]
142. Chung, Y.S.; Lee, M. Genotoxicity assessment of erythritol by using short-term assay. *Toxicol. Res.* **2013**, *29*, 249–255. [CrossRef] [PubMed]

143. Kawanabe, J.; Hirasawa, M.; Takeuchi, T.; Oda, T.; Ikeda, T. Noncariogenicity of erythritol as a substrate. *Caries Res.* **1992**, *26*, 358–362. [CrossRef] [PubMed]
144. Makinen, K.K.; Saag, M.; Isotupa, K.P.; Olak, J.; Nommela, R.; Soderling, E.; Makinen, P.L. Similarity of the effects of erythritol and xylitol on some risk factors of dental caries. *Caries Res.* **2005**, *39*, 207–215. [CrossRef] [PubMed]
145. Hashino, E.; Kuboniwa, M.; Alghamdi, S.A.; Yamaguchi, M.; Yamamoto, R.; Cho, H.; Amano, A. Erythritol alters microstructure and metabolomic profiles of biofilm composed of *Streptococcus gordonii* and *Porphyromonas gingivalis*. *Mol. Oral Microbiol.* **2013**, *28*, 435–451. [CrossRef]
146. Runnel, R.; Mäkinen, K.K.; Honkala, S.; Olak, J.; Mäkinen, P.L.; Nõmmela, R.; Vahlberg, T.; Honkala, E.; Saag, M. Effect of three-year consumption of erythritol, xylitol and sorbitol candies on various plaque and salivary caries-related variables. *J. Dent.* **2013**, *41*, 1236–1244. [CrossRef]
147. Honkala, S.; Runnel, R.; Saag, M.; Olak, J.; Nommela, R.; Russak, S.; Makinen, P.L.; Vahlberg, T.; Falony, G.; Makinen, K.; et al. Effect of erythritol and xylitol on dental caries prevention in children. *Caries Res.* **2014**, *48*, 482–490. [CrossRef]
148. Den Hartog, G.J.; Boots, A.W.; Adam-Perrot, A.; Brouns, F.; Verkooijen, I.W.; Weseler, A.R.; Haenen, G.R.; Bast, A. Erythritol is a sweet antioxidant. *Nutrition* **2010**, *26*, 449–458. [CrossRef]
149. Yokozawa, T.; Kim, H.Y.; Cho, E.J. Erythritol attenuates the diabetic oxidative stress through glucose metabolism and lipid peroxidation in streptozotocin-induced diabetic rats. *J. Agric. Food Chem.* **2002**, *50*, 5485–5489. [CrossRef]
150. Roberts, A.C.; Porter, K.E. Cellular and molecular mechanisms of endothelial dysfunction in diabetes. *Diabetes Vasc. Dis. Res.* **2013**, *10*, 472–482. [CrossRef]
151. Boesten, D.M.P.H.J.; Berger, A.; de Cock, P.; Dong, H.; Hammock, B.D.; den Hartog, G.J.M.; Bast, A. Multi-targeted mechanisms underlying the endothelial protective effects of the diabetic-safe sweetener erythritol. *PLoS ONE* **2013**, *8*, e65741. [CrossRef]
152. Flint, N.; Hamburg, N.; Holbrook, M.; Dorsey, P.; LeLeiko, R.; Berger, A.; de Cock, P.; Bosscher, D.; Vita, J. Effects of erythritol on endothelial function in patients with type 2 diabetes mellitus: A pilot study. *Acta Diabetol.* **2013**, *51*, 513–516. [CrossRef] [PubMed]
153. Boesten, D.M.; den Hartog, G.J.; de Cock, P.; Bosscher, D.; Bonnema, A.; Bast, A. Health effects of erythritol. *Nutrafoods* **2015**, *14*, 3–9. [CrossRef]
154. Dobbs, C.M.; Bell, L.N. Storage stability of tagatose in buffer solutions of various compositions. *Food Res. Int.* **2010**, *43*, 382–386. [CrossRef]
155. Kruger, C.L.; Whittaker, M.H.; Frankos, V.H.; Schroeder, R.E. Developmental toxicity study of D-tagatose in rats. *Regul. Toxicol. Pharm.* **1999**, *29 Pt 2*, S29–S35. [CrossRef]
156. Kruger, C.L.; Whittaker, M.H.; Frankos, V.H.; Trimmer, G.W. 90-Day oral toxicity study of D-tagatose in rats. *Regul. Toxicol. Pharm.* **1999**, *29 Pt 2*, S1–S10. [CrossRef]
157. Saunders, J.P.; Donner, T.W.; Sadler, J.H.; Levin, G.V.; Makris, N.G. Effects of acute and repeated oral doses of D-tagatose on plasma uric acid in normal and diabetic humans. *Regul. Toxicol. Pharm.* **1999**, *29 Pt 2*, S57–S65. [CrossRef]
158. Boesch, C.; Ith, M.; Jung, B.; Bruegger, K.; Erban, S.; Diamantis, I.; Kreis, R.; Bär, A. Effect of oral D-tagatose on liver volume and hepatic glycogen accumulation in healthy male volunteers. *Regul. Toxicol. Pharm.* **2001**, *33*, 257–267. [CrossRef]
159. Donner, T.W. The metabolic effects of dietary supplementation with D-tagatose in patients with type 2 diabetes. *Diabetes* **2006**, *55* (Suppl. 1), 461.
160. Buemann, B.; Toubro, S.; Raben, A.; Astrup, A. Human tolerance to single, high dose of D-tagatose. *Regul. Toxicol. Pharm.* **1999**, *29*, S66–S70. [CrossRef]
161. World Health Organization. *Evaluation of Certain Food Additives Food Additives, Sixty-First Report of the Joint FAO/WHO Expert Committee on Food Additives*; WHO Technical Report Series; World Health Organization: Geneva, Switzerland, 2004; p. 922.
162. EFSA. Scientific opinion on the revised exposure assessment of Steviol glycosides (E 960) for the proposed uses as a food additive. *EFSA J.* **2014**, *12*, 3639.
163. Samuel, P.; Ayoob, K.T.; Magnuson, B.A.; Wölwer-Rieck, U.; Jeppesen, P.B.; Rogers, P.J.; Rowland, I.; Mathews, R. Stevia leaf to Stevia sweetener: Exploring its science, benefits, and future potential. *J. Nutr.* **2018**, *148*, 1186S–1205S. [CrossRef] [PubMed]

164. WHO Expert Committee on Food Additives, & World Health Organization (JECFA). *82nd Joint FAO/WHO Expert Committee on Food Additives (JECFA) Meeting—Food Additives (Summary and Conclusions)*; World Health Organization: Geneva, Switzerland, June 2016.
165. Food Standards Australia New Zealand (FSANZ). Final Assessment Report Application A.540 Steviol Glycosides as Intense Sweeteners. August 2008. Available online: https://www.foodstandards.gov.au/code/applications/documents/FAR_A540_Steviol_glycosides.pdf (accessed on 6 July 2020).
166. EFSA. Statement of EFSA Revised exposure assessment for steviol glycosides for the proposed uses as a food additive on request from the European Commission, Question No. EFSA-Q-2010-01214. *EFSA J.* **2011**, *9*, 1–19.
167. Matsui, M.; Matsui, K.; Kawasaki, Y.; Oda, Y.; Noguchi, T.; Kitagawa, Y.; Sawada, M.; Hayashi, M.; Nohmi, T.; Yoshihira, K.; et al. Evaluation of the genotoxicity of stevioside and steviol using six in vitro and one in vivo mutagenicity assays. *Mutagenesis* **1996**, *11*, 573–579. [CrossRef] [PubMed]
168. Pezzuto, J.M.; Nanayakkara, N.D.; Compadre, C.M.; Swanson, S.M.; Kinghorn, A.D.; Guenthner, T.M.; Sparnins, V.L.; Lam, L.K. Characterization of bacterial mutagenicity mediated by 13-hydroxy-ent-kaurenoic acid (steviol) and several structurally-related derivatives and evaluation of potential to induce glutathione S-transferase in mice. *Mutat. Res. Genet. Toxicol.* **1986**, *169*, 93–103. [CrossRef]
169. Klongpanichpak, S.; Temcharoen, P.; Toskulkao, C.; Apibal, S.; Glinsukon, T. Lack of mutagenicity of stevioside and steviol in Salmonella typhimurium TA 98 and TA 100. *J. Med. Assoc. Thail.* **1997**, *80*, 121–128.
170. Suttajit, M.; Vinitketkaumnuen, U.; Meevatee, U.; Buddhasukh, D. Mutagenicity and human chromosomal effect of stevioside, a sweetener from Stevia rebaudiana Bertoni. *Environ. Health Perspect.* **1993**, *101*, 53–56.
171. Brusick, D. A critical review of the genetic toxicity of steviol and steviol glycosides. *Food Chem. Toxicol.* **2008**, *46*, S83–S91. [CrossRef]
172. Mizushina, Y.; Akihisa, T.; Ukiya, M.; Hamasaki, Y.; Murakami-Nakai, C.; Kuriyama, I.; Takeuchi, T.; Sugawara, F.; Yoshida, H. Structural analysis of isosteviol and related compounds as DNA polymerase and DNA topoisomerase inhibitors. *Life Sci.* **2005**, *77*, 2127–2140. [CrossRef]
173. Melis, M. Effects of chronic administration of *Stevia rebaudiana* on fertility in rats. *J. Ethnopharmacol.* **1999**, *67*, 157–161. [CrossRef]
174. Aze, Y.; Toyoda, K.; Imaida, K.; Hayashi, S.; Imazawa, T.; Hayashi, Y.; Takahashi, M. Subchronic oral toxicity study of stevioside in F344 rats. *Eisei Shikenjo Hokoku* **1991**, *109*, 48–54.
175. Saenphet, K.; Aritajat, S.; Saenphet, S.; Manosroi, J.; Manosroi, A. Safety evaluation of aqueous extracts from Aegle marmelos and Stevia rebaudiana on reproduction of female rats. *Southeast Asian J. Trop. Med. Public Health* **2006**, *37*, 203–205. [PubMed]
176. Geuns, J.M. Safety evaluation of Stevia and stevioside. In *Studies in Natural Products Chemistry (Part H)*, 1st ed.; Elsevier Science: Amsterdam, The Netherlands, 2002; pp. 299–319.
177. Barriocanal, L.A.; Palacios, M.; Benitez, G.; Benitez, S.; Jimenez, J.T.; Jimenez, N.; Rojas, V. Apparent lack of pharmacological effect of steviol glycosides used as sweeteners in humans. A pilot study of repeated exposures in some normotensive and hypotensive individuals and in Type 1 and Type 2 diabetics. *Regul. Toxicol. Pharm.* **2008**, *51*, 37–41. [CrossRef] [PubMed]
178. Abbas Momtazi-Borojeni, A.; Esmaeili, S.A.; Abdollahi, E.; Sahebkar, A. A review on the pharmacology and toxicology of steviol glycosides extracted from *Stevia rebaudiana*. *Curr. Pharm. Des.* **2017**, *23*, 1616–1622. [CrossRef] [PubMed]
179. Ahmad, J.; Khan, I.; Blundell, R.; Azzopardi, J.; Mahomoodally, M.F. *Stevia rebaudiana* Bertoni.: An updated review of its health benefits, industrial applications and safety. *Trends Food Sci. Technol.* **2020**, *100*, 177–189. [CrossRef]
180. Zhang, Q.; Yang, H.; Li, Y.; Liu, H.; Jia, X. Toxicological evaluation of ethanolic extract from *Stevia rebaudiana* Bertoni leaves: Genotoxicity and subchronic oral toxicity. *Regul. Toxicol. Pharm.* **2017**, *86*, 253–259. [CrossRef]
181. Barclay, A.; Sandall, P.; Shwide-Slavin, C. *The Ultimate Guide to Sugars and Sweeteners: Discover the Taste, Use, Nutrition, Science, and Lore of Everything from Agave Nectar to Xylitol*, 1st ed.; The Experiment: New York, NY, USA, 2014; pp. 209–249.
182. Roohbakhsh, A.; Iranshahy, M.; Iranshahi, M. Glycyrrhetinic acid and its derivatives: Anti-cancer and cancer chemopreventive properties, mechanisms of action and structure-cytotoxic activity relationship. *Curr. Med. Chem.* **2016**, *23*, 498–517. [CrossRef]

183. Kim, Y.S.; Kim, J.J.; Cho, K.H.; Jung, W.S.; Moon, S.K.; Park, E.K.; Kim, D.H. Biotransformation of ginsenoside Rb1, crocin, amygdalin, geniposide, puerarin, ginsenoside Re, hesperidin, poncirin, glycyrrhizin, and baicalin by human fecal microflora and its relation to cytotoxicity against tumor cells. *J. Microbiol. Biotechnol.* **2008**, *18*, 1109–1114.
184. Yu, K.; Chen, F.; Li, C. Absorption, disposition, and pharmacokinetics of saponins from Chinese medicinal herbs: What do we know and what do we need to know more? *Curr. Drug Metab.* **2012**, *13*, 577–598. [CrossRef]
185. Kim, D.H.; Hong, S.W.; Kim, B.T.; Bae, E.A.; Park, H.Y.; Han, M.J. Biotransformation of glycyrrhizin by human intestinal bacteria and its relation to biological activities. *Arch. Pharm. Res.* **2000**, *23*, 172–177. [CrossRef]
186. Yim, J.S.; Kim, Y.S.; Moon, S.K.; Bae, H.S.; Kim, J.J.; Park, E.K.; Dim, D.H. Metabolic activities of ginsenoside Rb1, baicalin, glycyrrhizin and geniposide to their bioactive compounds by human intestinal microflora. *Biol. Pharm. Bull.* **2004**, *10*, 1580–1583. [CrossRef]
187. Kinghorn, D.A.; Kaneda, N.; Baek, N.; Kennelly, E.J. Noncariogenic intense natural sweeteners. *Med. Res. Rev.* **1998**, *18*, 347–360. [CrossRef]
188. Hsu, H.W.; Vavak, D.L.; Satterlee, L.D.; Miller, G.A. A multienzyme technique for estimating protein digestibility. *J. Food Sci.* **1977**, *42*, 1269–1273. [CrossRef]
189. WHO Expert Committee on Food Additives, & World Health Organization (JECFA). *Evaluation of Certain Food Additives and Contaminants: Twenty-Ninth Report of the Joint FAO*; World Health Organization: Geneva, Switzerland, 1986.
190. Higginbotham, J.; Snodin, D.; Eaton, K.; Daniel, J. Safety evaluation of thaumatin (talin protein). *Food Chem. Toxicol.* **1983**, *21*, 815–823. [CrossRef]
191. Zemanek, E.C.; Wasserman, B.P. Issues and advances in the use of transgenic organisms for the production of thaumatin, the intensely sweet protein from *Thaumatococcus daniellii*. *Crit. Rev. Food Sci. Nutr.* **1995**, *35*, 455–466. [CrossRef] [PubMed]
192. EFSA–The Panel on Additives and Products or Substances used in Animal Feed. Scientific opinion on the safety and efficacy of thaumatin for all animal species. *EFSA J.* **2011**, *9*, 2354–2363.

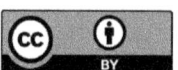

© 2020 by the authors. Licensee MDPI, Basel, Switzerland. This article is an open access article distributed under the terms and conditions of the Creative Commons Attribution (CC BY) license (http://creativecommons.org/licenses/by/4.0/).

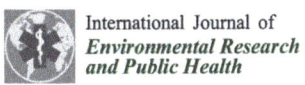

Review

Microbial Biofilms in the Food Industry—A Comprehensive Review

Conrado Carrascosa [1,*], Dele Raheem [2], Fernando Ramos [3,4], Ariana Saraiva [1] and António Raposo [5,*]

1 Department of Animal Pathology and Production, Bromatology and Food Technology, Faculty of Veterinary, Universidad de Las Palmas de Gran Canaria, Trasmontaña s/n, 35413 Arucas, Spain; ariana_23@outlook.pt
2 Northern Institute for Environmental and Minority Law (NIEM), Arctic Centre, University of Lapland, 96101 Rovaniemi, Finland; braheem@ulapland.fi
3 Pharmacy Faculty, University of Coimbra, Azinhaga de Santa Comba, 3000-548 Coimbra, Portugal; framos@ff.uc.pt
4 REQUIMTE/LAQV, R. D. Manuel II, Apartado 55142 Oporto, Portugal
5 CBIOS (Research Center for Biosciences and Health Technologies), Universidade Lusófona de Humanidades e Tecnologias, Campo Grande 376, 1749-024 Lisboa, Portugal
* Correspondence: conrado.carrascosa@ulpgc.es (C.C.); antonio.raposo@ulusofona.pt (A.R.)

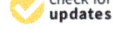

Citation: Carrascosa, C.; Raheem, D.; Ramos, F.; Saraiva, A.; Raposo, A. Microbial Biofilms in the Food Industry—A Comprehensive Review. *Int. J. Environ. Res. Public Health* **2021**, *18*, 2014. https://doi.org/10.3390/ijerph18042014

Academic Editor: Paul B. Tchounwou

Received: 26 December 2020
Accepted: 7 February 2021
Published: 19 February 2021

Publisher's Note: MDPI stays neutral with regard to jurisdictional claims in published maps and institutional affiliations.

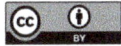

Copyright: © 2021 by the authors. Licensee MDPI, Basel, Switzerland. This article is an open access article distributed under the terms and conditions of the Creative Commons Attribution (CC BY) license (https://creativecommons.org/licenses/by/4.0/).

Abstract: Biofilms, present as microorganisms and surviving on surfaces, can increase food cross-contamination, leading to changes in the food industry's cleaning and disinfection dynamics. Biofilm is an association of microorganisms that is irreversibly linked with a surface, contained in an extracellular polymeric substance matrix, which poses a formidable challenge for food industries. To avoid biofilms from forming, and to eliminate them from reversible attachment and irreversible stages, where attached microorganisms improve surface adhesion, a strong disinfectant is required to eliminate bacterial attachments. This review paper tackles biofilm problems from all perspectives, including biofilm-forming pathogens in the food industry, disinfectant resistance of biofilm, and identification methods. As biofilms are largely responsible for food spoilage and outbreaks, they are also considered responsible for damage to food processing equipment. Hence the need to gain good knowledge about all of the factors favouring their development or growth, such as the attachment surface, food matrix components, environmental conditions, the bacterial cells involved, and electrostatic charging of surfaces. Overall, this review study shows the real threat of biofilms in the food industry due to the resistance of disinfectants and the mechanisms developed for their survival, including the intercellular signalling system, the cyclic nucleotide second messenger, and biofilm-associated proteins.

Keywords: biofilms; food industry; food microbiology; food safety

1. Introduction

Typically, bacteria bind to surfaces and form spatially structured communities inside a self-produced matrix, which consist of extracellular polymeric substances (EPS) known as biofilms [1,2]. Biofilms imply major challenges for the food industry because they allow bacteria to bind to a range of surfaces, including rubber, polypropylene, plastic, glass, stainless steel, and even food products, within just a few minutes, which is followed by mature biofilms developing within a few days (or even hours) [3].

Since ancient times, this sessile life form has been followed as an excellent survival technique for microorganisms, given the protective barrier generated and physiological changes made by the biofilm matrix, while it fights against the adverse environmental circumstances faced typically by bacteria in man-made and natural settings, even in food-processing facilities [4,5]. Hence, biofilms are believed responsible for damaged equipment, more expensive energy costs, outbreaks, and food spoilage [5–8]. Biofilms have become more robust to disinfections in many wide-ranging food industries, such as processing seafood, brewing, dairy processing, and meat and poultry processing [9] There is compelling evidence for biofilm lifestyle making them more resilient to antimicrobial agents, particularly compared to planktonic cells (Figures 1 and 2). This entails having to remove them from surfaces of food processing plants, which poses a massive task [10–12].

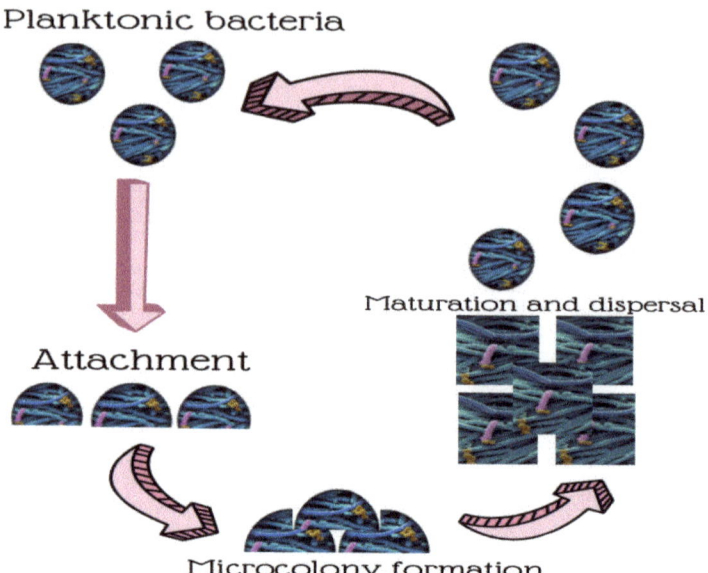

Figure 1. Biofilm formation and development stages.

Microbiological surface management is relevant for assessing and making decisions as to whether residual microbial species are found at a suitable level, and if harmful microorganisms are removed. The obtained results will allow criteria to be set, such as how to clean surfaces and food product quality [13,14].

Sensory tests that involve visually inspecting surfaces with good lighting, smelling unpleasant odours, and feeling encrusted or greasy surfaces are run as a process regulation to instantly overcome visible sanitation defects, while microbiological evaluations are often made to guarantee consistency with microbial standards and to make improvements to sanitation procedures [15]. The fact that visual inspection cannot coincide with bacterial counts has been well-documented [16]. The hygienic conditions of food-contact surfaces must be properly examined for all of the above-cited purposes. Lack of convergence between the various approaches followed to detect and quantify biofilms does, however, make it more difficult for the food industry to locate the most effective ones [17]. The Hazard Analysis and Critical Control Points (HACCP) system and good manufacturing practices have been developed to regulate food safety and quality. Bacterial biofilms are not directly mentioned in the HACCP system employed on food processing facilities. Hence, an updated HACCP system that contemplates evaluating biofilms in food environments, and establishes an apt sanitation plan, is expected to provide much clearer contamination information, and to facilitate production in the food industry's biofilm-free processing systems [18]. The importance and impact of biofilms on the food industry have become clear in several works where the cross-contamination is common among these food products, with a wide range of pathogens, including *Listeria monocytogenes*, *Yersinia enterocolitica*, *Campylobacter jejuni*, *Salmonella* spp., *Staphylococcus* spp., *Bacillus cereus*, and *Echerichia coli* O157:H7 [19].

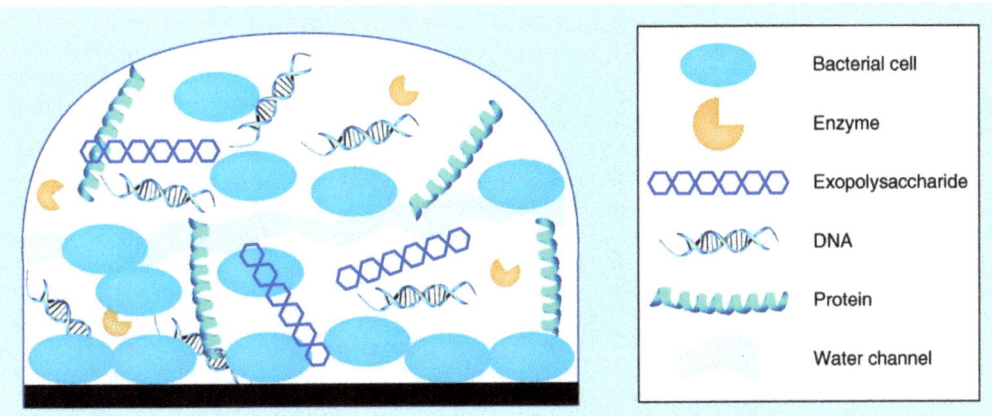

Figure 2. Biofilm structure in the growth and maturation stages [20].

The main objectives of this review were to identify the most important biofilm examples in the food industry and to present methods to visualise in situ biofilm production, how to avoid this production, and methods to remove biofilms. This study focused on the microbial biofilms that affect the food industry and provides an overview of their importance in cross-contamination when food comes into contact with surfaces. Although going into detail in each discipline, specific to microbiology for biofilm isolation and identification, is not the object of this work, it contributes new knowledge about techniques to control and eradicate biofilms in the food industry from food safety and quality perspectives.

2. Biofilm Development in Food Processing Environments

Modern food processing lines are a suitable environment for biofilms to form on food contact surfaces, primarily due to manufacturing plants' complexity, long production periods, mass product generation, and large biofilm growth areas [21]. Many food-borne bacteria may, therefore, bind to the contact surfaces present in these areas, which could contribute to increase the risk of bacterial food-borne diseases. By way of example, 80% of bacterial infections in the USA are believed to be related specifically to food-borne pathogens in biofilms [9].

Mixed-species biofilm production is extremely dynamic and depends on the attachment surface's characteristics [22], food matrix components [23], environmental conditions [24], and involved bacterial cells [8,25].

Attachment surface properties, such as hydrophobicity, electrostatic charging, interface roughness, and topography impact biofilm formation and, thus, affect the overall hygiene status of the surface [22,26]. Nevertheless, the precise consequence of some parameters vastly varies under specific laboratory conditions. Some experiments have revealed that bacterial attachment is more likely to happen on rougher surfaces [22,27], while others have found no association between roughness and bacterial attachment [28]. Hydrophobic surfaces tend to attract more bacteria, but studies that have tested the hydrophobicity effect present opposing results [29,30], and other experiments indicate that hydrophilic surfaces enable more bacterial adherence than hydrophobic equivalents [27,28]. The fact that clear results are lacking might lie in the various methods and bacterial strains employed, and in overall attachment likely being established for several reasons. The most popular food contact material in the food industry is stainless steel type 304 because it is chemically inert, easy to clean, and extremely corrosion-resistant at a range of processing temperatures. Given its continuous usage, this material's topography typically displays crevices and cracks that protect bacteria from sanitising treatments and mechanical cleaning methods.

The food matrix components in food processing environments also influence bacterial attachment [31]; e.g., food waste, such as milk and meat exudates enriched in fats, proteins, and carbohydrates, facilitate microorganism growth and multiplication, and favour dual-species biofilm development by *E. Coli* and *Staphylococcus aureus* [32]. Milk lactose improves biofilm production by both *Bacillus subtilis*, by activating the LuxS-mediated quorum-sensing system [33], and *S. aureus* through intercellular polysaccharide adhesion development [34]. Improved biofilm production by *Geobacillus* spp. in milk results in high concentrations of free Ca^{2+} and Mg^{2+} [35].

Microbial cell properties, especially hydrophobicity, cellular membrane components (e.g., protein and lipopolysaccharide), appendages (e.g., pili, flagella, fimbriae) and bacteria-secreted EPS, also play a key role in stimulating biofilm production [22]. Fluctuations in biofilm-forming capability among species or strains of different genotypes and serotypes have been identified, which reveals the evolution of enhanced biofilm formation from various genetic backgrounds [8,36]. Similar species can also impact one another in a mixed microbial community, which culminates in the co-colonisation of certain species.

3. Examples of the Most Relevant Biofilms in the Food Industry

In the food industry, biofilm-forming species appear in factory environments and can be pathogenic to humans because they develop biofilm structures. The processing environments of the food industry, e.g., wood, glass, stainless steel, polyethylene, rubber, polypropylene, etc., act as artificial substrates for these pathogens [37,38]. The characteristics of the bacterial growth form on food in a processing environment involve different behaviours when considering cleaning and disinfection processes. Controlling biofilm formations in the food industry can prove difficult when having to decide the right strategy.

Examples of these relevant biofilm-forming pathogens for the food industry are briefly described in Table 1.

3.1. Bacillus Cereus

Bacillus cereus is a Gram-positive anaerobic or facultative anaerobic spore-forming bacterium that can grow in various environments at wide-ranging temperatures (4 °C–50 °C). It is resistant to chemicals, heat treatment, and radiation [39]. *B. cereus* is a frequently isolated soil inhabitant from food and food products, such as rice, dairy products, vegetables and meat. It secretes toxins that can cause sickness and diarrhoea symptoms in humans.

B. cereus is responsible for biofilm formation on food contact surfaces, such as stainless steel pipes, conveyor belts and storage tanks. It can also form floating or immersed biofilms, which can secrete a vast array of bacteriocins, metabolites, surfactants, as well as enzymes, such as proteases and lipases, in biofilms, which can affect food sensorial qualities [40]. Motility by bacterial flagella confers access to suitable biofilm formation surfaces, and is required for biofilms to spread on non-colonised surfaces. However, *B. cereus* flagella have not been found to be directly involved in adhesion to glass surfaces, but can play a key role in biofilm formation via their motility [55].

3.2. Campylobacter Jejuni

Campylobacter spp., mainly *C. jejuni*, are Gram-negative spiral, rod-shaped, or curved thermophilic and bipolar flagellated motile bacteria [41]. *C. jejuni*, also known as an anaerobic bacterium, can develop biofilms under both microaerophilic (5% O_2 and 10% CO_2) and aerobic (20% O_2) conditions [56]. Despite it being a fastidious organism, *C. jejuni* can survive outside the avian intestinal tract before it reaches a human host. A range of environmental elements initiates the formation of biofilms, which are then affected by a set of intrinsic factors [57]. The European Union One Health 2018 Zoonoses Report classifies *C. jejuni* as an opportunistic pathogen that is believed to be the causative agent of most bacterial gastroenteritis cases, and has been regarded as a common commensal of food animals and poultry, with turkeys and hens in particular [42]. When the preparation and processing areas of food products or water become contaminated, such as unpasteurised milk, *C. jejuni* reaches the human host by infecting and colonising the gastrointestinal tract to cause disease [43].

Table 1. Biofilm-forming pathogens in the food industry.

Pathogen	Characteristics	Contaminated Food	Examples of Harmful Spoilage Effects	References
Bacillus cereus	Gram-positive, spore-forming, anaerobic, facultative anaerobic	dairy products, rice, vegetables, meat	diarrhoea and vomiting symptoms	[39,40]
Campylobacter jejuni	Gram-negative, aerobic and anaerobic	animals, poultry, unpasteurised milk	bloody diarrhoea, fever, stomach cramp, nausea and vomiting	[41–43]
Escherichia coli	Gram-negative, rod-shaped	raw milk, fresh meat, fruits and vegetables	diarrhoea outbreaks and haemolytic uremic syndrome	[44]
Listeria monocytogenes	Gram-positive, rod-shaped, facultative anaerobic	dairy products, meat, ready-to-eat products, fruit, soft cheeses, ice cream, unpasteurised milk, candied apples, frozen vegetables, poultry	listeriosis in the elderly, pregnant women and immune-compromised patients	[45,46]
Salmonella Enterica	Gram-negative, rod-shaped, flagellate, facultative aerobic	Poultry meat, bovine, ovine, porcine, fish	can cause gastroenteritis or septicaemia	[47,48]
Staphylococcus aureus	Gram-positive, non-spore forming, non-motile, facultative anaerobic	meat products, poultry, egg products, dairy products, salads, bakery products, especially cream-filled pastries and cakes, and sandwich fillings	methicillin resistance, can cause vomiting and diarrhoea	[49,50]
Pseudomonas spp.	psychrotrophic, motile, Gram-negative rod-shaped	fruits, vegetables, meat surfaces and low-acid dairy products	produces blue discolouration on fresh cheese.	[17]
Geobacillus stearothermophilus	thermophilic, Gram-positive, spore-forming, aerobic or facultative anaerobic	dried dairy products	production of acids or enzymes leading to off-flavours	[51,52]
Anoxybacillus flavithermus	thermophilic organism, Gram-positive, spore-forming, facultatively anaerobic, non-pathogenic	dried milk powder	an indicator of poor hygiene	[53,54]
Pectinatus spp.	Gram-negative, non-spore-forming, anaerobic	beer and brewery environment	rapid cell growth makes beer turbid and smells like rotten eggs due to production of sulphur compounds	[23]

3.3. Enterohaemorrhagic Escherichia coli (EHEC)

Escherichia coli is a Gram-negative and rod-shaped bacterium. Most *E. coli* strains form part of human intestinal microbiota and pose no health problem. However, the virulence types of *E. coli* include enterotoxigenic (ETEC), enteroinvasive (EIEC), enteropathogenic (EPEC), and Vero cytotoxigenic (VTEC). O157:H7 EHEC is the most frequent serotype associated with EHEC infections in humans in the USA [58]. Widespread *E. coli* dissemination in natural environments is, to a great extent, due to its ability to grow as a biofilm. It is worth considering that several *E. coli* strains may cause disease in humans, and that Enterohaemorrhagic *E. coli* (EHEC) strains are the most relevant for the food industry. EHEC serotype O157:H7 is the human pathogen responsible for bloody diarrhoea outbreaks and haemolytic uremic syndrome (HUS) worldwide. They can be transmitted by raw milk, drinking water or fresh meat, fruit, and vegetables; e.g., melons, tomatoes, parsley, coriander, spinach, lettuce, etc. [44].

E. coli can employ pili, flagella and membrane proteins to initiate attachment to inanimate surfaces when flagella are lost after attachment and bacteria start producing an extracellular polymeric substance (EPS) that helps to confer bacteria better resistance to disinfectants [59]. There are reports indicating that although EHEC can form biofilms on different food industry surfaces, neither an effective means to prevent EHEC biofilm formation nor an effective treatment for its infections exists because antibiotic treatment tends to increase the risk of haemolytic-uremic syndrome and kidney failure [60].

3.4. Listeria Monocytogenes

Listeria monocytogenes is a Gram-positive bacterium and a ubiquitous food-borne pathogen that can appear in soil, food, and water. Its ingestion can result in abortions in pregnant women, and other serious complications in the elderly and children. The pathogen can be transmitted to several food types, such as dairy products, seafood, meat, fruit, ready-to-eat meals, ice cream, soft cheeses, unpasteurised milk, frozen vegetables, candied apples, and poultry [45,46], but it is not known to be resistant to pasteurisation treatments [61]. The pathogen proliferates at low temperature, and is able to form pure culture biofilms or grow in multispecies biofilms [62]. *L. monocytogenes* can survive under acidic conditions for lengthy periods and can form biofilms that grow without oxygen. Its numbers are likely to rise or lower in biofilms depending on the competing microbes present [63].

Given the presence of pili, flagella and membrane proteins, prevalent *L. monocytogenes* strains possess good adhesion ability in food processing environments [64].

3.5. Salmonella Enterica

Salmonella enterica is a Gram-negative, rod-shaped, flagellate and facultative aerobic bacterium, and a species of the genus *Salmonella* [65].

It can cause gastroenteritis or septicaemia (in some serovars) [66]. *Salmonella* spp. express proteinaceous extracellular fibres known as curli, which are involved in surface and cell-cell contacts, and in promoting community behaviour and host colonisation [67]. Besides curli, different fimbrial adhesins have been identified with biofilm formation implications that are serotype-dependent [40]. *S. enterica* serovar Enteritidis is the most frequent serotype to cause fever, vomiting, nausea diarrhoea, and abdominal pain as main symptoms [47]. Poultry meat is a frequent reservoir for these bacteria in processed food, whose importance as a food pathogen has been demonstrated by the fact that *S. enterica* biofilm formation on food surfaces was the first reported case in 1966 to possess complex multicellular structures [48].

When contaminating a food pipeline biofilm, *S. enterica* may cause massive outbreaks, and even death in infants and the elderly. It can grow on stainless steel surfaces to form a three-dimensional (3D) structure with several call layers of different morphologies depending on available nutrients, such as the reticular shaped ones generated when cultured on tryptic soy broth (TSB) medium [68].

3.6. Staphylococcus Aureus

Staphylococcus aureus is a Gram-positive, non-spore-forming, non-motile, facultative anaerobic bacterium capable of producing enterotoxins from 10–46 °C. *S. aureus* can multiply on the skin and mucous membranes of food handlers, and can become a major issue in food factories [49]. These enterotoxins are heat-stable and can be secreted during *S.*

aureus growth in foods contaminated by food handlers. The bacterium grows well in high salt- or sugar-content foods with little water activity. The foods frequently implicated in Staphylococcal food-borne disease are meat and meat products, poultry and egg products, milk and dairy products, bakery products, salads, and particularly cream-filled cakes and pastries and sandwich fillings [50]. *S. aureus* is known for its numerous enteric toxins. These enterotoxins bind to class II MHC (major histocompatibility complex) in T-cells, which results in their activation that can lead to acute toxic shock with sickness and diarrhoea [69].

3.7. Pseudomonas spp.

Pseudomonas is a heterotrophic, motile, Gram-negative rod-shaped bacterium. Pseudomonads are generally ubiquitous psychrotrophic spoilage organisms that are often found in food processing environments, including floors and drains, and also on fruit, vegetables, and meat surfaces, and in low-acid dairy products [17,62]. The extracellular filamentous appendages produced by motile microorganisms result in both the attachment process and the interaction with surfaces in different ways. Flagella and pili have been thoroughly studied [70].

When biofilms develop and their regulation by quorum sensing is considered, *Pseudomonas aeruginosa* can be taken as a model organism [71], which is about 1–5 µm long and 0.5–1.0 µm wide. A facultative aerobe grows via aerobic and anaerobic respiration with nitrate as the terminal electron acceptor [71].

Pseudomonas spp. produce huge amounts of EPS and are known to attach and form biofilms on stainless steel surfaces. They can co-exist with other pathogens in biofilms to form multispecies biofilms, which make them more resistant and stable [62]. These biofilms can be accompanied by a distinct blue discolouration (pyocyanin) on fresh cheese produced by *P. fluorescens* [72].

3.8. Geobacillus stearothermophilus

Geobacillus stearothermophilus is a Gram-positive, thermophilic, aerobic, or facultative anaerobic bacterium [73]. Thermophiles, such as *G. Stearothermophilus*, formerly known as *Bacillus stearothermophilus*, can attach to stainless steel surfaces on processing lines in evaporators and plate heat exchangers, which allows them to grow and produce biofilms, which implies the potential release of single cells or aggregates of cells into the final dry product [74]. *B. stearothermophilus* are able to form biofilms on clean stainless steel surfaces and to release bacteria into milk during dairy industry processing [75]. The above-cited authors observed that the conditions for a biofilm in a laminar flow milk system were more adequate for the growth of spore-forming bacteria, which are thermophilic. Their growth as a culture medium in milk is quite difficult [75].

3.9. Anoxybacillus flavithermus

Anoxybacillus flavithermus is another Gram-positive, thermophilic, and spore-forming organism that is facultatively anaerobic and non-pathogenic [76]. *A. flavithermus* is a potential contaminant of dairy products, and poses a problem for the milk powder processing industry, as high levels will reduce milk powder acceptability for both local and international markets [77]. *A. flavithermus* spores are very heat-resistant and their vegetative cells can grow at temperatures up to 65 °C with a significant increase in bacterial adhesion on stainless steel surfaces in the presence of skimmed milk. This indicates that milk positively influences these species' biofilm formation [78]. In the dairy industry, the commonest biofilm-forming isolates are thermophilic genera [79]. In many parts of the world, *A. flavithermus* and *G. stearothermophilus* are regarded as the most dominant thermophilic microbial contaminants of milk powders [78].

3.10. Pectinatus spp.

Pectinatus is Gram-negative, non-spore-forming, and anaerobic bacteria that have been linked with a high concentration of biofilms in breweries due to sanitation problems [80].

Spoilage bacteria were first isolated from a brewery in the USA in unpasteurised beer stored at 30 °C [81]. *P. cerevisiiphilus* have also been isolated from many breweries in Germany, Spain, Norway, Japan, the Netherlands, Sweden, and France [80].

3.11. Synergistic Pathogens

A combination of several pathogens can synergistically interact to form biofilms in the food industry. In food-processing environments, bacteria are able to exist as multispecies biofilms, from where both spoilage and pathogenic bacteria can contaminate food [82]. For instance in the fishing industry, fresh fish products can suffer from biofilm formation by mixed pathogenic species (*Aeromonas hydrophila*, *L. monocytogenes*, *S. enterica*, or *Vibrio* spp.), which can imply significant health and economic issues [83]. Synergistic interactions have been observed in a fresh-cut produce processing plant, where *E. coli* interacted with *Burkholderia caryophylli* and *Ralstonia insidiosa* to form mixed biofilms. Acylhomoserine lactones (AHLs) can control biofilm formation in synergistic interactions among mixed species. Interference of AHLs is manifested by AHL lactonases and acylases, both of which are present in Gram-positive and Gram-negative bacteria [60].

Bacteria use quorum sensing to coordinate biofilm production and dispersion, when bacteria attach to a biotic or abiotic surface, and cell-to-cell attachment engages in communication via a quorum sensing (QS)-based extracellular cell signalling system [84]. The importance of cell signalling for bacterial biofilm formation has been further confirmed by the control of exopolysaccharide synthesis by quorum-sensing signals, as in *Vibrio cholera* [85].

Synergistic pathogens are found in several works, where biofilm levels of the four-species consortia have been further examined and compared to the biofilm production levels of each isolate under monospecies conditions. They have revealed that *P. aeruginosa* and *A. junii* isolated from different samples to contribute as best biofilm producers, including poor or non-biofilm-producing isolates, which increases the overall biofilm formation in the included consortia [86]. Several authors [87] have found positive synergistics in other studies by investigating mixed species of biofilms, such as *Candida albicans*.

In food industries, biofilm-related effects (pathogenicity, corrosion of metal surfaces, and alteration to organoleptic properties due to the secretion of proteases or lipases) are critically important. For example, in the dairy industry several processes and structures (pipelines, raw milk tanks, butter centrifuges, pasteurisers, cheese tanks, packing tools) can act as surface substrates for biofilm formation at different temperatures and involve several mixed colonising species. Thus, it is essential that accurate methods to visualise biofilms in situ be set up to avoid contamination and to ensure food safety in the food industry.

4. Biofilm Control and Elimination

It is well-known that biofilm bacteria present a distinct phenotype with a genotype as regards gene transcription and growth rates under very particular conditions that differ from planktonic conditions [88]. Biofilms are capable of adhering to a very wide diversity of surfaces with distinct biotic and abiotic compositions, including human tissue and medical devices. Once biofilms form, they are a major threat because they cause infectious diseases and economic loss. In the 1940s, several authors produced further research works into biofilm evolution and surface relations for marine microorganisms [89] and seawater [90]. Nevertheless, marked progress has been made given the incorporation of the electron microscope, which allows high-resolution photomicroscopy at much higher magnifications than light microscopy [85]. Indeed, the most revealing discovery of the relation with biofilm elimination was a description of its structure, the surrounding matrix material, and the cells enclosed in these biofilms were polysaccharides, as by special stains revealed [85]. Doubtlessly, disinfectants have proven more efficient in fighting against biofilms since 1973, while Characklis (1973) [91] showed marked persistence and resistance to disinfectants, such as chlorine.

4.1. Biofilm Elimination in the Food Industry

Biofilm formation has been investigated in food industry and hospital environments. Perhaps, in the research conducted, hospitals, to eliminate biofilms, have been more successful, thanks to the easier applications and special surface compositions (antibiofilm activity) in medical surroundings, such as implants, prostheses, tools, and surfaces for operating theatres.

To date, many efforts have been made to reduce biofilm formation on food industry surfaces, but those works were based mainly on new disinfectants with different efficacies. These results have improved in line with specific mechanisms for initial surface attachment, developing a group structure and ecosystem, and detachments [75] with dissimilar results.

Nowadays, disinfectants are the best ally to eliminate biofilms. However, other research fields, such as the composition of surfaces for materials to prevent bacterial adhesion and developing phages to combat biofilm-forming bacteria, have obtained favourable results. Doubtlessly, most research works have focused on the bacteriological biofilm, without discussing the hypothesis of filamentous fungi being responsible for biofilm formation. Several authors [92,93] support this theory, where the presence of Aspergillus fumigatus has been presented as biofilm-responsible. In this case, the marked similitude of bacteriological and filamentous fungi biofilms is based on morphological changes, the presence of an extracellular polymeric matrix, differential gene expression, and distinct sensitivity to antifungal drugs compared to diffuse or loosely associated (planktonic) colonies [94,95].

Before we go on to explain several factors that could influence bacterial adhesion and biofilm formation, we should bear the food industry's hygiene design in mind. In order to prevent microorganisms entering food production, factories, and the employed hygienic equipment should be designed to limit microorganisms from accessing. Aseptic equipment must be isolated from microorganisms and foreign particulates. To prevent microorganism growth, equipment should be designed to prevent any areas where microorganisms can harbour and grow, along with gaps, crevices, and dead areas. This is also important during production, when microorganisms can grow very quickly under favourable conditions [96].

According to such premises, food companies have the capacity to apply innovation to design the industry and its equipment. In both the USA and the European Union (EU), the trend in regulations in this field is not so much command and control by government regulators, but lies more in self-determination by the food industry. In particular, hazard analysis and critical control points (HACCP) systems provide the skills to replace detailed regulatory requirements with the overall goals to be fulfilled [97]. The Food and Drug Administration (FDA) and the United States Department of Agriculture (USDA) Food Safety Inspection Service (FSIS) share primary responsibility for regulating food safety in the USA. One example is the recommendation for equipment and process controls: "Seams on food-contact surfaces shall be smoothly bonded or maintained to reduce accumulation of food particles, dirt, and organic matter and thus minimise the opportunity for growth of microorganisms" [85].

European Union (EU) statutory instruments include EC regulation no. 852/2004 (Hygiene of Foodstuffs) and EC regulation no. 853/2004 (Specific Rules Food of Animal Origin), which expect food manufacturers to control food safety risks by HACCP systems.

In short, the performance of a cleaning and disinfection programme (CDP) to avoid biofilm formation should start by aptly designing the hygiene of equipment, surfaces, and devices. Today the CDP is a proven effective measure in fighting against biofilms.

4.2. Factors Associated with Bacteria

Several factors associated with surfaces or bacteria can influence adhesion from the planktonic phase and biofilm evolution, such as:

Surfaces:

- Surface charge: the adhesion sequence can be influenced by the particle surface charge in combination with the electrode's surface charge.

- Hydrophobicity: adsorption of surface-active organics influences the surface's hydrophobic or hydrophilic character, and changes surface tension [98].
- Temperature: temperature and contact time impact the bacterial adhesion and biofilm formation process, and increasing the formulation of mathematical models is necessary to assess how both factors and their interactions influence the process [99].
- Presence of substrates: adsorption of electrolyte components and the particle surface are equally important. Adsorption of surface-active organics impacts the surface's hydrophobic or hydrophilic character, and also changes surface tension [98].

Bacterial cellular surface components:
Hydrophobic interactions tend to increase with the enhanced non-polar nature of one involved surface or more, and most bacteria are negatively charged [85]. This means that the cell surface's hydrophobicity is a relevant factor during adhesion.

- Fimbria, pili, and flagella: fimbriae, non-flagellar appendages other than those implicated in the transfer of viral or bacterial nucleic acids (known as pili) are responsible for cell surface hydrophobicity. Most investigated fimbriae contain a high proportion of hydrophobic amino acid residues [100]. Fimbriae include adhesins that attach to some sort of substratum so that bacteria can withstand shear forces and obtain nutrients. Therefore, fimbriae play a role in cell surface hydrophobicity and attachment, presumably by overcoming the initial electrostatic repulsion barrier between the cell and the substratum [101].

Studies' responses surface methods are used to not only develop and optimise models for food processing systems and operations, but also to better elucidate bacterial adhesion and biofilm formation processes. The response surface method provides valuable information to help decision making about disinfection and cleaning procedures for the utensils, equipment and containers employed in the food industry [102]. Hence, surfaces and materials of equipment, plus floors and walls, also impact biofilms, along with dead spaces, crevices, porous and rough material surfaces, which must be eliminated to avoid biofilm formation [12].

The most adopted strategies for controlling biofilms are sanitation procedures that combine detergents and disinfectants. Alkaline detergent eliminates organic and inorganic acid detergent waste from surfaces, while disinfectants reduce spoilage microorganisms, and diminish or eliminate pathogens, to safe levels [12]. Enzymatic detergents have replaced traditional alkaline and acid detergents, because enzymes (proteases, lipases, amylases) can remove biofilms in the food industry [102] as enzymes reduce the physical integrity of PS by weakening the structural bonds of the lipids, proteins, and carbohydrates that form its structure [103]. Other advantages over detergents include low-toxicity and biodegradability, but application costs and requirements (temperature, time) are higher than detergents. This is why several detergent manufacturers have marketed a synergetic combination of enzymes, chelating agents, surfactants, and solvents.

4.3. Disinfectants and Biofilm Resistance

The most widely used disinfectants in the food industry's disinfection programmes are quaternary ammonium compounds (QAC), amphoteric compounds, hypochlorites, peroxides (peracetic acid and hydrogen peroxide) [15], aldehydes (formaldehyde, glutaraldehyde, paraformaldehyde), and phenolics. This product list remains unchanged after 18 years. Today, alkyl amines, chlorine dioxide and quaternary ammonium blends are incorporated into disinfection programmes. Besides these, alcohols, phenolic compounds, aldehydes, and chlorhexidine are also resorted to, but mostly in health services. In the food processing industry, disinfectants can remain on surfaces for longer due to microorganisms' prolonged exposure to the employed disinfectant, which improves their efficacy [104].

1. Sodium hypochlorite (NaOCl):

It is one of the most widespread disinfectants in the food industry despite its disadvantages and the growing use of new products on the market. Its desirable reaction produces both hypochlorous acid (HOCl) and the hypochlorite ion (-OCl), which are strong oxidising agents that eliminate cells given their ability to cross the cell membrane, and to oxidise the sulfhydryl groups of certain enzymes participating on the glycolytic pathway [97]. It has been described to react with wide-ranging biological molecules, such as proteins [105], amino acids [106], lipids [107], peptides [108], and DNA [109] under physiological pH conditions [110].

However, sodium hypochlorite may be affected by organic matter because free chlorine might react with natural organic matter and be converted into inorganic chloramines to generate trihalomethanes, by reducing antimicrobial activity against biofilms [111], and it is known to be less reactive than free chlorine. Peracetic acid is reported as being the most effective sanitiser against biofilms because it is a strong oxidising agent that does not interact with organic matter waste [112,113].

2. Quaternary ammonium:

QACs, such as benzalkonium chloride, cetrimide, didecyldimethylammonium chloride, and cetylpyridinium chloride, are cationic detergents (surfactants or surface-active agents). They reduce surface tension and form micelles to lead to dispersion in a liquid. This property is resourceful for removing microorganisms. They are membrane-active agents that interact with not only the cytoplasmic membrane of bacteria, but with the plasma membrane of yeast. Their hydrophobic activity also makes them effective against lipid-containing viruses. QACs interact with intracellular targets and bind to DNA [114]. However, their efficacy is still questioned given the appearance of relatively high resistance to *Listeria monocytogenes* (10%), *Staphylococcus* spp. (13%), and *Pseudomonas* spp. (30%), and lower resistance to lactic acid the bacteria (1.5%) and coliforms (1%) isolated from food and the food processing industry [115].

3. Peracetic acid:

In the last decade, peracetic acid (PAA) has been widely used by the food industry in water and wastewater treatment, even in paper machines [116], to control biofilms. Its antimicrobial effect is probably due to the oxidation of thiol groups in proteins, disruption of membranes [117], or damage to bases in DNA [118]. Its use has been shown to increase the sensitivity of bacterial spores to heat [119]. The efficacy and environmental safety of peracetic acid make it an attractive disinfecting agent for industrial use.

Bacterial regrowth after oxidant treatment (peracetic acid and free chlorine) depends on the absence or presence of organic matter. The oxidation-reduction (redox) potential of PAA (1.385 V vs. standard hydrogen electrode or standard hydrogen electrode (SHE) for the redox couple of $CH_3COOOH(aq)/(CH_3COO^-_{(aq)} + H_2O_{(l)}))$ comes close to that of free chlorine (1.288 V vs. SHE for the redox couple of $HOCl_{(aq)}/Cl^-_{(aq)}$) under biochemical standard state conditions (pH 7.0, 25 °C, 101.325 Pa) [120]. For this reason, acid peracetic and free chlorine may have similar efficiencies in preventing planktonic bacteria regrowth in the absence of organic matter. As PAA reacts with organic matter more slowly than free chlorine, its self-decomposition is slower [121].

Resistance to Disinfectants

Bacterial resistance to disinfectants in the planktonic phase can hardly be compared to biofilm resistance. Yet several studies have shown contrary results to widespread belief, such as the existence of wide interspecific variability of resistance to disinfectants. Gram-positive strains generally appear to better resist than Gram-negative strains. This resistance is also variable among strains of the same species [122].

Given the growing interest in knowing biofilm resistance to chlorine, quaternary ammonium and peracetic acid, many studies have been conducted [123]. The bacteria in mature biofilms are 10- to 1000-fold more resistant to antibiotics than the bacteria in the planktonic phase [124], and this resistance appears against biocides. However, this natural resistance is still unknown, and probably depends on many factors, mainly of structural biofilm barriers and genetic factors for adaptation. To explain this resistance, several authors [125] have suggested three possible causes by three hypotheses: the first is based on the slow or incomplete diffusion of antibiotics into inner biofilm layers. The second lies in the changes taking place in the biofilm microenvironment as some biofilm bacteria fall into a slow growth state due to lack of nutrients or given the accumulation of harmful metabolites and, therefore, survive [126]. Finally, the third hypothesis indicates a subpopulation of cells in the biofilm whose differentiation resembles the spore formation process. They have a unique and highly resistant phenotype to protect them from the effects of antibiotics, and are a biologically programmed response to the sessile life form of bacteria [127].

In addition, aquatic fauna is less affected by PAA than by chlorine [128]. Therefore, PAA is considered a green alternative to chlorine for disinfection purposes, and its disinfection performance is currently being investigated [120].

As previously mentioned, there are two very different situations for action against biofilm formation: the food industry and the health field. There is still a lot to do in both fields, but it is true that CDP is practically the only implementation in the food industry. The health field has witnessed much more progress: phages [129], aerosolisation [130], sonication brush [131], and metal ion solutions (silver, copper, platinum, gold, and palladium) [132].

In short, some authors [133] establish two strategies for fighting biofilms in the food industry: structural modification of surfaces or application of antibacterial or antibiofilm coatings [134]. Thus, several alternative products to classic disinfectants (chlorine, quaternary ammonium, etc.), such as, plant-derived antimicrobials (essential oils: orange-sorrel, lemon, lavender, chamomile, peppermint, oregano), with thymol and carvacrol being the compounds that display more significant antimicrobial action in shorter action times.

4.4. Alternative Methods to Eliminate Biofilms

Phages: bacteriophages are specific "viruses" of microbial cells that are specific to the different serotypes or strains of microbial species, and are obligate parasites with a genetic parasitism [135]. Bacteriophages inject their DNA and force the cell to produce the bacteriophage genome and structures (e.g., capsid and tail). When phages are complete, they lyse cells, which means that bacteriophage infection can destroy the entire colony [136,137]. In the last few years, the FDA/USA approved preparing bacteriophages (LISTEX P100) to combat the direct presence of *L. monocytogenes* in foods [138,139].

Aerosolisation: a disinfection method with different disinfectants applied to working areas by pulverisation. Several authors [138] have shown its efficacy as a biofilm control method in the food industry and hospitals by using hydrogen peroxide [140], sodium hypochlorite, and peracetic acid [141].

Knowledge about the resistance mechanisms associated with biofilm evolution could be primordial to develop new actions or strategies by biocides and antibiotics [142], such as modified wound dressings with phyto-nanostructured coatings to prevent staphylococcal and pseudomonal biofilm development [143].

Involving bacterial adherence: in recent years, new biochemistry methods have been studied to prevent biofilm formation. The most efficient strategy would interfere with bacterial adherence, as this first step is paramount in biofilm formation, performed by the direct blockage of surface receptors [144] or by a non-specific strategy, which normally involves compounds with anti-adherence properties [145]. Another biofilm inhibition form would be to impede communication processes between bacteria to enter the biofilm by employing different natural or artificially synthesised compounds [146]. One example of this is *P. aeruginosa*, which uses quorum sensing for modular biofilm evolution, and proposes that agents are capable of blocking quorum sensing (QS), and could be useful for avoiding biofilm formation [144].

The role of the QS in biofilms includes controlling the cell-to-cell communicating system in response to small diffusible signal molecules, such as N-acyl-homoserine lactones (AHLs), produced by Gram-negative bacteria [147]. It has been shown to play crucial roles in biofilm formation by activating the transcription of related genes [148]. Specifically, different AHLs have been detected in biofilm reactors and several bacterial species have been identified to possess the capacity to produce AHLs [149]. Thus, AHLs-based QS has been widely reported to regulate many microbial behaviours, including EPS expression, nitrogen transformation, organic pollutant degradation and microbial community construction [150].

Current advances in nanoscience nanotechnology and nanosensors [151] have emerged for applications to detect microorganisms and biofilms [152] with high sensitivity and good spatial resolution on nanoscale scopes [153]. Recent works have been published on imaging approaches of biofilm microprocesses [154], in-situ surface-enhanced Raman Scattering (SERS) analyses, biofilm visualisation [155] and biosensors of bacteria in foods [156]. The enormous advantages and great potential observed in bioassays based on multifunctional optical nanosensors are promising to continue with a view to ensure and promote food safety and quality. From the detection targets perspective, QS detection might become a new biofilm research trend based on evidence that biofilm formation can be inhibited by blocking QS [151].

5. Biofilm Identification Techniques and Methods to Visualise Biofilms In Situ

5.1. General Aspects of Biofilm Study Techniques

Doubtlessly, biofilms can pose a major challenge in both clinical microbiology and hygiene food areas. In the latter area, several authors consider them a real threat. Currently, methods aim to analyse biofilm formation and development, which have not yet been standardised. Different methods have been followed to qualitatively and quantitatively evaluate biofilms, and each one is useful for estimating one peculiar biofilm lifestyle aspect [157]. Nevertheless, research to identify and acquire knowledge of biofilms has allowed distinct techniques to be developed and adapted from microbiology or cell histology. It is essential to evaluate biofilm formation for a sensitive, specific and reproducible methodology for biofilm quantification to become available.

Different approaches classify the methods followed to detection biofilms on very distinct surfaces: (i) the simplest classification of methods is direct or indirect [17]. (ii) Rapid tests of hygienic control, and methods for microscopic, biomolecular, extracellular polymeric, physical, or chemical substances (EPS) are another possible classification [158]. (iii) A recent publication [159] only refers to the technology of the referred methods being classified as physics, physico-chemistry or chemistry, and recommends three effective approaches for testing biofilms: (a) observations by various microscopic methods with different view fields at the same point; (b) in-depth data analyses during microscopic image processing; (c) a combination study using atomic force microscopy (AFM) and chemical analysis. Perhaps this is the most advanced and appropriate methodology for biofilm analyses, where the detailed image of the surface will help to build a relation among the biofilm matrix, interactions and other factors like pH, surfaces [159]. However, there is another case in which bacterial species can help to reduce biofilms, where *Bacillus licheniformis* can express hydrolytic enzymes capable of reducing detrimental biofilms [160].

Therefore, depending on the set objectives, that is, what we wish to achieve with the biofilm, we should choose a technique according to our study. Not all techniques are suitable for a certain purpose, but might be compatible. Thus, some methods are suited for quantifying the biofilm matrix, while others are able to evaluate both living and dead cells, or exclusively quantify viable cells in biofilms.

By considering the complexity and heterogeneity of the biofilm structure, the exact research objective should be set. The amount of EPS, the total number of bacterial cells embedded in biofilms, or the actual number of living bacteria in biofilms must be considered to be different targets that require distinct experimental approaches [157]. We should bear in mind that the biofilm volume is constituted mainly by an extracellular matrix (95–65% range), which is composed mostly of proteins (>2%), and other constituents, such as polysaccharides (1–2%), DNA molecules (<1%), RNA (<1%), ions (bound and free), and finally 97% water [161]. Thus, the biofilm research methodology should address the identification of bacteria and other matrix constituents.

In order to obtain a fundamental understanding of the formation and presence of bacterial biofilms, our analysis should include the detection of bacteria and the matrix. The most frequently followed methods to assess biofilm heterogeneity are direct microscopic imaging of the local biofilm morphology or microscopic measurements of local biofilm thickness [162]. For many applications, time-lapse microscopy with Confocal Laser Scanning Microscopy (CLSM) is an ideal tool for monitoring at a spatial resolution in the order of micrometres, and it allows the non-destructive study of biofilms by examining all layers at different depths. In this way, it is possible to reconstruct a three-dimensional structure [163]. Matrix detection can be achieved by a double-staining technique combined with CLSM, which allows the simultaneous imaging of bacterial cells and glycocalyx in biofilms [164].

5.2. Colorimetric Methods

5.2.1. Evaluating the Biofilm Matrix

Staining the biofilms grown in microtiter plates wells is widely utilised by researchers to screen and compare biofilm formation by different bacteria or under various conditions [165]. Of the methods described in the literature, crystal violet (CAS number 931418 92 7) [166] is the most widespread for biofilm biomass quantification [167,168]. This basic dye binds negatively charged molecules and, thus, stains are able to dye both bacteria and the surrounding biofilm matrix. Acetic acid can be used as the extraction solvent and be measured by absorbance at 700–600 nm. Safranin staining can also be employed for biofilm biomass quantification [165,169], but results in lower optical densities than crystal violet staining and, therefore, may not be as sensitive to detect small amounts of biofilm [165].

Crystal violet staining tests the concentration of the dye incorporated into bacterial cell walls, and depends on cells' integrity, but not on viability. However, other methods like ATP bioluminescence report the cell's metabolic status and drops to undetectable limits within minutes after cell death. Resorting to both methods can provide supplementary information on the cell exposed to disinfectant. The results can indicate that, despite the drastic drop in viable cell numbers in the biofilm after disinfectant treatment, a significant number of intact cells, or cellular debris, may still be capable of retaining the dye. This observation leads to the question about the reliability of crystal violet staining as a method to monitor biofilm disinfection [170].

Another colorimetric method for living cells is fluorescein diacetate (CAS number 596 09 8), which employs a useful live-cell fluorescent stain that is hydrolysed to fluorescent fluorescein in live cells. The signal can be spectrophotometrically measured. This is suitable for cell viability assays with intact membranes as dead cells are unable to metabolise fluorescein diacetate. Thus, there is no fluorescent signal [157].

5.2.2. Cell Staining

Visualising a cell with fluorescent compounds provides a wide variety of information to analyse cell functions. Various activities and cell structures can be targeted for staining with fluorescent compounds [171]. These cell components are mostly cell membranes, nucleotides, and proteins. The stain can pass to cells depending on the molecule charge, hydrophobicity, or reactivity. Thus, small neutral and positively charged fluorescent compounds can normally reach mitochondria for dyeing. Negatively charged molecules cannot pass through viable cell membranes. Ester is a suitable functional group for staining viable cells because it can pass through viable cell membranes, where it is hydrolysed by cellular esterases into a negatively charged compound [171].

Other complementary techniques can be run to examine the performances of advanced microscopic techniques employed to study microbial biofilms (i.e., confocal laser scanning microscopy, mass spectrometry, electron microscopy, Raman spectroscopy) [157].

Spectrofluorometric assays for the quantification of biofilms of gram-negative and gram-positive bacteria is a method that utilises the specific binding of the wheat germ agglutinin-Alexa Fluor 488 conjugate (WGA) to N-acetylglucosamine in biofilms [172]. This lectin conjugate also binds to N-acetylneuraminic acid on the peptidoglycan layer of gram-positive bacteria. WGA specifically binds to polysaccharide adhesin (poly N-acetylglucosamine), which is involved in biofilm formation by both gram-positive and gram-negative bacteria. Burton et al. [172] compared the colorimetric assay with the spectrofluorometric assay, whose results revealed that WGA staining may be a more specific means of *E. coli* and *Staphylococcus epidermidis* biofilm detection and quantification.

5.2.3. LIVE/DEAD

This method is based on employing two different nucleic acid binding stains. The first dye is green fluorescent (Syto9, λ_{ex} 486 nm and λ_{em} 501 nm), which is able to cross all bacterial membranes and bind to the DNA of both Gram-positive and Gram-negative bacteria. The second dye is red-fluorescent (propidium-iodide (PI), CAS number 25535-16-4, λ_{ex} 530 nm and λ_{em} 620 nm), which crosses only damaged bacterial membranes. Stained samples are observed under a fluorescent optical microscopy to evaluate live and dead bacterial populations (see Figures 3–5). In fact, live bacteria fluoresce in green and dead bacteria fluoresce in orange/red [173]. The efficiency of both stains is conditioned by some factors, such as the reagent's binding affinity to cells [169], physiological cell state [174], reagent concentration [175], and temperature and incubation time [176].

Both stains are suitable for use in fluorescence microscopy, confocal laser scanning microscopy, fluorometry flow and cytometry, and can be employed as a nuclear counterstain. LIVE/DEAD staining cannot be performed for the direct staining of biofilms on surfaces because of interference between the stain and polysaccharides of the biofilm matrix and slime [177].

This method's main downside involves having to observe a statistically relevant portion of the sample, which is representative of the whole population. Overall, the method provides only semiquantitative results because the total count of bacterial cells is not possible [178]. Nevertheless, this inconvenience can be prevented by employing imaging software, such as cellSens®, which can count and measure cells depending on the staining cell.

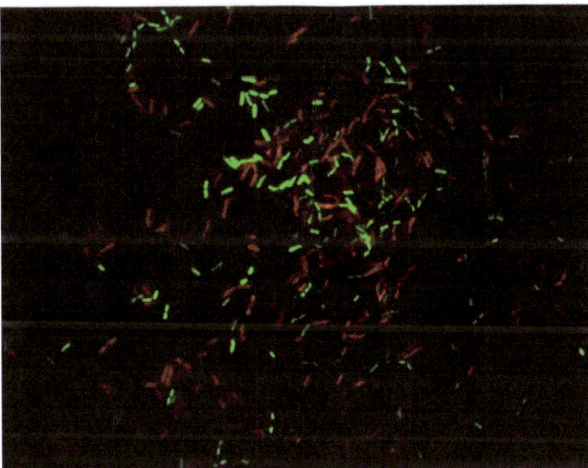

Figure 3. Planktonic state of *Pseudomonas fluorescens* stained with LIVE/DEAD (SYTO 9 and propidium iodine) after treatment with sodium hypochlorite (500 ppm) for 15 min. Viable bacteria (green) and damaged bacteria (red). Magnification ×100.

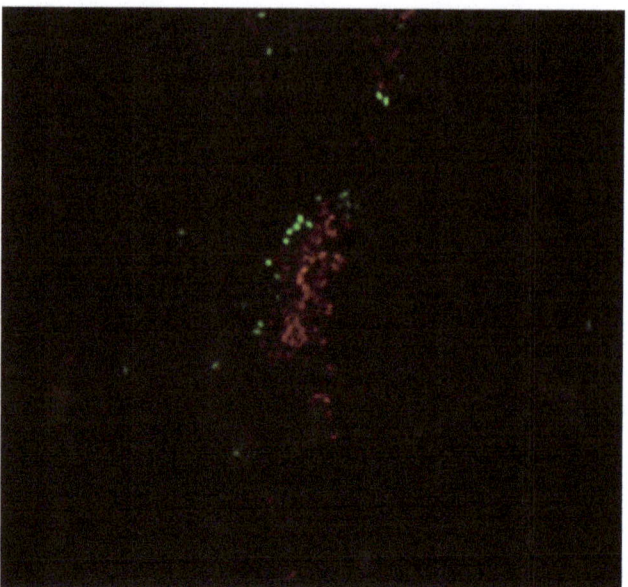

Figure 4. Planktonic state of *Pseudomonas fluorescens* stained with LIVE/DEAD (SYTO 9 and propidium iodine) after treatment with peracetic acid (250 ppm) for 15 min. Viable bacteria (green) and damaged bacteria (red). Magnification ×100.

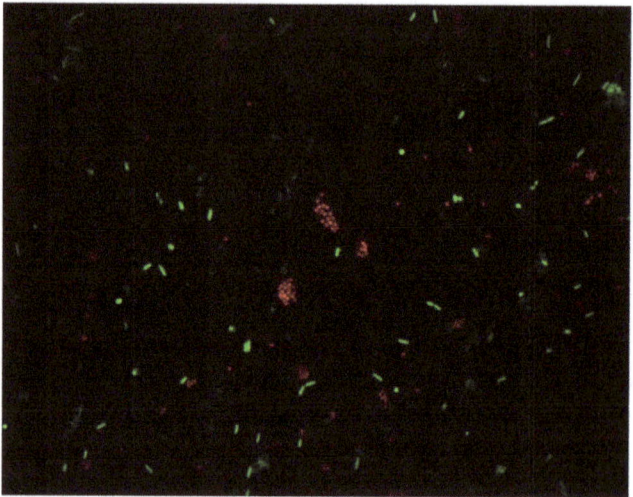

Figure 5. Planktonic state of *Pseudomonas fluorescens* stained with LIVE/DEAD (SYTO 9 and propidium iodine) after treatment with Sodium hypochlorite (350 ppm) for 15 min. Viable bacteria (green) and damaged bacteria (red). Magnification ×100.

5.2.4. Different Fluorescents Stainings

The application of fluorescent stains to cells and food soil can be useful for the quantitative analysis of surface cleanability. Thus, the stain combination and working concentration are essential for assessing the hygienic conditions of surfaces [179] or testing disinfectant efficacy against bacteria. Different methods can be followed to visualise and differentiate cells and organic matter. The staining techniques to measure surface coverage by the two stains by image analysis are highlighted [180] using DAPI and Rhodamine B, DAPI and Fluorescein, or non-specific stains, such as acridine orange, and are also available and specific for particular organic matter [180], and/or for microorganisms [181].

The use of different staining types can be explained by the results obtained in each study after checking the best biofilm and cells staining. These results depend on bacterial species, residual organic matter on surfaces, pH, disinfectant, etc. Whitehead et al. [182] conducted a large study with different dyeing, and concluded that the best combination was DAPI (CAS no. 28718-90-3, λ_{ex} 340 nm, λ_{em} 488 nm, blue) and Rhodamine B (CAS no. 81-88-9, λ_{ex} 553 nm, λ_{em} 627 nm, red), as it allowed the quantitative determination of *L. monocytogenes* and whey on a surface with fluorescent staining under epifluorescence microscopy. It is also useful for demonstrating the hygienic status of surfaces (Figures 7 and 8). The other tested staining procedures were unsatisfactory, or only slightly so, for distinguishing between viable and dead cells [182].

DAPI staining is suitable for studying cell viability in planktonic situations (initial attachment) and biofilms attached to surfaces (proliferation and growth–maturation) (Figure 6). Nevertheless, coculture biofilm studies need to spatially discriminate between species, and classic methods, such as crystal violet (CV), SYTO9/propidium iodide, and DAPI staining are insufficient given their non-specific nature [183], and selectively bind to each species. This burden can be overcome by applications, such as mutants expressing green fluorescent protein (GFP) [182,184], fluorescently labelled antibodies [185], and fluorescence in situ hybridisation (FISH).

The DAPI/Rhodamine B combination in biofilms offers the best resolution and quantification power between cells and organic matter (Figures 6–8). Several authors, such as Almeida et al. [183], have applied peptide nucleic acid fluorescence in situ hybridization (PNA FISH) combined with DAPI as a steady method to evaluate, validate, quantify, and characterise the initial adhesion and biofilm formation of three microorganisms: *Salmonella enterica*, *Listeria monocytogenes* and *Escherichia coli*.

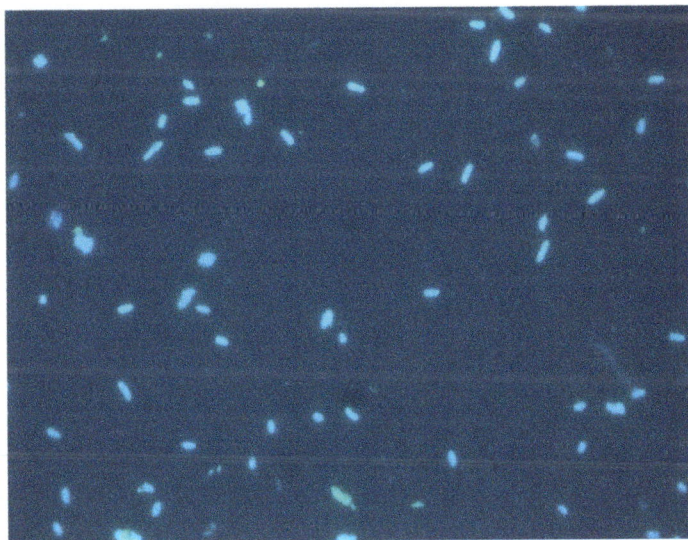

Figure 6. *Pseudomonas aeruginosa* biofilm on the stainless steel coupons. Stained with DAPI (0.1 mg/mL; 10 µL) (Magnification ×100).

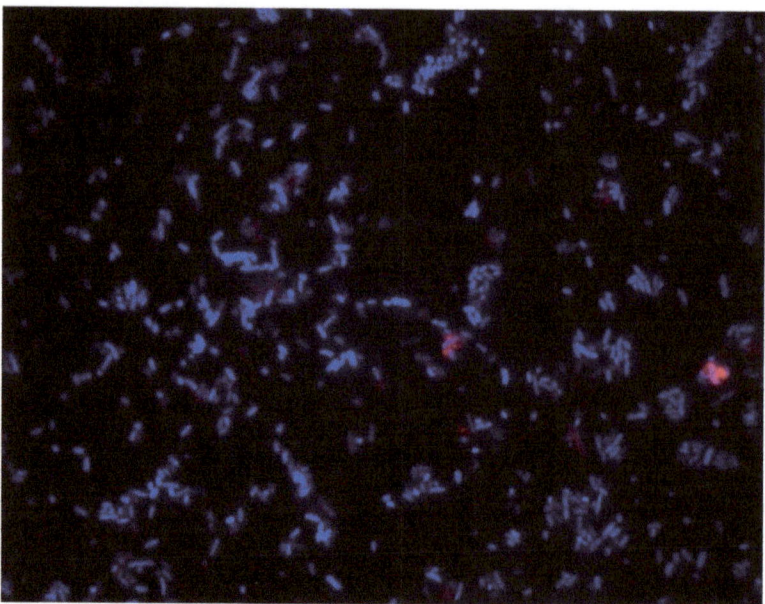

Figure 7. *Pseudomonas fluorescens* biofilm (24 h) on the stainless steel. Coupons stained with DAPI (0.1 mg/mL; 10 µL) and Rhodamine B (0.1 mg/mL; 10 µL) (Magnification ×100).

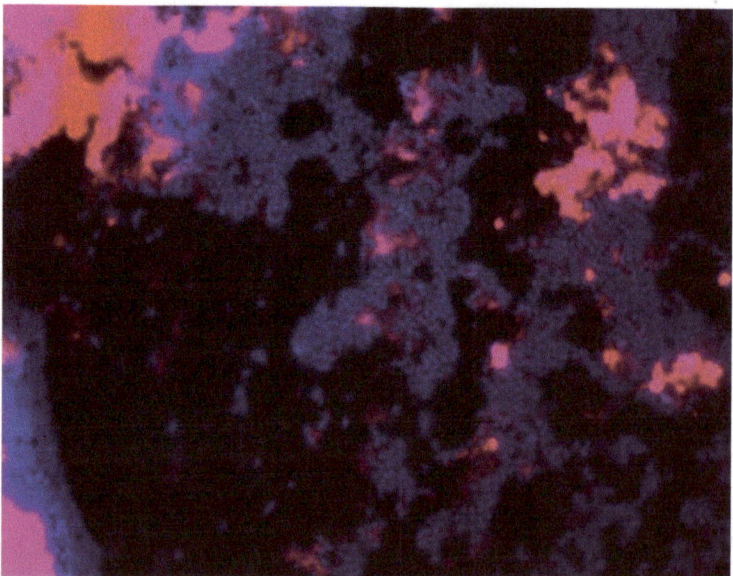

Figure 8. *Pseudomonas fluorescens* biofilm (7 days) on the stainless steel. Coupons stained with DAPI (0.1 mg/mL; 10 µL) and Rhodamine B (0.1 mg/mL; 10 µL) (Magnification ×100).

5.2.5. Confocal Laser Scanning Microscopy (CLSM)

Confocal laser scanning microscopy (CLSM) is an optical microscope equipped with a laser beam that is particularly useful for examining thick samples like microbial biofilms. Samples are stained with specific fluorescent dye insofar as the fluorescent light from the illuminated spot is collected on the objective and transformed by a photodiode into an electrical signal to be computer-processed [160] given the complexity of the microbial biofilm's extracellular matrix formed by heterogeneous compounds: polysaccharide, lipids, enzymes, extracellular DNA, and proteins [186].

However, no fluorescence labelling method is currently available for visualising the whole biofilm matrix owing to its different compositions, which depend on each bacterium and environmental condition, which means that each matrix component must be individually stained. Unfortunately, however, a general stain for polysaccharides does not exist because the chemical structure of matrix polysaccharides differs between distinct bacteria: Gram + and Gram− [186].

Extracellular DNA has been related to bacterial attachment and early biofilm formation stages in many species across the phylogenetic tree. These findings were discovered by employing combined stains, such as PicoGreen® and SYTOX®, PI, 1,3-dichloro-7-hydroxy-9,9-dimethyl-2(9H)-acridinone (DDAO), TOTO®-1, TO-PRO® 3. Most reports employed DDAO for staining eDNA in biofilms after the first publications by Allesen-Holm et al. [187] and Conover et al. [188]. Excellent efficacy has been reported for TOTO®-1, SYTOX® Green, while PI provides the most reliable results. TO-PRO®-3 and DDAO are not completely cell-impermeant [189].

With biofilm proteins, which may sometimes be more important than polysaccharides, this occurs in cell wall-anchored proteins in *Staphylococcus aureus* and *S. epidermidis,* and contributes to aggregation by homophilic interactions [190], or interacts with matrix components that originate from the host, such as fibronectin, collagen, or fibrin [191]. These biofilm proteins can be visualised with strains FilmTracer™ SyPro® [192]. Several proteins also play a key role in the *P. aeruginosa* biofilm matrix, such as CdrA and others, perform functions that range from nutrient acquisition to protection from oxidative stress [193]. Moreover, serine-protease inhibitor ecotin has been identified as a matrix protein that binds to Psl [194].

Nowadays, confocal microscopy is a relevant tool for studying the structure of biofilms thanks to its excellent real-time visualisation capability of fully hydrated living samples. The limitation of light microscopy's spatial resolution is improved by a fluorescence technique and by coupling CLSM with other imaging techniques [157]. The PNA FISH and CLSM combination allows the spatial organisation of and changes in specific members of complex microbial populations to be studied without disturbing the biofilm structure [195,196].

5.3. Raman Microscopy (RM)

This non-destructive analytical technique provides fingerprint spectra with the spatial resolution of an optical microscope [197]. This original technique permits the quantitative, label-free, non-invasive, and rapid monitoring of biochemical changes in complex biofilm matrices with high sensitivity and specificity [198]. Raman spectra studies are characterised by high specificity, and by usually revealing sharper clearer bands than IR spectra, and a small water background. Compared to IR microscopy, excitation with visible light can be employed in Raman spectroscopy, which allows standard optics to be utilised. Other advantages include its application to characterise and identify different biological systems (fungi, bacteria, yeasts) because all biologically associated molecules (e.g., nucleic acids, proteins, lipids, carbohydrates) exhibit distinct spectral features [197]. Therefore, Ivleva et al. [197] analysed seven different specific microorganisms by RM to characterise microorganisms in biofilms.

Another author evaluated the antibiotic effect on biofilms [198], and the oxidation of graphene as antibacterial activity against the *Pseudomonas putida* biofilm with variable ages [199].

5.4. Scanning Electron Microscopy (SEM)

Scanning electron microscopy (SEM) provides useful information about size, shape, and localisation in the biofilms of single bacteria, and in biofilm formation process steps about bacterial interactions and EPS production [200]. Surface topography has been widely discussed as a parameter that influences microbial adhesion. In line with this, the experiments by Kouider et al. [201], which employed SEM to establish the effect of stainless steel surface roughness on *Staphylococcus aureus* adhesion, revealed that the adhesion level largely depends on substrate roughness with a maximum at Ra = 0.025 µm and a minimum at Ra = 0.8 µm. [202]. Mallouki et al. studied the anti-adhesive effect of fucans by SEM and a MATLAB programme to determine the number and characteristics of adhered cells [203].

SEM has been extensively used to qualitatively observe biofilm disruption owing to its high resolution, and is usually applied in combination with biological assays of biofilm removal efficiency [204,205]. With SEM images, simple thresholding cannot often be implemented because biofilm normal surface intensity values are similar due to the same effective contrast seen by SEM. Rough (textured) biomaterial surfaces complicate image analyses, and advanced segmentation methods, such as semi-supervised machine-learning techniques, are usually needed [206]. The biofilm might be segmented from the surface using the Trainable Weka Segmentation plugin, which utilises a collection of machine-learning algorithms for segmentation purposes [207].

As with other previously mentioned techniques, SEM is a widely used resource for confirming the presence of bacteria and the exopolysaccharide matrix when studying biofilms (Figures 9–11). These studies usually obtain SEM results and are supplemented with the results of other techniques like confocal [208,209], surface-enhanced Raman scattering (SERS) spectroscopy [210], epifluorescence microscopy (DAPI/Rhodamine B), and contact plates [211].

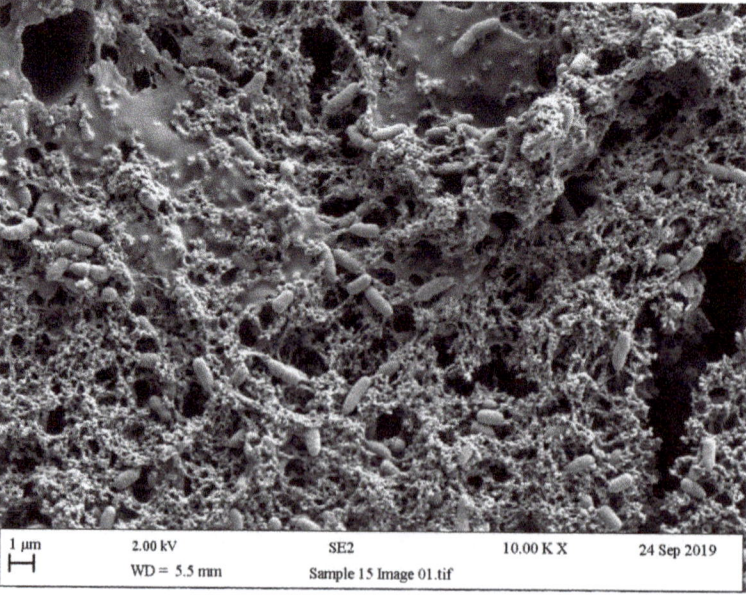

Figure 9. Scanning electronic microscopy (SEM) images of stainless steel of 3-day biofilms formed by *Pseudomonas fluorescens*.

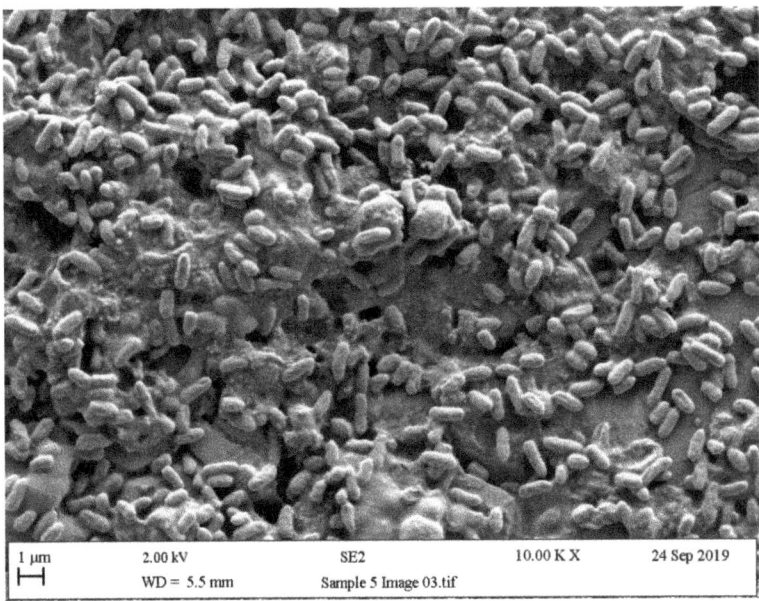

Figure 10. Scanning electronic microscopy (SEM) images of stainless steel of 7-day biofilms formed by *Pseudomonas fluorescens*.

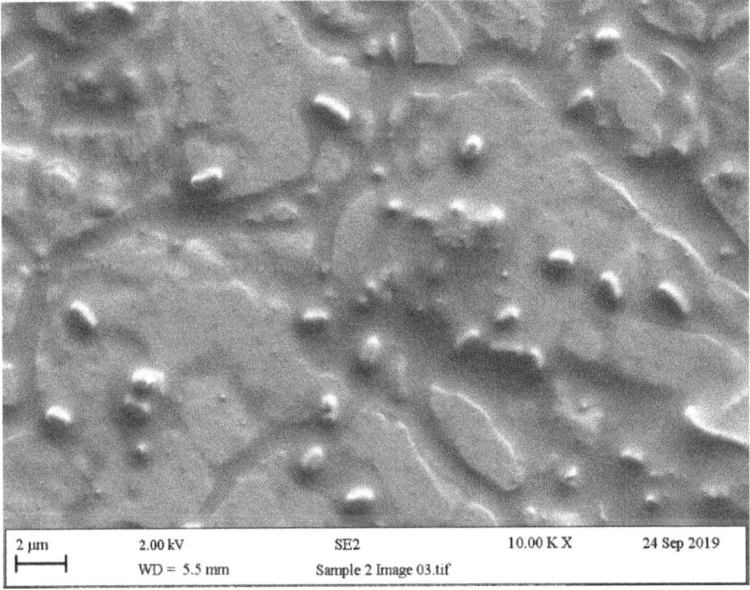

Figure 11. Scanning electronic microscopy (SEM) images of stainless steel of 7-day biofilms formed by *Pseudomonas fluorescens* after treatment with peracetic acid (250 ppm) for 15 min.

5.5. Microbiological Methods

The estimation of the total number of organisms (total viable count) is the most widely used technique to estimate biofilm viable cells. This count is done on agar media and its result is colony-forming units (CFU). Based on the serial dilution series approach followed to quantify microorganisms, this technique is easy and requires no special equipment [158]. Surface samples (stainless steel, plastic, rubber coupons) with biofilms are analysed by swab or sonication, and transferred to agar plates. This culture medium can be specific for either the studied species or non-specific species (plate count agar media).

Several authors like [212] discovered that some bacterial species can enter a distinct state called the viable, but non-culturable (VBNC) state. These living cells have lost the ability to grow on plate agar media. However, this method has serious drawbacks and limitations [213]: (i) the fraction of detached live cells may not be representative of the initial biofilm population; (ii) a subpopulation of biofilm cells can be viable, but non-culturable (VBNC), and cannot be detected by the CFU approach for the CFU estimation of the recovery and quantification of viable biofilm cells. Several authors, such as Cerca et al. [214] and Olivera et al. [215], have proposed applying flow cytometry coupled with a few possible fluorophores as an alternative to the total viable count from biofilms because flow cytometry solves both CFU counting limitations by distinguishing total, dead, and VBNC.

The total viable count technique is fundamental for the evolution of biofilm studies, as are studies about the efficacy of industrial disinfectants and increased resistance to the application of different disinfectants. Table 2 shows some results of disinfectant efficacy against several bacterial species.

Table 2. Resistance of several bacterial species to disinfectant on different material surfaces.

Bacterial Species	Disinfectant	ppm or %	Surfaces	Biofilm. Log Reduction CFU	Reference
S. aureus	Sodium hypochlorite	250	Stainless steel/PP	4.5/4.4	[212]
Cronobacter Sakazakii	Sodium hypochlorite	250	Stainless steel/PP	3.7/3.9	[216]
S. Typhimurium	Sodium hypochlorite	250	Stainless steel/PP	5.82/6.1	[216]
S. aeruginosa	Sodium hypochlorite	250, 500	Stainless steel 316	2/100%	[217]
S. aeruginosa	Sodium hypochlorite	750, 1000	Stainless steel 316	100%/100%	[217]
B. cereus	NaOH and HNO$_3$, 65 °C	1%	CIP dairy	2	[218]
Enterococcus faecium	Sodium hypochlorite	100	Stainless steel	3	[98]
E. faecium	Peracetic acid	300	Stainless steel	4	[98]
Rhodococcus erythropolis	Alkyl amine	1–1.3%	Stainless steel	>5	[103]
R. erythropolis	Peracetic acid	0.2%	Stainless steel	0.48	[103]
R. erythropolis	Sodium hypochlorite	0.5–1%	Stainless steel	4.51	[103]
R. erythropolis	QAC	200	Stainless steel	>5	[103]
Sphingomonas sp.	Alkyl amine	1–1.3%	Stainless steel	>5	[103]
Sphingomonas sp.	Peracetic acid	0.2%	Stainless steel	>5	[103]
Sphingomonas sp.	Sodium hypochlorite	0.5–1%	Stainless steel	>5	[103]
Sphingomonas sp.	QAC	200	Stainless steel	>5	[103]
Methylobacterium rhodesianum	Alkyl amine	1–1.3%	Stainless steel	4.48	[103]
M. rhodesianum	Peracetic acid	0.2%	Stainless steel	>5	[103]
M. rhodesianum	Sodium hypochlorite	0.5–1%	Stainless steel	0.01	[103]
M. rhodesianum	QAC	200	Stainless steel	0.64	[103]
L. monocytogenes	Sodium hydroxide	0.5%	Rubber	0.66	[112]
L. monocytogenes	QAC	0.5%	Rubber	1.72	[112]
L. monocytogenes	Sodium hypochlorite	0.5%	Rubber	1.79	[112]
L. monocytogenes	Peracetic acid	0.5%	Rubber	5.10	[112]
L. monocytogenes	Sodium hydroxide	0.5%	Polypropylene	1.20	[112]
L. monocytogenes	QAC	0.5%	Polypropylene	2.57	[112]
L. monocytogenes	Sodium hypochlorite	0.5%	Polypropylene	2.74	[112]
L. monocytogenes	Peracetic acid	0.5%	Polypropylene	6.62	[112]
L. monocytogenes	Sodium hydroxide	0.5%	Stainless steel	1	[112]
L. monocytogenes	QAC	0.5%	Stainless steel	4.06	[112]
L. monocytogenes	Sodium hypochlorite	0.5%	Stainless steel	1.97	[112]
L. monocytogenes	Peracetic acid	0.5%	Stainless steel	6.63	[112]
L. monocytogenes	Sodium hydroxide	0.5%	Aluminium foil	0.52	[112]
L. monocytogenes	QAC	0.5%	Aluminium foil	5.1	[112]
L. monocytogenes	Sodium hypochlorite	0.5%	Aluminium foil	3.84	[112]
L. monocytogenes	Peracetic acid	0.5%	Aluminium foil	6.54	[112]
L. monocytogenes	Benzalkonium chloride	100–10,000	Polystyrene	1–7	[112]
L. monocytogenes	Benzalkonium chloride	10	Polystyrene	100%	[170]

Colony-forming units (CFU); cleaning-in-place (CIP); polypropylene (PP); quaternary ammonium compounds (QAC).

6. Conclusions

Biofilms have become a major environmental microbiology concern in the food industry over the last 30 years. This topic is prominent due to the potential for contamination of food from biofilms; they are responsible for more than 20% of food poisoning cases and for being up to 1000-fold more tolerant to antibiotics than their planktonic counterparts [219].

Many bacterial species have the ability to form biofilms, such as microbial subsistences (when faced with hostilities from the environment), antibiotics, and disinfectants. For these reasons, cleaning and disinfecting in the food industry must bring about changes that favour eliminating biofilms, because once they form, the resulting costs and risks will be very high. As previously discovered in many publications, the ability of bacteria to form biofilms is greater than the discoveries. Thus, they must be eliminated. The advancement of new, non-destructive technologies (e.g., laser dissection) to study biofilms and their results should be applied to biofilm diagnoses in the food industry, to better understand the physiological anatomy of microbes and biofilms, and future applications in the food industry.

Author Contributions: Conceptualization, A.S., C.C., D.R., F.R., and A.R.; methodology, A.S., C.C., D.R., F.R., and A.R.; software, A.S., C.C., D.R., F.R., and A.R.; validation, A.S., C.C., D.R., F.R., and A.R.; formal analysis, A.S., C.C., D.R., F.R., and A.R.; investigation, A.S., C.C., D.R., F.R., and A.R.; resources, A.S., C.C., D.R., F.R., and A.R.; data curation, A.S., C.C., D.R., F.R., and A.R.; writing—original draft preparation, A.S., C.C., D.R., F.R., and A.R.; writing—review and editing, A.S., C.C., D.R., F.R., and A.R.; visualization, A.S., C.C., D.R., F.R., and A.R.; supervision, A.S., C.C., D.R., F.R., and A.R.; project administration, A.S., C.C., D.R., F.R., and A.R. All authors have read and agreed to the published version of the manuscript.

Funding: This research received no external funding.

Institutional Review Board Statement: Not applicable.

Informed Consent Statement: Not applicable.

Data Availability Statement: Not applicable.

Acknowledgments: The authors are very grateful to their families and friends for all of the support they provided.

Conflicts of Interest: The authors declare no conflict of interest.

References

1. Satpathy, S.; Sen, S.K.; Pattanaik, S.; Raut, S. Review on bacterial biofilm: An universal cause of contamination. *Biocatal. Agric. Biotechnol.* **2016**, *7*, 56–66. [CrossRef]
2. Flemming, H.C.; Wingender, J. The biofilm matrix. *Nat. Rev. Microbiol.* **2010**, *8*, 623–633. [CrossRef] [PubMed]
3. Hall-Stoodley, L.J.; Costerton, W.; Stoodley, P. Bacterial biofilms: From the natural environment to infectious diseases. *Nat. Rev. Microbiol.* **2004**, *2*, 95–108. [CrossRef]
4. Acker, H.V.; Dijck, P.V.; Coenye, P.V. Molecular mechanisms of antimicrobial tolerance and resistance in bacterial and fungal biofilms. *Trends Microbiol.* **2014**, *22*, 326–333. [CrossRef]
5. Alvarez-Ordóñez, A.L.; Coughlan, M.; Briandet, R.; Cotter, P.D. Biofilms in food processing environments: Challenges and opportunities. *Annu. Rev. Food Sci. Technol.* **2019**, *10*, 173–195. [CrossRef]
6. Brooks, J.D.; Flint, S.H. Biofilms in the food industry: Problems and potential solutions. *Int. J. Food Sci. Technol.* **2008**, *43*, 2163–2176. [CrossRef]
7. Møretrø, M.; Langsrud, S. Residential bacteria on surfaces in the food industry and their implications for food safety and quality. *Compr. Rev. Food Sci. Food Saf.* **2017**, *16*, 1022–1041. [CrossRef]
8. Yuan, L.; Sadiq, F.A.; Burmølle, M.; Liu, T.; He, G. Insights into bacterial milk spoilage with particular emphasis on the roles of heat-stable enzymes, biofilms, and quorum sensing. *J. Food Prot.* **2018**, *81*, 1651–1660. [CrossRef]
9. Srey, S.; Jahid, I.K.; Ha, S.D. Biofilm formation in food industries: A food safety concern. *Food Control* **2013**, *31*, 572–585. [CrossRef]
10. Anwar, H.; Strap, J.L.; Costerton, J.W. Establishment of aging biofilms: Possible mechanism of bacterial resistance to antimicrobial therapy. *Antimicrob. Agents Chemother.* **1992**, *36*, 1347. [CrossRef]
11. Costerton, J.W.; Ellis, B.; Lam, K.; Johnson, F.; Khoury, A.E. Mechanism of electrical enhancement of efficacy of antibiotics in killing biofilm bacteria. *Antimicrob. Agents Chemother.* **1994**, *38*, 2803–2809. [CrossRef]

12. Simoes, M.; Simoes, L.; Vieira, M. A review of current and emergent biofilm control strategies. *LWT Food Sci. Technol.* **2010**, *43*, 573–583. [CrossRef]
13. Fung, D.Y.C. Rapid methods and automation in microbiology: A review. *Ir. J. Agric. Food Res.* **2000**, *39*, 301–307. [CrossRef]
14. Bouix, M.; Leveau, J.Y. Les applications de la cytometrie en flux en microbiologie. *L'Eurobiologiste* **2002**, *36*, 31–43.
15. Holah, J.T.; Taylor, J.H.; Dawson, D.J.; Hall, K.E. Biocide use in the food industry and the disinfectant resistance of persistent strains of *Listeria monocytogenes* and *Escherichia Coli*. *J. Appl. Microbiol.* **2002**, *92*, 111S–120S. [CrossRef] [PubMed]
16. Kassa, H. An outbreak of Norwalk-like viral gastroenteritis in a frequently penalized food service operation: A case for mandatory training of food handlers in safety and hygiene. *J. Environ. Health.* **2001**, *64*.
17. González-Rivas, F.; Ripolles-Avila, C.; Fontecha-Umaña, F.; Ríos-Castillo, A.G.; Rodríguez-Jerez, J.J. Biofilms in the Spotlight: Detection, Quantification, and Removal Methods. *Compr. Rev. Food Sci. Food Saf.* **2018**, *17*, 1261–1276. [CrossRef]
18. Shi, X.; Zhu, X. Biofilm formation and food safety in food industries. *Trends Food Sci. Technol.* **2009**, *20*, 407–413. [CrossRef]
19. Anand, S.; Singh, D.; Avadhanula, M.; Marka, S. Development and control of bacterial biofilms on dairy processing membranes. *Compr. Rev. Food Sci. Food Saf.* **2014**, *13*, 18–33. [CrossRef]
20. Rabin, N.; Zheng, Y.; Opoku-Temeng, C.; Du, Y.; Bonsu, E.; Sintim, H.O. Biofilm formation mechanisms and targets for developing antibiofilm agents. *Future Med. Chem.* **2015**, *7*, 493–512. [CrossRef]
21. Lindsay, D.; von Holy, A. What food safety professionals should know about bacterial biofilms. *Br. Food J.* **2006**, *108*, 27–37. [CrossRef]
22. Tang, L.; Pillai, S.; Revsbech, N.P.; Schramm, A.; Bischoff, C.; Meyer, R.L. Biofilm retention on surfaces with variable roughness and hydrophobicity. *Biofouling* **2011**, *27*, 111–121. [CrossRef] [PubMed]
23. Van Houdt, R.; Michiels, C.W. Biofilm formation and the food industry, a focus on the bacterial outer surface. *J. Appl. Microbiol.* **2010**, *109*, 1117–1131. [CrossRef]
24. Govaert, M.; Smet, C.; Baka, M.; Janssens, T.; Van Impe, J. Influence of incubation conditions on the formation of model biofilms by Listeria monocytogenes and Salmonella Typhimurium on abiotic surfaces. *J. Appl. Microbiol.* **2018**, *125*, 1890–1900. [CrossRef] [PubMed]
25. Makovcova, J.; Babak, V.; Kulich, P.; Masek, J.; Slany, M.; Cincarova, L. Dynamics of mono- and dual-species biofilm formation and interactions between Staphylococcus aureus and gramnegative bacteria. *Microb. Biotechnol.* **2017**, *10*, 819–832. [CrossRef]
26. Araújo, E.A.; de Andrade, N.J.; da Silva, L.H.M.; de Carvalho, A.F.; da Silva, C.A.; Ramos, A.M. Control of microbial adhesion as a strategy for food and bioprocess technology. *Food Bioprocess Technol.* **2010**, *3*, 321–332. [CrossRef]
27. Dhowlaghar, N.; Bansal, M.; Schilling, M.W.; Nannapaneni, R. Scanning electron microscopy of Salmonella biofilms on various food-contact surfaces in catfish mucus. *Food Microbiol.* **2018**, *74*, 143–150. [CrossRef] [PubMed]
28. Jindal, S.; Anand, S.; Metzger, L.; Amamcharla, J. A comparison of biofilm development on stainless steel and modified-surface plate heat exchangers during a 17-h milk pasteurization run. *J. Dairy Sci.* **2018**, *101*, 2921–2926. [CrossRef] [PubMed]
29. Gomes, L.C.; Silva, L.N.; Simoes, M.; Melo, L.F.; Mergulhao, F.J. Escherichia coli adhesion, biofilm development and antibiotic susceptibility on biomedical materials. *J. Biomed. Mater. Res.* **2015**, *103*, 1414–1423. [CrossRef] [PubMed]
30. Veluz, G.A.; Pitchiah, S.; Alvarado, C.Z. Attachment of *Salmonella* serovars and *Listeria monocytogenes* to stainless steel and plastic conveyor belts. *Poult. Sci.* **2012**, *91*, 2004–2010. [CrossRef] [PubMed]
31. Iñiguez-Moreno, M.M.; Gutiérrez-Lomelí, A.; Avila-Novoa, M.G. Kinetics of biofilm formation by pathogenic and spoilage microorganisms under conditions that mimic the poultry, meat, and egg processing industries. *Int. J. Food Microbiol.* **2019**, *303*, 32–41. [CrossRef] [PubMed]
32. Dutra, T.V.; Fernandes, M.D.; Perdoncini, M.R.F.G.; dos Anjos, M.M.; Abreu Filho, B.A.D. Capacity of *Escherichia coli* and *Staphylococcus aureus* to produce biofilm on stainless steel surfaces in the presence of food residues. *J. Food Process. Preserv.* **2018**, *42*, e13574. [CrossRef]
33. Duanis-Assaf, D.; Steinberg, D.; Chai, Y.; Shemesh, M. The LuxS based quorum sensing governs lactose induced biofilm formation by Bacillus subtilis. *Front. Microbiol.* **2016**, *6*, 1517. [CrossRef]
34. Xue, T.; Chen, X.; Shang, F. Effects of lactose and milk on the expression of biofilm-associated genes in Staphylococcus aureus strains isolated from a dairy cow with mastitis. *J. Dairy Sci.* **2014**, *97*, 6129–6134. [CrossRef] [PubMed]
35. Somerton, B.; Lindsay, D.; Palmer, J.; Brooks, J.; Flint, S. Changes in sodium, calcium, and magnesium ion concentrations that inhibit Geobacillus biofilms have no effect on Anoxybacillus flavithermus biofilms. *Appl. Environ. Microbiol.* **2015**, *81*, 5115–5122. [CrossRef]
36. Wang, R.; Kalchayanand, N.; Bono, J.L. Sequence of colonization determines the composition of mixed biofilms by *Escherichia coli* O157:H7 and O111:H8 strains. *J. Food Prot.* **2015**, *78*, 1554–1559. [CrossRef]
37. Abdallah, M.; Khelissa, O.; Ibrahim, A.; Benoliel, C.; Heliot, L.; Dhulster, P.; Chihib, N.E. Impact of growth temperature and surface type on the resistance of *Pseudomonas aeruginosa* and *Staphylococcus aureus* biofilms to disinfectants. *Int. J. Food Microbiol.* **2015**, *214*, 38–47. [CrossRef]
38. Colagiorgi, A.; Bruini, I.; Di Ciccio, P.A.; Zanardi, E.; Ghidini, S.; Ianieri, A. Listeria Monocytogenes Biofilms in the Wonderland of Food Industry. *Pathogens* **2017**, *6*, 41. [CrossRef] [PubMed]
39. Bottone, E.J. Bacillus Cereus, a Volatile Human Pathogen. *Clin. Microbiol. Rev.* **2010**, *23*, 382–398. [CrossRef]
40. Grigore-Gurgu, L.; Bucur, F.I.; Borda, D.; Alexa, E.A.; Neagu, C.; Nicolau, A.I. Biofilms Formed by Pathogens in Food and Food Processing Environments. In *Bacterial Biofilms*; IntechOpen: London, UK, 2019.

41. Klančnik, A.; Šimunović, K.; Sterniša, M.; Ramić, D.; Smole Možina, S.; Bucar, F. Anti-Adhesion Activity of Phytochemicals to Prevent Campylobacter Jejuni Biofilm Formation on Abiotic Surfaces. *Phytochem. Rev.* **2020**. [CrossRef]
42. EFSA; European Food Safety Authority and European Centre for Disease Prevention and Control (EFSA and ECDC). The European Union One Health 2018 Zoonoses Report. *EFSA J.* **2019**, *17*, e05926.
43. Chlebicz, A.; Śliżewska, K. Campylobacteriosis, Salmonellosis, Yersiniosis, and Listeriosis as Zoonotic Foodborne Diseases: A Review. *Int. J. Environ. Res. Public Health* **2018**, *15*, 863. [CrossRef] [PubMed]
44. Galié, S.; García-Gutiérrez, C.; Miguélez, E.M.; Villar, C.J.; Lombó, F. Biofilms in the Food Industry: Health Aspects and Control Methods. *Front. Microbiol.* **2018**, 898. [CrossRef]
45. CDC. Centre for Disease Control, USA: Listeria (Listeriosis). 2017. Available online: https://www.cdc.gov/listeria/outbreaks/index.html (accessed on 29 November 2020).
46. Rothrock, M.J.; Davis, M.L.; Locatelli, A.; Bodie, A.; McIntosh, T.G.; Donaldson, J.R.; Ricke, S.C. Listeria Occurrence in Poultry Flocks: Detection and Potential Implications. *Front. Vet. Sci.* **2017**, *4*. [CrossRef]
47. Nguyen, H.D.N.; Yang, Y.S.; Yuk, H.G. Biofilm Formation of Salmonella Typhimurium on Stainless Steel and Acrylic Surfaces as Affected by Temperature and PH Level. *LWT Food Sci. Technol.* **2014**, *55*, 383–388. [CrossRef]
48. Duguid, J.P.; Anderson, E.S.; Campbell, I. Fimbriae and Adhesive Properties in Salmonellae. *J. Pathol. Bacteriol.* **1966**, *92*, 107–137. [CrossRef]
49. Giaouris, E.; Heir, E.; Desvaux, M.; Hébraud, M.; Møretrø, T.; Langsrud, S.; Doulgeraki, A.; Nychas, G.-J.; Kačániová, M.; Czaczyk, K.; et al. Intra- and Inter-Species Interactions within Biofilms of Important Foodborne Bacterial Pathogens. *Front. Microbiol.* **2015**, *6*. [CrossRef]
50. Kadariya, J.; Smith, T.C.; Thapaliya, D. Staphylococcus Aureus and Staphylococcal Food-Borne Disease: An Ongoing Challenge in Public Health. *Biomed Res. Int.* **2014**. [CrossRef]
51. Hammer, B.K.; Bassler, B.L. Quorum sensing controls biofilm formation in Vibrio cholerae. *Mol. Microbiol.* **2003**, *50*, 101–114. [CrossRef]
52. Otto, M. Staphylococcal infections: Mechanisms of biofilm maturation and detachment as critical determinants of pathogenicity. *Annu. Rev. Med.* **2013**, *64*, 175–188. [CrossRef] [PubMed]
53. Morgan, R.; Kohn, S.; Hwang, S.H.; Hassett, D.J.; Sauer, K. BdlA, a chemotaxis regulator essential for biofilm dispersion in *Pseudomonas aeruginosa*. *J. Bacteriol.* **2006**, *188*, 7335–7343. [CrossRef] [PubMed]
54. Somerton, B.; Flint, S.; Palmer, J.; Brooks, J.; Lindsay, D. Preconditioning with cations increases the attachment of Anoxybacillus flavithermus and Geobacillus species to stainless steel. *Appl. Environ. Microbiol.* **2013**, *79*, 4186–4190. [CrossRef]
55. Houry, A.; Briandet, R.; Aymerich, S.; Gohar, M. Involvement of Motility and Flagella in Bacillus Cereus Biofilm Formation. *Microbiology* **2010**, *156*, 1009–1018. [CrossRef]
56. Téllez, S. Biofilms and their impact on food industry. In *VISAVET Outreach Journal*; Complutense University: Madrid, Spain, 2010.
57. Tram, G.; Day, C.J.; Korolik, V. Bridging the Gap: A Role for Campylobacter Jejuni Biofilms. *Microorganisms* **2020**, *8*, 452. [CrossRef]
58. Gould, L.H.; Mody, R.K.; Ong, K.L.; Clogher, P.; Cronquist, A.B.; Garman, K.N.; Lathrop, S.; Medus, C.; Spina, N.L.; Webb, T.H.; et al. Increased recognition of non-O157 Shiga toxin-producing *Escherichia coli* infections in the United States during 2000–2010: Epidemiologic features and comparison with *E. coli* O157 infections. *Foodborne Pathog. Dis.* **2013**, *10*, 453–460. [CrossRef] [PubMed]
59. Lim, E.S.; Koo, O.K.; Kim, M.J.; Kim, J.S. Bio-enzymes for inhibition and elimination of Escherichia coli O157: H7 biofilm and their synergistic effect with sodium hypochlorite. *Sci. Rep.* **2019**, *9*, 9920. [CrossRef] [PubMed]
60. Lee, J.; Bansal, T.; Jayaraman, A.; Bentley, W.E.; Wood, T.K. Enterohemorrhagic Escherichia Coli Biofilms Are Inhibited by 7-Hydroxyindole and Stimulated by Isatin. *Appl. Environ. Microbiol.* **2007**, *73*, 4100–4109. [CrossRef]
61. Milillo, S.R.; Friedly, E.C.; Saldivar, J.C.; Muthaiyan, A.; O'bryan, C.; Crandall, P.G.; Johnson, M.G.; Ricke, S.C. A Review of the Ecology, Genomics, and Stress Response of Listeria Innocua and Listeria Monocytogenes. *Crit. Rev. Food Sci. Nutr.* **2012**, *52*, 712–725. [CrossRef]
62. Chmielewski, R.A.N.; Frank, J.F. Biofilm Formation and Control in Food Processing Facilities. *Compr. Rev. Food Sci. Food Saf.* **2003**, *2*, 22–32. [CrossRef]
63. Raheem, D. Outbreaks of Listeriosis Associated with Deli Meats and Cheese: An Overview. *Aims Microbiol.* **2016**, *2*, 230–250. [CrossRef]
64. Lemon, K.P.; Higgins, D.E.; Kolter, R. Flagellar Motility Is Critical for Listeria Monocytogenes Biofilm Formation. *J. Bacteriol.* **2007**, *189*, 4418–4424. [CrossRef] [PubMed]
65. Giannella, R.A.; Baron, S.; Albrecht, T.; Castro, G.; Couch, R.B.; Davis, C.P.; Dianzani, F.; Mcginnis, M.R.; Niesel, D.W.; Woods, G.W. Salmonella. In *Baron's Medical Microbiology*, 4th ed.; University of Texas Medical Branch: Galveston, TX, USA, 1996.
66. Lamas, A.; Miranda, J.M.; Regal, P.; Vázquez, B.; Franco, C.M.; Cepeda, A. A Comprehensive Review of Non-Enterica Subspecies of Salmonella Enterica. *Microbiol. Res.* **2018**, 60–73. [CrossRef]
67. Ćwiek, K.; Bugla-Płoskońska, G.; Wieliczko, A. Salmonella Biofilm Development: Structure and Significance. *Postepy Hig. I Med. Dosw.* **2019**, 937–943. [CrossRef]
68. Wang, H.; Ding, S.; Wang, G.; Xu, X.; Zhou, G. In situ characterization and analysis of Salmonella biofilm formation under meat processing environments using a combined microscopic and spectroscopic approach. *Int. J. Food Microbiol.* **2013**, *167*, 293–302. [CrossRef]

69. Schelin, J.; Susilo, Y.; Johler, S. Expression of Staphylococcal Enterotoxins under Stress Encountered during Food Production and Preservation. *Toxins* **2017**, *9*, 401. [CrossRef]
70. Amina, M.; Bensoltane, A. Review of Pseudomonas Attachment and Biofilm Formation in Food Industry Pseudomonas Biofilm; Chemotaxis and Motility View Project. *Poult. Fish Wildl. Sci.* **2015**, *3*, 1. [CrossRef]
71. Golovlev, E.L. The Mechanism of Formation of Pseudomonas Aeruginosa Biofilm, a Type of Structured Population. *Microbiology* **2002**, 249–254. [CrossRef]
72. Carrascosa, C.; Millán, R.; Jaber, J.R.; Lupiola, P.; del Rosario-Quintana, C.; Mauricio, C.; Sanjuán, E. Blue Pigment in Fresh Cheese Produced by *Pseudomonas fluorescens*. *Food Control* **2015**, *54*, 95–102. [CrossRef]
73. Wu, P.; Guo, Y.; Golly, M.K.; Ma, H.; He, R.; Luo, S.; Zhang, C.; Zhang, L.; Zhu, J. Feasibility Study on Direct Fermentation of Soybean Meal by *Bacillus Stearothermophilus* under Non-sterile Conditions. *J. Sci. Food Agric.* **2019**, *99*, 3291–3298. [CrossRef]
74. Flint, S.; Palmer, J.; Bloemen, K.; Brooks, J.; Crawford, R. The Growth of Bacillus Stearothermophilus on Stainless Steel. *J. Appl. Microbiol.* **2001**, *90*, 151–157. [CrossRef]
75. Palmer, J.S.; Flint, S.H.; Schmid, J.; Brooks, J.D. The Role of Surface Charge and Hydrophobicity in the Attachment of Anoxybacillus Flavithermus Isolated from Milk Powder. *J. Ind. Microbiol. Biotechnol.* **2010**, *37*, 1111–1119. [CrossRef]
76. Strejc, J.; Kyselova, L.; Cadkova, A.; Matoulkova, D.; Potocar, T.; Branyik, T. Experimental Adhesion of Geobacillus Stearothermophilus and Anoxybacillus Flavithermus to Stainless Steel Compared with Predictions from Interaction Models. *Chem. Pap.* **2020**, *74*, 297–304. [CrossRef]
77. Murphy, P.M.; Lynch, D.; Kelly, P.M. Growth of Thermophilic Spore Forming Bacilli in Milk during the Manufacture of Low Heat Powders. *Int. J. Dairy Technol.* **1999**, *52*, 45–50. [CrossRef]
78. Sadiq, F.A.; Flint, S.; Yuan, L.; Li, Y.; Liu, T.J.; He, G.Q. Propensity for Biofilm Formation by Aerobic Mesophilic and Thermophilic Spore Forming Bacteria Isolated from Chinese Milk Powders. *Int. J. Food Microbiol.* **2017**, *262*, 89–98. [CrossRef]
79. Burgess, S.A.; Brooks, J.D.; Rakonjac, J.; Walker, K.M.; Flint, S.H. The Formation of Spores in Biofilms of *Anoxybacillus Flavithermus*. *J. Appl. Microbiol.* **2009**, *107*, 1012–1018. [CrossRef] [PubMed]
80. Paradh, A.D.; Mitchell, W.J.; Hill, A.E. Occurrence of Pectinatus and Megasphaera in the Major UK Breweries. *J. Inst. Brew.* **2011**, *117*, 498–506. [CrossRef]
81. Lee, S.Y.; Mabee, M.S.; Jangaard, N.O. Pectinatus, a New Genus of the Family Bacteroidaceae. *Int. J. Syst. Bacteriol.* **1978**, *28*, 582–594. [CrossRef]
82. Sterniša, M.; Klančnik, A.; Smole Možina, S. Spoilage Pseudomonas biofilm with *Escherichia coli* protection in fish meat at 5 °C. *J. Sci. Food Agric.* **2019**, *99*, 4635–4641. [CrossRef]
83. Mizan, M.F.R.; Jahid, I.K.; Ha, S.D. Microbial Biofilms in Seafood: A Food-Hygiene Challenge. *Food Microbiol.* **2015**, 41–55. [CrossRef]
84. Toushik, S.H.; Mizan, M.F.R.; Hossain, M.I.; Ha, S.D. Fighting with Old Foes: The Pledge of Microbe-Derived Biological Agents to Defeat Mono- and Mixed-Bacterial Biofilms Concerning Food Industries. *Trends Food Sci. Technol.* **2020**, 413–425. [CrossRef]
85. González, J.E.; Keshavan, N.D. Messing with Bacterial Quorum Sensing. *Microbiol. Mol. Biol. Rev.* **2006**, *70*, 859–875. [CrossRef] [PubMed]
86. Zupančič, J.; Raghupathi, P.K.; Houf, K.; Burmølle, M.; Sørensen, S.J.; Gunde-Cimerman, N. Synergistic interactions in microbial biofilms facilitate the establishment of opportunistic pathogenic Fungi in household dishwashers. *Front. Microbiol.* **2018**, *9*, 21. [CrossRef] [PubMed]
87. Pammi, M.; Liang, R.; Hicks, J.; Mistretta, T.A.; Versalovic, J. Biofilm extracellular DNA enhances mixed species biofilms of *Staphylococcus epidermidis* and *Candida Albicans*. *BMC Microbiol.* **2013**, *13*, 257. [CrossRef]
88. Donlan, R.M.; Piede, J.A.; Heyes, C.D.; Sanii, L.; Murga, R.; Edmonds, P.; El-Sayed, I.; El-Sayed, M.A. Model System for Growing and Quantifying Streptococcus Pneumoniae Biofilms in Situ and in Real Time. *Appl. Environ. Microbiol.* **2004**, *70*, 4980–4988. [CrossRef] [PubMed]
89. Heukelekian, H.; Heller, A. Relation between food concentration and surface forbacterial growth. *J. Bacteriol.* **1940**, *40*, 547–558. [CrossRef] [PubMed]
90. Zobell, C.E. The effect of solid surfaces on bacterial activity. *J. Bacteriol.* **1943**, *46*, 39–56. [CrossRef] [PubMed]
91. Characklis, W.G. Attached microbial growths-II. Frictional resistance due to microbial slimes. *Water Res.* **1973**, *7*, 1249–1258. [CrossRef]
92. Moreno-García, J.; García-Martinez, T.; Moreno, J.; Mauricio, J.C.; Ogawa, M.; Luong, P.; Bisson, L.F. Impact of yeast flocculation and biofilm formation on yeast-fungus coadhesion in a novel immobilization system. *Am. J. Enol. Vitic.* **2018**, *69*, 278–288. [CrossRef]
93. Ogawa, M.; Bisson, L.F.; García-Martínez, T.; Mauricio, J.C.; Moreno-García, J. New Insights on Yeast and Filamentous Fungus Adhesion in a Natural Co-Immobilization System: Proposed Advances and Applications in Wine Industry. *Appl. Microbiol. Biotechnol.* **2019**, *103*, 4723–4731. [CrossRef] [PubMed]
94. Mowat, E.; Lang, S.; Williams, C.; McCulloch, E.; Jones, B.; Ramage, G. Phase-dependent antifungal activity against *Aspergillus fumigatus* developing multiculluar filamentous biofilms. *J. Antimicrob. Chemother.* **2008**, *62*, 1281–1284. [CrossRef]
95. Mowat, E.; Butcher, J.; Lang, S.; Williams, C.; Ramage, G. Development of a simple model for studying the effects of antifungal agents on multicellular communities of *Aspergillus fumigatus*. *J. Med. Microbiol.* **2007**, *56*, 1205–1212. [CrossRef]

96. European Hygienic Engineering and Design Group (EHEDG). *Hygienic Design Principles*, 3rd ed.; EHEDG Guidelines; European Hygienic Engineering & Design Group: Naarden, The Netherlands, 2018.
97. Fortin, N.D. *Regulatory Requirements in the United States on Hygiene Control in the Design, Construction, and Renovation of Food Processing Factories*. Chapter 4 in Hygiene Control in the Design, Construction and Renovation of Food Processing Factories; Lelieveld, H.L.M., Holah, J., Eds.; Woodhead Publishing Ltd., 2011. Available online: https://ssrn.com/abstract=2497425 (accessed on 25 November 2020).
98. Plieth, W. *Electrochemistry for Materials Science*; Elsevier: Amsterdam, The Netherlands, 2008; Chapter 12.
99. Rosado-Castro, M.; da Silva Fernandes, M.; Kabuki, D.Y.; Kuaye, A.Y. Biofilm Formation of *Enterococcus Faecium* on Stainless Steel Surfaces: Modeling and Control by Disinfection Agents. *J. Food Process Eng.* **2018**, *41*, 1–9. [CrossRef]
100. Rosenberg, M.; Kjelleberg, S. Hydrophobic interactions in bacterial adhesion. *Adv. Microb. Ecol.* **1986**, *9*, 353–393.
101. Corpe, W.A. Microbial surface components involved in adsorption of microorganisms onto surfaces. In *Adsorption of Microorganisms to Surfaces*; Bitton, G., Marshall, K.C., Eds.; John Wiley & Sons: New York, NY, USA, 1980; pp. 105–144.
102. Peña, W.E.L.; Andrade, N.J.; Soares, N.F.F.; Alvarenga, V.O.; Rodrigues Junior, S.; Granato, D.; Zuniga, A.D.G.; de Souza Sant'Ana, A. Modeling *Bacillus cereus* adhesion on stainless steel surface as affected by temperature, pH and time. *Int. Dairy J.* **2014**, *34*, 153–158. [CrossRef]
103. Furukawa, S.; Akiyoshi, Y.; Komoriya, M.; Ogihara, H.; Morinaga, Y. Removing *Staphylococcus aureus* and *Escherichia coli* biofilms on stainless steel by cleaning-in-place (CIP) cleaning agents. *Food Control* **2010**, *21*, 669–672. [CrossRef]
104. Bore, E.; Langsrud, S. Characterization of Micro-Organisms Isolated from Dairy Industry after Cleaning and Fogging Disinfection with Alkyl Amine and Peracetic Acid. *J. Appl. Microbiol.* **2005**, *98*, 96–105. [CrossRef]
105. Hawkins, C.L.; Davies, M.J. Hypochlorite-induced oxidation of proteins in plasma: Formation of chloramines and nitrogen-centred radicals and their role in protein fragmentation. *Biochem. J.* **1999**, *340*, 539–548. [CrossRef] [PubMed]
106. Nightingale, Z.D.; Lancha, A.H., Jr.; Handelman, S.K.; Dolnikowski, G.G.; Busse, S.C.; Dratz, E.A.; Blumberg, J.B.; Handelman, G.J. Relative reactivity of lysine and other peptide-bound amino acids to oxidation by hypochlorite. *Free Radic. Biol. Med.* **2000**, *29*, 425–433.
107. Heinecke, J.W.; Li, W.; Daehnke, H.; Goldstein, J.A. Dityrosine, a specific marker of oxidation, is synthesized by the myeloperoxidase-hydrogen peroxide system of human neutrophils and macrophages. *J. Biol. Chem.* **1993**, *268*, 4069–4077. [CrossRef]
108. Spickett, C.M.; Jerlich, A.; Panasenko, O.M.; Arnhold, J.; Pitt, A.R.; Stelmaszynska, T.; Schaur, R.J. The reactions of hypochlorous acid, the reactive oxygen species produced by myeloperoxidase, with lipids. *Acta Biochim. Pol.* **2000**, *47*, 889–899. [CrossRef]
109. Prutz, W.A. Interactions of hypochlorous acid with pyrimidine nucleotides, and secondary reactions of chlorinated pyrimidines with GSH, NADH, and other substrates. *Arch. Biochem. Biophys.* **1998**, *349*, 183–191. [CrossRef] [PubMed]
110. Fukuzaki, S. Mechanisms of actions of sodium hypochlorite in cleaning and disinfection processes. *Biocontrol Sci.* **2006**, *11*, 147–157. [CrossRef] [PubMed]
111. Fernandes, M.S.; Fujimoto, G.; Souza, L.P.; Kabuki, D.Y.; Silva, M.J.; Kuaye, A.Y. Dissemination of *Enterococcus faecalis* and *Enterococcus faecium* in a ricotta processing plant and evaluation of pathogenic and antibiotic resistance profiles. *J. Food Sci.* **2015**, *80*, M765–M775. [CrossRef] [PubMed]
112. Skowron, K.; Hulisz, K.; Gryń, G.; Olszewska, H.; Wiktorczyk, N.; Paluszak, Z. Comparison of selected disinfectants efficiency against *Listeria monocytogenes* biofilm formed on various surfaces. *Int. Microbiol.* **2018**, *21*, 23–33. [CrossRef] [PubMed]
113. Ibusquisa, P.A.; Herrera, J.J.R.; Cabo, M.L. Resistance to benzalkonium chloride, peracetic acid and nisin during formation of mature biofilms by *List. Monocytogenes*. *Food Microbiol.* **2011**, *28*, 418–428. [CrossRef]
114. Eterpi, M.; McDonnell, G.; Thomas, V. Disinfection efficacy against parvoviruses compared with reference viruses. *J. Hosp. Infect.* **2009**, *73*, 64–70. [CrossRef]
115. Langsrud, S.; Sidhu, M.S.; Heir, E.; Holck, A.L. Bacterial Disinfectant Resistance—A Challenge for the Food Industry. *Int. Biodeterior. Biodegrad.* **2003**, *51*, 283–290. [CrossRef]
116. Rasimus, S.; Kolari, M.; Rita, H.; Hoornstra, D.; Salkinoja-Salonen, M. Biofilm-Forming Bacteria with Varying Tolerance to Peracetic Acid from a Paper Machine. *J. Ind. Microbiol. Biotechnol.* **2011**, *38*, 1379–1390. [CrossRef] [PubMed]
117. Russell, A.D. Similarities and differences in the responses of microorganisms to biocides. *J. Antimicrob. Chemother.* **2003**, *52*, 750–763. [CrossRef]
118. Block, S.S. Peroxygen compounds. In *Disinfection, Sterilization, and Preservation*, 5th ed.; Lippincott Williams & Wilkins: Philadelphia, PA, USA, 2001; pp. 185–204.
119. Marquis, R.E.; Rutherford, G.C.; Faraci, M.M.; Shin, S.Y. Sporicidal action of peracetic acid and protective eVects of transition metal ions. *J. Ind. Microbiol.* **1995**, *15*, 486–492. [CrossRef]
120. Dunkin, N.; Weng, S.; Schwab, K.J.; McQuarrie, J.; Bell, K.; Jacangelo, J.G. Comparative inactivation of murine norovirus and MS2 bacteriophage by peracetic acid and monochloramine in municipal secondary wastewater effluent. *Environ. Sci. Technol.* **2017**, *51*, 2972–2981136. [CrossRef]
121. Zhang, C.; Brown, P.J.B.; Miles, R.J.; White, T.A.; Grant, D.A.G.; Stalla, D.; Hu, Z. Inhibition of Regrowth of Planktonic and Biofilm Bacteria after Peracetic Acid Disinfection. *Water Res.* **2019**, *149*, 640–649. [CrossRef] [PubMed]
122. Bridier, A.; Briandet, R.; Thomas, V.; Dubois-Brissonnet, F. Comparative biocidal activity of peracetic acid, benzalkonium chloride and ortho-phthalaldehyde on 77 bacterial strains. *J. Hosp. Infect.* **2011**, *78*, 208–213. [CrossRef] [PubMed]

123. Vázquez-Sánchez, D.; Cabo, M.L.; Ibusquiza, P.S.; Rodríguez-Herrera, J.J. Biofilm-forming ability and resistance to industrial disinfectants of *Staphylococcus aureus* isolated from fishery products. *Food Control.* **2014**, *39*, 8–16. [CrossRef]
124. Mah, T.F.C.; O'Toole, G.A. Mechanisms of biofilm resistance to antimicrobial agents. *Trends Microbiol.* **2001**, *9*, 34–39. [CrossRef]
125. Marić, S.; Vraneš, J. Characteristics and Significance of Microbial Biofilm Formation. *Period. Biol.* **2007**, *109*, 115–121.
126. Beveridge, T.J.; Makin, S.A.; Kadurugamuwa, J.L.; Li, Z. Interactions between biofilms and the environment. *FEMS Microbiol. Rev.* **1997**, *20*, 291–303. [CrossRef]
127. Flemming, H.C. Biofilms and environmental protection. *Water Sci. Technol.* **1993**, *27*, 1–10. [CrossRef]
128. Da Costa, J.B.; Rodgher, S.; Daniel, L.A.; Espíndola, E.L.G. Toxicity on aquatic organisms exposed to secondary effluent disinfected with chlorine, peracetic acid, ozone and UV radiation. *Ecotoxicology* **2014**, *23*, 1803–1813. [CrossRef]
129. Ferriol-González, C.; Domingo-Calap, P. Phages for Biofilm Removal. *Antibiotics* **2020**, *9*, 268. [CrossRef]
130. Hiom, S.J.; Lowe, C.; Oldcorne, M. Assessment of surface bioburden during hospital aseptic processing. *Int. J. Pharm. Pract.* **2003**, *11*, R62.
131. Wang, Y.; Tan, X.; Xi, C.; Phillips, K.S. Removal of Staphylococcus aureus from skin using a combination antibiofilm approach. *NPJ Biofilms Microbiomes.* **2018**, *4*, 1–9. [CrossRef]
132. Vaidya, M.Y.; McBain, A.J.; Butler, J.A.; Banks, C.E.; Whitehead, K.A. Antimicrobial efficacy and synergy of metal ions against *Enterococcus faecium, Klebsiella pneumoniae* and *Acinetobacter baumannii* in planktonic and biofilm phenotypes. *Sci. Rep.* **2017**, *7*, 1–9. [CrossRef] [PubMed]
133. Miao, J.; Liang, Y.; Chen, L.; Wang, W.; Wang, J.; Li, B.; Li, L.; Chen, D.; Xu, Z. Formation and development of Staphylococcus biofilm: With focus on food safety. *J. Food Saf.* **2017**, *37*, e12358. [CrossRef]
134. Cacciatore, F.A.; Brandelli, A.; Malheiros, P.D.S. Combining natural antimicrobials and nanotechnology for disinfecting food surfaces and control microbial biofilm formation. *Crit. Rev. Food Sci. Nutr.* **2020**, 1–12. [CrossRef] [PubMed]
135. Iacumin, L.; Manzano, M.; Comi, G. Phage Inactivation of Listeria Monocytogenes on San Daniele Dry-Cured Ham and Elimination of Biofilms from Equipment and Working Environments. *Microorganisms* **2016**, *4*, 4. [CrossRef] [PubMed]
136. Greer, G.G. Bacteriophage control of foodborne bacteria. *J. Food Prot.* **2011**, *68*, 1102–1111. [CrossRef]
137. Soni, K.A.; Nannapaneni, R. Bacteriophage significantly reduces *L. monocytogenes* on raw salmon fillet tissue. *J. Food Prot.* **2010**, *73*, 32–38. [CrossRef]
138. Gironés, R.R.G.; Simmons, M.M. Evaluation of the safety and efficacy of ListexTM P100 for reduction of pathogens on different ready-to-eat (RTE) food products. *EFSA J.* **2016**, *14*, 4565.
139. Marsden, J.L. *The Effectiveness of Listex P100 in Reducing Listeria monocytogenes in RTE Food*; Food Science Institute, Kansas State University; Available online: https://www.foodsafetynews.com/files/2013/05/Listex-P100-Final-Report-1-2.pdf (accessed on 1 December 2020).
140. Choi, N.Y.; Baek, S.Y.; Yoon, J.H.; Choi, M.R.; Kang, D.H.; Lee, S.Y. Efficacy of aerosolized hydrogen peroxide-based sanitizer on the reduction of pathogenic bacteria on a stainless steel surface. *Food Control.* **2012**, *27*, 57–63. [CrossRef]
141. Park, S.H.; Cheon, H.L.; Park, K.H.; Chung, M.S.; Choi, S.H.; Ryu, S.; Kang, D.H. Inactivation of biofilm cells of foodborne pathogen by aerosolized sanitizers. *Int. J. Food Microbiol.* **2012**, *154*, 130–134. [CrossRef]
142. Del Pozo, J.L.; Patel, R. The challenge of treating biofilm-associated bacterial infections. *Clin. Pharmacol. Ther.* **2007**, *82*, 204–209. [CrossRef] [PubMed]
143. Anghel, I.; Holban, A.M.; Grumezescu, A.M.; Andronescu, E.; Ficai, A.; Anghel, A.G.; Maganu, M.; Lazăr, V.; Chifiriuc, M.C. Modified wound dressing with phyto-nanostructured coating to prevent staphylococcal and pseudomonal biofilm development. *Nanoscale Res. Lett.* **2012**, *7*, 1–8. [CrossRef] [PubMed]
144. De Kievit, T.R.; Iglewski, B.H. Bacterial quorum sensing in pathogenic relationships. *Infect. Immun.* **2000**, *68*, 4839–4849. [CrossRef]
145. Sajjan, U.; Moreira, J.; Liu, M.; Humar, A.; Chaparro, C.; Forstner, J.; Keshavjee, S. A novel model to study bacterial adherence to the transplanted airway: Inhibition of *Burkholderia cepacia* adherence to human airway by dextran and xylitol. *J. Heart Lung Transplant.* **2012**, *23*, 1382–1391. [CrossRef]
146. Singh, P.K.; Schaefer, A.L.; Parsek, M.R.; Moninger, T.O.; Welsh, M.J.; Greenberg, E.P. Quorum-sensing signals indicate that cystic fibrosis lungs are infected with bacterial biofilms. *Nature* **2000**, *407*, 762–764. [CrossRef] [PubMed]
147. Xiong, F.; Zhao, X.; Wen, D.; Li, Q. Effects of N-acyl-homoserine lactones-based quorum sensing on biofilm formation, sludge characteristics, and bacterial community during the start-up of bioaugmented reactors. *Sci. Total Environ.* **2020**, *735*, 139449. [CrossRef]
148. Schuster, M.; Joseph Sexton, D.; Diggle, S.P.; Peter Greenberg, E. Acyl-homoserine lactone quorum sensing: From evolution to application. *Annu. Rev. Microbiol.* **2013**, *67*, 43–63. [CrossRef]
149. Wang, J.; Liu, Q.; Ma, S.; Hu, H.; Wu, B.; Zhang, X.X.; Ren, H. Distribution characteristics of N-acyl homoserine lactones during the moving bed biofilm reactor biofilm development process: Effect of carbon/nitrogen ratio and exogenous quorum sensing signals. *Bioresour. Technol.* **2019**, *289*, 121591. [CrossRef]
150. Maddela, N.R.; Sheng, B.; Yuan, S.; Zhou, Z.; Villamar-Torres, R.; Meng, F. Roles of quorum sensing in biological wastewater treatment: A critical review. *Chemosphere* **2019**, *221*, 616–629. [CrossRef]
151. Pu, H.; Xu, Y.; Sun, D.-W.; Wei, Q.; Li, X. Optical nanosensors for biofilm detection in the food industry: Principles, applications and challenges. *Crit. Rev. Food Sci. Nutr.* **2020**, 1–18. [CrossRef]

152. Jayan, H.; Pu, H.; Sun, D.-W. Recent development in rapid detection techniques for microorganism activities in food matrices using bio-recognition: A review. *Trends Food Sci. Technol.* **2020**, *95*, 233–246. [CrossRef]
153. Lv, M.; Liu, Y.; Geng, J.; Kou, X.; Xin, Z.; Yang, D. Engineering nanomaterials-based biosensors for food safety detection. *Biosens. Bioelectron.* **2018**, *106*, 122–128. [CrossRef] [PubMed]
154. Zhang, P.; Chen, Y.P.; Qiu, J.H.; Dai, Y.Z.; Feng, B. Imaging the microprocesses in biofilm matrices. *Trends Biotechnol.* **2019**, *37*, 214–226. [CrossRef]
155. Ivleva, N.P.; Kubryk, P.; Niessner, R. Raman microspectroscopy, surface-enhanced Raman scattering microspectroscopy, and stable-isotope Raman microspectroscopy for biofilm characterization. *Anal. Bioanal. Chem.* **2017**, *409*, 4353–4375. [CrossRef]
156. Vanegas, D.C.; Gomes, C.L.; Cavallaro, N.D.; Giraldo-Escobar, D.; McLamore, E.S. Emerging biorecognition and transduction schemes for rapid detection of pathogenic bacteria in food. *Compr. Rev. Food Sci. Food Saf.* **2017**, *16*, 1188–1205. [CrossRef] [PubMed]
157. Pantanella, F.; Valenti, P.; Natalizi, T.; Passeri, D.; Berlutti, F. Analytical Techniques to Study Microbial Biofilm on Abiotic Surfaces: Pros and Cons of the Main Techniques Currently in Use. *Ann. Ig. Med. Prev. E Comunità* **2013**, *25*, 31–42. [CrossRef]
158. Azeredo, J.; Azevedo, N.F.; Briandet, R.; Cerca, N.; Coenye, T.; Costa, A.R.; Desvaux, M.; Di Bonaventura, G.; Hébraud, M.; Jaglic, Z.; et al. Critical Review on Biofilm Methods. *Crit. Rev. Microbiol.* **2017**, *43*, 313–351. [CrossRef] [PubMed]
159. Huang, Y.; Chakraborty, S.; Liang, H. Methods to Probe the Formation of Biofilms: Applications in Foods and Related Surfaces. *Anal. Methods* **2020**, *12*, 416–432. [CrossRef]
160. Nijland, R.; Hall, M.J.; Burgess, J.G. Dispersal of biofilms by secreted, matrix degrading, bacterial DNase. *PLoS ONE* **2010**, *5*, e15668. [CrossRef] [PubMed]
161. Jamal, M.; Ahmad, W.; Andleeb, S.; Jalil, F.; Imran, M.; Nawaz, M.A.; Hussain, T.; Ali, M.; Rafiq, M.; Kamil, M.A. Bacterial Biofilm and Associated Infections. *J. Chin. Med. Assoc.* **2018**, *81*, 7–11. [CrossRef]
162. Ansari, M.A.; Khan, H.M.; Khan, A.A.; Cameotra, S.S.; Alzohairy, M.A. Anti-biofilm efficacy of silver nanoparticles against MRSA and MRSE isolated from wounds in a tertiary care hospital. *Indian J. Med. Microbiol.* **2015**, *33*, 101. [CrossRef]
163. Lawrence, J.R.; Neu, T.R. Confocal laser scanning microscopy for analysis of microbial biofilms. *Methods Enzymol.* **1999**, *310*, 131–144. [PubMed]
164. Kania, R.E.; Lamers, G.E.; Vonk, M.J.; Huy, P.T.B.; Hiemstra, P.S.; Bloemberg, G.V.; Grote, J.J. Demonstration of bacterial cells and glycocalyx in biofilms on human tonsils. *Arch. Otolaryngol. Head Neck Surg.* **2007**, *133*, 115–121. [CrossRef]
165. Ommen, P.; Zobek, N.; Meyer, R.L. Quantification of Biofilm Biomass by Staining: Non-Toxic Safranin Can Replace the Popular Crystal Violet. *J. Microbiol. Methods* **2017**, *141*, 87–89. [CrossRef]
166. Stepanović, S.; Vuković, D.; Dakić, I.; Savić, B.; Švabić-Vlahović, M. A Modified Microtiter-Plate Test for Quantification of Staphylococcal Biofilm Formation. *J. Microbiol. Methods* **2000**, *40*, 175–179. [CrossRef]
167. Doll, K.; Jongsthaphongpun, K.L.; Stumpp, N.S.; Winkel, A.; Stiesch, M. Quantifying Implant-Associated Biofilms: Comparison of Microscopic, Microbiologic and Biochemical Methods. *J. Microbiol. Methods* **2016**, *130*, 61–68. [CrossRef]
168. Extremina, C.I.; Costa, L.; Aguiar, A.I.; Peixe, L.; Fonseca, A.P. Optimization of processing conditions for the quantification of enterococci biofilms using microtitreplates. *J. Microbiol. Methods* **2010**. [CrossRef]
169. Stiefel, P.; Rosenberg, U.; Schneider, J.; Mauerhofer, S. Is biofilm removal properly assessed? Comparison of different quantification methods in a 96-well plate system. *Appl. Microbiol. Biotechnol.* **2016**, *100*, 4135–4145. [CrossRef]
170. Romanova, N.A.; Gawande, P.V.; Brovko, L.Y.; Griffiths, M.W. Rapid Methods to Assess Sanitizing Efficacy of Benzalkonium Chloride to Listeria Monocytogenes Biofilms. *J. Microbiol. Methods* **2007**, *71*, 231–237. [CrossRef] [PubMed]
171. Cell Staining. 2019. Available online: https://www.dojindo.com/ (accessed on 2 December 2020).
172. Burton, E.; Yakandawala, N.; LoVetri, K.; Madhyastha, M.S. A Microplate Spectrofluorometric Assay for Bacterial Biofilms. *J. Ind. Microbiol. Biotechnol.* **2007**, *34*, 1–4. [CrossRef]
173. Deng, Y.; Wang, L.; Chen, Y.; Long, Y. Optimization of Staining with SYTO 9/Propidium Iodide: Interplay, Kinetics and Impact on Brevibacillus Brevis. *BioTechniques* **2020**, *69*, 89–99. [CrossRef]
174. Shi, L.; Gunther, S.; Hubschmann, T.; Wick, L.Y.; Harms, H.; Muller, S. Limits of propidium iodide as a cell viability indicator for environmental bacteria. *Cytom. A* **2007**, *71*, 592–598. [CrossRef] [PubMed]
175. Munukka, E.; Leppäranta, O.; Korkeamäki, M.; Vaahtio, M.; Peltola, T.; Zhang, D.; Hupa, L.; Ylänen, H.; Salonen, J.I.; Viljanen, M.K.; et al. Bactericidal effects of bioactive glasses on clinically important aerobic bacteria. *J. Mater. Sci. Mater. Med.* **2008**, *19*, 27–32. [CrossRef] [PubMed]
176. Larrosa, M.; Truchado, P.; Espin, J.C.; Tomás-Barberán, F.A.; Allende, A.; García-Conesa, M.T. Evaluation of *Pseudomonas aeruginosa* (PAO1) adhesion to human alveolar epithelial cells A549 using SYTO 9 dye. *Mol. Cell. Probes* **2012**, *26*, 121–126. [CrossRef] [PubMed]
177. Maukonen, J.; Mattila-Sandholm, T.; Wirtanen, G. Metabolic Indicators for Assessing Bacterial Viability in Hygiene Sampling Using Cells in Suspension and Swabbed Biofilm. *LWT Food Sci. Technol.* **2000**, *33*, 225–233. [CrossRef]
178. Tawakoli, P.N.; Al-Ahmad, A.; Hoth-Hannig, W.; Hannig, M.; Hannig, C. Comparison of different live/dead stainings for detection and quantification of adherent microorganisms in the initial oral biofilm. *Clin. Oral Investig.* **2013**, *17*, 841–850. [CrossRef]
179. Verran, J. Biofouling in food processing: Biofilm or biotransfer potential? *Food Bioprod. Process.* **2002**, *80*, 292–298. [CrossRef]

180. Verran, J.; Whitehead, K.A. Assessment of organic materials and microbial components on hygienic surfaces. *Food Bioprod. Process.* **2006**, *84*, 260–264. [CrossRef]
181. Declerck, P.; Verelst, L.; Duvivier, L.; Van Damme, A.; Ollevier, F. A detection method for *Legionella* spp. in (cooling) water: Fluorescent in situ hybridisation (FISH) on whole bacteria. *Water Sci. Technol.* **2003**, *47*, 143–146. [CrossRef] [PubMed]
182. Whitehead, K.A.; Benson, P.; Verran, J. Differential fluorescent staining of *Listeria monocytogenes* and a whey food soil for quantitative analysis of surface hygiene. *Int. J. Food Microbiol.* **2009**, *135*, 75–80. [CrossRef] [PubMed]
183. Almeida, C.; Azevedo, N.F.; Santos, S.; Keevil, C.W.; Vieira, M.J. Discriminating Multi-Species Populations in Biofilms with Peptide Nucleic Acid Fluorescence in Situ Hybridization (PNA FISH). *PLoS ONE* **2011**, *6*. [CrossRef] [PubMed]
184. Hansen, S.K.; Rainey, P.B.; Haagensen, J.A.; Molin, S. Evolution of species interactions in a biofilm community. *Nature* **2007**, *445*, 533–536. [CrossRef] [PubMed]
185. Gu, F.; Lux, R.; Du-Thumm, L.; Stokes, I.; Kreth, J.; Anderson, M.H.; Wong, D.T.; Wolinsky, L.; Sullivan, R.; Shi, W. In situ and noninvasive detection of specific bacterial species in oral biofilms using fluorescently labeled monoclonal antibodies. *J. Microbiol. Methods* **2005**, *62*, 145–160. [CrossRef]
186. Schlafer, S.; Meyer, R.L. Confocal Microscopy Imaging of the Biofilm Matrix. *J. Microbiol. Methods* **2017**, *138*, 50–59. [CrossRef]
187. Allesen-Holm, M.; Barken, K.B.; Yang, L.; Klausen, M.; Webb, J.S.; Kjelleberg, S.; Molin, S.; Givskov, M.; Tolker-Nielsen, T. A characterization of DNA release in *Pseudomonas aeruginosa* cultures and biofilms. *Mol. Microbiol.* **2006**, *59*, 1114–1128. [CrossRef]
188. Conover, M.S.; Mishra, M.; Deora, R. Extracellular DNA is essential for maintaining Bordetella biofilm integrity on abiotic surfaces and in the upper respiratory tract of mice. *PLoS ONE* **2011**, *6*, e16861. [CrossRef]
189. Okshevsky, M.; Meyer, R.L. Evaluation of fluorescent stains for visualizing extracellular DNA in biofilms. *J. Microbiol. Methods* **2014**, *105*, 102–104. [CrossRef]
190. Schaeffer, C.R.; Woods, K.M.; Longo, G.M.; Kiedrowski, M.R.; Paharik, A.E.; Büttner, H.; Christner, M.; Boissy, R.J.; Horswill, A.R.; Rohde, H.; et al. Accumulation-associated protein enhances Staphylococcus epidermidis biofilm formation under dynamic conditions and is required for infection in a rat catheter model. *Infect. Immun.* **2015**, *83*, 214–226. [CrossRef]
191. Büttner, H.; Mack, D.; Rohde, H. Structural basis of *Staphylococcus epidermidis* biofilm formation: Mechanisms and molecular interactions. *Front. Cell. Infect. Microbiol.* **2015**, *5*, 14. [CrossRef]
192. Frank, K.L.; Patel, R. Poly-N-acetylglucosamine is not a major component of the extracellular matrix in biofilms formed by icaADBC-positive *Staphylococcus lugdunensis* isolates. *Infect. Immun.* **2007**, *75*, 4728–4742. [CrossRef]
193. Toyofuku, M.; Roschitzki, B.; Riedel, K.; Eberl, L. Identification of proteins associated with the Pseudomonas aeruginosa biofilm extracellular matrix. *J. Proteome Res.* **2012**, *11*, 4906–4915. [CrossRef]
194. Tseng, B.S.; Reichhardt, C.; Merrihew, G.E.; Araujo-Hernandez, S.A.; Harrison, J.J.; MacCoss, M.J.; Parsek, M.R. A biofilm matrix-associated protease inhibitor protects Pseudomonas aeruginosa from proteolytic attack. *MBio* **2018**, *9*. [CrossRef]
195. Dige, I.; Nyengaard, J.R.; Kilian, M.; Nyvad, B. Application of stereological principles for quantification of bacteria in intact dental biofilms. *Oral Microbiol. Immunol.* **2009**, *24*, 69–75. [CrossRef] [PubMed]
196. Malic, S.; Hill, K.E.; Hayes, A.; Percival, S.L.; Thomas, D.W.; Williams, D.W. Detection and identification of specific bacteria in wound biofilms using peptide nucleic acid fluorescent in situ hybridization (PNA FISH). *Microbiology* **2009**, *155*, 2603–2611. [CrossRef]
197. Ivleva, N.P.; Wagner, M.; Horn, H.; Niessner, R.; Haisch, C. Towards a Nondestructive Chemical Characterization of Biofilm Matrix by Raman Microscopy. *Anal. Bioanal. Chem.* **2009**, *393*, 197–206. [CrossRef] [PubMed]
198. Jung, G.B.; Nam, S.W.; Choi, S.; Lee, G.-J.; Park, H.-K. Evaluation of Antibiotic Effects on *Pseudomonas aeruginosa* Biofilm Using Raman Spectroscopy and Multivariate Analysis. *Biomed. Opt. Express* **2014**, *5*, 3238. [CrossRef]
199. Fallatah, H.; Elhaneid, M.; Ali-Boucetta, H.; Overton, T.W.; El Kadri, H.; Gkatzionis, K. Antibacterial effect of graphene oxide (GO) nano-particles against *Pseudomonas putida* biofilm of variable age. *Environ. Sci. Pollut. Res.* **2019**, *26*, 25057–25070. [CrossRef]
200. Vuotto, C.; Donelli, G. Field Emission Scanning Electron Microscopy of Biofilm-Growing Bacteria Involved in Nosocomial Infections. In *Microbial Biofilms. Methods in Molecular Biology (Methods and Protocols)*; Donelli, G., Ed.; Humana Press: New York, NY, USA, 2014. [CrossRef]
201. Kouider, N.; Hamadi, F.; Mallouki, B.; Bengoram, J.; Mabrouki, M.; Zekraoui, M.; Ellouali, M.; Latrache, H. Effect of stainless steel surface roughness on Staphylococcus aureus adhesion. *Int. J. Pure Appl. Sci.* **2010**, *4*, 17.
202. Mallouki, B.; Latrache, H.; Mabrouki, M.; Outzourhit, A.; Hamadi, F.; Muller, D.; Ellouali, M. The inhibitory effect of fucans on adhesion and production of slime of Staphylococcus Aureus. *Microbiol. Hygiène Aliment.* **2007**, *19*, 6471.
203. El Abed, S.; Ibnsouda, S.K.; Latrache, H.; Hamadi, F. Scanning electron microscopy (SEM) and environmental SEM: Suitable tools for study of adhesion stage and biofilm formation. In *Scanning Electron Microscopy*; Intechopen: London, UK, 2012.
204. Agarwal, A.; Jern Ng, W.; Liu, Y. Removal of biofilms by intermittent low-intensity ultrasonication triggered bursting of microbubbles. *Biofouling* **2014**, *30*, 359–365. [CrossRef] [PubMed]
205. Fricke, K.; Koban, I.; Tresp, H.; Jablonowski, L.; Schröder, K.; Kramer, A.; Weltmann, K.D.; von Woedtke, T.; Kocher, T. Atmospheric Pressure Plasma: A High-Performance Tool for the Efficient Removal of Biofilms. *PLoS ONE* **2012**, *7*, e42539. [CrossRef] [PubMed]
206. Chan, T.F.; Esedoglu, S.; Nikolova, M. Algorithms for finding global minimizers of image segmentation and denoising models. *Siam. J. Appl. Math.* **2002**, *66*, 1632–1648. [CrossRef]
207. Vyas, N.; Sammons, R.L.; Addison, O.; Dehghani, H.; Walmsley, A.D. A quantitative method to measure biofilm removal efficiency from complex biomaterial surfaces using SEM and image analysis. *Sci. Rep.* **2016**, *6*, 32694. [CrossRef]

208. Hu, H.; Johani, K.; Gosbell, I.B.; Jacombs, A.S.W.; Almatroudi, A.; Whiteley, G.S.; Deva, A.K.; Jensen, S.; Vickery, K. Intensive care unit environmental surfaces are contaminated by multidrug-resistant bacteria in biofilms: Combined results of conventional culture, pyrosequencing, scanning electron microscopy, and confocal laser microscopy. *J. Hosp. Infect.* **2015**, *91*, 35–44. [CrossRef]
209. Mohmmed, S.A.; Vianna, M.E.; Penny, M.R.; Hilton, S.T.; Mordan, N.; Knowles, J.C. Confocal laser scanning, scanning electron, and transmission electron microscopy investigation of *Enterococcus faecalis* biofilm degradation using passive and active sodium hypochlorite irrigation within a simulated root canal model. *Microbiologyopen* **2017**, *6*, e00455. [CrossRef] [PubMed]
210. Bodelón, G.; Montes-García, V.; Costas, C.; Pérez-Juste, I.; Pérez-Juste, J.; Pastoriza-Santos, I.; Liz-Marzán, L.M. Imaging bacterial interspecies chemical interactions by surface-enhanced Raman scattering. *ACS Nano* **2017**, *11*, 4631–4640. [CrossRef]
211. Whitehead, K.A.; Saubade, F.; Akhidime, I.D.; Liauw, C.M.; Benson, P.S.; Verran, J. The detection and quantification of food components on stainless steel surfaces following use in an operational bakery. *Food Bioprod. Process.* **2019**, *116*, 258–267. [CrossRef]
212. Xu, H.S.; Roberts, N.; Singleton, F.L.; Attwell, R.W.; Grimes, D.J.; Colwell, R.R. Survival and viability of nonculturable *Escherichia coli* and *Vibrio cholerae* in the estuarine and marine environment. *Microb. Ecol.* **1982**, *8*, 313–323. [CrossRef]
213. Li, L.; Mendis, N.; Trigui, H.; Oliver, J.D.; Faucher, S.P. The importance of the viable but non-culturable state in human bacterial pathogens. *Front. Microbiol.* **2014**, *5*, 258. [CrossRef]
214. Cerca, F.; Andrade, F.; França, Â.; Andrade, E.B.; Ribeiro, A.; Almeida, A.A.; Cerca, N.; Pier, G.; Azeredo, J.; Vilanova, M. *Staphylococcus epidermidis* biofilms with higher proportions of dormant bacteria induce a lower activation of murine macrophages. *J. Med. Microbiol.* **2011**, *60*, 1717–1724. [CrossRef]
215. Oliveira, F.; Lima, C.A.; Brás, S.; França, Â.; Cerca, N. Evidence for interand intraspecies biofilm formation variability among a small group of coagulase-negative staphylococci. *FEMS Microbiol. Lett.* **2015**, 362. [CrossRef]
216. Bayoumi, M.A.; Kamal, R.M.; Abd El Aal, S.F.; Awad, E.I. Assessment of a regulatory sanitization process in Egyptian dairy plants in regard to the adherence of some food-borne pathogens and their biofilms. *Int. J. Food Microbiol.* **2012**, *158*, 225–231. [CrossRef] [PubMed]
217. Khaddouj, A.; Fatima, H.; Rachida, M.; Hassan, L.; Khadija, A.; Youssef, N.; Mustapha, M. Evaluation of sodium hypochlorite efficiency on the elimination of *Pseudomonas aeruginosa* biofilm using two methods. *Russ. Open Med. J.* **2019**, *8*, e0302.
218. Bremer, P.J.; Fillery, S.; McQuillan, A.J. Laboratory scale Clean-In-Place (CIP) studies on the effectiveness of different caustic and acid wash steps on the removal of dairy biofilms. *Int. J. Food Microbiol.* **2006**, *106*, 254–262. [CrossRef] [PubMed]
219. Lebeaux, D.; Ghigo, J.M.; Beloin, C. Biofilm-related infections: Bridging the gap between clinical management and fundamental aspects of recalcitrance toward antibiotics. *Microbiol. Mol. Biol. Rev.* **2014**, *78*, 510–543. [CrossRef] [PubMed]

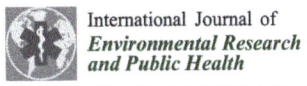

Review

Texture-Modified Food for Dysphagic Patients: A Comprehensive Review

Dele Raheem [1], Conrado Carrascosa [2,*], Fernando Ramos [3,4], Ariana Saraiva [2] and António Raposo [5,*]

1. Northern Institute for Environmental and Minority Law (NIEM), Arctic Centre, University of Lapland, 96101 Rovaniemi, Finland; braheem@ulapland.fi
2. Department of Animal Pathology and Production, Bromatology and Food Technology, Faculty of Veterinary, Universidad de Las Palmas de Gran Canaria, Trasmontaña s/n, 35413 Arucas, Spain; ariana_23@outlook.pt
3. Pharmacy Faculty, University of Coimbra, Azinhaga de Santa Comba, 3000-548 Coimbra, Portugal; framos@ff.uc.pt
4. REQUIMTE/LAQV, R. D. Manuel II, Apartado 55142, 4051-401 Porto, Portugal
5. CBIOS (Research Center for Biosciences and Health Technologies), Universidade Lusófona de Humanidades e Tecnologias, Campo Grande 376, 1749-024 Lisboa, Portugal
* Correspondence: conrado.carrascosa@ulpgc.es (C.C.); antonio.raposo@ulusofona.pt (A.R.)

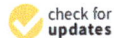

Citation: Raheem, D.; Carrascosa, C.; Ramos, F.; Saraiva, A.; Raposo, A. Texture-Modified Food for Dysphagic Patients: A Comprehensive Review. *Int. J. Environ. Res. Public Health* **2021**, *18*, 5125. https://doi.org/10.3390/ijerph18105125

Academic Editor: Alberto Mantovani

Received: 5 March 2021
Accepted: 8 May 2021
Published: 12 May 2021

Publisher's Note: MDPI stays neutral with regard to jurisdictional claims in published maps and institutional affiliations.

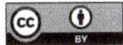

Copyright: © 2021 by the authors. Licensee MDPI, Basel, Switzerland. This article is an open access article distributed under the terms and conditions of the Creative Commons Attribution (CC BY) license (https://creativecommons.org/licenses/by/4.0/).

Abstract: Food texture is a major food quality parameter. The physicochemical properties of food changes when processed in households or industries, resulting in modified textures. A better understanding of these properties is important for the sensory and textural characteristics of foods that target consumers of all ages, from children to the elderly, especially when food product development is considered for dysphagia. Texture modifications in foods suitable for dysphagic patients will grow as the numbers of elderly citizens increase. Dysphagia management should ensure that texture-modified (TM) food is nutritious and easy to swallow. This review addresses how texture and rheology can be assessed in the food industry by placing particular emphasis on dysphagia. It also discusses how the structure of TM food depends not only on food ingredients, such as hydrocolloids, emulsifiers, and thickening and gelling agents, but also on the applied processing methods, including microencapsulation, microgels as delivery systems, and 3D printing. In addition, we address how to modify texture for individuals with dysphagia in all age groups, and highlight different strategies to develop appropriate food products for dysphagic patients.

Keywords: dysphagia; the elderly; food industry; food products; nutrition; processing; rheology; texture

1. Introduction

Food colloids are multi-component, multi-phase systems, involving a complex mixture of water, proteins, polysaccharides, lipids, and many minor constituents that contribute to food textures [1]. While eating and swallowing food, sensory tasks require the tongue's motor behavior to explore, squeeze, or move a bolus to ascertain its flow properties [2]. However, eating and swallowing food can pose problems that result in dysphagia; those with this condition are dysphagic patients.

Dysphagia refers to difficulty in swallowing, or sometimes the impossibility of swallow liquid or semisolid/solid food [3]. This condition affects almost 580 million people worldwide, especially infants and the elderly, and it leads to nutritional deficiencies [4,5]. As populations in many developed countries age, the number of dysphagic patients is likely to rise. Approximately 2 billion people will be aged 60 and over by 2050, in many countries, (e.g., Japan, Germany and Korea); around 15% of their populations will be over 80 years old [6]. The older population is the global population's fastest growing segment. Average life expectancy at birth is expected to rise from the present 70 years to 77 years by 2045, with more than 400 million individuals older than 80 years by 2050 [7]. Hence, urgent attention must be paid to the food and nutrition requirements of the elderly, particularly those who are very old and frail. This creates an excellent opportunity for food scientists to respond by formulating food products that meet this demand [8]. Apart from the elderly, and infants whose muscle mass and strength—related to swallowing foods—are weak, those with other medical conditions, such as trauma, cancer, surgery, cerebral palsy, stroke, and other neurological conditions in any age group, may also suffer dysphagia.

Modifying food texture and liquid thickness, without compromising nutritional quality, will play a key role in dysphagia management to ensure that patients can meet their nutritional requirements [9]. For example, studies on bolus rheology by Ishihara et al. [10] suggest that bolus viscoelasticity balance is important to ease swallowing. Other researchers recommended that food texture for dysphagia diets be soft, smooth, moist, elastic, and easy to swallow [11,12]. Handling viscous food components will involve more studies on their rheological parameters. However, a general understanding of the parameters defining texture-modified (TM) food for dysphagia patients worldwide is generally lacking. One extremely important matter for dysphagia management and treatment is to implement the same terminology for it to be universally accepted. A classification system for food viscosity and texture based on sound empirical evidence to help with dysphagia management is necessary. There is a gap in communicating and collaborating among experts in food services and clinical staff. To bridge this gap, in 2012, the International Dysphagia Diet Standardization Initiative (IDDSI) was founded to provide a globally standardized terminology and definitions for TM food and liquids that are applicable to dysphagia individuals of all ages, in all care settings, and for all cultures [13]. We need to conduct more studies to maintain a valid and quantitatively defined scale for different food/fluid textures that can be tested under clinical conditions. Likewise, developing standard recipes for TM food and fluid is also important. For example, in order to provide foods with suitable textures to dysphagic patients, healthcare personnel will have to communicate what this texture is to food producers.

Texture is a sensory multiparameter attribute. It includes all the attributes of the rheological and structural properties of a food product, perceptible by mechanical, visual, auditory and tactile preceptors [14,15]. The roots of the multiparameter attributes of texture lies in its molecular, microscopic, or macroscopic structure. Moreover, certain texture aspects can be seen by the naked eye (e.g., coarse or fine cake texture) or heard by ears (e.g., sounds made when biting on a crunchy celery stalk or a crisp piece of toast) [16]. Dysphagic patients need nutritious foods; such foods need to be of the right texture to improve their consumption and deliver the required nutrients. The need for better intervention strategies is addressed in previous works that target elderly hospitalized patients; this is important because it has the potential to improve patient treatments and outcomes [17]. There are concerns that some TM strategies, such as the IDDSI, do not address the nutritional aspects of foods [9].

Food industries are concerned about variations in taste that come about with changes in viscosity and flow behavior. For instance, evidence suggests that increasing solution viscosity in regular syrup substantially lowers taste intensity, while an increased non-Newtonian flow property observed in light syrup diminishes taste intensity [18]. A better understanding of rheological properties would allow the systemic development of food products to be designed for desired texture and taste interactions. Texture, for many food materials, is a key quality factor. Knowledge gained from the rheological and mechanical properties of various food systems will be relevant for designing flow processes to ensure quality, and to predict storage and stability measurements. Rheological behavior is directly associated with sensory qualities, which significantly influence taste, mouth feel, and stable shelf life. Hence, there is a need for caterers and food scientists to formulate suitable food products for aging populations, which requires a classification system based on rheological properties, consistency, and texture for dysphagia management. These products can be developed for dysphagic patients by blending food ingredients according to personalized recipes for TM food and fluids [19]. To supply dysphagic patients with appropriately textured food, healthcare personnel have to communicate this texture to food service providers by utilizing the same terminology in dysphagia management and treatment [20].

In order to overcome this dilemma, a guide for TM food was developed, in collaboration with dieticians, speech and language pathologists, and a food company specialized in TM diets (Table 1). The purpose of this guide was to develop different food texture definitions based on several Swedish documents. This guide was influenced by the guidelines developed by the British Dietetic Association in collaboration with the Royal College of Speech and Language Therapists [21,22]. It was a pioneering work in the early years (2000–2002), which objectively defined and quantified categories of texture-modified food by conducting rheological measurements and sensory analyses [23]. However, there are limitations in the work, as analyses were conducted on 15 representative TM sample food items. Moreover, individual medical research will be needed to provide diet recommendations to dysphagic patients.

Table 1. Descriptions of the consistencies in the texture guide [23].

Category	Description	Example
Regular or cut	Normal texture, possibly cut into smaller pieces.	Whole or cut meat, whole fish, meat or sausage dishes, vegetables, potatoes and gravy. Fresh fruit or canned fruit with whipped cream or ice cream.
Coarse pâtés	Grainy, porous soft texture with coarse grains, such as a juicy and soft meatloaf. Easy to cut with a fork.	Coarse meat pâté or whole steamed fish, coarse vegetable pâté or well-cooked vegetables, whole or pressed potatoes, and gravy. Canned fruit in pieces with whipped cream or ice cream.
Timbales	Smooth, soft, short, and uniform consistency, similar to an omelet. Can be eaten with a fork or spoon.	Meat or fish timbale/soufflé, vegetable timbale/purée, mashed/pressed potatoes, and gravy. Fruit mousse with whipped cream or ice cream.
Jellied products	Soft and slippery food, such as mousse. Can be eaten with a fork or spoon.	Cold jellied meat or fish, vegetable purée or cold jellied vegetables, mashed potatoes, and thick gravy. Jellied fruits with whipped cream or ice cream.
Liquids	Smooth and liquid consistency, such as tomato soup. Fluid runs off the spoon. Cannot be eaten with a fork.	Enriched meat, fish or vegetable soup with whipped cream or crème fraîche. Fruit soup with whipped cream or ice cream.
Thickened liquids	Smooth and viscous, such as sour cream. Fluid drops off the spoon. Cannot be eaten with a fork.	Enriched viscous meat, fish or vegetable soup with whipped cream or crème fraîche. Viscous fruit soup with whipped cream or ice cream.

Today, the literature on the impacts of TM food, developed by food scientists, on food swallowing, remains scarce. Food processing industries are adopting various treatments—including thermal and non-thermal treatments—to modify texture. Future trends will likely include a combination of three-dimensional (3D) printing and drying to design foods, and to enhance textural and sensory characteristics for dysphagic patients [24]. A good starting point to develop these new food products is to gain a better understanding on sensory and rheological characteristics (see Table 1), which will be useful for modifying food texture. The objectives of this review article are to raise awareness about the importance of texture modification in the foods provided to dysphagic patients, describe methods to assess viscosity and texture properties in TM food for dysphagia, and compile those aspects that are related to the nutritional quality of foods for dysphagia. Section 2 describes various textural properties by highlighting methods to assess texture in general, particularly referring to dysphagia. Section 3 describes the varying effects of ingredients and processing methods on food texture. Section 4 discusses texture modification for dysphagic patients. Section 5 offers some food examples developed for dysphagic patients. Finally, Section 6 concludes this review.

2. Methods to Assess Texture in the Food Industry

The International Organization of Standardization (ISO) recognizes texture as both a sensory quality attribute and a multiparameter attribute. The commonly accepted ISO defines texture as all rheological and structural (geometric and surface) attributes of a food product perceptible by means of mechanical, tactile and, wherever appropriate, visual and auditory preceptors [14].

Texture and rheology are important parameters that need to be assessed when developing food products. One of the physical properties in food technological and sensory analyses that agrees with the ISO definition related to food texture is given by Szczesniak [25] as: "the sensory and functional manifestation of the structural, mechanical and surface properties of foods detected through the senses of vision, hearing, touch and kinesthetics". Texture is one of the key food attributes that is used to define product quality and acceptability [26], and even shelf life. This characteristic is present in all food, can affect its handling and processing, and can even be decisive for both shelf life and consumer acceptance. It will depend on the analyzed food type. Thus raw material food, handling and processing conditions, such as storage temperature, can have a significant influence on, for example, meat textural properties [27]. To understand this physical food property, we should understand the role of rheology in food. It was defined by Steffe [28] as "a branch of physics that studies the deformation and flow of matter". This means that it is the condition under which materials respond to an applied force or deformation, despite the fact that many authors relate rheology to liquid or semiliquid food sensory properties rather than to solids. In cases where swallowing food is difficult, hydrocolloids, which exhibit many functionalities in foods, including thickening, gelling, water-holding, dispersing, stabilizing, film-forming, and foaming agents are useful [29]. They have been used as a texture modifiers in almost all kinds of processed food products [29]. All materials have rheological properties that can be employed to assess raw materials and process characteristics, as well as their behavior and stability, throughout storage time until they are eaten to determine their customer acceptance [30]. This means that rheological analyses are necessary to identify the most suitable foods in accordance with final consumer requirements and to ensure the uniformity of different batches over time [30].

Food rheology has been defined as "the science of the deformation and flow of matter" [31]. Therefore, food texture characterization is no new science. Founded in 1929, the American Society of Rheology has already considered experimental foodstuff rheology [30] and consumers previously employed the food rheology/texture as food quality parameters. Conscientious interest has always been shown in its analysis, which has led it to be characterized in the past with senses by means of sensorial techniques. Nevertheless, this analysis is completely subjective and, thus, it is apt and necessary to perform instrumental analyses, which can relate their results to sensorial tests [32].

Matter starts deforming or flowing only when it is acted upon by forces that may be applied deliberately or accidentally; moreover, there is the all-pervading force of gravity that causes "soft" bodies to flow and lose shape. Rheology is, thus, mainly concerned with forces, deformations, and time [31]. Time matters in many ways, but it is often introduced into measuring rates of changes of deformations and forces. The passage of time does not actually bring about changes in materials. Chemical changes in foodstuff often occur with time, but can be studied by rheological methods. Temperature is also important and frequently appears in rheological equations [31].

In 1958, Blair [31] classified the frequently used instrumental techniques to measure texture into three main groups:

- Empirical tests to measure some physical properties under well-defined conditions;
- Imitative tests to simulate the conditions to which a material is subjected in mouths;
- Fundamental tests to measure physical properties, such as viscosity and elasticity.

A widely used imitative test today in the food technology field is the so-called Texture Profile Analysis (TPA). The TPA is not only widespread, but also convenient for rapid food texture evaluations [33], although texture can be measured by expert people with sensorial analyses. This test involves double compression to determine food textural properties. Any food texture identity is rarely a simple matter of understanding a singular characteristic, such as toughness or cohesion. The texture of each food is versatile and related to consumers' sensory expectations. It is not enough to deliver food with the target hardness and elasticity if consumers do not like it and it does not meet their expectations for that food type [34].

Food oral processing is described as a complex and dynamic pathway that involves mechano/chemoreceptors, mixing with saliva, temperature, friction, etc. When thickening formulas for dysphagia are considered, imitation by means of instrumental techniques is difficult as the physico-chemical features of each specific hydrocolloid or food involved in diet will be differently perceived in the mouth [35]. Viscosity is a fundamental property that is obtained from rheological measurements, and is used as the most important criterion in developing thickeners for dysphagia patients. The American Dietetic Association reached an agreement, which was published in the National Dysphagia Diet T [36], and categorizes foods according to their viscosity (at 50 s^{-1}) shear rate range values. The categories are: (1) nectar-like (51–350 cP); (2) honey-like (351–1750 cP); (3) spoon thick (>1750 cP)) to ensure safe swallowing and to facilitate palliative care procedures for different types of patient needs, although the categorization does not consider very relevant sensory aspects. Although viscosity values are obtained at 50 s^{-1}, no consensus has been reached by the scientific community about the shear rate value of the swallowing process [36]. A study that considered rheological and tribological responses of biopolymer-based thickening solutions incorporated into different food matrices for dysphagic patients observed that an increase in the biopolymer concentration significantly affected rheological properties as xanthan gum showed the highest viscosity, pseudoplasticity, and viscoelasticity, followed by flaxseed gum [37].

ISO 11036:2020 [38] sensory profiling methods can be used for these attributes. This ISO document specifies a method for developing a texture profile of food products (solids, semisolids, liquids). This method is one approach to the sensory texture profile analysis. Chemical composition determines the basic physical structure of foods which, in turn, influences their texture. An understanding of textural properties will, therefore, require studying the physical structure of foods. Other methods based on physical structure that can offer a description of a product's textural attributes include light and/or electron microscopy, and an X-ray diffraction analysis that provides information about crystalline structure. Differential scanning calorimetry provides information about melting, solidification, and other phase or state transitions, while a particle size analysis and sedimentation methods offer information on particle size distribution and particle shape [39]. Conventional profiling via QDA®, flash profiling and projective mapping performed by panels were used by Albert et al. [40] to describe foods with complex textures. The application of QDA®, flash profiling and projective mapping using panels with different degrees of training helps to overcome issues in the sensory description of served hot food with a complex texture [40].

However, a qualitative empirical method on test conditions that can better measure viscosity is lacking, as the literature on dysphagia indicates [41]. Researchers have used a quick empirical test, the line spread test (LST), to compare relative viscosities of several similar products. It measures the consistency of a liquid using the distance that a standard amount of liquid spreads over a horizontal surface when released from a confined chamber [42].

Dr. Szczesniak developed and improved sensory descriptions for the texture of specific food while searching for more universal descriptors to be applied to a broader array of food. One of the goals was to develop a common lexicon and a set of procedures to allow objective and repeatable sensory texture evaluation tests to be run in different laboratories, with several operators, and for many distinct food types [34]. These experiments described and introduced food sensory analyses as five basic independent mechanical parameters: hardness, cohesiveness, adhesiveness, viscosity, elasticity, and into three more dependent parameters (brittleness, chewiness, gumminess) [34]. These mechanical parameters [34] can be read from the curve and compared to the observed sensory characteristics. A high correlation between the measurements taken by this technique and sensory evaluations has been shown.

Figure 1 shows a typical TPA graph for food, which is a popular double-compression test run to establish textural food material properties [25] and to quantify mechanical parameters from recorded force-deformation curves.

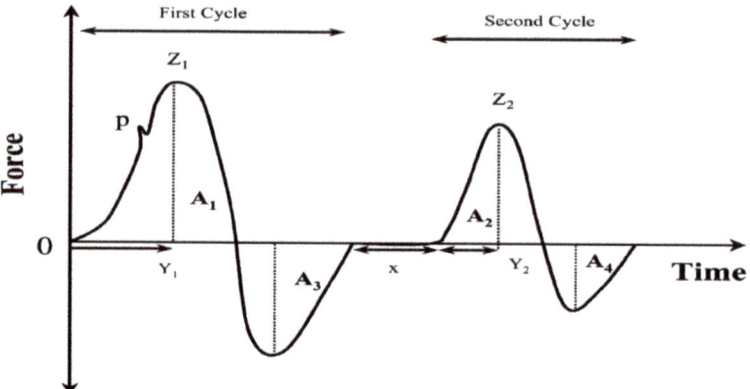

Figure 1. Generalized instrumental texture profile curve modified from Szczesniak [25]. A_1: positive force area during first compression; A_2: positive force area during second compression; A_3: negative force area during first compression; A_4: negative force area during second compression; Z_1: height of the maximum force during first compression; Z_2: height of the maximum force during second compression; Y_1: time of maxime force during first compression; Y_2: time of maxime force during second compression; x: time between the first and second compression.

Generally, the parameters observed in the texture profile analysis, i.e., hardness, adhesiveness, and cohesiveness, are used to compare the sensory attributes and rheological properties of various foods. They are employed to examine the material properties of commercial oral moisturizers and denture adhesives, which are relevant to dysphagia [43].

In the curves generated in the two TPA cycles, when foods are chewed over time, as shown in Figure 1, hardness (N/m^2): the peak force in the first compression cycle (Z_1); adhesiveness: negative force area A_3 for the first bite; cohesiveness (J/m^3): the ratio between the positive force area during the second compression and that during the first compression (A_2/A_1); springiness: Y_2/Y_1.

It is important to emphasize that TPA has not been broadly used in texture measurements for dysphagia as it does not assess some of the core attributes that are relevant to their foods, which are important; they include slipperiness, humidity, and mouth coating. However, other new tests were developed to help complete the knowledge about the physicochemical properties of food in different analytical fields, such as microscopic, submicroscopic, and molecular [44]. This technical progress was assisted by computer science. Indeed, without computer aid, modern spectroscopy, calorimetry, microscopy, and rheological equipment would not have been able to help texture analyses [44].

Nowadays, new texture analyses include a range of food texture-related parameters: firmness, hardness, consistency, fibrosity, tenderness, elasticity, resistance, gel strength, stickiness, adhesiveness, spreadability, bloom force, extensibility, cohesiveness, chewiness extrudability, texture profile analyses, rubberiness, and resilience. Touch characteristics can be classified as mechanical, which measure chewing effort, geometric, related to shape, and others, such as moisture and fat content. Therefore, most of these characteristics are perceived in the mouth if we bear in mind that texture includes all the steps from the first bite to swallowing [45]. Food mastication covers different processes, including deformation and flow (rheology), size reduction (comminution), and mixing and hydration with saliva. Other physical behaviors that can also be relevant for texture are changes in temperature and surface roughness (rugosity). Food researchers should run rheological tests to describe only a portion of the physical properties sensed in our mouth while chewing [46].

An assessment of rheological properties, particularly in relation to the dysphagia field, includes tests on the flowability or consistency of food. For these tests, a Bostwick Consistometer can be applied to assess the slump of sauces and condiments using a volume of 75 mL, which is released to flow along a channel. The distance traveled by the liquid over 30 s is used to classify consistency [47]. An adaptation of slumping with a reference to dysphagia drinks is called the line-spread test. The IDDSI flow test can be applied using a standard 10 mL Luer slip tip syringe as the "funnel". This test classifies consistency based on the volume of the residual liquid in the syringe after a period of a 10 s flow. The resulting levels are then defined as level 0 thin (0–1 mL liquid remaining), level 1 slightly-thick (1–4 mL), level 2 mildly thick (4–8 mL) and level 3, moderately thick (8–10 mL) [48]. The new International Dysphagia Diet Standardization Initiative (IDDSI) classification system considers practical measurements for liquids that could be used in kitchens, bedsides and in laboratories. In addition, devices capable of modeling human swallowing will provide more accurate measurement information on shear rates during swallowing in dysphagic patients. Clinicians can employ either manometry or video-fluoroscopy for this purpose. With a manometry, a probe is inserted into the patient's pharynx, which obstructs the bolus flow and causes discomfort [49]. During video-fluoroscopic analyses, swallowing of fluids is monitored by X-ray imaging and the entire swallowing process is recorded, which, therefore, enables the examiner to follow the swallowing sequence frame by frame [50].

Studies about food texture rheological properties have been systematically conducted since the early 1950s, while the rheological properties of several food types have been studied, and are summarized in many publications, e.g., for roast turkey breast muscle [51]; Japanese sweets [52], the rheology of food dispersion [53]; and food rheology [54]. Many variables can influence rheological properties, including ripeness, processing methods, temperature, composition, time, instrumental techniques, and analytical assumptions and methods), and modify the results obtained by one test [54]. However, not all tests focus on solving the swallowing problem. Suebsaen et al. [55] prepared banana gels from hydrocolloids for the elderly with dysphagia, modified texture and hardness, to obtain a dessert. This product had different characteristics in instrumental rheology, texture properties, and sensory attributes terms. To improve the swallowing ability of foodstuff, different thickeners are added to normal food and drinks, which may be gum- or starch-based [56].

Food technologists are interested in the mastication process, rheological changes, and other textural properties that occur during this process [46]. For dysphagic patients, sensory tasks that require motor behaviors of the tongue to explore, squeeze, or move a bolus to ascertain its flow properties are challenging tasks related to eating and swallowing foods. In addition to taste receptors in the mouth, trigeminal nerve receptors in the mouth and tongue are capable of detecting both static and dynamic characteristics of items placed in the mouth, such as shape, size, volume, mass, location, temperature, two-point discrimination, and flow or movement [57]. It is, therefore, interesting to understand the sensory function of the tongue for tasks that may be relevant for detecting differences in the flow characteristics of swallowing.

Most of the available information on rheological properties of ready-to-eat dysphagia-oriented products only focuses on viscosity [10]. However, new tests on hardness will be necessary to reveal the effect of elastic modulus on the swallowing ability of solid foods for dysphagia [29].

Several aspects could be considered in the foods for dysphagic patients: the positive effect of dysphagia-oriented products on the quality of life of dysphagic patients; improve their nutritional status and prevent more weight loss. Designing standardized diets for each type of dysphagia is proposed as a desirable approach in rheological studies that are related to the management of dysphagia [29].

2.1. Gels: Rheological Characterization

Some of the most popular foods, such as gelatin desserts, cooked egg whites, frankfurters, surimi-based seafood analogs, and fruit jellies, can be considered gels. In short, they are solid-in-liquid, and the solid phase immobilizes to the liquid phase [54].

Rheological properties can be measured by (a) puncture test, which is one of the simplest methods to obtain a stress strain curve, and is widely used in both solid and semisolid foods; (b) the torsion test, a method that applies shear stress to samples in a twisting fashion; (c) the folding test, which can be used to measure the binding structure of gels, especially surimi gels, and can be interpreted in cohesiveness terms; (d) the oscillatory test, dynamic rheological testing that evaluates the properties of gel systems, which are suitable for testing the characteristics of gels, gelation, and melting; (e) the stress relaxation test, namely rapid deformation applied to food samples [54]. It can be done while under compression, extension, or shear; (f) yield stress, used for predicting how products respond to processing and/or how they endure performance; (g) rheological characterization of time-dependent fluids, it analyzes the flow behavior (or viscosity) of liquid and semi-liquid food. It is an intrinsic parameter and a measure of fluids' resistance to flow when shearing stress is applied [54].

2.2. Emulsions: Rheology of Food Emulsions

Emulsions are dispersions of one liquid phase in the form of fine droplets in another immiscible liquid phase. The immiscible phases are usually oil and water, so emulsions can be broadly classified as oil in water or water in oil emulsions, depending on the dispersed phase (mild cream, ice cream, butter, margarine, salad dressing, and meat emulsions) [58], although the rheology of food emulsions is mainly dependent on the strength of inter-droplet interactions and dilute emulsions (that is, milk) have a low-viscosity Newtonian behavior. Nevertheless, concentrated food emulsions show gel-like rheological characteristics [59].

2.3. Rheological Measurements: Equipment

The rheometer, or viscometer, measures resistance to flow when a known force or stress is produced by a known amount of flow, and is crucial equipment in food rheological studies. Such equipment can be capillary viscometers, falling-ball viscometers, and rotational and oscillatory rheometers, which are used to take rheological measurements [54]. Tests must be carried out under certain conditions for samples, such as steady flow, laminar flow, and uniform temperature [60]. Figure 2 shows the different tests used in rheology.

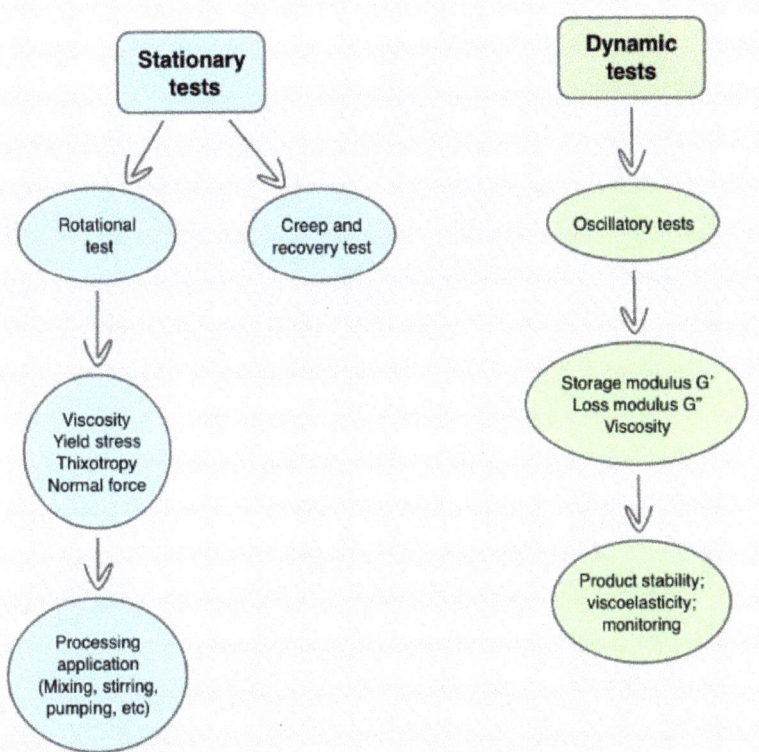

Figure 2. Rheological tests used in food characterization [54].

These rheological measurements use experimentation with and observation of sampled food to compare data, whose main goals are to analyze materials' mechanical properties and identify molecular interactions and foodstuff composition [61]. Nevertheless, these results should be tested with people. Currently, there are two method groups for rheological studies [29], and both are based on measuring force and deformation according to time:

- Empirical: instrumental-dependent and specified to test a hypothesis;
- Fundamental tests: based on known concepts and equations of physics and fundamental rheology. The European Society for Swallowing Disorders (ESSD) stressed in its published White Paper the importance of rheological parameters, such as shear rate, non-Newtonian fluids properties, yield stress, elasticity, and density [50].

Lack of oral cavity control, poor bolus preparation, or a delayed swallowing response are some reasons for using thicker food and drink for dysphagic patients because thickened foods change the speed at which they are transported through the throat, which is related to delayed swallowing response and, therefore, reduces the aspiration risk [62]. Thickeners, which are typically gum- or starch-based, are added to food to slow down the flow of the bolus. Thickened liquids are highly recommended for dysphagic patients as slowing down the flow rate can provide the time required to close airways [63]. However, excessively thickened food may require much more force on the tongue and pharynx during swallowing [63].

Moreover, we should take into account the texture profile panel, which is a valuable tool for describing and quantifying textural characteristics of food products when the panel is carefully selected, trained, and maintained [64]. Nor should we forget the application from trained panelists or consumer panels in these tests. Thus Saldaña et al. [65] obtained suitable results when sensory hardness correlated positively with instrumental springiness in light mortadella analyses. Other authors, such as Yates [66], performed a descriptive analysis of Gouda cheese texture by a sensory panel and Barden et al. [67] did so on cheddar cheese.

3. The Effects of Processing Methods and Ingredients on Food Texture

The structure of modified foods depends very much on the ingredients making it up, and also on the processes involved in their development [68]. Based on these premises, it should be noted that the main building blocks for developing most TM food items are carbohydrates, lipids, and proteins [69]

When heated, globular proteins unfold and denature, which increases liquid viscosity (e.g., in protein drinks). They can self-assemble as nano-sized aggregates and fibrils upon additional heating, and eventually become the network chains of gels [70]. Proteins are appreciated not only for these structural applications, but also for certain essential amino acids (e.g., leucine), whose high hydrolysate content tends to facilitate muscle protein synthesis during aging [71].

Polysaccharides have been used as gelling agents to thicken aqueous food dispersions, and to stabilize emulsions and foams [72]. Nishinari et al. [73] offer an exceptional overview of the rheological properties of polysaccharide solutions and gels associated with tasting and swallowing of TM foods. Dextrins include viscous clear solutions that are often employed as thickening agents and encapsulating matrices for nutrients, colorants, flavors, enzymes, and antioxidants, along with starch and gum [74]. Dietary fiber, such as cellulose derivatives (e.g., microcrystalline cellulose), or resistant starch, which may alleviate constipation, can be added directly to food [75]. Although typically used to thicken liquids, starch has been underexploited as a texture-modifier in the pastes and gels utilized as TM food [76]. As starch granules accumulate large quantities of water during gelatinization, they can be preloaded during this process with water-soluble micronutrients and bioactives [77]. Starch can also be partially gelatinized so that various glycemic responses are elicited [78].

Given their amphiphilic nature, phospholipids and monoglycerides can be used as emulsifiers in interfaces or self-associated with a plurality of nano-sized structures (e.g., vesicles and micelles) as bioactive and nutrient delivery vehicles. Triacylglycerol molecules crystallize from a molten state and cluster to form aggregates and, ultimately, a fat network to occlude parts of liquid fat, which ends in a plastic matrix [79]. Food nano- and microemulsion, a topic reviewed recently by McClements [80], can be used to encapsulate and deliver hydrophobic components, such as nutraceuticals, vitamins, and flavors. Oleogels, formed by a liquid lipid process trapped inside a stable gel network, are involved in drug delivery applications as carriers of unsaturated fats and increase food texture [81].

In order to develop TM foods, with a view to retain the overall flavor and appearance of whole pieces while softening their structure, several known technologies achieve this texture-softening effect: freeze-thawing (with/without enzyme infusion), enzyme impregnation, high-pressure processing, pulsed electric fields, and sonication [6]. The regular supervision of process variables maintains the color and flavor of food products, while adjusting their soft texture to various degrees.

Many technologies contribute to small particles and may have applications in TM foods. The food industry has long since been aware of the aggregation and microparticulation of proteins and products employed as thickening agents and fat replacers for beverages and semisolid food [82]. Technologies focus primarily on globular proteins' capacity to undergo denaturation and aggregation in solution, which results in several morphologies (e.g., spherical particles, fibrils, and flexible strands), whose main dimensions range from approximately 10 nm to a few microns [83].

The aim of another group of techniques is developing fibers and soft particles from biopolymer solutions. Microgels are small soft and stable particles (e.g., sizes from

<1–100 mm) and come with a wide variety of shapes, sizes, and textural properties that can be tuned to structures [84]. Microgel formation is often performed by direct gelling, often under shear, in a particle or fiber shape, or by reducing bulk gel size by mechanical means. Microgel suspension is typically free-flowing as opposed to bulk gels with prevailing viscoelastic behavior [85].

Apart from their function as texture modifiers, microgels have been proposed as delivery vehicles for non-polar compounds, such as vitamins, flavors antimicrobials and antioxidants, which can be spread in tiny micelles or more functional liposomes (20 nm and a few hundred mm) in the aqueous phase [86]. Given their soft texture and flowability, micron-sized hydrocolloid gel particles with their high water content (e.g., >95%) are very appealing to be employed as structuring agents to consolidate dispersed phases, and also as soup and sauce thickeners. These hydrocolloid microparticles are generally formed by shear gelling or preformed droplet gelation [87]. A recent study showed that a combination of 0.5% Alcalase, and two-step heating at 37 °C and 90 °C was useful for improving the physico-functional properties of a novel surimi gel for people with dysphagia [88].

Some innovative micro-technology techniques have recently emerged and may lead to revolutionary TM food design and manufacturing applications [89–99]. In channels with cross-sections of a few hundred microns, microfluidic systems handle minute quantities of fluids. Systems have been developed to produce foams and emulsions of identical size and different shapes with a monodispersed discontinuous phase and gel microspheres [92]. 3D printing is a rapid prototyping technique based on digitally-controlled material depositing and layer-by-layer stacking. From "printable" mixtures of carbohydrates it is possible to obtain lipids and proteins, and complex food structures based on liquid deposition or powder binding. According to Kouzani et al. [100], 3D printing reduced design, and fabrication time, improved the consistency and repeatability of 3D printed tuna fish (consisting of tuna, puréed pumpkin, and puréed beetroot), and optimized sensory characteristics of this puréed food for dysphagic patients. Electrospinning employs a high-voltage electrical field to create biopolymer solution electrically-charged jets that become nanofibers upon solvent evaporation. During the encapsulation of bioactives and probiotics, electrospun protein fibers (e.g., <1 μm in diameter) are used as dietary supplements, and also confer food mouthfeel and texture. The nanofibers employed to encapsulate bioactives or as entangled mats to simulate meat are suggested electrospinning technology applications to manufacture TM food [96–98]. Electro-spraying is another electrohydrodynamic manufacturing technique whereby near-spherical droplets are produced from a jet flowing through a nozzle submitted to an external electrical field that yields micro- or nanoparticles upon solvent evaporation. Microencapsulation matrices used to protect biologically active compounds is a suggested use for electro-spraying technology in TM food manufacturing [99].

The relevant role thickeners play in TM food while swallowing, slowing down the flow of liquids and stopping them from being aspired via the airway is highlighted [4]. Currently, starch and gums are the most popular commercial choices. Thus increasing the availability of thickeners to be employed in TM food and extending their properties can be challenging [29].

Gel microparticles are excellent alternatives to tailor food rheological properties thanks to their small tunable size, soft texture and free-flowing state [101]. To be able to change their texture perception and flow behavior, they can be blended into thin liquids or incorporated into purées. They evoke a stronger aroma during mouth breakdown if filled with flavors and supplied with a thin delicate texture [102]. Artificial caviars introduced by molecular cuisine proved to be the most innovative use of soft gel particles. Tiny spheres with a soft core and a tough outer layer were formed by dipping droplets in a calcium bath of colored and flavored alginate solutions [103]. Artificial caviars are now often featured in main dishes, desserts, drinks, etc., and are offered in contemporary restaurants [104,105]. Using tiny "gelatinous" beads and other light-molecular cooking creations (i.e., foam or "air") has been proposed to inspire the elderly to produce attractive TM foods [106].

Recently, the extensive literature on gel microparticles essentially endorses employing them as encapsulating agents and delivery systems rather than applying them to alter texture or to act as major nutritional functions [107,108]. For example, by adding protein microparticles, the texture control of matrices can be achieved [109] and elderly people are likely to try protein-enriched foods if they need a higher protein intake [110]. Conversely, by introducing a dispersed gas phase into bubble form, softness and density can be adjusted [111], which provides the added beneficial effect of a higher perceived intensity of tastants in the gel phase [112]. Insoluble fiber can be filled with gelled microparticles to increase fecal bulk and to prevent constipation, while partially masking the insipid fiber flavor and its rough texture [75,113]. Lastly, emulsion gels are food items in which lipid droplets are enclosed inside a soft biopolymer matrix (e.g., sauces, yogurt, frankfurters, etc.). Gelled emulsion microparticles are small biphasic structures in which a lipid phase offers many opportunities [114]. The incorporation of whey protein isolate (WPI)-based gelled microspheres loaded with lipids into food bars, soups, and other food systems has been suggested by Egan et al. [115]. These microparticles can also be employed as delivery systems for bioactive lipophilic ingredients (fatty acid ω-3, phytosterols, carotenoids, etc.), tastants, and fat-soluble aromas [116]. WPI microgels can lower the plasma insulin peak and postpone the postprandial amino acid profile in relation to protein powder in the interface with drugs [117].

4. Modifying Texture for Dysphagic Patients

Food contains several phases and hierarchical structures that vary from nanoscopic to microscopic length scales [118]. The configurations offer some features like texture control and nutritional value, or support for processing and shelf-life stability [101]. Texture control and alteration are common ways to control dysphagia. Modified diets are believed to minimize the risk of choking and the need for chewing or oral food processing [119]. Eating thickened fluids is indicated to help safe swallowing as the act of swallowing is delayed and the transit time of food with an altered consistency in modified foods is typically longer than for non-modified foods. This gives the glottis more time to close and avoids food or fluid aspiration to the lungs of dysphagic patients [120].

Food texture can be modulated and altered to meet consumers' nutritional demands. Texture modification and thickening of fluids are normal features of dysphagia evaluation and therapy [121]. TM foods can be defined based on many variables, such as viscosity, density, and fluid flow rate. However, using viscosity to describe thickened beverages for dysphagia management has been questioned as no viscosity measurements are available for most clinicians and caregivers [122].

When designing healthy foods for the elderly, significant factors need to be addressed. TM foods prescribed for seniors' dysphagia management and dietary intake should be soft, moist, smooth, elastic, and simple to swallow [5]. One important key for designing texture and bolus rheology is understanding dynamic food structure changes during oral processing. This rheological state should allow the more cohesively mass flow of bolus throughout the pharyngeal phase to help to improve easy swallowing in dysphagic patients [10].

The IDDSI framework provides standardized terms and descriptions to classify TM food and thickened liquids for dysphagia patients [122]. The IDDSI framework consists in a continuum of eight levels (0–7), as shown in Figure 3. In addition, the syringe flow test classifies IDDSI levels from 0 to 3 based on the flow rate, while a fork pressure test is best used to assess the foods of levels 4 to 7 [5].

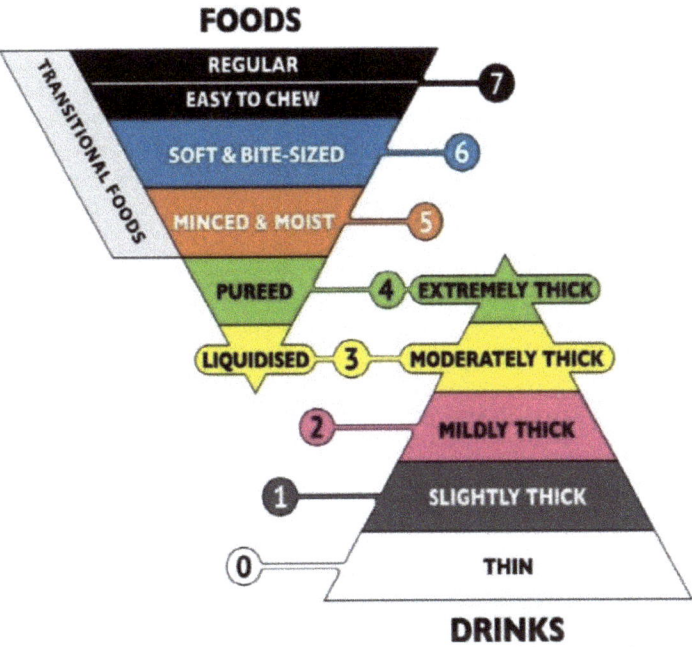

Figure 3. The IDDSI Framework for the TM food and thickened liquids used with dysphagic individuals from all age groups, in all healthcare facilities and of all cultures [122]. Note. 0: thin; 1: slightly thick; 2: slightly thick; 3: liquidized/moderately thick; 4: puréed/extremely thick; 5: minced and moist; 6: soft and bite-sized; 7: easy to chew/regular.

It is worth noting that foods classified as levels 4 to 7 are texture-modified foods for dysphagic patients [5]. Sungsinchai et al. [5] described the various levels as follows: puréed foods at level 4 do not require chewing, and include products like potato purée, carrot purée, and avocado purée; level 5 (minced and moist) represents soft and moist food with no separate thin liquid; small lumps (of 2–4 mm in size) may be visible in food and minimal chewing is required. Level 5 foodstuff includes items like minced meat and fish, mashed fruit, fully softened cereal, and rice (not sticky or glutinous); level 6 (soft and bite-sized) food that can be mashed and broken down by applying pressure with forks, spoons, or chopsticks that are soft, tender, and moist throughout, but with no separate thin liquid. Chewing is required for this food class, which include cooked tender meat, cooked fish, and steamed or boiled vegetables. Level 7 is regular food with various textures (that can be hard, crunchy and naturally soft).

An example of the TM foods defined in the IDDSI framework is puréed food at the fourth level of the IDDSI framework. Puréed foods are typically ground and/or mixed in a form that involves less chewing and oral manipulation. A cohesive swallowable mass, referred to as 'bolus,' is formed that is easy to push with the tongue to the pharynx [123], which can make swallowing simpler and avoid bolus regurgitation, which causes dysphagia aspiration. Other examples of dysphagia-specific standardized scales when considering TM foods for dysphagia include the Penetration-Aspiration Scale [124] SWAL-QOL and SWAL-CARE [125], the Dysphagia Outcome Severity Scale [126], and the Functional Oral Intake Scale [127].

Using thickeners to improve bolus viscosity in post-stroke oral dysphagia has been proposed as a countervailing clinical technique against aspiration. Nonetheless, this strategy has been questioned because the number of experiments is limited and methodologies vary [128]. One experiment has indicated improved safe swallowing when patients received altered starch and xanthan gum thickeners with 'spoon-thick' viscosity. The therapeutic effect of these thickeners was due to a counterbalancing process that brought about no major change in swallow reaction timing [129]. Another research study revealed that enhanced bolus viscosity promotes safe swallowing and lowers mid-term pneumonia in patients with oral dysphagia [130]. Some studies have demonstrated that elevated viscosity impairs swallowing effectiveness in oral dysphagia by increasing oropharyngeal residue. Other studies argue that the effect of thickeners on swallow reaction physiology is still not fully understood [129]. Analyzing the effect of augmented bolus viscosity on swallowing safety in patients with dysphagia poses a research challenge. However, novel naturally sourced thickeners from food biopolymers are drawing significant attention and enable on-demand dysphagia management, where fluidal food must be adequately thickened for patients. A recent study investigated the rheological behaviors of a novel thickener with a carboxymethylated curdlan potential for dysphagia, which was a traditional food thickener of konjac glucomannan and its mixtures in both water and model nutrition emulsions. It reported both the efficacy and applicability of these thickened fluids and compared them to those of xanthan gum, taken as the reference. It showed that carboxymethylated curdlan, which is similar to xanthan, displayed a unique viscosity-enhancing ability in both water and emulsions, and proved promising feasible as a novel dysphagia-oriented thickener [131]. Furthermore, the modification of viscosity with thickeners was used as a strategy to circumvent oropharyngeal dysphagia patients' swallowing problems. Generally, the formulations of commercial food products with thickening properties often contain xanthan and starch. However, flaxseed gum was found to improve rheological behavior in liquid foods and can be considered a potential thickener with additional health benefits [132]. These results offer the opportunity to tailor the rheological characteristics of food systems by adding and combining natural ingredients to improve technological and nutritional properties.

Hydrocolloids are often used by the food industry to enhance consistency and cohesiveness, and to reduce TM foods syneresis. Enhanced food consistency and cohesiveness make it safe to swallow [133]. Although all hydrocolloids can be used as thickeners, they are not all capable of forming a cross-linked gel network to be employed to confer modified food solidity. Food mixture thickening that involves hydrocolloids is mainly the result of polymer chains that entangle while their concentration rises. Entanglements in dilute systems are less common, and polymer chains are free to move and viscosity is minimum. After eating thickened food mixtures, saliva dilutes and breaks, which leads to substantially reduced viscosity. Lower viscosity is a problem, particularly when starch-based thickeners are used because saliva contains α-amylase that breaks down amylopectin and amylose [134]. Non-starch gums can be employed to reduce this, even though they do not completely remove undesirable viscosity declination. When non-starch biopolymer gums are resorted to as thickeners, non-specific entanglement can come into play which, above a given concentration, can increase stickiness, which impairs the ability to swallow. Hydrocolloids in TM food have been reported to have an effect on particle breakdown, microstructure, deformation force during mastication, mouth coating, and bolus lubrication [133]. These properties have an implication for oral processing and sensory food perception. Thickened liquids have also been reported to be considerably less palatable than their non-thick counterparts [135]. It is also necessary to produce new thickening agents that are well-defined in terms of sensory properties, and can be employed to enhance swallowing while preserving palatability. This will include a plan to control dysphagia in order to avoid the detrimental effects of decreased palatability and increasing residual viscosity when complying with therapy. In order to increase palatability, TM foods need to be homogeneous in appearance, and particular attention must be paid to their flavor and odor. Adapting the sensory characteristics of dishes to dysphagia in association with cerebral palsy was possible by the check all-that-apply (CATA) method [136]. CATA is faster, more economical, and does not require trained judges. It is sufficiently robust to obtain the profile of a wide range of food products to be developed.

When modifying texture for dysphagic patients, the influence of two natural different hydrocolloids (apple and citrus pectin) on physical, rheological, and textural parameters, bioactive compounds, and antioxidant activity of courgette (*Cucurbita pepo*) purée was studied. Pectin was added within the 0.1–0.3% range to courgette purée and ohmically heated at 20 V/cm for 3 min. Ohmic heating was utilized to improve and preserve the main properties of purées. Antioxidant activity has also increased with ohmic heating, up to 58% compared to the control sample [137]. The study shows the potential of this treatment for ready-to-eat courgettes as food that can be developed for dysphagic patients.

It should be noted that although several hydrocolloids can be used, they have different physicochemical properties, and even different behavior when preparation variables, such as temperature, shearing, and pressure, are applied.

5. Developed Food Products for Dysphagic Patients

People usually eat raw or cooked foods, but swallowing is the key issue. It starts during the mastication process in the mouth, and passes from oropharyngeal safe food transfer to the esophagus to reach the stomach, where the gastro intestinal digestion process starts to allow nutritional food use [138].

Processing food to increase ease of swallowing requires modifications to texture, and also to physicochemical and rheological properties. For instance, plasma processing is effective in improving the cooking properties of brown rice. Swelling of starch granules due to water uptake not only cuts cooking time, but also softens the cooked rice texture and makes it easier to chew. Bran layer fissure significantly improves water absorption and reduces cooking time [5].

Calorie and nutrient requirements diets for dysphagic patients are similar to those presented by persons of the same age and sex, unless co-existent diseases are present [139]. Just like all people, dysphagic patients require suitable food. As previously mentioned in the introduction, this suitability is not only related to food texture, which needs to be appropriate, but should also offer nutritional value and adequate palatability/acceptability and, if at all possible, it must be visually appealing. Combining all of these characteristics is truly challenging [140].

Thus, if we consider not only hospitalized patients, but also the number of older people [141] living in institutionalized settings, and those with dysphagic problems, the major role of food and pharmaceutical industries in developing TM foods is a welcoming development [142,143] The main food texture characteristics that affect dysphagia management can be classified as [138]: adhesiveness (effort made to overcome food adhering to the palate), cohesiveness (if food is deformed or sheared when compressed), firmness (force needed to compress semisolid food), "fracturability" (force required to break solid food), hardness (force required to compress food to attain a certain deformation), springiness (rate or degree that food goes back to its original shape after being compressed), viscosity (rate of flow per unit of force) and yield stress (minimum shear stress applied before flow begins) [134]. The recommended food texture of dysphagic diets must be, at least, smooth, moist, soft and elastic if we contemplate that these attributes should combine TM food rheological properties and patients' difficulty swallowing [29,119].

The IDDSI framework shown in Figure 3 is a useful guide when a dysphagic patient's diet is considered. Variations based on individual circumstances may exist. The Functional Diet Scale, in addition to this framework (IDDSI–FDS), permits levels 2–5 as being suitable food and drinks for dysphagic patients. In a Canadian study with adults living in long-term care institutions, IDDSI Functional Diet Scale scores were derived based on diet orders and were compared between residents with and without dysphagia. The IDDSI–FDS for residents with no dysphagia risk ranged from 4 to 8, which reflects the lack of severe diet texture restrictions, while the probability of having an IDDSI–FDS score of <5 was significantly higher in individuals at dysphagia risk [142]. When foods are prepared or formulated for dysphagic patients, it is important for the bolus to be swallowed safely if it is not chewed. Thus particle size and moisture content of food are key criteria, especially for minced and moist foods at level 5. Simple and inexpensive tests at home and in residential care or nursing settings recommended by the IDDSI are: the spoon tilt test to ensure that food is not too dry or sticky; the fork drip test to guarantee that the food is not too runny [9]. In many German nursing homes, minced and moist texture diets are available, which are easy to produce because only a blender and no special knowledge are needed. In these settings, the puréed texture is the most elaborate because they should be lump-free and require special equipment (e.g., a bowl cutter) for several food types (e.g., meat) because of natural fiber content [144].

In one intervention study conducted in a long-term care facility in Canada, the presentation to dysphagic patients of developed foods based on texture and shape resulted in increased body weight, and higher energy and nutrient intake, after 12 weeks in residents receiving reshaped TM diets compared to a control group on unshaped TM diets. Another study in the USA showed a 15% higher food intake after changing to the 3D preparation of puréed foods [145]. This shows that reshaping food components enhances the visual appeal of meals significantly and they are more likely to be eaten. Therefore, it is essential that either liquid or solid food is modified for them to offer appropriate nutritional properties to make swallowing easy for dysphagic patients. Different strategies have been applied to achieve this goal. The main ones can be summarized by following thermal processing and non-thermal technologies, and employing thickeners [139,146].

The simplest form of thermal processing is using hot water, which is known to be effective in transforming hard food into soft food. It is also known that some nutrients are especially heat-sensitive and using thermal processing leads to marked vitamin loss, especially in food rich in these essential nutrients like fruit and vegetables [147]. It is noteworthy that this thermal processing type is often used at home and in industry. To solve this problem, food and pharmaceutical industries usually apply two strategies: first, addition of the micronutrients lost from processing; second, using non-thermal technologies. The most widespread thermal technologies applied to obtain TM food are pulsed electric field, high-pressure processing, high hydrodynamic pressure, ultrasound, and gamma-irradiation [5].

The above-mentioned non-thermal technologies can be applied to meat [148], fish, or its by-products [11], rice [63], starch, and carbohydrate-based products [149], or fruit [150] and vegetables [151]. The use of non-thermal technologies helps to maintain bioactive compounds (especially heat-labile compounds) in food and, thus, promotes health benefits for dysphagic patients. As dysphagic patients benefit from soft food that is safe for swallowing, the characteristics and gel properties of starch play an important role in the desired final product quality.

Irradiation can increase gelatinization temperature, water solubility, water absorption capacity, and oil absorption capacity, but can lower peak, trough, final breakdown, and setback viscosities in starch-based foods. Irradiation has been shown to induce the depolymerization and destruction of the crystalline structure of chickpea flour, which resulted in gamma-irradiated flour being cooked more easily with less retrogradation [5].

The texture of solid food can be generally classified into four grades, as shown in Figure 3. Nevertheless, if regular/unmodified everyday food is not considered, then only three categories are useful for dysphagic patients: (i) "soft"—food is naturally soft (e.g., ripe banana) or cooked or cut to alter food texture; (ii) "minced and moist"—food easily forms into bolus using only the tongue; (iii) "smooth puréed"—food is cohesive enough to maintain its shape on a spoon, similar to the consistency of commercial puddings [152].

No international harmonized terminology is available for thickened liquids, although four or five categories have been defined according to respective viscosity values [4]. However, if the so-called water-like viscosity (<50 cP) is excluded, in a very simplistic form, and according to the "fork test" [63], it is possible to classify thickeners into three texture grades: (i) "nectar"—can be drunk in a cup or with the help of a straw (51-350 cP); (ii) "honey"—can be drunk in a cup, but not with a straw (351–1750 cP); (iii) "pudding"—should be eaten with a spoon (>1750 cP). [4,139].

Commercial TM food was developed to improve nutritional intervention in dysphagic patients. To minimize the risk of aspiration and dehydration, ready-to-serve commercially packaged pre-thickened (CPPT) and instant food thickeners (IFT) are used to modify beverage consistency in dysphagia management [20]. The test of masticating and swallowing solids (TOMASS), an international study that performs quantitative solid bolus ingestion assessments [153], and in vitro testing, such as that performed by Mathieu and co-workers [154] or by Qazi et al. [155], are relevant tools that contribute to assess that these food types do not require further preparation by patients' families and/or caregivers.

Thus, in commercial terms, food and pharmaceutical companies have made different product types available on the market, which can be summarized as:

(i) Thickeners to be added to liquids and food—the main compounds used to obtain suitable rheological characteristics are gum-based thickeners and starch-based thickeners. The most widespread are carrageenan (E407), modified corn (E1442), xanthan gum (E415), guar gum (E412), and tara gum (E417). Other compounds include calcium citrate (E333) and potassium chloride (E508), used as thickener additives [156–158];
(ii) Nutritional supplements with a pudding texture [159];
(iii) Lyophilized or dehydrated powdered products, and pasteurized or sterilized ready to eat or to be reconstituted with both the desired texture, and savory and sweet flavors as purées, or cereals, compotes, and puddings, to eat as breakfasts, snacks, and desserts [139,160]. Examples of commercially developed food products for dysphagia from starch and gum are Nutilis®(Nutricia, Milupa GmbH., Fulda, Germany) and Resource®(Resource, Nestlé Portugal S.A., Linda-a-Velha, Portugal). Both products are presented as white powder that easy to dissolve and can instantly thicken clear liquids. Nutilis®is composed of maltodextrin, modified maize starch (E-1442), tara gum, xanthan gum, and guar gum, while Resource®contains only modified maize starch (E-1442). In both cases, the employed modified starch was hydroxypropyl distarch phosphate [161].

The variety and supply of TM foods targeted at elderly consumers in Asian countries is more promising. The market in Japan is steadily expanding; in South Korea, the market value of the "senior-friendly" food industry in 2010 was around USD 4 million and growing at a rate of 11% per year [6]. The guidelines for TM foods in Japan have been issued by several initiatives, such as food for special dietary uses (FOSDU), the dysphagia diet 2013, and "Smile-Care" foods [6]. Several companies have a special product line that consists mainly in thickened beverages and purées for individuals with swallowing disorders. TM foods offer food companies the opportunity to tailor-make products with soft textures because the products for this market segment have been slow to appear in Europe [162].

Finally, diets should be as varied as possible, and ought to supply sufficient energy and protein. In addition, dishes ought to be pleasantly presented to encourage whetting people's appetite. Servings should be small and frequent rather than a few copious meals a day. For such purposes, molecular gastronomy [163] and 3D printing technology [100] have been used to produce food from various raw material sources with a variety of textures to enhance diet and to make them more palatable and esthetically appealing. In order to apply 3D printing to food, it is necessary for the food material to possess suitable rheological characteristics to allow its extrusion and for it to be cohesive enough to maintain its shape. However, further research into the application of selected non-thermal technologies as a means to modify food texture for subsequent 3D printing will be worthwhile [5]. In the future, it is envisaged that the food industry will advance toward convergence technology by the utilization of digital solutions, such as machine learning to food systems, as shown in the results of a recent study. This suggests a pioneering framework to identify the rheological levels of foods for the elderly by combining experimental results with machine learning technology in the food application domain [164].

6. Conclusions

Food texture modifications are essential to suit the nutritional diets of dysphagic patients. It is necessary to gain a better understanding of the complex factors that influence the colloidal food matrix from a multidisciplinary perspective. Individual and household food service operators, including nursing homes, need to acquire better knowledge about food texture, nutrition, and sensory properties. The elderly and dysphagic patients require a sourcing of special foods that are not only soft and easy and safe to swallow, but are also nutritious and tasty. This is vital for them to achieve their nutritional needs. Current food product development initiatives on the TM foods industrial scale also need to employ novel technologies to ensure dysphagic patients' access to appropriate TM food products. Additional quality criteria and clinical guidelines that target dysphagic patients, and based on the rheological parameters discussed in this review, need to be introduced by the food industry, and healthcare and catering services. In the very near future, it is hoped that more food processors will engage in the commercialization of cost-effective TM foods to put innovative technologies in this field to the best possible use.

Author Contributions: Conceptualization, A.S., C.C., D.R., F.R. and A.R.; methodology, A.S., C.C., D.R., F.R. and A.R.; software, A.S., C.C., D.R., F.R. and A.R.; validation, A.S., C.C., D.R., F.R. and A.R.; formal analysis, A.S., C.C., D.R., F.R. and A.R.; investigation, A.S., C.C., D.R., F.R. and A.R.; resources, A.S., C.C., D.R., F.R. and A.R.; data curation, A.S., C.C., D.R., F.R. and A.R.; writing—original draft preparation, A.S., C.C., D.R., F.R. and A.R.; writing—review and editing, A.S., C.C., D.R., F.R. and A.R.; visualization, A.S., C.C., D.R., F.R. and A.R.; supervision, A.S., C.C., D.R., F.R., and A.R.; project administration, A.S., C.C., D.R., F.R. and A.R. All authors have read and agreed to the published version of the manuscript.

Funding: This research received no external funding.

Institutional Review Board Statement: Not applicable.

Informed Consent Statement: Not applicable.

Data Availability Statement: Not applicable.

Acknowledgments: The authors are very grateful to their families and friends for all of the support they provided.

Conflicts of Interest: The authors declare no conflict of interest.

References

1. Sullo, A.; Norton, I.T. Food Colloids and Emulsions. In *Encyclopedia of Food and Health*; Caballero, B., Finglas, P.M., Toldrá, F., Eds.; Elsevier: Amesterdam, The Netherlands, 2016; pp. 7–15.
2. Bourne, M. *Food Texture and Viscosity: Concept and Measurement*, 2nd ed.; Academic Press, Elsevier: New York, NY, USA, 2002.
3. Loret, C. Using sensory properties of food to trigger swallowing: A review. *Crit. Rev. Food Sci. Nutr.* **2015**, *55*, 140–145. [CrossRef] [PubMed]
4. Cichero, J.A.Y.; Steele, C.; Duivestein, J.; Clavé, P.; Chen, J.; Kayashita, J.; Dantas, R.; Lecko, C.; Speyer, R.; Lam, P.; et al. The need for international terminology and definitions for texture-modified foods and thickened liquids used in dysphagia management: Foundations of a global initiative. *Curr. Phys. Med. Rehabil. Rep.* **2013**, *1*, 280–291. [CrossRef] [PubMed]
5. Sungsinchai, S.; Niamnuy, C.; Wattanapan, P.; Charoenchaitrakool, M.; Devahastin, S. Texture modification technologies and their opportunities for the production of dysphagia foods: A review. *Compr. Rev. Food Sci. Food Saf.* **2019**, *18*, 1898–1912. [CrossRef] [PubMed]
6. Aguilera, J.M.; Park, D.J. Texture-modified foods for the elderly: Status, technology and opportunities. *Trends Food Sci. Technol.* **2016**, *57*, 156–164. [CrossRef]
7. UN. World Population Prospects: The 2015 Revision, Key Findings and Advance Tables. Department of Economic and Social Affairs, Population Division (2015) Working Paper No. ESA/P/WP.241. 2015. Available online: https://population.un.org/wpp/publications/files/key_findings_wpp_2015.pdf (accessed on 1 September 2020).
8. IUFoST. Meeting the Food Needs of the Ageing Population. Implications for Food Science and Technology. 2014. Available online: http://www.iufost.org/iufostftp/IUF.SIB.Meeting%20the%20Food%20Needs%20of%20the%20Ageing%20Population.pdf (accessed on 1 September 2020).

9. Cichero, J.A.Y.; Lam, P.; Steele, C.M.; Hanson, B.; Chen, J.; Dantas, R.O.; Duivestein, J.; Kayashita, J.; Lecko, C.; Murray, J.; et al. Development of international terminology and definitions for texture-modified foods and thickened fluids used in dysphagia management: The IDDSI framework. *Dysphagia* **2017**, *32*, 293–314. [CrossRef]
10. Ishihara, S.; Nakauma, M.; Funami, T.; Odake, S.; Nishinari, K. Swallowing profiles of food polysaccharide gels in relation to bolus rheology. *Food Hydrocoll.* **2011**, *25*, 1016–1024. [CrossRef]
11. Yoshioka, K.; Yamamoto, A.; Matsushima, Y.; Hachisuka, K.; Ikeuchi, Y. Effects of high pressure on the textural and sensory properties of minced fish meat gels for the dysphagia diet. *Food Nutr. Sci.* **2016**, *7*, 732–742. [CrossRef]
12. Miles, A.; Liang, V.; Sekula, J.; Broadmore, S.; Owen, P.; Braakhuis, A.J. Texture-modified diets in aged care facilities: Nutrition, swallow safety and mealtime experience. *Australas. J. Ageing* **2020**, *39*, 31–39. [CrossRef]
13. Lam, P.; Stanschus, S.; Zaman, R.; Cichero, J.A. The international dysphagia diet standardisation initiative (IDDSI) framework: The Kempen pilot. *Br. J. Neurosci. Nurs.* **2017**, *13*, S18–S26. [CrossRef]
14. ISO. *Sensory Analysis Vocabulary, Part 4*; International Organization for Standardization: Geneva, Switzerland, 1981.
15. Thybo, A.K.; Martens, M. Analysis of sensory assessors in texture profiling of potatoes by multivariate modelling. *Food Qual. Prefer.* **2000**, *11*, 283–288. [CrossRef]
16. Szczesniak, A.S. Textural perceptions and food quality. *J. Food Qual.* **1991**, *14*, 75–85. [CrossRef]
17. Bomze, L.; Dehom, S.; Lao, W.P.; Thompson, J.; Lee, N.; Cragoe, A.; Luceno, C.; Crawley, B. Comorbid Dysphagia and Malnutrition in Elderly Hospitalized Patients. *Laryngoscope* **2021**. [CrossRef]
18. Herh, P.K.; Colo, S.M.; Roye, N.; Hedman, K. Rheology of foods: New techniques, capabilities, and instruments. *Am. Lab.* **2000**, *32*, 16–21.
19. Cuomo, F.; Angelicola, M.; De Arcangelis, E.; Lopez, F.; Messia, M.C.; Marconi, E. Rheological and Nutritional Assessment of Dysphagia—Oriented New Food Preparations. *Foods* **2021**, *10*, 663. [CrossRef]
20. Adeleye, B.; Rachal, C. Comparison of the rheological properties of ready-to-serve and powdered instant food–thickened beverages at different temperatures for dysphagic patients. *J. Am. Diet. Assoc.* **2007**, *107*, 1176–1182. [CrossRef]
21. Socialstyrelsen. *Näringsproblem i Vård och Omsorg. Prevention och Behandling (SoS Rapport 2000:11)*; Socialstyrelsen: Stockholm, Sweden, 2020. Available online: http://www.socialstyrelsen.se/Lists/Artikelkatalog/Attachments/11653/2000-3-11_0003012.pdf (accessed on 2 March 2021).
22. BDA. The British Dietetic Association and the Royal College of Speech and Language Therapists. National Descriptors for Texture Modification in Adults. May 2002. Available online: https://www.acquiredbraininjury-education.scot.nhs.uk/wp-content/uploads/National-Descriptors-Texture-Modification-Adults-2009.pdf (accessed on 2 March 2021).
23. Wendin, K.; Ekman, S.; Bülow, M.; Ekberg, O.; Johansson, D.; Rothenberg, E.; Stading, M. Objective and quantitative definitions of modified food textures based on sensory and rheological methodology. *Food Nutr. Res.* **2010**, *54*, 5134. [CrossRef]
24. Hemsley, B.; Palmer, S.; Kouzani, A.; Adams, S.; Balandin, S. Review informing the design of 3D food printing for people with swallowing disorders: Constructive, conceptual, and empirical problems. In *HICSS 52: Proceedings of the 52nd Annual Hawaii International Conference on System Sciences*; University of Hawaii at Manoa: Honolulu, HI, USA, 2019; pp. 5735–5744.
25. Szczesniak, A.S. Texture is a sensory property. *Food Qual. Prefer.* **2002**, *13*, 215–225. [CrossRef]
26. Torrico, D.D.; Fuentes, S.; Viejo, C.G.; Ashman, H.; Dunshea, F.R. Cross-cultural effects of food product familiarity on sensory acceptability and non-invasive physiological responses of consumers. *Food Res. Int.* **2019**, *115*, 439–450. [CrossRef]
27. Farag, K.W.; Lyng, J.G.; Morgan, D.J.; Cronin, D.A. Effect of low temperatures (−18 to +5 °C) on the texture of beef lean. *Meat Sci.* **2009**, *81*, 249–254. [CrossRef]
28. Steffe, J.F. *Rheological Methods in Food Process Engineering*; Freeman Press: East Lansing, MI, USA, 1996.
29. Zargaraan, A.; Rastmanesh, R.; Fadavi, G.; Zayeri, F.; Mohammadifar, M.A. Rheological aspects of dysphagia-oriented food products: A mini review. *Food Sci. Hum. Wellness* **2013**, *2*, 173–178. [CrossRef]
30. Anonymous. Food Rheolgy. 2021. Available online: https://www.anton-paar.com/es-es/reologia-de-los-alimentos/ (accessed on 2 March 2021).
31. Scott-Blair, G. Rheology in food research. *Adv. Food Res.* **1958**, *8*, 1–56.
32. Chen, L.; Opara, U.L. Texture measurement approaches in fresh and processed foods—A review. *Food Res. Int.* **2013**, *51*, 823–835. [CrossRef]
33. Nishinari, K.; Kohyama, K.; Kumagai, H.; Funami, T.; Bourne, M.C. Parameters of texture profile analysis. *Food Sci. Technol. Res.* **2013**, *19*, 519–521. [CrossRef]
34. Anonymous. Overview of Texture Profiles Analysis. Chapter II. 2020. Available online: https://texturetechnologies.com/resources/texture-profile-analysis (accessed on 2 March 2021).
35. Martínez, O.; Vicente, M.S.; De Vega, M.C.; Salmerón, J. Sensory perception and flow properties of dysphagia thickening formulas with different composition. *Food Hydrocoll.* **2019**, *90*, 508–514. [CrossRef]
36. National Dysphagia Diet Task Force. *National Dysphagia Diet: Standardization for Optimal Care*; American Dietetic Association: Chicago, IL, USA, 2002.
37. Vieira, J.M.; Oliveira, F.D., Jr.; Salvaro, D.B.; Maffezzolli, G.P.; de Mello, J.D.B.; Vicente, A.A.; Cunha, R.L. Rheology and soft tribology of thickened dispersions aiming the development of oropharyngeal dysphagia-oriented products. *Curr. Res. Food Sci.* **2020**, *3*, 19–29. [CrossRef]

38. ISO 11036:2020. Sensory Analysis—Methodology—Texture Profile. 2020. Available online: https://www.iso.org/standard/76668 (accessed on 2 March 2021).
39. Levine, H.; Finley, J.W. Texture. In *Principles of Food Chemistry*; Springer: Cham, Switzerland, 2018; pp. 329–336. [CrossRef]
40. Albert, A.; Varela, P.; Salvador, A.; Hough, G.; Fiszman, S. Overcoming the issues in the sensory description of hot served food with a complex texture. Application of QDA®, flash profiling and projective mapping using panels with different degrees of training. *Food Qual. Prefer.* **2011**, *22*, 463–473. [CrossRef]
41. O'Leary, M.; Hanson, B.; Smith, C.H. Variation of the apparent viscosity of thickened drinks. *Int. J. Lang. Commun. Disord.* **2011**, *46*, 7–29. [CrossRef]
42. Nicosia, M.A.; Robbins, J. The usefulness of the line spread test as a measure of liquid consistency. *Dysphagia* **2007**, *22*, 306–311. [CrossRef]
43. Fujimoto, K.; Minami, N.; Goto, T.; Ishida, Y.; Watanabe, M.; Nagao, K.; Ichikawa, T. Hardness, cohesiveness, and adhesiveness of oral moisturizers and denture adhesives: Selection criteria for denture wearers. *Dent. J.* **2016**, *4*, 34. [CrossRef]
44. Karel, M. Food research tasks at the beginning of the new millennium—A personal vision. In *Water Management in the Design and Distribution of Quality of Foods*; Roos, Y.H., Leslie, R.B., Lillford, P.J., Eds.; Technomic Publishing: New York, NY, USA, 1999; pp. 535–559.
45. Stone, H.; Sidel, J.L. 6–Descriptive Analysis, Sensory Evaluation Practices. In *Food Science and Technology*, 3rd ed.; Academic Press: Cambridge, MA, USA, 2004; pp. 201–245.
46. Bourne, M.C. Is rheology enough for food texture measurement? *J. Texture Stud.* **1975**, *6*, 259–262. [CrossRef]
47. Barbon, C.E.A.; Steele, C.M. Thickened Liquids for Dysphagia Management: A Current Review of the Measurement of Liquid Flow. *Curr. Phys. Med. Rehabil. Rep.* **2018**, *6*, 220–226. [CrossRef] [PubMed]
48. Hanson, B.; Jamshidi, R.; Redfearn, A.; Begley, R.; Steele, C.M. Experimental and Computational Investigation of the IDDSI Flow Test of Liquids Used in Dysphagia Management. *Ann. Biomed. Eng.* **2019**, *47*, 2296–2307. [CrossRef] [PubMed]
49. Reginelli, A.; D'Amora, M.; Del Vecchio, L.; Monaco, L.; Barillari, M.R.; Di Martino, N.; Barillari, U.; Motta, G.; Cappabianca, S.; Grassi, R. Videofluoroscopy and oropharyngeal manometry for evaluation of swallowing in elderly patients. *Int. J. Surg.* **2016**, *33* (Suppl. 1), S154–S158. [CrossRef] [PubMed]
50. Stading, M.; Waqas, M.Q.; Holmberg, F.; Wiklund, J.; Kotze, R.; Ekberg, O. A Device that Models Human Swallowing. *Dysphagia* **2019**, *34*, 615–626. [CrossRef]
51. Myhan, R.; Białobrzewski, I.; Markowski, M. An approach to modeling the rheological properties of food materials. *J. Food Eng.* **2012**, *111*, 351–359. [CrossRef]
52. Wang, Z.; Hirai, S. Modeling and estimation of rheological properties of food products for manufacturing simulations. *J. Food Eng.* **2011**, *102*, 136–144. [CrossRef]
53. Rao, M.A. Flow and functional models for rheological properties of fluid foods. In *Rheology of Fluid, Semisolid, and Solid Foods*; Springer: Boston, MA, USA, 2014; pp. 27–61.
54. Tabilo-Munizaga, G.; Barbosa-Cánovas, G.V. Rheology for the food industry. *J. Food Eng.* **2005**, *67*, 147–156. [CrossRef]
55. Suebsaen, K.; Suksatit, B.; Kanha, N.; Laokuldilok, T. Instrumental characterization of banana dessert gels for the elderly with dysphagia. *Food Biosci.* **2019**, *32*, 100477. [CrossRef]
56. Seo, C.W.; Yoo, B. Steady and dynamic shear rheological properties of gumbased food thickeners used for diet modification of patients with dysphagia: Effect of concentration. *Dysphagia* **2013**, *28*, 205–211. [CrossRef]
57. Steele, C.M.; Hill, L.; Stokely, S.; Peladeau-Pigeon, M. Age and strength influences on lingual tactile acuity. *J. Texture Stud.* **2014**, *45*, 317–323. [CrossRef]
58. Barbosa-Cánovas, G.V.; Kokini, J.L.; Ma, L.; Ibarz, A. The rheology of semiliquid foods. *Adv. Food Nutr. Res.* **1996**, *39*, 1–69.
59. Gallegos, C.; Franco, J.M. Rheology of food emulsions. In *Rheology Series*; Elsevier: Amsterdam, The Netherlands, 1999; Volume 8, pp. 87–118.
60. Barringer, S.; Ratanatriwong, P. Rheometers. In *Encyclopedia of Agricultural, Food, and Biological Engineering*; Marcel Dekker, Inc.: New York, NY, USA, 2003; pp. 862–865.
61. Dobraszczyka, B.J.; Morgenstern, M.P. Rheology and the breadmaking process. *J. Cereal Sci.* **2003**, *38*, 229–245. [CrossRef]
62. Riso, S.; Baj, G.; D'Andrea, F. Thickened beverages for dysphagic patients. Data and myth. *Mediterr. J. Nutr. Metab.* **2008**, *1*, 15–17. [CrossRef]
63. Park, D.J.; Han, J.A. Quality controlling of brown rice by ultrasound treatment and its effect on isolated starch. *Carbohydr. Polym.* **2016**, *137*, 30–38. [CrossRef]
64. Civille, G.V.; Czczesniak, A.S. Guidelines to training a texture profile panel. *J. Texture Stud.* **1973**, *4*, 204–223. [CrossRef]
65. Saldaña, E.; Behrens, J.H.; Serrano, J.S.; Ribeiro, F.; de Almeida, M.A.; Contreras-Castillo, C.J. Microstructure, texture profile and descriptive analysis of texture for traditional and light mortadella. *Food Struct.* **2015**, *6*, 13–20. [CrossRef]
66. Yates, M.D.; Drake, M.A. Texture properties of Gouda cheese. *J. Sens. Stud.* **2007**, *22*, 493–506. [CrossRef]
67. Barden, L.M.; Osborne, J.A.; McMahon, D.J.; Foegeding, E.A. Investigating the filled gel model in Cheddar cheese through use of Sephadex beads. *J. Dairy Sci.* **2015**, *98*, 1502–1516. [CrossRef]
68. Chen, J.; Rosenthal, A. Food texture and structure. In *Modifying Food Texture*; Chen, J., Rosenthal, A., Eds.; Woodhead Publishing: Cambridge, UK, 2015; Volume 1, pp. 3–24.

69. Aguilera, J.M. Seligman lecture 2005 food product engineering: Building the right structures. *J. Sci. Food Agric.* **2006**, *86*, 1147–1155. [CrossRef]
70. Chen, L.; Remondetto, G.E.; Subirade, M. Food protein-based materials as nutraceutical delivery systems. *Trends Food Sci. Technol.* **2006**, *17*, 272–283. [CrossRef]
71. Katsanos, C.S.; Kobayashi, H.; Sheffield-Moore, M.; Aarsland, A.; Wolfe, R.R. A high proportion of leucine is required for optimal stimulation of the rate of muscle protein synthesis by essential amino acids in the elderly. *Am. J. Physiol. Endocrinol. Metab.* **2006**, *291*, E381–E387. [CrossRef] [PubMed]
72. Funami, T.; Ishihara, S.; Nakauma, M.; Kohyama KNishinari, K. Texture design for products using food hydrocolloids. *Food Hydrocoll.* **2012**, *26*, 412–420. [CrossRef]
73. Nishinari, K.; Takemasa, M.; Brenner, T.; Su, L.; Fang, Y.; Hirashima, M.; Yoshimura, M.; Nitta, Y.; Moritaka, H.; Tomczynska-Mleko, M.; et al. The food colloid principle in the design of elderly food. *J. Texture Stud.* **2016**, *47*, 284–312. [CrossRef]
74. Ray, S.; Raychaudhuri, U.; Chakraborty, R. An overview of encapsulation of active compounds used in food products by drying technology. *Food Biosci.* **2016**, *13*, 76–83. [CrossRef]
75. Elleuch, M.; Bedigian, D.; Roiseux, O.; Besbes, S.; Blecker, C.; Attia, H. Dietary fibre and fibre-rich by-products of food processing: Characterisation, technological functionality and commercial applications: A review. *Food Chem.* **2011**, *124*, 411–421. [CrossRef]
76. Chung, C.; Degner, B.; McClements, D.J. Creating novel food textures: Modifying rheology of starch granule suspensions by cold-set whey protein gelation. *LWT Food Sci. Technol.* **2013**, *54*, 336–345. [CrossRef]
77. Zhang, L.; Cai, W.; Shan, J.; Zhang, S.; Dong, F. Physical properties and loading capacity of gelatinized granular starches. *Ind. Crops Prod.* **2014**, *53*, 323–329. [CrossRef]
78. Parada, J.; Aguilera, J.M. Starch matrices and the glycemic response. *Food Sci. Technol. Int.* **2011**, *17*, 187–204. [CrossRef]
79. Marangoni, A.G.; Wesdorp, L.H. *Structure and Properties of Fat Crystal Networks*, 2nd ed.; CRC Press: Boca Raton, FL, USA, 2012.
80. McClements, D.J. Nanoscale nutrient delivery systems for food applications: Improving bioactive dispersibility, stability, and bioavailability. *J. Food Sci.* **2015**, *80*, N1602–N1611. [CrossRef]
81. Marangoni, A.G. Organogels: An alternative edible oil-structuring method. *J. Am. Oil Chem. Soc.* **2012**, *89*, 749–780. [CrossRef]
82. Singer, N.S.; Dunn, J.M. Protein microparticulation: The principle and the process. *J. Am. Coll. Nutr.* **1990**, *9*, 388–397. [CrossRef]
83. Nicolai, T.; Durand, D. Controlled food protein aggregation for new functionality. *Curr. Opin. Colloid Interface Sci.* **2013**, *18*, 249–256. [CrossRef]
84. Nicolai, T. Formation and functionality of self-assembled whey protein microgels. *Colloids Surf. B* **2016**, *137*, 32–38. [CrossRef]
85. Dickinson, E. Microgels—An alternative colloidal ingredient for stabilization of food emulsions. *Trends Food Sci. Technol.* **2015**, *43*, 178–188. [CrossRef]
86. Zhang, Z.; Zhang, R.; Tong, Q.; Decker, E.A.; McClements, D.J. Food-grade filled hydrogels for oral delivery of lipophilic active ingredients: Temperature-triggered release microgels. *Food Res. Int.* **2015**, *69*, 274–280. [CrossRef]
87. Burey, P.; Bhandari, B.R.; Howes, T.; Gidley, M.J. Hydrocolloid gel particles: Formation, characterization, and application. *Crit. Rev. Food Sci. Nutr.* **2008**, *48*, 361–377. [CrossRef]
88. Okita, A.; Takahashi, K.; Itakura, M.; Horio, A.; Yamamoto, R.; Nakamura, Y.; Osako, K. A novel soft surimi gel with functionality prepared using alcalase for people suffering from dysphagia. *Food Chem.* **2021**, *344*, 128641. [CrossRef]
89. Marquis, M.; Davy, J.; Cathala, B.; Fang, A.; Renard, D. Microfluidics assisted generation of innovative polysaccharide hydrogel microparticles. *Carbohydr. Polym.* **2015**, *116*, 189–199. [CrossRef]
90. Neethirajan, S.; Kobayashi, I.; Nakajima, M.; Wu, D.; Nandagopal, S.; Lin, F. Microfluidics for food, agriculture and biosystems industries. *Lab Chip* **2011**, *11*, 1574–1586. [CrossRef]
91. Amici, E.; Tetradis-Meris, G.; de Torres, C.P.; Jousse, F. Alginate gelation in microfluidic channels. *Food Hydrocoll.* **2008**, *22*, 97–104. [CrossRef]
92. Skurtys, O.; Aguilera, J.M. Applications of microfluidic devices in food engineering. *Food Biophys.* **2008**, *3*, 1–15. [CrossRef]
93. Sun, J.; Peng, Z.; Zhou, W.; Fuh, J.Y.; Hong, G.S.; Chiu, A. A review on 3D printing for customized food fabrication. *Procedia Manuf.* **2015**, *1*, 308–319. [CrossRef]
94. Godoi, F.C.; Prakash, S.; Bhandari, B.R. 3d printing technologies applied for food design: Status and prospects. *J. Food Eng.* **2016**, *179*, 44–54. [CrossRef]
95. Goole, J.M.; Amighi, K. 3D printing in pharmaceutics: A new tool for designing customized drug delivery systems. *Int. J. Pharm.* **2016**, *499*, 376–394. [CrossRef]
96. Ghorani, B.; Tucker, N. Fundamentals of electrospinning as a novel delivery vehicle for bioactive compounds in food nanotechnology. *Food Hydrocoll.* **2015**, *51*, 227–240. [CrossRef]
97. Nieuwland, M.; Geerdink, P.; Brier, P.; van den Eijnden, P.; Henket, J.T.M.M.; Langelaan, M.L.P.; Stroeks, N.; van Deventer, H.C.; Martin, A.H. Food-grade electrospinning of proteins. *Innov. Food Sci. Emerg. Technol.* **2013**, *20*, 269–275. [CrossRef]
98. Stijnman, A.C.; Bodnar, I.; Tromp, R.H. Electrospinning of food-grade polysaccharides. *Food Hydrocoll.* **2011**, *25*, 1393–1398. [CrossRef]
99. Gómez-Mascaraque, L.G.; Lagarón, J.M.; López-Rubio, A. Electrosprayed gelatin submicroparticles as edible carriers for the encapsulation of polyphenols of interest in functional foods. *Food Hydrocoll.* **2015**, *49*, 42–52. [CrossRef]
100. Kouzani, A.Z.; Adams, S.; Whyte, D.J.; Oliver, R.; Hemsley, B.; Palmer, S.; Balandin, S. 3D printing of food for people with swallowing difficulties. *Knowl. Eng.* **2017**, *2*, 23–29. [CrossRef]

101. Stokes, J.R.; Boehm, M.W.; Baier, S.K. Oral processing, texture and mouthfeel: From rheology to tribology and beyond. *Curr. Opin. Colloid Interface Sci.* **2013**, *18*, 349–359. [CrossRef]
102. Kalviainen, N.; Roininen, K.; Tuorila, H. Sensory characterisation of high viscosity gels made with different thickeners. *J. Texture Stud.* **2007**, *31*, 407–420. [CrossRef]
103. Barham, P.; Skibsted, L.H.; Bredie, W.L.; Bom Frøst, M.; Møller, P.; Risbo, J.; Snitkjær, P.; Mortensen, L.M. Molecular gastronomy: A new emerging scientific discipline. *Chem. Rev.* **2010**, *110*, 2313–2365. [CrossRef]
104. Vega, C.; Castells, P. Spherification. In *The Kitchen as the Laboratory*; Vega, C., Ubbink, J., van der Linden, E., Eds.; Columbia University Press: New York, NY, USA, 2012; pp. 25–32.
105. Yuasa, M.; Tagawa, Y.; Tominaga, M. The texture and preference of "mentsuyu (Japanese noodle soup base) caviar" prepared from sodium alginate and calcium lactate. *Int. J. Gastron. Food Sci.* **2019**, *18*, 100178. [CrossRef]
106. Kim, S.; Joo, N. The study on development of easily chewable and swallowable foods for elderly. *Nutr. Res. Pract.* **2015**, *9*, 420–424. [CrossRef]
107. Oh, J.K.; Lee, D.I.; Park, J.M. Biopolymer-based microgels/nanogels for drug delivery applications. *Prog. Polym. Sci.* **2009**, *34*, 1261–1282. [CrossRef]
108. Joye, I.J.; McClements, D.J. Biopolymer-based nanoparticles and microparticles: Fabrication, characterization, and application. *Curr. Opin. Colloid Interface Sci.* **2014**, *19*, 417–427. [CrossRef]
109. Purwanti, N.; Peters, J.P.C.M.; van der Goot, A.J. Protein micro-structuring as a tool to texturize protein foods. *Food Funct.* **2013**, *4*, 277–282. [CrossRef]
110. Van der Zanden, L.D.T.; van Kleef, E.; de Wijk, R.A. Examining heterogeneity in elderly consumers' acceptance of carriers for protein-enriched food: A segmentation study. *Food Qual. Prefer.* **2015**, *42*, 130–138. [CrossRef]
111. Zuñiga, R.N.; Aguilera, J.M. Aerated food gels: Fabrication and potential applications. *Trends Food Sci. Technol.* **2008**, *19*, 176–187. [CrossRef]
112. Goh, S.M.; Leroux, B.; Groeneschild, C.A.G.; Busch, J.L.H.C. On the effect of tastant excluded fillers on sweetness and saltiness of a model food. *J. Food Sci.* **2010**, *75*, S245–S249. [CrossRef]
113. Debusca, A.; Tahergorabi, R.; Beamer, S.K.; Matak, K.E.; Jaczynski, J. Physicochemical properties of surimi gels fortified with dietary fiber. *Food Chem.* **2014**, *148*, 70–76. [CrossRef] [PubMed]
114. Dickinson, E. Emulsion gels: The structuring of soft solids with protein-stabilized oil droplets. *Food Hydrocoll.* **2012**, *28*, 224–241. [CrossRef]
115. Egan, T.; Jacquier, J.C.; Rosenberg, Y.; Rosenberg, M. Cold-set whey protein microgels for the stable immobilization of lipids. *Food Hydrocoll.* **2013**, *31*, 317–324. [CrossRef]
116. Lesmes, U.; McClements, D.J. Structure–function relationships to guide rational design and fabrication of particulate food delivery systems. *Trends Food Sci. Technol.* **2009**, *20*, 448–457. [CrossRef]
117. Pouteau, E.B.; Bovetto, L.; Schlup-Ollivier, G.; Grathwohl, D.; Beaumont, M.; Macé, C. PP226-MON microgel formation of whey protein reduces its insulinogenic index without modifying glycemic response in healthy men. *Clin. Nutr. Suppl.* **2012**, *1*, 227–228. [CrossRef]
118. Munialo, C.D. *Energy Storage and Dissipation in Deformed Protein-based Networks on Seconds Time Scale is Controlled by Submicron Length Scales*; Wageningen University: Wageningen, The Netherlands, 2015.
119. Sukkar, S.G.; Maggi, N.; Travalca Cupillo, B.; Ruggiero, C. Optimizing texture modified foods for oro-pharyngeal dysphagia: A difficult but possible target? *Front. Nutr.* **2018**, *5*, 68. [CrossRef]
120. Steele, C.M. The blind scientists and the elephant of swallowing: A review of instrumental perspectives on swallowing physiology. *J. Texture Stud.* **2015**, *46*, 122–137. [CrossRef]
121. Langmore, S.E.; Miller, R.M. Behavioral treatment for adults with oropharyngeal dysphagia. *Arch. Phys. Med. Rehabil.* **1994**, *75*, 1154–1160. [CrossRef]
122. IDDSI. International Dysphagia Diet Standardisation Initiative (IDDSI). Complete IDDSI Framework (Detailed Definitions). 2019. Available online: https://iddsi.org/IDDSI/media/images/Complete_IDDSI_Framework_Final_31July2019.pdf (accessed on 2 March 2021).
123. Hotaling, D.L. Nutritional considerations for the pureed diet texture in dysphagic elderly. *Dysphagia* **1992**, *7*, 81–85. [CrossRef] [PubMed]
124. Rosenbek, J.C.; Robbins, J.A.; Roecker, E.B.; Coyle, J.L.; Wood, J.L. A penetration-aspiration scale. *Dysphagia* **1996**, *11*, 93–98. [CrossRef]
125. McHorney, C.A.; Robbins, J.; Lomax, K.; Rosenbek, J.C.; Chignell, K.; Kramer, A.E.; Bricker, D.E. The SWAL–QOL and SWAL–CARE outcomes tool for oropharyngeal dysphagia in adults: III. Documentation of reliability and validity. *Dysphagia* **2002**, *17*, 97–114. [CrossRef]
126. O'Neil, K.H.; Purdy, M.; Falk, J.; Gallo, L. The dysphagia outcome and severity scale. *Dysphagia* **1999**, *14*, 139–145. [CrossRef]
127. Crary, M.A.; Mann, G.D.C.; Groher, M.E. Initial psychometric assessment of a functional oral intake scale for dysphagia in stroke patients. *Arch. Phys. Med. Rehabil.* **2005**, *86*, 1516–1520. [CrossRef]
128. Munialo, C.D.; Kontogiorgos, V.; Euston, S.R.; Nyambayo, I. Rheological, tribological and sensory attributes of texture-modified foods for dysphagia patients and the elderly: A review. *Int. J. Food Sci. Technol.* **2020**, *55*, 1862–1871. [CrossRef]

129. Vilardell, N.; Rofes, L.; Arreola, V.; Speyer, R.; Clavé, P. A comparative study between modified starch and xanthan gum thickeners in post-stroke oropharyngeal dysphagia. *Dysphagia* **2016**, *31*, 169–179. [CrossRef]
130. Kuhlemeier, K.V.; Palmer, J.B.; Rosenberg, D. Effect of liquid bolus consistency and delivery method on aspiration and pharyngeal retention in dysphagia patients. *Dysphagia* **2001**, *16*, 119–122. [CrossRef]
131. Wei, Y.; Guo, Y.; Li, R.; Ma, A.; Zhang, H. Rheological characterization of polysaccharide thickeners oriented for dysphagia management: Carboxymethylated curdlan, konjac glucomannan and their mixtures compared to xanthan gum. *Food Hydrocoll.* **2021**, *110*, 106198. [CrossRef]
132. Vieira, J.M.; Cristiane Conte Paim Andrade, T.P.; Santos, P.K.; Okuro, S.T.; Garcia, M.I.; Rodrigues, A.A.V.; Cunha, R.L. Flaxseed gum-biopolymers interactions driving rheological behaviour of oropharyngeal dysphagia-oriented products. *Food Hydrocoll.* **2021**, *111*, 106257. [CrossRef]
133. Sharma, M.; Duizer, L. Characterizing the Dynamic Textural Properties of Hydrocolloids in Pureed Foods—A Comparison Between TDS and TCATA. *Foods* **2019**, *8*, 184. [CrossRef]
134. Butterworth, P.J.; Warren, F.J.; Ellis, P.R. Human α-amylase and starch digestion: An interesting marriage. *Starch-Stärke* **2011**, *63*, 395–405. [CrossRef]
135. Yver, C.M.; Kennedy, W.P.; Mirza, N. Taste acceptability of thickening agents. *World J. Otorhinolaryngol. Head Neck Surg.* **2018**, *4*, 145–147. [CrossRef]
136. Garcia, J.M.; Chambers, E. Managing dysphagia through diet modifications. *Am. J. Nurs.* **2010**, *110*, 26–33. [CrossRef]
137. Merino, G.; Marín-Arroyo, M.R.; Beriain, M.J.; Ibañez, F.C. Dishes Adapted to Dysphagia: Sensory Characteristics and Their Relationship to Hedonic Acceptance. *Foods* **2021**, *10*, 480. [CrossRef]
138. Olaru, L.D.; Nistor, O.V.; Andronoiu, D.G.; Ghinea, I.O.; Barbu, V.; Botez, E. Effect of added hydrocolloids on ready-to-eat courgette (Cucurbita pepo) puree ohmically treated. *J. Food Sci. Technol.* **2021**. [CrossRef]
139. De Luis, D.A.; Aller, R.; Izaola, O. Menú de textura modificada y su utilidade en pacientes con situaciones de riesgo nutricional. *Nutr Hosp.* **2014**, *29*, 751–759.
140. Mendes, C.; Bohn, D.M. Expanding horizons: Encouraging cross-campus student collaboration to develop a novel food product for individuals experiencing dysphagia. *J. Food Sci. Educ.* **2020**, *19*, 36–40. [CrossRef]
141. WHO—World Health Organization. Nutrition for Older Persons. Ageing and Nutrition: A Growing Global Challenge. 2020. Available online: https://www.who.int/nutrition/topics/ageing/en/ (accessed on 31 October 2020).
142. Fernández, A.C.; de la Maza, B.P.; Casariego, A.V.; Taibo, R.V.; Fondo, A.U.; Rodríguez, I.C.; Pomar, M.D.B. Características técnicas de los productos alimentarios específicos para el paciente con disfagia. *Nutr. Hosp.* **2015**, *32*, 1401–1407.
143. Baijens, L.W.J.; Clavé, P.; Cras, P.; Ekberg, O.; Forster, A.; Kolb, G.F.; Leners, J.-C.; Masiero, S.; Mateos-Nozal, J.; Ortega, O.; et al. European Society for Swallowing Disorders—European Union Geriatric Medicine Society white paper: Oropharyngeal dysphagia as a geriatric syndrome. *Clin. Interv. Aging* **2016**, *11*, 1403–1428. [CrossRef]
144. Burger, C.; Kiesswetter, E.; Alber, R.; Pfannes, U.; Arens-Azevedo, U.; Volkert, D. Texture modified diet in German nursing homes: Availability, best practices and association with nursing home characteristics. *BMC Geriatr.* **2019**, *19*, 284. [CrossRef]
145. Cassens, D.; Johnson, E.; Keelan, S. Enhancing taste, texture, appearance, and presentation of pureed food improved resident quality of life and weight status. *Nutr Rev.* **1996**, *54 Pt 2*, S51–S54. [CrossRef]
146. Hadde, E.K.; Chen, W.; Chen, J. Cohesiveness visual evaluation of thickened fluids. *Food Hydrocoll.* **2020**, *101*, 105522. [CrossRef]
147. Sucupira, N.R.; Xerez, A.C.P.; Sousa, P.H.M. Losses of vitamins in heat treatment of foods. *UNOPAR Cient Ciênc Biol. Saúde* **2012**, *14*, 121–128.
148. Rus-Polski, V.; Koutchma, T.; Xue, J.; Defelice, C.; Balamurugan, S. Effects of high hydrostatic pressure processing parameters and NaCl concentration on the physical properties, texture and quality of white chicken meat. *Innov. Food Sci. Emerg. Technol.* **2015**, *30*, 31–42. [CrossRef]
149. Singh, S.; Singh, N.; Ezekiel, R.; Kaur, A. Effects of gamma-irradiation on the morphological, structural, thermal and rheological properties of potato starches. *Carbohydr. Polym.* **2011**, *83*, 1521–1528. [CrossRef]
150. Jin, T.Z.; Yu, Y.; Gurtler, J.B. Effects of pulsed electric field processing on microbial survival, quality change and nutritional characteristics of blueberries. *LWT Food Sci. Technol.* **2017**, *77*, 517–524. [CrossRef]
151. Nayak, C.A.; Suguna, K.; Narasimhamurthy, K.; Rastogi, N.K. Effect of gamma irradiation on histological and textural properties of carrot, potato and beetroot. *J. Food Eng.* **2007**, *79*, 765–770. [CrossRef]
152. Cichero, J.A.Y.; Atherton, M.; Bellis-Smith, N.; Suter, M. Texture-modified foods and thickened fluids as used for individuals with dysphagia: Australian standardised labels and definitions. *Nutr Diet.* **2007**, *64* (Suppl. 2), S53–S76.
153. Huckabee, M.-L.; McIntosh, T.; Fuller, L.; Curry, M.; Thomas, P.; Walshe, M.; McCague, E.; Battel, I.; Nogueira, D.; Frank, U.; et al. The Test of Masticating and Swallowing Solids (TOMASS): Reliability, validity and international normative data. *Int. J. Lang. Commun. Disord.* **2018**, *53*, 144–156. [CrossRef]
154. Mathieu, V.; de Loubens, C.; Thomas, C.; Panouillé, M.; Magnin, A.; Souchon, I. An experimental model to investigate the biomechanical determinants of pharyngeal mucosa coating during swallowing. *J. Biomech.* **2018**, *72*, 144–151. [CrossRef]
155. Qazi, W.M.; Ekberg, O.; Wiklund, J.; Kotze, R.; Stading, M. Assessment of the food-swallowing process using bolus visualization and manometry simultaneously in a device that models human swallowing. *Dysphagia* **2019**, *34*, 821–833. [CrossRef]
156. Casanovas, A.; Hernández, M.J.E.; Martí-Bonmatí, E.; Dolz, M. Cluster classification of dysphagia-oriented products considering flow, thixotropy and oscillatory testing. *Food Hydrocoll.* **2011**, *25*, 851–859. [CrossRef]

157. Payne, C.; Methven, L.; Fairfield, C.; Bell, A. Consistently inconsistent: Commercially available starch-based dysphagia products. *Dysphagia* **2011**, *26*, 27–33. [CrossRef]
158. Bolivar-Prados, M.; Rofes, L.; Arreola, V.; Guida, S.; Nascimento, W.V.; Martin, A.; Vilardell, N.; Fernández, O.O.; Ripken, D.; Lansink, M.; et al. Effect of a gum-based thickener on the safety of swallowing in patients with poststroke oropharyngeal dysphagia. *Neurogastroenterol. Motil.* **2019**, *31*, e13695. [CrossRef]
159. Gómez-Busto, F.; Muñoz, V.A.; Sarabia, M.; Ruiz de Alegría, L.; González de Viñaspre, I.; López-Molina, N.; Cabo Santillán, N. Suplementos nutricionales gelatinizados: Una alternativa válida para la disfagia. *Nutr Hosp.* **2011**, *26*, 775–783.
160. Lee, H.S.; Lee, J.-J.; Kim, M.-G.; Kim, K.-T.; Cho, C.-W.; Kim, D.-D.; Lee, J.-Y. Sprinkle formulations—A review of commercially available products. *Asian J. Pharm. Sci.* **2020**, *15*, 292–310. [CrossRef] [PubMed]
161. Moret-Tatay, A.; Rodríguez-García, J.; Martí-Bonmatí, E.; Hernando, I.; Hernández, M.J. Commercial thickeners used by patients with dysphagia: Rheological and structural behaviour in different food matrices. *Food Hydrocoll.* **2015**, *51*, 318–326. [CrossRef]
162. Scott-Thomas, C. R&D Challenge: Developing Texture-Modified Foods For The Elderly. 2012. Available online: http://www.foodnavigator.com/Science/R-D-challenge-Developing-texture-modified-foods-for-the-elderly (accessed on 19 March 2021).
163. Reilly, R.; Frankel, F.; Edelstein, S. Molecular gastronomy: Transforming diets for dysphagia. *J. Nutr. Health Food Sci.* **2013**, *1*, 1.
164. Jeong, S.; Kim, H.; Lee, S. Rheology-Based Classification of Foods for the Elderly by Machine Learning Analysis. *Appl. Sci.* **2021**, *11*, 2262. [CrossRef]

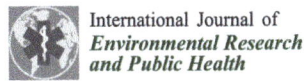

Article

Exploring the Roles of Green Food Consumption and Social Trust in the Relationship between Perceived Consumer Effectiveness and Psychological Wellbeing

Jianming Wang [1], Ninh Nguyen [2,3] and Xiangzhi Bu [4,*]

1. School of Business Administration, Zhejiang University of Finance & Economics, Hangzhou 310018, China; sjwjm@zufe.edu.cn
2. Department of Economics, Finance and Marketing, La Trobe Business School, La Trobe University, Melbourne 3086, Australia; ninh.nguyen@latrobe.edu.au or ninhnguyen@tmu.edu.vn
3. Business Sustainability Research Group, Thuongmai University, Hanoi 100000, Vietnam
4. Department of Business Administration, Business School, Shantou University, Shantou 515063, China
* Correspondence: buxiangzhistu@yahoo.com

Received: 11 June 2020; Accepted: 27 June 2020; Published: 29 June 2020

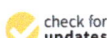

Abstract: Green food consumption is a core issue that contributes to solving environmental pollution and achieving sustainable development. This study aims to investigate the mediating role of green food consumption and social trust in the relationship between perceived consumer effectiveness and psychological wellbeing to provide new insights into green food consumption, based on social ideal theory and social trust theory. Using a sample data of 514 consumers in China, the results of structural equation modeling showed that perceived consumer effectiveness was positively related to psychological wellbeing. Furthermore, green food consumption mediated the relationship between perceived consumer effectiveness and psychological wellbeing. In addition, social trust moderated the relationship between perceived consumer effectiveness and green food consumption. Social trust also moderated the indirect effect of perceived consumer effectiveness on psychological wellbeing through green food consumption. The findings of this study enrich the extant literature relating to green food consumption and have practical implications for business managers and policymakers.

Keywords: perceived consumer effectiveness; green food consumption; social trust theory; social ideal theory; psychological wellbeing; China

1. Introduction

Global warming and climate change have generated a tremendous challenge to our society in the last decades [1]. The challenge of reducing environmental pollution and obtaining sustainable development is an important issue for governments, organizations, researchers, and practitioners [2]. Green purchases and green food consumption are core issues that contribute to such a challenge [3].

Various studies have examined the issue of green purchases and green food consumption in the current literature. For example, Mohd et al. [4] explored the factors and mechanisms that motivate consumers to engage in green consumption behavior. He et al. [5] determined the relationship between tourists' perceptions and relational quality with their environmentally responsible behaviors. Li et al. [1] investigated gender inequality that affects a household's decision to adopt green consumption. Zhang et al. [6] determined the impact of haze pollution on residents' green consumption behavior. Rustam et al. [3] examined the relationship between corporate environmental sustainability disclosure and green consumption behavior with the moderating role of environmental awareness. Furthermore, several studies have determined socioeconomic factors (e.g., gender, age, family size, and income) that influence green food purchase behavior [1,4]. Prior studies have provided substantial evidence on the factors that influence green purchases and green food consumption. However, further research should explore additional factors and mechanisms that affect green food consumption and their impact on human physiological and psychological outcomes [3,4,7].

Social ideal theory believes that an individual expects an ideal society [8–10]. People who expect an ideal society often think and act in ways that generate benefits and bring goodwill to society [9]. For example, those people tend to engage in charitable donation and philanthropy behavior [10]. Furthermore, perceived consumer effectiveness reflects an individual's belief about his or her ability to improve environmental and social problems [11]. This perception may affect consumers' behavior toward green food consumption, which may influence their psychological outcomes [12,13]. For example, those who hold high perceptions of effectiveness tend to engage in recycling behavior and purchase environmentally friendly products [11,12]. Unfortunately, how perceived consumer effectiveness affects green food consumption and psychological outcomes has not been determined in the current literature. Therefore, this study investigates the relationship between perceived consumer effectiveness and psychological wellbeing with the mediating role of green food consumption, drawing upon the theoretical foundation of social ideal theory.

In addition, social trust theory states that people who hold a high level of social trust tend to be optimistic about the future and confident in society, and they tend to trust in others [14,15]. Consequently, social trust may play an important role in enhancing people's perceptions of their ability to solve environmental and social problems. Social trust may also influence people's behavior toward consuming green products [16,17]. Unfortunately, the role of social trust has been ignored in the current literature. Thus, this study also investigates the moderating role of social trust in the relationship between perceived consumer effectiveness and green food consumption. Moreover, this study examines the moderating role of social trust in the indirect effect of perceived consumer effectiveness on psychological wellbeing through green food consumption.

In sum, this study focusses on social ideal theory and social trust theory to investigate the mediating role of green food consumption and the moderating role of social trust in the relationship between perceived consumer effectiveness and psychological wellbeing. The objective is to provide new insights into the antecedent and consequence of green food consumption.

The structure of this paper is organized as follows. Section 2 reviews the current literature and develops hypotheses. Section 3 discusses the research design and sample procedure. Section 4 presents the empirical results. Sections 5 and 6 provide discussions and implications.

2. Literature and Hypotheses

2.1. Perceived Consumer Effectiveness

Perceived consumer effectiveness is defined as an individual's belief about his or her ability to improve environmental and social problems [11]. Nevertheless, perceived consumer effectiveness reflects an individual's belief that their actions can make a difference in solving social and environmental pollution [18]. People who hold high perceptions of effectiveness tend to believe that they can influence and improve environmental and social problems. Hence, they tend to be highly confident and engage in socially responsible behavior [19]. For example, Roberts [20] suggested that green consumption is often associated with consumers' perceptions of effectiveness. Webb et al. [21] and Cojuharenco et al. [22] reported that perceived consumer effectiveness is an important predictor of socially responsible behavior. Jaiswal and Kant [12] found that consumers who believe in their effectiveness tend to hold high intention to purchase green products. He and Zhan [23] demonstrated that perceived consumer effectiveness positively predicts consumers' intention to adopt environmentally electric vehicles. Wang and Chen [24] found that perceived effectiveness of fair trade consumers tends to hold high intention to purchase fair trade products. Higueras-Castillo et al. [13] also reported that perceived consumer effectiveness is an important predictor of consumers' attitudes toward electromobility.

In sum, prior studies have provided substantial evidence to explain the predictive ability of perceived consumer effectiveness on socially responsible behavior.

2.2. Psychological Wellbeing

Wellbeing refers to a physical, mental, and psychological state in which individuals experience a sense of happiness, satisfaction, and pleasure [25,26]. Research in the last decades focused on psychological wellbeing. Three important scientific disciplines have been critical for the study of psychological wellbeing: developmental psychology often studies the psychological wellbeing of human life across different lifespans [25]. Personality psychology focuses on the relationship between self-actualization, individuation, and maturity with psychological wellbeing [27]. Clinical psychology emphasizes the association between mental illness and psychological wellbeing [28]. Moreover, several researchers have identified social life satisfaction as a core indicator of psychological wellbeing [29]. Social life satisfaction is the way in which individuals present their emotions and feelings and satisfaction with social relationships, goal achievement, self-concepts, and self-perceived ability to cope with an individual's daily life [30]. Several studies have reported important factors that affect life satisfaction, including personality, self-esteem, age, experience, personal values, culture, family, and career [25,29–31]. In this study, social life satisfaction is treated as a key factor that reflects the psychological wellbeing of consumers [26,28,30].

2.3. Perceived Consumer Effectiveness and Psychological Wellbeing

Social ideal theory states that people tend to expect an ideal society in which they can enjoy justice, goodwill, and wellbeing [8–10]. Social ideal theory provides directions and guidelines to drive people's attitudes and behavior toward positive activities that are beneficial to society [32]. People who hold high expectations about an ideal society often favor living in a harmonious and peaceful environment. They tend to engage in activities that create a high value for the environment and society [33]. Furthermore, those who hold the belief of an ideal society often show positive emotions and feelings about the social world. They also are highly confident, enjoyable, and optimistic about their lives because they are often motivated by hope and expectation about a better future [8].

From the logic of social ideal theory, consumers who hold high perceptions of their effectiveness often believe that they can change the social world. That is, they are optimistic about their capability to improve and solve environmental problems [10]. When consumers perceive their effectiveness to improve environmental and social problems, they may actively engage in activities that generate benefits for their society [12,23]. For example, consumers may believe that if they engage in recycling activities, purchase environmentally friendly products, and reduce their consumption of electricity and water, then they will contribute to solving environmental pollution [13]. Thus, these consumers tend to be satisfied with their social life because they may believe that they create good things for society. In other words, perceived consumer effectiveness enhances consumers' positive emotions and wellbeing because they are optimistic and believe that they can contribute to the goodwill of their society. They have contributed to building an ideal society [9]. Thus, the following hypothesis is proposed.

Hypothesis (H1): *Perceived consumer effectiveness is positively related to psychological wellbeing.*

2.4. Mediating Role of Green Food Consumption

Green consumption is a broad concept in the current literature. Van Raaij and Verhallen [34] identified energy consumption behavior as the key activity of green consumption. Clark et al. [35] suggested that consumers engaging in a green electricity program are considered a green consumption behavior. Gilg et al. [36] defined green consumption as consumer purchasing products that have a less negative impact on the environment. Hartmann and Apaolaze-Ibanez [37] stated that consumers' intention to purchase green energy brands could also be viewed as green consumption. Guo et al. [38]

explained residential electricity consumption as a major type of green consumption based on the theory of planned behavior. In a broader concept, Mohd et al. [4] identified green consumption as an entire process of selection, use, and disposal of resources that generate impacts on the environment and society. Green food consumption is often viewed as a type of green consumption, which reflects consumers' purchase behavior toward green food products that are perceived as healthy, safe, and environmentally friendly [39].

Social ideal theory can provide a solid theoretical foundation to explain the relationship between perceived consumer effectiveness, green food consumption, and psychological wellbeing. According to social ideal theory [8–10], consumers who hold high perceptions of effectiveness tend to engage in activities that create values and benefits the society because they believe that their behavior will contribute to building an ideal society [8]. With the idea of a better world, these consumers may invest time, energy, and effort to address environmental and social issues. For example, consumers may engage in donations to help other people. They also engage in green consumption behaviors, such as purchasing environmentally friendly products [12], using electric vehicles [23], consuming organic foods [39], and adopting electromobility to replace traditional polluted cars [13]. Furthermore, when consumers engage in green consumption behavior, they likely obtain additional benefits from such behavior. For example, the behavior of consumers purchasing and consuming organic and green foods contributes to their health because these types of foods provide additional nutrition and are safe to human health than traditional foods. Green food consumption also reduces the negative impact of farming and processing on the environment [39]. Consequently, when consumers perceive that their green food consumption contributes to the goodwill of human health, environment, and society, they tend to feel happy and satisfied with their behavior and lives [40]. Therefore, perceived consumer effectiveness will likely motivate consumers to engage in green food consumption, which in turn increases consumers' positive emotions and wellbeing toward their lives. The following hypothesis is proposed.

Hypothesis (H2): *Green food consumption positively mediates the relationship between perceived consumer effectiveness and psychological wellbeing.*

2.5. Moderating Role of Social Trust

Social trust theory states the tendency that people hold a positive belief about the social world. These people tend to be optimistic and trust others in their society [14,15]. Social trust reflects an individual's general belief that people will avoid behaving in ways that disadvantage others and take actions that benefit others [41]. Social trust may not be a stable trait, but it can be affected by several factors from an individual's internal and external environment, such as social interaction and individual experiences [42]. Social trust is a broad concept that has not been defined in a consistent way [43]. However, this study followed Day and Settersten Jr.'s [16] suggestions and focused on several aspects of social trust, including confidence in society, optimism about the future, and general trust in others. Furthermore, social trust theory states that beliefs about society shape and influence a person's view about the benevolence of other human beings [17]. People who hold different perceptions of social trust tend to think and act differently [16]. For example, people with low social trust are likely to be pessimistic, uncooperative, and egoistic. These people are less likely to help others [44]. By contrast, trusting people tend to be optimistic, cooperative, tolerant, and altruistic. They often engage in activities that bring benefits and positive results for others [45].

According to social trust theory, the influence of perceived consumer effectiveness on green food consumption may differ between people who trust and do not trust their society. Considering that people who hold a high level of social trust tend to be optimistic and altruistic, they may believe that they are useful, and their actions will bring benefits to the environment, society, and other people [46]. Hence, these people may actively engage in green food consumption because they believe that their green food consumption will create additional values for society [4,47]. For example, when consumers trust their society and other people, consumers may think that if they purchase environmentally friendly foods, then their purchase behavior will generate goodwill for the society. Consequently, consumers may actively engage in such consumption activities [8,12,23]. By contrast, people who hold a low level of social trust may be pessimistic and lack confidence. These people may believe that they are not able to contribute to society. Hence, the lack of trust people may behave in egoistic manners and even take actions that harm others and society [44,47]. In other words, when people hold a low level of social trust, they do not believe in their ability to improve social and environmental issues. They may not engage in green food consumption because they lack confidence and may perceive green food consumption as unnecessary activities [47]. Therefore, the influence of perceived consumer effectiveness on green food consumption will likely vary between people who hold a high level of social trust as compared with those who hold a low level of social trust. The following hypothesis is proposed.

Hypothesis (H3): *Social trust moderates the relationship between perceived consumer effectiveness and green food consumption such that the relationship is strong when social trust is high and vice versa.*

This study proposed a research model, as shown in Figure 1. As stated above, green food consumption is argued to have a mediating effect on the relationship between perceived consumer effectiveness and psychological wellbeing. Moreover, social trust is hypothesized to moderate the relationship between perceived consumer effectiveness and green food consumption. Thus, social trust will moderate the indirect effect of perceived consumer effectiveness on psychological wellbeing through green food consumption. The following hypothesis is proposed.

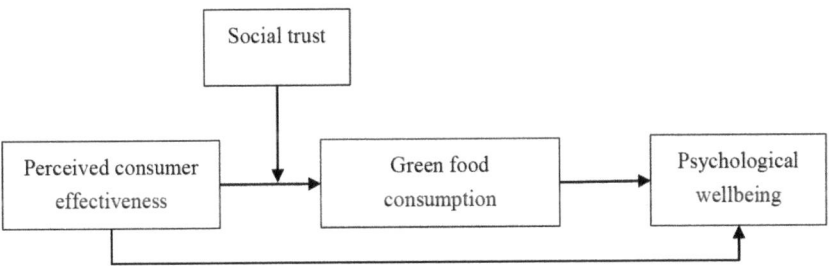

Figure 1. Conceptual framework of the study.

Hypothesis (H4): *Social trust moderates the indirect effect of perceived consumer effectiveness on psychological wellbeing through green food consumption such that the indirect effect is strong when social trust is high and weaker when social trust is low.*

3. Methods

3.1. Measures of Variables

This study adopted measurement items of variables in prior studies. Perceived consumer effectiveness was measured using four items from Straughan and Robert [48]. Green food consumption was measured using four items from Mohd et al. [4]. These constructs were measured using a five-point Likert scale from 1 (strongly disagree) to 5 (strongly agree). Moreover, social trust was measured using two items from Day and Setterstern Jr. [16]. This construct was measured using a five-point scale from 1 (never) to 5 (every day). Psychological wellbeing was measured using four items from Diener et al. [49]. This construct was measured using a five-point Likert scale from 1 (strongly disagree) to 5 (strongly agree). Table 1 shows the details of the items and variables.

Table 1. Items and constructs of measures.

Construct	Items	Source
Perceived consumer effectiveness	What I purchase as a consumer affects the nation's environmental problem. Each consumer's behavior can affect how companies treat their employees. Each consumer can have a positive effect on society by purchasing products sold by socially responsible companies. Given that one person cannot have any effect on pollution and natural resource problems, what I do doesn't make any difference (r).	[48]
Green food consumption	I always buy green food. I always try to buy food with green labels. I buy green food even at higher prices. I recommend green food that I have consumed to my relatives and friends.	[4]
Social trust	In the last month, how often did you feel that the way our society works makes sense to you. In the last month, how often did you feel that our society is becoming a better place.	[16]
Psychological wellbeing	In most ways, my social life is close to my ideal. I am satisfied with my social life. So far, I have the important things that I want in my social life. If I could live my social life again, then I would change almost nothing.	[49]

3.2. Sample Procedure

This study used a questionnaire survey to collect data. We recruited professional translators to translate the measures. A forward and backward language translation was conducted to ensure the meaning of measurement items. Moreover, a pilot test was conducted at a large supermarket with the participation of 30 consumers. The purpose of this pilot test is to modify and ensure the clarity of the questionnaire. In the formal survey stage, we recruited a team to distribute questionnaires at different physical stores in Shanghai city. We randomly selected 10 physical stores to collect the sample data. The research team conveniently approached consumers and invited them to complete the questionnaire. We adopted a systematic sampling technique in which one of the three consumers was selected, considering that the list of consumers was not available. Consumers voluntarily participated in the survey. The survey was conducted from October 2019 to January 2020. Among the 800 questionnaires distributed, 520 were returned, and 514 were valid, with a response rate of 64.25%. Only six questionnaires were invalid and excluded from the final sample because of missing values. Kline [50] noted that the sample size should comply with N:q rule (N is the number item of the measurement scales, q is the number of cases). The ideal sample size should be 1:10 (1 measurement item requires 10 cases). In this study, the total measurement is was 14; hence, the number of sample sizes should be 140 cases. Thus, the sample size of 514 is considered adequate in this study.

3.3. Ethical Considerations

This study conducted a survey that involves human activity. Considering ethical standards, this study was conducted with the approval of the Major Project of The National Social Science Fund of China (20ZDA084). Consumers voluntarily participated in the survey and provided the measures with an anonymous questionnaire. Therefore, this study ensured the privacy and security of the respondents.

3.4. Analytical Methods

This study used SPSS statistical software (IBM, Armonk, NY, United States) to analyze the descriptive statistics and reliability of the measures. Furthermore, partial least square structural equation modeling (PLS-SEM) was adopted to perform the measurement model, which is used to test the validity of the measures. In addition, PLS-SEM was used to test the hypotheses in this study. Specifically, basic PLS-SEM was used to perform a confirmatory factor analysis (CFA). Based on the results of this CFA, the values of composite reliability (CR), the average variance extracted (AVE), and square roots of AVE were calculated to test the convergent and discriminant validity. Furthermore, PLS-SEM with the maximum likelihood estimation method was used to test all hypotheses in a single model. Structural equation modeling (SEM) is a combination of path and factor analyses. Several multiple regression analyses were combined into a single model so that the standard errors were controlled in SEM. PLS-SEM has been widely used in business and management studies [50].

4. Results

4.1. Sample Characteristics and Descriptive Statistics

Table 2 presents the basic information and characteristics of the respondents in this study: (1) most of the respondents were female (65.6%); (2) more than half of the respondents aged between 20 and under 30 (58.0%); (3) the majority of the respondents were not married (70.4%); (4) approximately 66.7% of the respondents had university education; (5) most of the respondents had monthly income between 500 and under 1000 USD (67.7%).

Table 2. Sample characteristics ($N = 514$).

Variable	Frequency	Percentage
Gender		
Male	177	34.4%
Female	337	65.6%
Age		
Under 20	102	19.8%
20–under 30	298	58.0%
30–under 40	66	12.8%
41 and above	48	9.3%
Marital status		
Married	150	29.2%
Not married	362	70.4%
Education		
High school and below	153	29.8%
University	243	66.7%
Master and above	18	3.5%
Income		
Under 500 USD	124	24.1%
500–under 1000 USD	348	67.7%
1000 USD or above	42	8.2%

Table 3 shows the descriptive statistics of all variables. Results show that perceived consumer effectiveness was positively associated with green food consumption ($r = 0.53$, $p < 0.01$) and psychological wellbeing ($r = 0.41$, $p < 0.01$). Furthermore, green food consumption was positively associated with psychological wellbeing ($r = 0.27$, $p < 0.01$). In addition, social trust was positively associated with green food consumption ($r = 0.51$, $p < 0.01$) and psychological wellbeing ($r = 0.47$, $p < 0.01$).

Table 3. Means, standard deviation, and Pearson correlation ($N = 514$).

Variable	Means	SD	1	2	3	4
Perceived consumer effectiveness	3.86	0.71	0.76			
Green food consumption	3.74	0.74	0.53 **	0.78		
Social trust	3.69	0.83	0.48 **	0.51 **	0.85	
Psychological wellbeing	3.59	0.78	0.41 **	0.27 **	0.47 **	0.74

** $p < 0.01$

4.2. Measurement Model

The results of the measurement model in this study indicate a good model fit of the hypothesized model. Specifically, all goodness of fit index of the measurement model met the required threshold:

χ^2/d.f. = 2.93 which was less than 3; Comparative Fit Index - CFI = 0.94, Goodness-of-fit Index-GFI = 0.91, and Tucker Lewis Index - TLI = 0.92 which were all greater than 0.90; and Root Mean Square Error of Approximation - RMSEA = 0.07 which was less than 0.08 [50].

This study used Cronbach's alpha to measure reliability. Results in Table 4 show that Cronbach's alpha of all variables ranged from 0.77 to 0.90, which exceeded the cutoff value of 0.60 [51]. Thus, the measures in this study show good reliability.

Table 4. Results of the measurement model (N = 514).

Variable	Items	Factor Loadings	CR Value	AVE Value	Cronbach's α
Perceived consumer effectiveness (PCE)	PCE1	0.65 ***	0.84	0.57	0.84
	PCE2	0.80 ***			
	PCE3	0.77 ***			
	PCE4	0.80 ***			
Green food consumption (GFC)	GFC1	0.81 ***	0.86	0.61	0.90
	GFC2	0.79 ***			
	GFC3	0.81 ***			
	GFC4	0.72 ***			
Social trust (STR)	STR1	0.85 ***	0.84	0.72	0.84
	STR2	0.85 ***			
Psychological wellbeing (PSW)	PSW1	0.62 ***	0.83	0.55	0.77
	PSW2	0.63 ***			
	PSW3	0.83 ***			
	PSW4	0.85 ***			

*** p <0.001.

Convergent validity was tested using CR and AVE in this study. Hair et al. [51] suggested that the CR value must be greater than 0.70, and AVE values must be greater than 0.50. Results indicate that CR and AVE values of all variables were all greater than the threshold value. Thus, the measures in this study have good convergent reliability.

Discriminant validity was tested by comparing the square roots of AVE and Pearson correlations of all variables. Hair et al. [51] suggested that square roots of AVE must be greater than all correlation coefficients of all variables. Table 3 shows that the square roots of AVE were greater than all Pearson correlation, thereby providing evidence for the good discriminant validity of the measures in this study.

4.3. Common Method Bias

Following Podsakoff et al. [52], this study conducted Harman's one-factor test to detect the problem of common method bias. Results of the unrotated solution of principle component analysis show that four factors emerged with 64.24% of the variance, and the first factor accounted for only 17.02% of the variance. Furthermore, results of one-factor model of CFA indicate a poor model fit (χ^2/d.f. = 11.47, CFI = 0.76, GFI = 0.74, TLI = 0.734, and RMSEA = 0.14). Thus, the common method bias may not seriously affect the results of hypothesis testing in this study.

4.4. Structural Model

This study used PLS-SEM to test the hypotheses. Results in Figure 2 show that perceived consumer effectiveness was positively related to psychological wellbeing (β = 0.119, p <0.01), thereby supporting Hypothesis (H1). Furthermore, perceived consumer effectiveness was positively related to green food consumption (β = 0.532, p < 0.001) which in turn was positively related to psychological wellbeing (β = 0.425, p < 0.001). We followed Preacher et al. [53] to conduct a bootstrap analysis with 1000 bootstrap samples to confirm this indirect effect. Results indicate that the indirect effect of perceived consumer effectiveness on psychological wellbeing through green food consumption was statistically significant (perceived consumer effectiveness → green food consumption → psychological wellbeing: $\beta = 0.328$, $p < 0.01$, 95% CI = [0.252, 0.419]). Thus, Hypothesis (H2) was supported. In addition, results in Figure 2 show that the interaction effect between perceived consumer effectiveness and social trust was positively related to green food consumption ($\beta = 0.043$, $p < 0.05$). Results in Figure 3 also indicate that the influence of perceived consumer effectiveness on green food consumption was strong when social trust was high and vice versa. In other words, the influence of perceived consumer effectiveness on green food consumption varied among different levels of social trust. Thus, Hypothesis (H3) was supported.

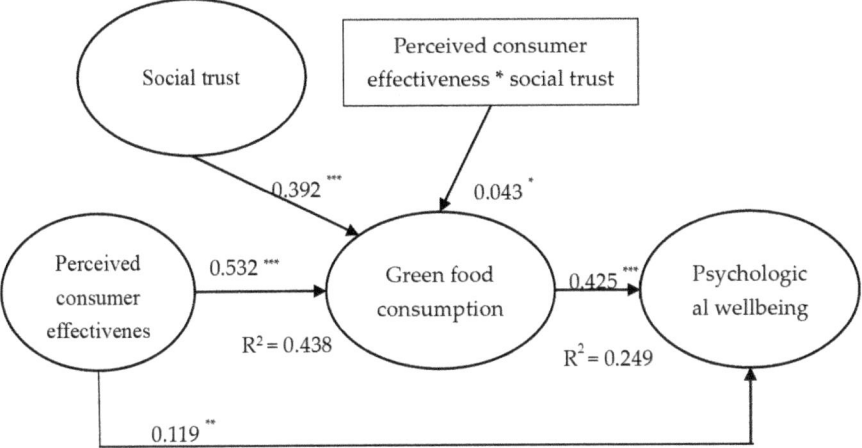

Figure 2. Results of hypothesis testing ($N = 514$). * $p < 0.05$, ** $p < 0.01$, *** $p < 0.001$.

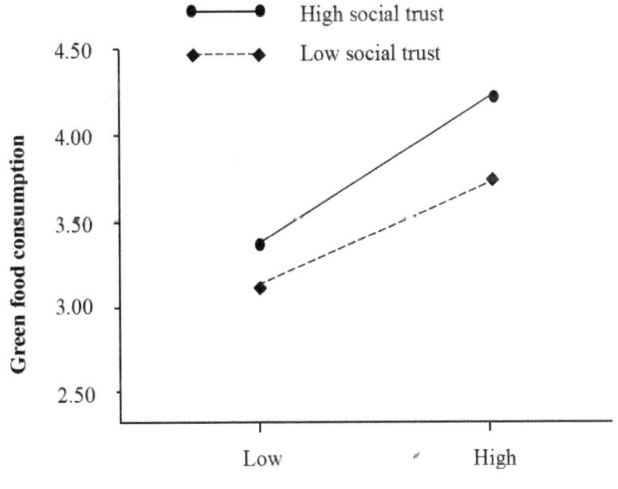

Figure 3. Moderating effect of social trust.

This study followed Edward and Lambert's [54] procedure to test the moderating effect of social trust on the indirect effect of perceived consumer effectiveness on psychological wellbeing through green food consumption. Table 5 shows that the indirect effect of perceived consumer effectiveness on psychological wellbeing through green food consumption varied among different groups of social trust ($\Delta\beta = 0.058$, $p < 0.01$). Thus, Hypothesis (H4) was supported.

Table 5. Moderating role of social trust ($N = 514$).

Moderator	Perceived Consumer Effectiveness (X) → Green Food Consumption (M) → Psychological Wellbeing (Y)				
	Stage		Effect		
	First (P_{XM})	Second (P_{MY})	Direct Effects (P_{XY})	Indirect Effects ($P_{XM}P_{MY}$)	Total Effects ($P_{XY} + P_{XM}P_{MY}$)
Low social trust	0.557 ***	0.391 ***	0.062 *	0.218 ***	0.280 **
High social trust	0.629 ***	0.438 **	0.098 *	0.276 ***	0.374 **
Differences	0.072 ***	0.047 ***	0.036	0.058 **	0.094 **

* $p < 0.05$, ** $p < 0.01$, *** $p < 0.001$; P_{XM}: path from independent variable to mediator; P_{MY}: path from mediator to dependent variable; P_{XY}: path from independent variable to dependent variable.

5. Discussion and Implications

This study aims to investigate the mediating role of green food consumption and social trust in the relationship between perceived consumer effectiveness and psychological wellbeing. The results provide important implications for researchers and managers.

5.1. Research Implications

First, this study argues for the direct influence of perceived consumer effectiveness on psychological wellbeing based on social ideal theory. Findings indicate that consumers who hold perceptions of effectiveness believe in their ability to solve social and environmental issues. Given this perception, they tend to feel satisfied with their social life because they may believe that they can contribute to the goodwill of their society [9]. The findings of this study provide new insights into the relationship between perceived consumer effectiveness and psychological wellbeing. To our best knowledge, this relationship has not been determined in prior literature. Thus, our study provides new knowledge and advances our understanding of the impact of perceived consumer effectiveness on psychological wellbeing.

Second, our findings demonstrate the mediating role of green food consumption in the relationship between perceived consumer effectiveness and psychological wellbeing. That is, according to social ideal theory, consumers who believe in their ability to change the social world tend to actively engage in green food consumption because they believe that their green food consumption is good behavior that contributes to building a better world [12]. Furthermore, green food consumption helps to protect the environment, solves social issues, and creates values for society [23,39]. Hence, when consumers contribute to bringing goodwill to society, they tend to feel satisfied with their social life [8]. Prior studies often determined the antecedents of green food consumption. However, this study extends social ideal theory and provides new evidence on the mediating mechanism of green food consumption into the relationship between perceived consumer effectiveness and psychological wellbeing. The findings of this study provide a theoretical foundation for researchers who may be interested in studying the role of social ideal theory in green food consumption.

Third, this study found the moderating role of social trust in the relationship between perceived consumer effectiveness and green food consumption. This finding indicates that consumers who trust other people in their society often feel optimistic and also tend to engage in altruistic activities [14,15]. These consumers may often believe in their ability to improve social and environmental problems. Consequently, they tend to engage in green food consumption behavior [4,47]. By contrast, consumers who hold a low level of social trust tend to be pessimistic and even engage in egoistic behavior. They are less likely to engage in green food consumption behavior due to the lack of confidence and beliefs in others [44,47]. Thus, the findings of this study provide new evidence on the moderating mechanism of social trust. This important effect of social trust has not been investigated in prior literature. Our findings help to extend social trust theory and clarify the role of social trust in green food consumption research.

Last, the research model in this study is unique and deals with the relationship among variables that have been greatly ignored in prior literature. The mediating mechanism of green food consumption behavior in the relationship between perceived consumer effectiveness and psychological wellbeing helps to advance our knowledge about the antecedent of green food consumption and the impact of green food consumption on consumers' psychological wellbeing. To our best knowledge, none of the prior studies have determined the influence of green food consumption on consumers' psychological wellbeing. Furthermore, the moderating mechanism of social trust is unique in our research model. Findings in this study clarify the role of social trust in enhancing consumers' beliefs and behavior toward their ability to improve social and environmental problems. Thus, the mediating and moderating mechanisms in this study provide new insight into our knowledge and understanding of green food consumption behavior in the current literature.

5.2. Practical Implications

Based on empirical findings, this study provides several suggestions for business managers and policymakers. When consumers hold the belief that they can improve and change social and environmental problems, they will actively engage in green food consumption behavior. Thus, business managers should plan and implement marketing strategies to integrate green food consumption with consumers' perceptions of effectiveness. For example, marketing advertising may trigger consumers' perceptions of environmental protection and combine this with their green food purchasing behavior (e.g., combining organic food consumption with environmental protection and bridging green food purchases with reducing pollution). Furthermore, policymakers should launch different strategies to persuade consumers to engage in green food consumption. For example, government agencies may use advertising to persuade consumers that if they purchase environmentally friendly food products, then they will contribute greatly to the improvement of the environment and society. In addition, policymakers should plan different strategies to enhance consumers' trust in society because when consumers trust their society, they will engage in positive activities that benefit the entire society. The findings of this study also provide implications for individual consumers. Individuals should trust our society and believe that each consumer can contribute to our society in solving environmental and social issues. We can experience a happy life and create value for our entire society by engaging in green food consumption.

6. Conclusions

To the best of the researchers' knowledge, this study is the first attempt to examine a mediating and moderating mechanism in the relationship between perceived consumer effectiveness and psychological wellbeing. Empirical results reveal several fresh insights. Perceived consumer effectiveness has a positive impact on psychological wellbeing. Green food consumption appears to have a mediating effect on the relationship between perceived consumer effectiveness and psychological wellbeing. Furthermore, social trust has a moderating effect on the relationship between perceived consumer effectiveness and green food consumption. Notably, social trust also moderates the indirect effect of perceived consumer effectiveness on psychological wellbeing through green food consumption.

Some limitations should be acknowledged and overcome in future research. For example, cross-sectional data may affect the causal relationship among variables in this study. Hence, future research should collect longitudinal data to validate such a relationship to overcome this limitation. Furthermore, cross-sectional data may generate a common method bias that influences the results of the hypothesis testing. We suggest that future research should obtain consumers' contact and collect data from them several times. In addition, this study analyzed data from consumers in China only, which may limit the generalizability of the results. Thus, future research should collect data from consumers in different emerging markets (e.g., Southeast Asia, Russia, and Brazil).

Author Contributions: Conceptualization: J.W., N.N., and X.B.; methodology: J.W., N.N., and X.B.; formal analysis: J.W. and X.B.; investigation: J.W. and X.B.; resources: J.W. and X.B.; writing—original draft preparation: J.W., N.N., and X.B.; writing—review and editing: J.W., N.N., and X.B. All authors have read and agreed to the published version of the manuscript.

Funding: This research received funding from the Major Project of The National Social Science Fund of China (20ZDA087).

Conflicts of Interest: The authors declare that they have no conflict of interest.

References

1. Li, J.; Zhang, J.; Zhang, D.; Ji, Q. Does gender inequality affect household green consumption behaviour in China? *Energy Policy* **2019**, *135*, 111071. [CrossRef]
2. Liu, J.; Zhang, D.; Cai, J.; Davenport, J. Legal Systems, National Governance and Renewable Energy Investment: Evidence from Around the World. *Br. J. Manag.* **2019**, *31*, 1875–1911. [CrossRef]
3. Rustam, A.; Wang, Y.; Zameer, H. Environmental awareness, firm sustainability exposure and green consumption behaviors. *J. Clean. Prod.* **2020**, *268*, 122016. [CrossRef]
4. Seo, Y.; Cruz, A.G.B.; Fam, K.S.; Suki, N.M.; Suki, N.M. Does religion influence consumers' green food consumption? Some insights from Malaysia. *J. Consum. Mark.* **2015**, *32*, 551–563. [CrossRef]
5. He, X.; Hu, D.; Swanson, S.R.; Su, L.; Chen, X. Destination perceptions, relationship quality, and tourist environmentally responsible behavior. *Tour. Manag. Perspect.* **2018**, *28*, 93–104. [CrossRef]
6. Zhang, L.; Guo, X.; Zhao, T.; Gong, S.; Xu, X.; Li, Y.; Luo, L.; Gui, K.; Wang, H.; Zheng, Y.; et al. A modelling study of the terrain effects on haze pollution in the Sichuan Basin. *Atmos. Environ.* **2019**, *196*, 77–85. [CrossRef]
7. Shiel, C.; Paço, A.; Alves, H. Generativity, sustainable development and green consumer behaviour. *J. Clean. Prod.* **2020**, *245*, 118865. [CrossRef]
8. Farrelly, C. *Contemporary Political Theory*; SAGE: Thousand Oaks, CA, USA, 2004.
9. Robeyns, I. Ideal Theory in Theory and Practice. *Soc. Theory Pr.* **2008**, *34*, 341–362. [CrossRef]
10. Stemplowska, Z. *What's Ideal About Ideal Theory? Theories of Justice*; Routledge: New York, NY, USA, 2017; pp. 205–232.
11. Kinnear, T.C.; Taylor, J.R.; Ahmed, S.A. Ecologically concerned consumers: Who are they? Ecologically concerned consumers can be identified. *J. Mark.* **1974**, *38*, 20–24. [CrossRef]
12. Jaiswal, D.; Kant, R. Green purchasing behaviour: A conceptual framework and empirical investigation of Indian consumers. *J. Retail. Consum. Serv.* **2018**, *41*, 60–69. [CrossRef]
13. Higueras-Castillo, E.; Liébana-Cabanillas, F.J.; Muñoz-Leiva, F.; García-Maroto, I. Evaluating consumer attitudes toward electromobility and the moderating effect of perceived consumer effectiveness. *J. Retail. Consum. Serv.* **2019**, *51*, 387–398. [CrossRef]
14. Barber, B. *The Logic and Limits of Trust*; Rutgers University Press: New Brunswick, NJ, USA, 1983.
15. Yamagishi, T.; Yamagishi, M. Trust and commitment in the United States and Japan. *Motiv. Emot.* **1994**, *18*, 129–166. [CrossRef]
16. Day, J.K.; Settersten, R.A. Less trusting and connected? Social trust and social integration among young adults during the recession. *Adv. Life Course Res.* **2018**, *37*, 57–68. [CrossRef]
17. Justwan, F.; Bakker, R.; Berejikian, J.D. Measuring social trust and trusting the measure. *Soc. Sci. J.* **2018**, *55*, 149–159. [CrossRef]
18. Ellen, P.S.; Wiener, J.L.; Cobb-Walgren, C. The Role of Perceived Consumer Effectiveness in Motivating Environmentally Conscious Behaviors. *J. Public Policy Mark.* **1991**, *10*, 102–117. [CrossRef]
19. Kang, J.; Liu, C.; Kim, S.-H. Environmentally sustainable textile and apparel consumption: The role of consumer knowledge, perceived consumer effectiveness and perceived personal relevance. *Int. J. Consum. Stud.* **2013**, *37*, 442–452. [CrossRef]
20. Roberts, J.A. Green consumers in the 1990s: Profile and implications for advertising. *J. Bus. Res.* **1996**, *36*, 217–231. [CrossRef]

21. Webb, D.J.; Mohr, L.A.; Harris, K.E. A re-examination of socially responsible consumption and its measurement. *J. Bus. Res.* **2008**, *61*, 91–98. [CrossRef]
22. Cojuharenco, I.; Cornelissen, G.; Karelaia, N. Yes, I can: Feeling connected to others increases perceived effectiveness and socially responsible behavior. *J. Environ. Psychol.* **2016**, *48*, 75–86. [CrossRef]
23. He, X.; Zhan, W. How to activate moral norm to adopt electric vehicles in China? An empirical study based on extended norm activation theory. *J. Clean. Prod.* **2018**, *172*, 3546–3556. [CrossRef]
24. Wang, E.S.-T.; Chen, Y.-C. Effects of perceived justice of fair trade organizations on consumers' purchase intention toward fair trade products. *J. Retail. Consum. Serv.* **2019**, *50*, 66–72. [CrossRef]
25. Ryff, C.D. Happiness is everything, or is it? Explorations on the meaning of psychological well-being. *J. Personal. Soc. Psychol.* **1989**, *57*, 1069–1081. [CrossRef]
26. Yang, H.; Ma, J. How an epidemic outbreak impacts happiness: Factors that worsen (vs. protect) emotional well-being during the coronavirus pandemic. *Psychiatry Res.* **2020**, *289*, 113045. [CrossRef] [PubMed]
27. Ryff, C.D.; Keyes, C.M. The structure of psychological well-being revisited. *J. Personal. Soc. Psychol.* **1995**, *69*, 719–727. [CrossRef]
28. Keyes, C.L.M. The mental health continuum: From languishing to flourishing in life. *J. Health Soc. Behav.* **2002**, *43*, 207–222. [CrossRef] [PubMed]
29. Sophie, G.; Philippe, C. Contributions of psychological well-being and social support to an integrative model of subjective health in later adulthood. *Ageing Int.* **2010**, *35*, 38–60.
30. Wu, C.-H.; Tsai, Y.-M.; Chen, L.H. How do Positive Views Maintain Life Satisfaction? *Soc. Indic. Res.* **2008**, *91*, 269–281. [CrossRef]
31. Cummins, R.A. Normative Life Satisfaction: Measurement Issues and a Homeostatic Model. *Soc. Indic. Res.* **2003**, *64*, 225–256. [CrossRef]
32. Valentini, L. Ideal vs. Non-ideal Theory: A Conceptual Map. *Philos. Compass* **2012**, *7*, 654–664. [CrossRef]
33. Li, C. The Confucian Ideal of Harmony. *Philos. East West* **2006**, *56*, 583–603. [CrossRef]
34. Van Raaij, W.; Verhallen, T.M. A behavioral model of residential energy use. *J. Econ. Psychol.* **1983**, *3*, 39–63. [CrossRef]
35. Clark, C.F.; Kotchen, M.J.; Moore, M.R. Internal and external influences on pro-environmental behavior: Participation in a green electricity program. *J. Environ. Psychol.* **2003**, *23*, 237–246. [CrossRef]
36. Gilg, A.; Barr, S.; Ford, N. Green consumption or sustainable lifestyles? Identifying the sustainable consumer. *Futures* **2005**, *37*, 481–504. [CrossRef]
37. Hartmann, P.; Apaolaza-Ibáñez, V. Consumer attitude and purchase intention toward green energy brands: The roles of psychological benefits and environmental concern. *J. Bus. Res.* **2012**, *65*, 1254–1263. [CrossRef]
38. Guo, Z.; Zhou, K.; Zhang, C.; Lu, X.; Chen, W.; Yang, S. Residential electricity consumption behavior: Influencing factors, related theories and intervention strategies. *Renew. Sustain. Energy Rev.* **2018**, *81*, 399–412. [CrossRef]
39. Wang, J.; Pham, T.L.; Dang, V.T. Environmental Consciousness and Organic Food Purchase Intention: A Moderated Mediation Model of Perceived Food Quality and Price Sensitivity. *Int. J. Environ. Res. Public Health* **2020**, *17*, 850. [CrossRef]
40. Xiao, J.J.; Li, H. Sustainable Consumption and Life Satisfaction. *Soc. Indic. Res.* **2010**, *104*, 323–329. [CrossRef]
41. Luhmann, N. Familiarity, Confidence, Trust: Problems and Alternatives. *Trust Mak. Break. Coop. Relat.* **2020**, *6*, 94–107.
42. Paxton, P.; Glanville, J.L. Is Trust Rigid or Malleable? A Laboratory Experiment. *Soc. Psychol. Q.* **2015**, *78*, 194–204. [CrossRef]
43. Hardin, R. *The Street-Level Epistemology of Trust. Organizational Trust: A Reader*; Oxford University Press: New York, NY, USA, 2006.
44. Rathbun, B.C. Before Hegemony: Generalized Trust and the Creation and Design of International Security Organizations. *Int. Organ.* **2011**, *65*, 243–273. [CrossRef]
45. Uslaner, E.M. *The Moral Foundations of Trust*; Cambridge University Press: London, UK, 2020.
46. Kaltenthaler, K.; Miller, W.J. Social Psychology and Public Support for Trade Liberalization. *Int. Stud. Q.* **2013**, *57*, 784–790. [CrossRef]
47. Han, L.; Sun, R.; Gao, F.; Zhou, Y.; Jou, M. The effect of negative energy news on social trust and helping behavior. *Comput. Hum. Behav.* **2019**, *92*, 128–138. [CrossRef]

48. Straughan, R.D.; Roberts, J.A. Environmental segmentation alternatives: A look at green consumer behavior in the new millennium. *J. Consum. Mark.* **1999**, *16*, 558–575. [CrossRef]
49. Diener, E.; Emmons, R.A.; Larsen, R.J.; Griffin, S. The Satisfaction with Life Scale. *J. Pers. Assess.* **1985**, *49*, 71–75. [CrossRef]
50. Kline, R.B. *Principles and Practice of Structural Equation Modeling*; The Guilford Press: New York, NY, USA, 2011.
51. Hair, J.F.; Black, W.C.; Babin, B.J.; Anderson, R.E. *Multivariate Data Analysis: A Global Perspective*, 7th ed.; Pearson: Upper Saddle River, NJ, USA, 2010.
52. Podsakoff, P.M.; MacKenzie, S.B.; Lee, J.Y.; Podsakoff, N.P. Common method biases in behavioral research: A critical review of the literature and recommended remedies. *J. Appl. Psychol.* **2003**, *5*, 879–903. [CrossRef]
53. Preacher, K.J.; Rucker, D.D.; Hayes, A.F. Addressing Moderated Mediation Hypotheses: Theory, Methods, and Prescriptions. *Multivar. Behav. Res.* **2007**, *42*, 185–227. [CrossRef]
54. Edwards, J.; Lambert, L.S. Methods for integrating moderation and mediation: A general analytical framework using moderated path analysis. *Psychol. Methods* **2007**, *12*, 1–22. [CrossRef]

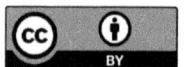
© 2020 by the authors. Licensee MDPI, Basel, Switzerland. This article is an open access article distributed under the terms and conditions of the Creative Commons Attribution (CC BY) license (http://creativecommons.org/licenses/by/4.0/).

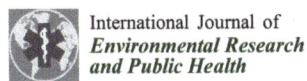 International Journal of *Environmental Research and Public Health*

Article

Food Sovereignty of the Indigenous Peoples in the Arctic Zone of Western Siberia: Response to COVID-19 Pandemic

Elena Bogdanova [1,*], Sergei Andronov [2], Ildiko Asztalos Morell [3], Kamrul Hossain [4], Dele Raheem [4,*], Praskovia Filant [5] and Andrey Lobanov [2]

1. Department of Economics and Management, Northern Arctic Federal University, 164500 Arkhangelsk, Russia
2. National Medical Research Center for Rehabilitation and Balneology, Ministry of Health of the Russia, 121099 Moscow, Russia; sergius198010@mail.ru (S.A.); alobanov89@gmail.com (A.L.)
3. Department of Urban and Rural Development, Swedish University of Agricultural Sciences, 75007 Uppsala, Sweden; ildiko.asztalos.morell@slu.se
4. Northern Institute of Environmental and Minority Law, Arctic Center of the University of Lapland, 96101 Rovaniemi, Finland; kamrul.hossain@ulapland.fi
5. Association of Reindeer Herders in YNAO, 629000 Salekhard, Russia; filant76@mail.ru
* Correspondence: e.n.bogdanova@narfu.ru (E.B.); bamidele.raheem@ulapland.fi (D.R.)

Received: 26 September 2020; Accepted: 15 October 2020; Published: 18 October 2020

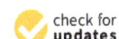

Abstract: This article presents the challenges facing reindeer herding as being both a profitable business and part of the traditional culture of the nomadic Indigenous peoples in the Arctic zone of Western Siberia which addresses substantial needs of the local population. Reindeer herding products are used as traditional nutrition, and as effective preventive means and remedies for adapting to the cold and geomagnetic activity in the High North. Export trends of traditional reindeer products have decreased local Indigenous peoples' access to venison and had a negative impact on their health. Due to the COVID-19 pandemic, it is especially urgent for the Indigenous peoples to have sufficient access to traditional food and be involved in policy decision-making to maintain this traditional business. We aim to analyze the dependencies of Indigenous peoples on the reindeer produce–exporting "food value chain" and explore how (1) the independence of reindeer herders could be increased in these export chains and (2) how provision of their products to local communities could be secured. The study takes a multidisciplinary approach based on policy and socioeconomic analyses with input from medical research. Primary sources include data collected from interviews and surveys of Indigenous peoples during expeditions to the Nyda settlement, the Nydinskaya tundra, the Tazovsky settlement, the Tazovskaya tundra, the Nakhodka tundra, the Gyda and Gydansky settlements, the Yavai-Salinskaya tundra, the Seyakha settlement, the Seyakhinskaya and Tambeyskaya tundras located along the southern coast of the Ob Bay, the northeast coast of the Yamal Peninsula, the Tazovsky and Gydansky Peninsulas, and the Shuryshkarsky district. Data were collected during the summers and winters of 2014–2020.

Keywords: food sovereignty; reindeer herding; food value chain; Indigenous peoples; COVID-19 pandemic; the Arctic; Western Siberia; Yamal-Nenets Autonomous Okrug

1. Introduction

Reindeer herding is deeply rooted in the traditional food culture of the Indigenous peoples in the Arctic zone of Western Siberia. Strengthening the position of reindeer herders in the food value chain could contribute to securing healthy, accessible, and culturally appropriate food for local communities and reindeer herders, while promoting the desired lifestyle of the given group. Food security for this group of Indigenous peoples cannot be addressed in isolation, but is linked to their economic security and food sovereignty. Therefore, both physical and economic access to reindeer meat in sufficient quantity is connected to their engagement in the export market and their participation in the food value chain. However, due to export trends in reindeer products, the needs and position of Indigenous peoples in the food value chain are jeopardized. Additionally, COVID-19 has brought yet other stressor for this group. As a result, the question of food sovereignty has emerged in evaluating how these people experience challenges to sovereignty over their own food system. Food sovereignty generally refers to a situation where local and Indigenous peoples possess the necessary control over the whole process of a food system. It is about "peoples' right to define their own policies and strategies for the sustainable production, distribution and consumption of food that guarantees the right to food for the entire population, on the basis of small- and medium-sized production, respecting their own cultures and the diversity of peasant, fishing and indigenous forms of agricultural production, marketing and management of rural areas, in which women play a fundamental role" (World Forum on Food Sovereignty, 2001) [1].

The Six Pillars of Food Sovereignty, developed by Nyéléni, 2007 (Food Secure Canada, 2012) [2], places people's need for food at the center of policy, and insists that food is more than just a commodity. Policy should be in line with "supporting sustainable livelihoods", "reducing the distance between suppliers and consumers", "placing control in the hands of local food suppliers", "recognizing the need to inhabit and share territories," building commodity production on traditional knowledge", and "maximizing the contributions of ecosystems" [2]. It is also strongly linked to food security related to food independence, the physical and economic accessibility of food, and the safety of available food (Rome Declaration on World Food Security and the World Food Summit Action Plan, 1996; Declaration of the World Summit on Food Security, 2009; Doctrine of Food Security of the Russian Federation, 2010).

The concept of food sovereignty challenges global food markets and empowers local actors [3]. It has special implications for Indigenous communities [4]. Taking the conditions of First Nation Indigenous people as a comparative point of analysis, Desmarais and Wittman (2014) identify that alarming problems of ill-health are closely related to food insecurity, which is in turn related to the decline of traditional food systems [5]. Among the reasons for this decline, the most important are disrupted access to land, traditional food, food trading and knowledge networks. Thus, traditional food, health and culture are tightly interconnected. The British Columbia Working Group on Indigenous Food Sovereignty defined the needs of Indigenous peoples to form sovereignty rights and the power of each nation in identifying the characteristics of their culture, as well as ways to enable Indigenous communities to "sustain traditional hunting, fishing, gathering, farming and distribution practices" [5]. Among the principles of culture, the most important element is the sacred nature of food: "Food sovereignty understands food as sacred, part of the web of relations with the natural world that define culture and community" (People's Food Policy Project, 2011) [6]. Thus, the sacred nature of food implies that "it cannot be treated as a commodity, manipulated into junk foods or taken from people's mouths to feed animals or vehicles" [7]. In the traditional food systems of Indigenous societies, reindeer form part of the culture and practices, with sacred and spiritual connotations [8]. The health of reindeer, nature and humans are tightly interrelated. So, a reindeer is utilized in a holistic manner. In contrast, when reindeer become goods on the free market, they are turned into a commodity, where utilization of body parts is compartmentalized.

Indigenous health and adaptation to the harsh conditions of the Arctic depend on the consumption of traditional products (local fish, reindeer meat, reindeer liver and blood, and wild plants) [9]. Reindeer meat has a specific health-promoting composition, and so is a necessary substance for maintaining a healthy diet in circumpolar circumstances and for decreasing the risk of chronic diseases [10–14]. It is the main tool for preventing cardiovascular and respiratory diseases, as well as metabolic disorders for the Indigenous peoples [15]. Dietary changes result in the declining health of the Indigenous population [16]. With the loss of traditional nutrition, hypertension, dyslipidemia, chronic bronchitis and obesity become even more prevalent problems among Indigenous peoples [17]. Maintenance of a traditional diet is closely related to the maintenance of the traditional food system, which is tightly interwoven with the culturally, socially and environmentally embedded practices of reindeer herding. Indigenous peoples and their traditional food systems emerged in harmony with nature and contain knowhow on the sustainable use of natural resources in ways that contribute to their health. New stressors related to the incorporation of reindeer exports in global markets force adjustments to the demands and infrastructure of markets. This implies the danger of new threats to the continued practice of environmentally, socially and economically sustainable Indigenous reindeer herding practices [12,18].

In meeting the nutritional needs of the Indigenous peoples in the Russian Arctic, it is vital that a major source of nutrition such as reindeer meat, which is readily available in the community, is well supported by all stakeholders. Reindeer meat offers a rich source of protein, minerals, and essential fatty acids, and is culturally acceptable in these Arctic communities [3]. Reindeer have contributed to the standard of living in these communities and served as a source of income from the sale of reindeer products (skin, meat, bones, velvet antlers, blood, etc.) which contribute to the value chain. The marketing of these products helps to create jobs and improve purchasing power for the suppliers, which makes other food products affordable. Food sovereignty emphasizes the promotion of small- and medium-sized production with particular respect for Indigenous cultures and traditional forms of agricultural production, management of land use and marketing [19]. The successful entrepreneurship of value addition in enhancing food sovereignty amongst the Indigenous peoples in the Russian Arctic zone of Western Siberia depends on collaboration amongst stakeholders. Recent trends of integration of reindeer herding producers from Western Siberia into global value chains have complemented national and Indigenous economies. However, increased exports from the area adversely impact the meat available locally and undermines the health of the Indigenous peoples and local communities. Challenges faced by most reindeer herders during the COVID-19 pandemic have accentuated these vulnerabilities.

In this study, we focus on integrating the different aspects of the reindeer food value chain in a multi-disciplinary approach to strengthen the food sovereignty of the Indigenous peoples in the Arctic zone of Western Siberia, and reflect on the main challenges of the COVID-19 pandemic.

2. Materials and Methods

2.1. Setting: The Yamal-Nenets Autonomous Okrug (YNAO): Geographic, Population and Ethnic Structure

YNAO, the geographic focus of our research, is an important region for the Indigenous peoples of Russia and is located in the circumpolar northwest of West Siberia (Figure 1). It has a population of 544,008 people [20] living in an area of 769,250 square kilometers [21]. The population density is 0.71 people per square kilometer. The location of YNAO significantly impacts the traditional occupations in this region (reindeer herding, hunting, fishery, etc.) as more than half of its territory is located beyond the Arctic Circle. It is a unique territory because almost half of the minority Indigenous population of the Russian Arctic (about 45,000 people) resides there, including the Nenets, the Khanty, the Selkups and the Komi-Zyryans [22]. Nearly half of the Indigenous residents are still nomadic. The culture, health and social well-being of Indigenous peoples are strongly linked to a traditional lifestyle that is the basis for meeting their vital needs and helping them survive in the severe Arctic areas.

2.2. Study Design

In this paper, we present the results of a quantitative and qualitative analysis of food sovereignty in reindeer herding communities living and practicing nomadism in the remote territories of the Yamal-Nenets Autonomous Okrug. We aimed to analyze the dependencies of Indigenous peoples on the reindeer produce exporting "food value chain" and to explore how the independence of reindeer herders could be increased in these export chains and how the provision of their products to local communities could be secured, while also addressing the challenges posed by the COVID-19 pandemic.

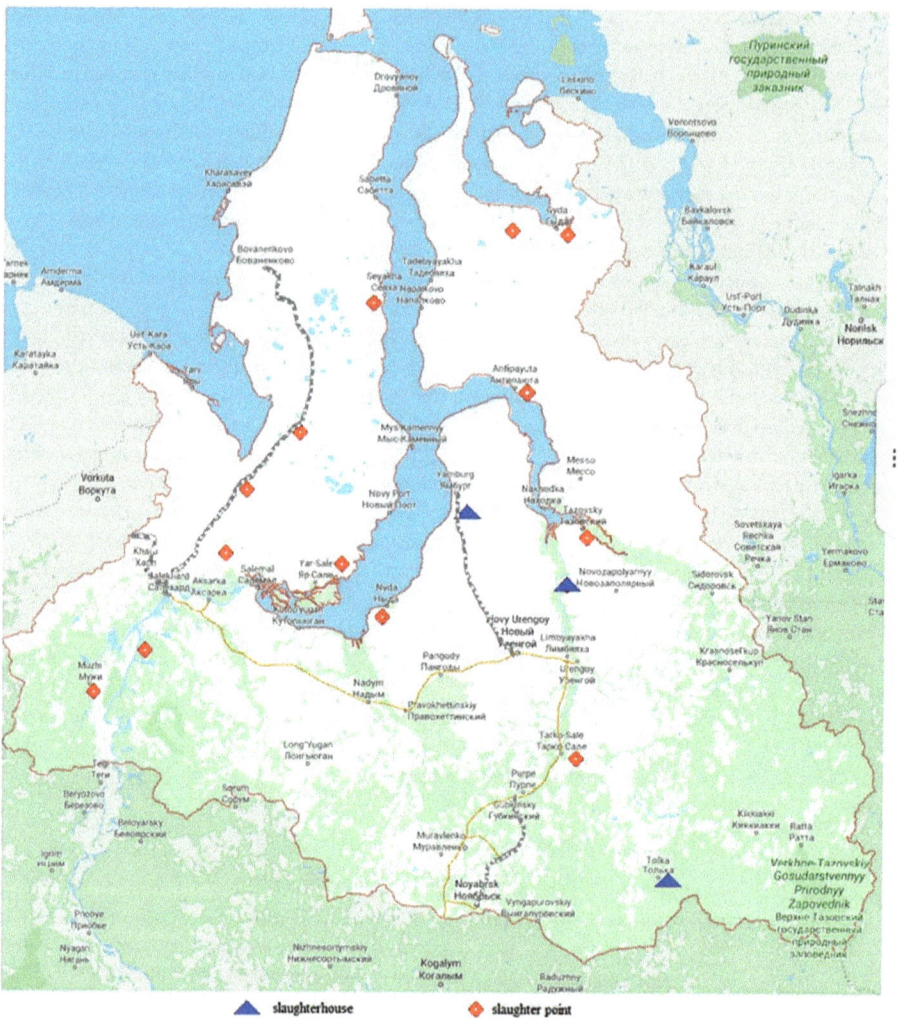

Source: Google Maps at https://maps.google.com. Map designer: Elena Bogdanova. Modification: logistic infrastructure (railways routes, slaughterhouses and slaughter points) is marked.

Figure 1. The territory of the Yamal-Nenets Autonomous Okrug.

2.3. Measurement Tools and Methodology

This study takes a multidisciplinary approach based on policy and socioeconomic analyses with input from medical research. The primary sources include data collected from interviews and surveys of Indigenous peoples during expeditions to the Nyda settlement, the Nydinskaya tundra, the Tazovsky settlement, the Tazovskaya tundra, the Nakhodka tundra, the Gyda and Gydansky settlements, the Yavai-Salinskaya tundra, the Seyakha settlement, the Seyakhinskaya and Tambeyskaya tundras located along the southern coast of the Ob Bay, the northeast coast of the Yamal Peninsula, the Tazovsky and Gydansky Peninsulas, and the Shuryshkarsky district. Data were collected in the summers and winters of 2014–2020. Fieldwork was conducted by researchers of the YNAO Arctic Scientific Research Centre, the National Medical Research Center for Rehabilitation and Balneology, the Northern Arctic Federal University and the Association of Reindeer Herders in YNAO (two of the researchers were Indigenous). Secondary sources used in the study consist of official information requested from local authorities, public statistical data and official government reports.

The methodology of the study is based on FAO's (Food and Agriculture Organization of the United Nations) sustainable food value chain (FVC) framework. The core FVC comprises the value chain actors who produce or procure products from the upstream level, add value to these products and then sell them on to the next level. These actors carry out four functions: production, aggregation, processing, and distribution (wholesale and retail). FVC actors are linked to each other and their wider operating environment through a governance structure [23]. Following this approach, we presented the food value chain as a network of stakeholders that includes those involved in reindeer herding husbandry (producers), people responsible for purchasing, storage, sanitary control and transportation of raw reindeer products to producers (brokers), processing (processors), and exporting, distributing and selling reindeer herding products (distributors) to consumers who shop for and consume this food. Also included as stakeholders are government, non-governmental organizations (NGOs), and regulators that monitor and regulate the entire reindeer food value chain from producers to consumers.

While collecting the information from local authorities, public statistical data and official government reports, we implemented quantitative methods of analysis to collect data on the number of different producers of reindeer products, the scale of reindeer livestock, and the results of slaughter campaigns and sale to local communities as well as national and international markets.

The data received from the semi-structured interviews showed the ways reindeer products are utilized and revealed the key issues of individual reindeer herders as stakeholders in the FVC, as well as the challenges raised by the COVID-19 pandemic.

Statistical analyses were performed using Microsoft Excel 2016 and SPSS Statistics 23.0 (IBM, Saint Petersburg, Russia). Significant differences were defined at a p-value <0.05.

2.4. Study Population

The participants in the study were asked to fill out the questionnaire and interviewed while undergoing a medical examination conducted by the YNAO Arctic Scientific Research Centre and the National Medical Research Center for Rehabilitation and Balneology at health care institutions—municipal hospitals and feldsher-midwife medical stations in remote settlements. The participants were also recruited during the fieldwork in summer 2020 to study the impact of the COVID-19 pandemic on reindeer herding activities. The inclusion criteria for the respondents were: aged over 18, of Indigenous origin, Indigenous language speaker, involved in reindeer herding, a nomadic or semi-nomadic lifestyle, and residing in the tundra or in the settlements of the Arctic zone of Western Siberia for over five years. The participants received information about the program both verbally and in writing. They also provided written informed consent. The consent form stated that participation was voluntary and assured the confidentiality of the participants, whose personal data were anonymized, numbered, and added to de-identified databases. The interviews were recorded and also included in the database.

2.5. Ethics Approval

The study was approved by the Ethics Committee of the Arctic Scientific Research Centre of Yamal-Nenets Autonomous Okrug, Salekhard, Russian Federation, on 18 January 2013 (approval protocol No. 01/1-13).

3. Results and Discussion

Two hundred and sixty-five semi-structured interviews were conducted based on the interview guide developed and approved by the Northern Arctic Federal University and YNAO Arctic Scientific Research Centre. Two hundred and fifty-two surveys with fixed questions were received.

Reindeer husbandry is the leading ethno-forming branch of the agro-industrial complex in the region. YNAO has the highest number of domesticated reindeer herds in the world, which has made it a prosperous reindeer herding area [24,25] with sustainable nomadic reindeer herding husbandry [26]. However, over the past two years, reindeer livestock has decreased by 11.3% from 2015 numbers (2015 numbers: 733; 2016: 465; 2017: 788; 2018: 690; 2019: 650) [27].

In YNAO, the network of stakeholders involved in producing, slaughtering, processing, distributing and consuming reindeer products forms the food value chain that is presented in Table 1.

Table 1. Food value chain of reindeer herding products in the Yamal-Nenets Autonomous Okrug (YNAO).

Stakeholder	1. Producers	2. "Brokers"	3. Processors	4. Distributors	5. Consumers
	Agricultural reindeer herding enterprises, peasantry farms, "national communities" (obschina), individual reindeer herders (families)	Gross purchasers (slaughterhouses, agricultural reindeer herding enterprises), trade points (faktoria), local merchants	Companies processing meat products and other by-products in YNAO, Russian and international producers	Export companies, shops, local merchants	Local Indigenous communities, other consumers
Role	Reindeer herding, trading to exporters and local communities	Purchase of reindeer products, storage, veterinary and sanitary control, transportation and delivery to processors or local consumers	Processing, value added processing, manufacturing, marketing and sales	Supplies to the consumer market	Shopping, consuming
Key issues	Dependence on "brokers" requirements and regulations, - high production costs due to insufficient logistics, deficit and remoteness of petroleum stations; low motivation towards business cooperation	High logistic costs; lack of innovative equipment for improved slaughter procedures	Low access to precious reindeer products of high quality (fat, skin and other by-products)	Low share of reindeer products distributed to the local market of YNAO	Low access to reindeer products for the Indigenous Peoples living in remote settlements of YNAO
	6. Government/NGOs/Regulators				
	Department of Agro-industrial Complex of YNAO Department of Natural Resources Regulation, Forest Relations and Development of the Oil and Gas Complex of the Yamal-Nenets Autonomous Okrug Department of Indigenous Minorities of the North of the Yamal-Nenets Autonomous Okrug Veterinary Service of the Yamal-Nenets Autonomous Okrug Associations of the Indigenous Peoples of YNAO etc. Role: Public policy on food security and support of reindeer herders				
Key issues	Limited access to subsidies for individual reindeer herders, insufficient legal and economic information support for reindeer herders and insufficient supplies of medications for reindeer, export-oriented economy of reindeer products in YNAO				

The producers of reindeer products in YNAO (different types of reindeer herding enterprises, "national communities" of the Indigenous peoples, peasant farms and individual reindeer herders) provide reindeer husbandry and trade food commodities, such as raw reindeer products (venison, blood, fat, skin, camus, antlers, velvet antlers, bones, and other by-products). In 2020, in YNAO, there were 19 agricultural enterprises, 447 national communities (obschina), 11 peasant farms specializing in reindeer herding and processing reindeer products, and 2839 individual reindeer herders (Table 2).

Table 2. Agricultural enterprises, national communities, peasantry farms and individual reindeer herders in YNAO* (on 1 January 2020).

District of YNAO	Agricultural Enterprises		National Communities of the Indigenous Peoples		Peasantry Farms		Individual Reindeer Herders	
	n	Reindeer	n	Reindeer	n	Reindeer	n	Reindeer
Salekhard	1	1200	1	580	0	0	0	0
Nadymsky	1	14,007	1	292	0	0	92	10,692
Purovsky	2	15,903	0	0	1	1710	137	14,052
Tazovsky	3	20,426	3	16,152	3	2730	1049	215,088
Shuryshkarsky	2	13,532	0	0	1	20	57	7682
Krasnosel'kupsky	2	1021	0	0	0	0	28	644
Yamalsky	6	25,756	436	88,526	3	14,033	761	97,142
Priural'sky	2	14,025	6	28,018	3	5062	715	47,957
Total	19	105,870	447	133,568	11	23,555	2839	393,257

* The data were received from the specialists of the Department of Agro-industrial Complex of YNAO [27] and collected from the Register of the main producers of the Yamal-Nenets Autonomous Okrug [28].

Collective reindeer herding in YNAO (agricultural reindeer herding enterprises, national communities and peasantry farms) is an effective organizational form for the Indigenous economy involved in producing, slaughtering and processing reindeer products. It is rooted in both the Soviet period (a state farm or sovkhoz) and traditional forms of Indigenous peoples' cooperation (national community or obschina [29,30], and peasantry farms [31,32] as joint family businesses). Anthropologist V. Vladimirova noticed that the cooperative organization of reindeer husbandry in the Russian North reproduces the economic and social patterns that were developed during the Soviet period, also adapting and incorporating elements of traditional indigenous social orders. "Such social arrangements and the accompanying moral values are embedded in the reindeer herding economy, and it is their persistence that Indigenous people achieve through adhering to cooperative values" [33]. This mixed culture-based approach to the collective organization of reindeer farming still provides sustainability for the sovkhoz in Western Siberia. Strong dependence of reindeer herding husbandry on the Indigenous traditional lifestyle and "democratic leadership" [34,35] also maintain such traditional forms of Indigenous peoples' self-organization in YNAO as a "national community" (obschina), a collaborative economy of family, clan and territorial neighbors that protect and maintain their traditional lifestyle, economic activities and culture [29].

The recognition of different forms of reindeer herding differs depending on the state. Indigenous reindeer herders' communities, unlike agricultural enterprises, are not strongly subsidized by the regional budget (apart from for producing reindeer meat). So some reindeer herders find transforming a national community into a peasantry farm or an agricultural production cooperative attractive because of access to government support, subsidies and future prospects for developing business. Bogdan O., a reindeer herder from the Laborovskaya tundra, thinks that "The head of a family with a reindeer herd will be able to register a peasant farm as an enterprise in the future if he wants to enlarge and offer new jobs to unite the farms of his relatives or neighbors into a cooperative."

However, individual reindeer herders are still the main producers of reindeer products in YNAO (60%) (see Table 1). They still prefer not to join any collective reindeer organizations and operate reindeer herding as individuals with their families—accompanied in the tundra by parents, spouses and children, and sometimes brothers, sisters, uncles and aunts. They are also cautious about any changes and paperwork. For example, the reindeer herder Ilia V. from the Laborovskaya tundra explains: "Joining peasant farms or entering a community to receive grants and subsidies? It is difficult because I cannot make documents and reports for grants well. My family and I are nomads in the tundra with my reindeer far away in the Karskoe Sea. I do not have time to go to the authorities and do not know how to run this business and what papers are needed. I finished seven years of formal schooling and escaped to the tundra. Reindeer herding is my life now." This reveals that reindeer herding husbandry in Western Siberia is still mostly focused on the subsistence economy combined with commodity production. In extreme climate conditions, societies do not use the revolutionary achievements of the Neolithic period: they do not strive to switch to a productive type of agriculture [36], since a herder interacts with the environment as a partner who feels like an equal part of it [37].

In the Arctic, most Indigenous communities belong to a mixed "subsistence-cash" economy [38]. In YNAO, individual reindeer herders, as part of Arctic communities, represent two types of social economy: commodity production—producing and sharing for sales to generate profit—and subsistence production—meeting the needs of reindeer herders and their families. The results of our research showed that the reindeer herders of the Tazovskaya, Messoyakhinskaya, Antipayutinskaya, the Tanamskaya tundras of the Tazovsky district, the Yamal and Gydan Peninsulas, and the Yamal'sky district of YNAO are mainly integrated into the commodity production of meat and velvet antlers thanks to relatively good logistics and presence of slaughterhouses. Subsistence farming, focused on providing a family with food and clothing, prevails in the northern part of the Gydan Peninsula, on the coast of the Yuratskaya Bay and other parts of the Tazovsky district, which are logistically remote from settlements, slaughterhouses and large oil and gas deposits. In the Priural'sky district, there is both commodity and subsistence reindeer production because of developed logistic complexes (Figure 1).

Reindeer herding is impacted annually by climate change [39–42], overgrazing of reindeer pastures [43,44], the growing cost of living in the tundra and changing government regulations for reindeer herding as a traditional occupation for Indigenous peoples. In 2020, the reindeer herding economy in YNAO has also been strongly affected by the COVID-19 pandemic since individual reindeer herders, as the main producers, are a vulnerable group faced with a number of issues due to: (1) limited access to food, fuel, medications, vaccination procedures for reindeer and slaughtering facilities; (2) increased production costs; and (3) dropping prices for reindeer products. This falls in line with global trends: the pandemic has impacted food security and food sovereignty, which are "greatly affected due to mobility restrictions, reduced purchasing power, and with a greater impact on the most vulnerable population groups" [45].

Reindeer herding in the Russian Arctic is mostly a subsidized business because of high productivity costs and low incomes. This makes the impact of COVID-19 very serious for reindeer herders who perceive the coronavirus, icing and anthrax as evil forces that "were fabricated to reduce the number of people in the tundra" [46]. It has made reindeer herders change their nomadic schedule and completely limited nomadic people's access to the settlements and cities where they can buy food, fuel and medications for reindeer. Alena V., a reindeer herder's wife, complained: "We usually buy products in April in Labytnangi at the base or 'from sledges.' But this year, due to the pandemic, my family did not have time to buy fuel, essential goods, food, or tarpaulin. We had to start the summer nomadic period earlier – in early April – and change our route. We bought food and went to the tundra with three other reindeer herding families." Other reindeer herding families made the decision to stay closer to the settlement during the period of pandemic limitations. For example, Venera S. noticed: "It is expensive to come to the city from the tundra—16,000 (*100 Russian Rubles = 1.12 € or 1.32 US$.) rubles one way. One also needs to buy food and live somewhere in the city. The reindeer stay with our relatives during this time. Our family was supposed to nomad during spring and summer this year, but because of the pandemic, it was impossible to go anywhere, and our family made the decision to stay close to the settlement".

Limited access to vaccines for reindeer during the COVID-19 pandemic has become a sensitive issue for food security. Most vaccination procedures are subsidized by the local government of YNAO to support reindeer herding and control the pandemic. However, in spring (from mid-February to April) only 40% of about 220,000 reindeer that were planned to be vaccinated against anthrax received a vaccine from the veterinary service of YNAO. The summer vaccination period in the Priural'sky, Yamal'sky, Tazovsky and Purovsky districts of YNAO was delayed and started in late June [47]. Timely preventive vaccination and treatment (against anthrax, salmonellosis, trichophytosis, colibacophytosis, brucellosis, erysipelas, classical swine flu, plague, rabies, edemagenosis, helminthiasis, etc.) are important for maintaining reindeer health and addressing the restrictions on slaughter since reindeer herders are not allowed to slaughter animals without a vaccination [48] and cannot get government donations for murrain [49]. Besides, some diseases result in production losses (loss of weight of a reindeer [28]) followed by decreased profit for reindeer herders at the slaughtery.

The medication for some other reindeer diseases (i.e., necrobacillosis) is not subsidized by the government. Thus, in summer 2020, during the period of limitations due to the COVID-19 pandemic, most nomadic reindeer herders suffered greatly because they could not get access to pharmacies in the cities and had to buy anti-necrobacillosis medications at the trading posts (faktoria) in remote areas and pay unfair prices. Viktoria Z., a reindeer herder from Aksarka, said: "It was very difficult to get medical supplies for reindeer during the summer period. Because of the coronavirus, it was impossible to buy them in pharmacies, and we were not given the medicine that reindeer really need when they limp—antibiotics. (...) Now we have not received any medications from the veterinary service. It used to be good: first-aid kits were given to us. Now, the veterinary service has only supplied us with a vaccine against gadflies." Bogdan A., the reindeer herder from the Laborovskaya tundra, noticed: "During the summer quarantine, < ... > I had to buy medicines for reindeer that were five times more expensive at the trading post. I paid 20,000 rubles for it." Moreover, reindeer herders sometimes could not find necessary products at the trade posts. Ilia S., the reindeer herder from the Laborovskaya tundra, recounted: *"On the way, we passed trading posts. Their prices were too high and the shops were almost empty."* Some other reindeer herders asked their relatives and friends in the city to buy and send necessary medications. Anna I., a reindeer herder from Aksarka, recalled: "I asked someone in Salekhard and kind people helped me get medications. Now I order them from Ekaterinburg." Challenges of delayed vaccination in the spring and summer could negatively impact the results of the slaughter campaign from November 2020 to January 2021 due to the possibility of decreased reindeer health and livestock approved for slaughter, and could make the reindeer herding business even less profitable for individuals.

High production costs were also a result of limited access to petroleum stations during the COVID-19 pandemic. Most individual reindeer herders had to cooperate and share logistical costs of hiring a taxi to get to petroleum stations close to the city and back to the tundra. However, this still increased their expenses for fuel by almost 50%. Mikhail V., a reindeer herder from the Priural'sky district, explained: "It was very difficult for us to get the fuel, which reindeer herders need most of all. Our petroleum station in Aksarka was also closed, so we had to go to Salekhard city and hire a taxi for 3000 rubles one way. If two or three people split the cost, then it was possible to buy more barrels of fuel since the cost was less. However, if only one reindeer herder was going, it was a very high price to pay." In YNAO, reindeer herding as commodity production strongly depends on the price of fuel and localization of logistic centers and slaughter facilities. The interviews of reindeer herders in the Tazovsky district of YNAO (n = 84) showed that the price of the delivery of fuel varied depending on distance from regional centers and petroleum stations. For example, in the Tazovsky settlement, the cost of petroleum AI-92 was 43 rubles per liter, in the trade point (faktoria) of Yuribei Gydansky, 94 rubles, in the Gyda settlement, 109 rubles, and on Oleniy Island, 138 rubles. Thus, the logistical expenses of reindeer herders increased in the remote areas and made them change their nomadic routes to pass by slaughter facilities or collaborate with other types of broker (i.e., local merchants).

Processors are supplied with reindeer products directly from the reindeer herding enterprises or via brokers who purchase them from individual reindeer herders or collective reindeer herders' farms, giving them a choice to sell their products to: (1) slaughterhouses; (2) state farms (sovkhoz); (3) local trade points (faktoria); or (4) local merchants in the tundra. These brokers have to take responsibility for sanitary (veterinary) control, appropriate storage and delivery of reindeer products to processors, and offer different terms of sale for reindeer herders who are also producers. As a result of the slaughter campaign in 2019, 1847 tons of reindeer meat were harvested (Department of Agro-industrial Complex of YNAO, 2020).

In YNAO, there are 13 slaughter complexes and three slaughter points (Figure 1) near logistical infrastructure—railway or marine logistical routes. In 2019, they slaughtered in total 46,033 reindeer

(1643 tons of venison), of which 26,259 (797.5 tons) came from agricultural enterprises, 16,281 (695.6 tons) from "national communities," 1662 (70.8 tons) from peasant farms, and 1831 (79 tons) from individual reindeer herders [27]. In 2020, 85% of the interviewed individual reindeer herders had faced some issues due to the COVID-19 pandemic: (1) slaughterhouses sorted out the meat in the most profitable manner to decrease the price; (2) a live reindeer was received by a slaughterhouse but reindeer herders were paid only for the meat, and they had to buy the skins and camuses if they wanted them back or accept the decreased price for the reindeer meat (category II instead of category I); and (3) reindeer herders had to wait up to three months to be paid for slaughtered meat. Sergei S., a reindeer herder, complained about the delayed payment for his products and an unfair deal with a slaughterhouse: "This year, we slaughtered meat at Antipayuta. If we slaughtered a lot of reindeer (more than 100 heads), the money was not paid immediately, but if we slaughtered much less reindeer, then the money was paid immediately. We delivered about a ton of meat and had to wait for the money for two months. We sold meat but skins and camuses were taken by slaughterhouses for nothing. And if you wanted to take them back, you had to buy them. Camuses cost 450 rubles in 2020, and 350 rubles in 2019." Larisa S., another reindeer herder, was unsatisfied with her dependence on slaughterhouse rules: "You bring a reindeer, they slaughter it and pay only for the meat. If you want to take the camus, then the meat will be cheaper; it will be accepted as of the second sort, and the second sort is phenous meat. That is, we have to sell reindeer and meat according to their terms and conditions." Slaughterhouses also dropped their prices for meat. In 2020, the average price of venison varied at the slaughterhouses in YNAO from 180 rubles for the second sort to up to 450 rubles for the first sort per kilogram. The reindeer herder Mikhail V. mentioned that the prices had not changed a lot during the past two years: "This year, slaughterhouses took meat for 450 rubles per kg, and the second sort of meat was taken for nothing—180 rubles—and they paid the money much later. In 2018, meat of the first sort was 220 rubles per kg and the second sort of meat cost 140 rubles." However, reindeer herders had to accept all the terms and conditions imposed by slaughterhouses because, in general, it was more profitable to slaughter a large number of reindeer, especially during the winter high slaughter season.

Due to the COVID-19 pandemic, delayed vaccination of reindeer, limited access to the slaughtery at the state farms (sovkhoz) along with complicated bureaucratic procedures and long waiting times for payment (up to six months), the sovkhoz was less attractive for individual reindeer herders (only 9% of our respondents ever sold their products to state farms). Elena O., a reindeer herder, explained: "While slaughtering reindeer at the state farm, there was no need to buy the camuses of our reindeer: the farm just slaughtered reindeer, took the carcasses, and gave us back the other parts. However, now it is more difficult to sell reindeer to a state farm: there are a lot of papers to fill out and we have to wait for our money for six months."

Regarding prices, trading posts (faktoria) and local merchants offered half the price for reindeer meat. For example, Venera S. noticed: "This year, the trading post bought reindeer meat for very cheap". The reindeer herder Iakov S. mentioned that the COVID-19 pandemic had dropped prices for velvet antlers: "This year, due to the coronavirus in the tundra, merchants bought the velvet antlers of the first sort for 1000 rubles per kg, the second sort for 800 rubles, and the third for 600 rubles." Venera S. compared current prices for velvet antlers with the previous years: "Last year, the price reached 2,700 rubles." However, collaboration with local merchants who arrived directly in the tundra was more convenient for reindeer herders and helped solve some COVID-19 related issues with supplies. Reindeer herders accepted the exchange of reindeer products for other goods (fuel, food, clothes, nets, spare parts for snowmobiles, diesel generators, pampers for babies, etc.), and they considered these sales as fair and more convenient, especially during the pandemic period, because they did not slaughter lots of reindeer (usually up to five for sustenance needs, i.e., food and making clothes) and could avoid production losses and the logistical costs associated with going to settlements or cities. The reindeer herder Nikolai S. mentioned: "Antipayuta was not on the way, and we had to nomad with the reindeer herd specifically to the slaughterhouse. This was bad because of weight loss by the reindeer. And it also depended on weather conditions—a lot of snow and ice." Thus, the COVID-19 pandemic could have an impact on decreasing the number of slaughtered reindeer during the winter due to unfair prices and could create delays until a later period. This could lead to a decline in profit and quality of life, especially for poor individual reindeer herders who are supported by the local government. In 2000, a member of a nomadic family earned 5000 rubles per month.

When slaughtered, YNAO reindeer products are exported by brokers to both primary and value added processors that process, manufacture, and market reindeer products, which are in high demand in the meat, pharmaceutical and beauty industries. However, processors are limited in the number of reindeer products they can process due to gaps in slaughter procedures. First, the quality of products depends on freezing facilities. If the rules of storage are violated, deterioration takes place several times faster [50,51]. Secondly, slaughterhouses are mostly focused on venison, and most other parts of the reindeer are thrown away or delivered as by-products of the third category. Due to the winter slaughter, it is almost impossible for industrial processors to get reindeer fat, reindeer skin and camuses of high quality. The collection of blood is a very complicated procedure that is implemented in YNAO only at state farms due to high technological requirements. This approach of utilizing meat differs completely from the Indigenous peoples' consumption of reindeer. Of those interviewed, 98% agreed that they use all parts of a reindeer for food and making clothes, shoes, tools, household items, handicrafts, etc. Andrei A. explained: "We eat the whole reindeer, and we eat it raw, sun-dried, boiled, or fried. My family likes hard boiled reindeer head with hoofs. It's very delicious. Only the reindeer skull is left. Our dogs eat the same food as we do." Based on the interviews, the ways of utilizing reindeer by reindeer herders and other stakeholders who process reindeer products are presented in Table 3.

The distributors, including wholesalers, market and sell reindeer products in YNAO, and export them to other regions of Russia and abroad. YNAO is the only region in Russia that officially exports reindeer products to the EU. In 2008, four tons of reindeer products from YNAO were exported to Sweden, Finland and Germany [27]. In 2019, the total export of YNAO reindeer products brought in an income of $29 million. A total of 440 tons (24%) of slaughtered reindeer meat and 11,000 reindeer skins from YNAO were exported to Finland and Germany [47]. Now, only three enterprises in YNAO—municipal enterprise Yamal'skie Oleni, municipal unitary enterprise Meat Processing Complex Payuta and LLC Vozrozhdenie—have certification as official exporters of reindeer meat and one more company—LLC Sibirsky olen—specializes in exporting reindeer skins and other by-products to the EU. In 2020, according to the national project "International Cooperation and Export," 400 tons of reindeer meat and 13,000 reindeer skins are planned to be exported to European countries [27]. Already this year, 270 tons of reindeer meat and 15 tons of other by-products of the third category have been exported to Finland and Germany [27], representing 50% of planned exports. By 2024, the government of YNAO plans to double exported reindeer products and to increase the number of consuming countries. Prospective reindeer products to be exported are bones and blood enriched with collagen, calcium, iron and protein. The COVID-19 pandemic has decreased the export of reindeer products. For example, Finland cancelled the import of 13,000 reindeer skins in March [27]. Tourists are the main consumers of the handicrafts made of skin, and the crisis in the tourism industry has resulted in a decline of demand for these products.

The COVID-19 pandemic has accentuated consumers' motivation "to protect themselves and their immune system by adopting healthier diets. The availability of bioactive ingredients of food and functional foods may become critical, as the demand for these products may increase" [52]. Due to the increasing export potential of reindeer products, local consumers (both Indigenous and non-Indigenous communities in YNAO) have low access to reindeer meat. Of the interviewed reindeer herders, 83% confirmed that they supply reindeer products to their relatives when they visit them, mostly during the winter period. A further 45% of interviewed individual reindeer herders sold some reindeer meat to local communities in the large settlements. According to official data from the Department of Agro-industrial Complex of YNAO, only 6% of all reindeer were sold to the local population: 2622 reindeer by agricultural enterprises and 2288 by national communities [27]. This has accentuated the trend of a dramatic decline of access to reindeer meat in the local communities. According to monitoring data received by the Arctic Research Scientific Centre, in 2012–2017 20% of the total volume of reindeer meat was consumed by the herders themselves, 18% was sold in Indigenous villages or transferred to relatives and 62% was exported outside the Yamal-Nenets Autonomous Okrug. On average, a family of nomadic Nenets reindeer herders consisting of two to four adults and three to seven children consumed no more than 10–12 reindeer per year. In addition, part of the meat was transported to relatives living in villages with an Indigenous population. A significant portion of reindeer meat was also sold in villages and towns with an Indigenous population or cities close to the herding routes [53].

Table 3. The utilization of the reindeer products of YNAO.

Product	Average Yield per one Reindeer		Utilization	
	Weight, kg	Yield, %	By Reindeer Herders	By Processors
Total reindeer	66.00	100.00		
Venison with carcass	33.00	50.00		
muscles	20.13	30.50	Raw, sun-dried, frozen ("stroganina"), boiled, fried meat—for food	Meat industry (canned, smoked, salted venison, sausages, chips)
fat	2.48	3.75	Raw—for remedies	Pharmaceutical industry (biologically active medications)
bones	6.93	10.50	Boiled—for food and making tools and household items	Animal feeding stuff
tendons and fascia	3.47	5.25		
Tongue	0.33	0.50	Boiled—for food	Meat industry
Blood	4.22	6.40	Raw—for food and remedies	Pharmaceutical industry (biologically active medications)
Heart	0.42	0.64	Raw and boiled—for food	Meat industry; animal feeding stuff (produced premium hypoallergenic dog and cat food)
Lungs	0.67	1.02		
Liver	0.70	1.06		
Kidneys	0.15	0.22		
Stomach:				
farding bag	3.06	4.64	For keeping fresh blood	Meat industry
honeycomb bag	0.37	0.56	Boiled—for food	
bible-bag	0.55	0.84		
rennet bag	0.36	0.54		
Intestine and esophagus	2.30	3.48		Animal feeding stuff
Gullet and larynx	0.18	0.28		
Antlers	1.06	1.60	Handicrafts, remedy, making tools and household items	Pharmaceutical industry (biologically active medications); beauty industry (cosmetic production enriched with collagen); handicrafts
Hoof	1.08	1.64	Boiled—for food	Beauty industry (cosmetic production enriched with collagen); animal feeding stuff
Skin, camus, forehead	6.97	10.56	Summer skin—for winter "chum" cover, coverage of the floor and "beds", making clothes, shoes handicrafts	Making clothes, shoes and handicrafts
Tail	0.12	0.18		
Cranial muscles and bones	3.30	5.00	Boiled—for food	Animal feeding stuff
Endocrine, enzymatic and special raw products	2.39	3.62	Raw and boiled—for food	Animal feeding stuff
Wastes (gastric and intestine contents etc.)	4.77	7.22	Boiled—for food	Animal feeding stuff

The COVID-19 pandemic almost completely limited the access of local communities to reindeer products; only 24% of the respondents could supply their relatives with reindeer meat in the settlements. This is because of food safety requirements as "a significant issue in order to avoid the spreading of the virus between producers, retailers, and consumers" [52]. People living in the remote territories of YNAO also had low access to reindeer products. The results of previous research also showed a dramatic decline of almost 50% in consumption of reindeer products by the Indigenous and non-Indigenous peoples in YNAO, and only one third of the studied population still eat venison once or twice daily [54]. This threatens the maintenance of their health since a diet enriched with venison significantly increases antiatherogenic blood lipid fractions, contributes to the maintenance of normal body weight, and improves microcirculation, tissue fluid exchange and antioxidant defense of the body against free radicals, which may explain the high prophylactic activity of venison [54] that has also shown a high efficiency in helping to adapt to cold stress [55] and geomagnetic activity in the Arctic [56]. It can be used as an effective remedy for reducing hypertension [10] and chronic nonobstructive bronchitis risk [13]. This makes reindeer products an important part of the local population's nutrition.

This systematic research into the reindeer food value chain in YNAO has revealed strong dependence of reindeer herders on other stakeholders—brokers, processors and government institutions,—which makes them a vulnerable group and establishes barriers to entering the global market. Individual reindeer herders are not involved in the complete processing of reindeer products and have to accept the rules imposed by wholesalers and other retailers. However, reindeer herders are keepers of precious traditional knowledge about utilizing reindeer. Strengthening the involvement of reindeer herders in the food value chain can contribute to Arctic Indigenous economies and maintain their traditional lifestyle.

The main strength of our study was using the unique data of quantitative and qualitative research collected from the reindeer herders and local authorities during expeditions that took place over seven years (2014–2020). Most similar studies remain fragmentary, and often hard to access. However, our study had several limitations. The studied population was recruited while undergoing a medical examination at health care institutions—municipal hospitals and feldsher-midwife medical stations in remote settlements. Participation was voluntary and did not include all representatives of the reindeer herding business (i.e., employees of the state farms and commercial agricultural enterprises) of the studied territories, which may limit the generalizability of findings. Future research could also benefit from exploring food security in reindeer herding, on utilizing reindeer in commodity production and on the impact of traditional reindeer products on the health and wellbeing of the local communities.

4. Conclusions

In the Arctic zone of Western Siberia, short- and long-term measures are needed to maintain a healthy lifestyle replete with traditional food as part of Indigenous peoples' food system. The economic position of reindeer herders in the food value chain, who are very dependent on other stakeholders, should be strengthened. This currently creates barriers for integration of reindeer herders into the global market and makes their positions insecure, and the situation is exacerbated by the COVID-19 pandemic. The strengthening the food sovereignty of reindeer herders (i.e., the improvement of their sovereignty over the use, sale and consumption of food) could be reached by improved economic sovereignty. This is also a key factor in solving food security for the local communities since this would mitigate the compulsive export sale of meat to obtain economic resources. Thus, this would improve the food security of the local communities while providing economic security for reindeer herders. Solutions could derive from an equilibrium between regulating and improving private business, state intervention, and cooperative mobilization of reindeer herders or local residents. State intervention is more feasible in some areas, bottom-up mobilization in other areas, while the maintenance of incentives of local private businesses need to be kept in mind. Apart from strengthening economic and food security for reindeer herders it is equally important to strengthen both traditional households and local businesses since they are central to improve the resilience of their communities facing economic, climate and pandemic challenges.

We propose the following:

Short-term measures:

- Organize a mobile economic and legal consulting service for nomadic and semi-nomadic reindeer herders to support business and establish cooperative reindeer husbandries.
- Encourage cooperative forms of reindeer husbandry and implement a new government program subsidizing peasant farms for purchase of slaughter, freezing and storage facilities (managed by reindeer herders' wives and elderly family members staying at the settlements with contribution the Indigenous and non-Indigenous people from the local communities) to contribute to reindeer herding as a traditional family business and increase year-round access of remote local communities to reindeer products.
- Organize veterinary facilities in the settlements and provide reindeer herders with medications for reindeer.
- Increase access of reindeer herders to reasonably priced fuel and basic food products near the settlements and trading spots.
- Organize mobile slaughter and supplemental reindeer feeding facilities in the tundra along the nomadic routes of reindeer herders.
- Extend the export potential of non-edible parts of reindeer (i.e., velvet antlers, reindeer skins, camuses) to support food sovereignty of the Indigenous peoples, while focusing government policies on improving access of the Indigenous communities to the edible and medicinal portions of the carcass.

Long-term measures

- Train Indigenous peoples to harvest and process reindeer products according to bioproduction standards and increase their involvement in the complete food value chain as producers, brokers, processors and distributors to strengthen food sovereignty among the Indigenous peoples.
- Subsidize medications for reindeer and fuel for reindeer herders and develop infrastructure to facilitate the economic empowerment of reindeer herders.
- Monitor the consumption of traditional food, as well as the health and social welfare of the Indigenous population in the Russian Arctic. Explore ways to maintain traditional nutrition in the local communities.

Author Contributions: Data curation: E.B. and S.A.; Formal analysis: E.B. and A.L.; Funding acquisition: D.R., E.B. and I.A.M.; Investigation: E.B. and A.L.; Methodology: E.B., D.R., I.A.M., A.L. and K.H.; Project administration: E.B.; Resources: A.L. and P.F.; Software: E.B.; Supervision: E.B.; Validation: S.A.; Writing—original draft: E.B., D.R., I.A.M.; Writing—review & editing: K.H. and A.L. All authors read the manuscript and approved this submission. All authors have read and agreed to the published version of the manuscript.

Funding: This study was funded by the Russian Foundation of Basic Research, grant number 18-010-00875.

Acknowledgments: We would like to thank the Indigenous communities of YNAO, the YNAO Arctic Scientific Research Centre, the Department of Health Care of YNAO and the health care institutions (municipal hospitals and feldsher-midwife medical stations in remote settlements) of YNAO for their assistance and sharing data. We are also grateful to the stakeholders of the networking project, "Indigenous food systems in transition: Comparative commodification practices and the future importance of reindeer for indigenous food supply and for the empowerment of reindeer herders within commodity chains in Sweden, Finland and Russia," supported by the SLU Future Food Foundation (No. 55950346) for their contribution to the discussion about the food value chain approach in the reindeer herding communities of the Arctic region.

Conflicts of Interest: The authors declare no conflict of interest.

References

1. WFFS. For the Peoples' Right to Produce, Feed Themselves and Exercise Their Food Sovereignty. In *Final Declaration of the World Forum on Food Sovereignty Havana, Cuba, 7 September 2001*; WFFS: Havana, Cuba, 2001.
2. *Declaration of the Forum for Food Sovereignty, Nyéléni (27 February 2007)*; Food Sovereignty Network: Sélingué, Mali, 2007.
3. Shelepov, V.G.; Uglov, V.A.; Boroday, E.V.; Poznyakovsky, V.M.; Rada, A.; Kosinsky, P.; Isachkova, O.A.; Ganichev, B.L.; Loginova, A.O.; Basalaev, Y.; et al. Chemical composition of indigenous raw meats. *Foods Raw Mater.* **2019**, *7*, 412–418. [CrossRef]
4. Herrmann, T.M.; Lamalice, A.; Coxam, V. Tackling the question of micronutrients intake as one of the main levers in terms of Inuit food security. *Curr. Opin. Clin. Nutr. Metab. Care* **2020**, *23*, 59–63. [CrossRef] [PubMed]
5. Desmarais, A.A.; Hannah, W. Farmers, foodies and First Nations: Getting to food sovereignty in Canada. *J. Peasant Stud.* **2014**, *41*, 1153–1173. [CrossRef]
6. Kneen, C. The People's Food Policy Project: Introducing Food Sovereignty in Canada 2012. Available online: https://foodsecurecanada.org/ (accessed on 27 August 2020).
7. Kneen, C. Food Secure Canada: Wqhere agriculture, environment, health, food and justice intersect. In *Food Sovereignty in Canada: Creating just and Sustainable Food Systems*; Fernwood Publishing: Halifax, UK, 2010; pp. 80–96.
8. Beach, H. *A Year in Lapland: Guest of the Reindeer Herders*; University of Washington Press: Seattle, WA, USA, 2000.
9. Yoshida, A. Food Culture of the Gydan Nenets (Interpretation and Social Adaptation): Abstract. Ph.D. Thesis, Institute of Ethnology and Anthropology RAS, Moscow, Russia, 1997.
10. Andronov, S.V.; Lobanov, A.A.; Kochkin, R.A.; Protasova, I.V.; Bogdanova, E.N.; Tokarev, S.A. Forecast of arterial hypertension in the inhabitants of the Arctic region of Western Siberia. *Curr. Probl. Public Health Med. Stat.* **2018**, *1*, 54–65.
11. Kozlov, A.; Vershubsky, G.; Kozlova, M. Indigenous peoples of Northern Russia: Anthropology and health. *Circumpolar Health* **2018**, *66* (Suppl. 1), 1–84.
12. Bogdanova, E.; Lobanov, A.; Andronov, S.; Popov, A.; Kochkin, R.; Morell, I.A. Traditional nutrition of Indigenous peoples in the Arctic zone of Western Siberia. Challenges and impact on food security and health. In *Food Security in the High North Contemporary Challenges Across the Circumpolar Region*; Taylor & Francis Group Series; Routledge Research in Polar Regions: London, UK, 2020. [CrossRef]
13. Andronov, S.; Lobanov, A.; Popov, A.; Lobanova, L.; Kochkin, R.; Bogdanova, E.; Protasova, I. The impact of traditional nutrition on reduction of the chronic nonobstructive bronchitis risk in the Indigenous peoples living in tundra of the Arctic zone in Western Siberia, Russia. *Eur. Respir. J.* **2018**, *52*, PA796. [CrossRef]
14. Lobanov, A.; Andronov, S.; Kochkin, R. The role of traditional nutrition of Indigenous people in the Arctic zone of Western Siberia in managing the risks of hypertension. *EFSA J. Suppl. Sci. Food Soc.* **2018**, 156–157. Available online: https://www.efsa.europa.eu/sites/default/files/event/180918-conference/conference18-EFSA_Journal_abstracts.pdf (accessed on 27 August 2020).
15. Lobanova, L.P.; Lobanov, A.A.; Andronov, S.V.; Popov, A.I. Nutrition as a key element of indigenous health. *Sci. Bull. Yamal-Nenets Auton. Okrug* **2014**, *5*, 6–9.
16. Andronov, S.; Lobanov, A.; Popov, A.; Luo, Y.; Shaduyko, O.; Fesyun, A.; Lobanova, L.; Bogdanova, E.; Kobel'kova, I. Changing diets and traditional lifestyle of Siberian Arctic Indigenous Peoples: Effects on health and well-being. *Ambio* **2020**. [CrossRef]
17. Lobanov, A.A.; Bogdanova, E.N.; Andronov, S.V.; Popov, A.I.; Kochkin, R.A.; Kostritsyn, V.V.; Lobanova, L.P.; Protasova, I.V.; Lobanova, E.A.; Kobelkova, I.V.; et al. A study of the traditional diet of the inhabitants of the Arctic zone of Western Siberia. *Nutr. Issues* **2018**, *87*, 31.
18. Forbes, B.C.; Kumpula, T.; Meschtyb, N.; Laptander, R.; Macias-Fauria, M.; Zetterberg, P.; Verdonen, M.; Skarin, A.; Kim, K.Y.; Boisvert, L.N.; et al. Sea ice, rain-on-snow and tundra reindeer nomadism in Arctic Russia. *Biol. Lett.* **2016**, *12*, 20160466. [CrossRef] [PubMed]
19. Hossain, K.; Raheem, D.; Cormier, S. *Food Security Governance in the Arctic-Barents Region*; Springer International Publishing AG: Cham, Switzerland, 2018.

20. Rosstat. Available online: http://rosstat.gov.ru/folder/12781?print=1 (accessed on 27 August 2020).
21. The Ministry of Foreign Affairs of the Russian Federation. Available online: https://www.mid.ru/vnesneekonomiceskie-svazi-sub-ektov-rossijskoj-federacii/-/asset_publisher/ykggrK2nCl8c/content/id/128534 (accessed on 27 August 2020).
22. SOTI. Tourist Information Exchange System. Available online: https://www.nbcrs.org/regions/yamalo-nenetskiy-avtonomnyy-okrug/etnicheskiy-sostav-naseleniya (accessed on 27 August 2020).
23. Sustainable Food Value Chains Knowledge Platform 2020. Available online: http://www.fao.org/sustainable-food-value-chains/what-is-it/en/ (accessed on 20 September 2020).
24. Forbes, B.C.; Stammler, F.; Kumpula, T.; Meschtyb, N.; Pajunen, A.; Kaarlejarvi, E. High resilience in the Yamal-Nenets social-ecological system, West Siberian Arctic, Russia. *Proc. Natl. Acad. Sci. USA* **2009**, *106*, 22041–22048. [CrossRef] [PubMed]
25. Klokov, K.B. Changes in reindeer population numbers in Russia: An effect of the political context or of climate? *Rangifer* **2011**, *32*, 19–33. [CrossRef]
26. Stammler, F. Oil Without Conflict? The Anthropology of Industrialisation in Northern Russia. In *Crude Domination: An Anthropology of Oil*; Berghahn Books: Oxford, UK, 2011; pp. 243–269.
27. Department of Agro-industrial Complex of YNAO. Available online: https://dapk.yanao.ru/ (accessed on 27 August 2020).
28. Department of Natural Resources Regulation, Forest Relations and Development of the Oil and Gas Complex of the Yamal-Nenets Autonomous Okrug. Available online: https://dprr.yanao.ru/documents/active/74512/ (accessed on 27 August 2020).
29. Federal Law "On non-profit organizations", Article 6.1. Communities of the Indigenous peoples of the Russian Federation. N 7-FL, 12 January 1996.
30. Law on reindeer husbandry in the Yamal-Nenets Autonomous Okrug. No. 34-ZAO, 6 June 2016.
31. Federal Law "On the peasantry farms". N 74-FL 2003, 11 June 2003.
32. Federal Law "On Agricultural Cooperation". N 193-FL, 8 December 1995.
33. Vladimirova, V. Producers' cooperation within or against cooperative agricultural institutions? The case of reindeer husbandry in Post-Soviet Russia. *J. Rural Stud.* **2017**, *53*, 247–258.
34. Golovnev, A. Indigenous Leadership in Northwestern Siberia: Traditional Patterns and Their Contemporary Manifestiations. *Arct. Anthropol.* **1997**, *34*, 149–166.
35. Khlomich, L.V. *Nentsy: Ocherki Traditsionnoi Kul'tury [The Nenets: Essays on Traditional Culture]*; Russkii Dvor: St. Petersburg, FL, USA, 1995.
36. Ivanova, A.A.; Stammler, F.M. The diversity of natural resource governance in the Russian Arctic. *Sib. Hist. Res. Sib. Istor. Issled.* **2017**, *4*, 210–225. [CrossRef]
37. Stammler, F. *Reindeer Nomads Meet the Market: Culture, Property and Globalisation at the End of the Land*; Lit Verlag: Münster, Germany, 2005.
38. Larsen, J.N.; Fondahl, G. *Arctic Human Development Report: Regional Processes and Global Linkages*; Nordisk Ministerrad: Copenhagen, Denmark, 2015.
39. Anisimov, O.; Orttung, R. Climate change in Northern Russia through the prism of public perception. *Ambio* **2019**, *48*, 661–671. [CrossRef]
40. Forbes, B.K.; Kumpula, T.; Messhtyb, N.; Laptander, R.; Masias-fauria, M.; Zetterberg, P.; Verdonen, M.; Skarin, A.; Kim, K.Y.; Boisvert, L.N.; et al. Influence of reduction of ice coverage in the Barents and Karskoe Seas on traditional reindeer husbandry of the Yamal Peninsula. *News Russ. Geogr. Soc.* **2018**, *150*, 3–19.
41. Glok, N.I.; Akexeev, G.; Vyazilova, A. Seasonal forecast of sea ice extent in the Barents sea. *Arct. Antarct. Res.* **2019**, *65*, 5–14. [CrossRef]
42. Golovnev, A. Challenges to Arctic Nomadism: Yamal Nenets Facing Climate Change Era Calamities. *Arct. Anthropol.* **2017**, *54*, 40–51. [CrossRef]
43. Golovnev, A. Yamal nomads: Facing risks and maneuvering. *Sib. Hist. Res. Sib. Istor. Issled.* **2016**, *4*, 154–171.
44. Loginov, V.G.; Ignatyeva, M.N.; Balashenko, V.V. Harm to the Resources of Traditional Nature Management and Its Economic Evaluation. *Ekon. Reg. Econ. Reg.* **2017**, *13*, 396–409. [CrossRef]
45. Siche, R. What is the impact of COVID-19 disease on agriculture? *Sci. Agropecu.* **2020**, *11*, 3–6. [CrossRef]
46. Stammler, F.M.; Ivanova, A. From spirits to conspiracy? Nomadic perceptions of climate change, pandemics and disease. *Anthropol. Today* **2020**, *36*, 12–18. [CrossRef]

47. Government of the Yamal-Nenets Autonomous Okrug. Available online: https://www.yanao.ru/presscenter/news/44271/ (accessed on 27 August 2020).
48. Order of the Ministry of agriculture of the Russian Federation "On the approval of the Rules in the field of veterinary medicine during the slaughter of animals and primary processing of meat and other products of slaughter of non-industrial production at slaughterhouses of medium and low power". N 72. 12 March 2014. Available online: https://jurescort.ru/en/cap--repair/pravila-zaboya-zhivotnyh-veterinarno-sanitarnye-pravila-vnutrihozyaistvennogo-uboya-skota-na-myaso-tr/ (accessed on 29 August 2020).
49. The Government Decree of the Yamal-Nenets Autonomous Okrug "Governing Subsidies from the District Budget for the Producing Reindeer Meat". N 1424-P, 26 December 2019.
50. Guryeva, K.B.; Ivanova, E.V. The biological value of proteins of frozen meat after storage. *Meat Technol.* **2012**, *3*, 46–59.
51. Rebezov, M.B.; Miroshnikova, E.P.; Bogatova, O.V.; Asenova, B.K.; Nurgazezova, A.N. *Physicochemical and Biochemical Principles of the Production of Meat and Meat Products*; Publishing Center of YuUrSU: Chelyabinsk, Russia, 2012.
52. Galanakis, C.M. The Food Systems in the Era of the Coronavirus (COVID-19) Pandemic Crisis. *Foods* **2020**, *9*, 523. [CrossRef] [PubMed]
53. Lobanov, A.A. Nutrition of the settlement and tundra indigenous population of the Taz region. In *Arctic Medicine, Ecology and Biology*; KIRA: Salekhard, Russia, 2017.
54. Lobanov, A.A.; Andronov, S.V.; Popov, A.I.; Kochkin, R.A.; Kostritsyn, V.V. *Traditional Food of the Indigenous Population of the Yamal-Nenets AO*; Arctic Research Scientific Centre of YNAO: Nadym, Russia, 2017; p. 78.
55. Kochkin, R.A.; Lobanov, A.A.; Andronov, S.V.; Kobelkova, I.V.; Nikityuk, D.B.; Bogdanova, E.N.; Popov, A.I.; Kostritsyn, V.V.; Protasova, I.V.; Lobanova, L.P.; et al. Influence of consumption of various types of fat on the stability of the central nervous system to cold stress. *Bull. New Med. Technol.* **2019**, *2*, 172–180.
56. Kochkin, R.A.; Lobanov, A.A.; Andronov, S.V.; Rapoport, S.I.; Popov, A.I.; Kostritsyn, V.V.; Protasova, I.V.; Lobanova, L.P.; Poskotinova, L.V.; Petrov, V.G.; et al. The ability of various dietary fats to enhance the adaptation of the central nervous system to geomagnetic disturbances in the Arctic. *Nutr. Issues* **2018**, *87*, 30.

Publisher's Note: MDPI stays neutral with regard to jurisdictional claims in published maps and institutional affiliations.

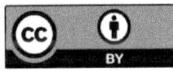

© 2020 by the authors. Licensee MDPI, Basel, Switzerland. This article is an open access article distributed under the terms and conditions of the Creative Commons Attribution (CC BY) license (http://creativecommons.org/licenses/by/4.0/).

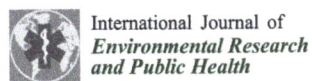

Article

The Effects of Epistemic Trust and Social Trust on Public Acceptance of Genetically Modified Food: An Empirical Study from China

Longji Hu, Rongjin Liu, Wei Zhang * and Tian Zhang

School of Public Administration, Central China Normal University, Wuhan 430079, China; hulongji@mail.ccnu.edu.cn (L.H.); liurongjing@mails.ccnu.edu.cn (R.L.); zhangtian@163.com (T.Z.)
* Correspondence: zhangwei2017@mail.ccnu.edu.cn; Tel.: +86-180-6200-9973

Received: 7 September 2020; Accepted: 20 October 2020; Published: 21 October 2020

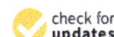

Abstract: Most studies exploring the public acceptance of genetically modified food (GMF) are based on social trust and the establishment of a causal model. The underlying premise is that social trust indirectly affects public acceptance of GMF through perceived risks and perceived benefits. The object of social trust is trust in people, organizations, and institutions. Different from the social trust, epistemic trust refers to people's trust in scientific knowledge behind the technology of concern. It has been shown that epistemic trust, like social trust, is also an important factor that affects the public perception of applicable risks and benefits. Therefore, it is necessary to incorporate epistemic trust into the causal model to derive a more complete explanation of public acceptance. However, such work has not been conducted to date. The causal model proposed in this paper integrated epistemic trust and social trust and divided social trust into trust in public organizations and trust in industrial organizations. A representative questionnaire survey (N = 1091) was conducted with Chinese adults. The model was analyzed by the partial least squares structural equation modeling (PLS-SEM) method. Three major findings were obtained: First, epistemic trust is an important antecedent of perceived risks and perceived benefits and exerts a significant indirect effect on the acceptance of GMF. Secondly, trust in industrial organizations negatively impacts perceived risks, while trust in public organizations positively impacts perceived benefits. Thirdly, contrary to the common opinion, trust in industrial organizations did not exert a significant direct effect on perceived benefits, and trust in public organizations did not demonstrate a significant direct effect on perceived risks. Therefore, trust in industrial organizations and trust in public organizations utilize different influence paths on GMF acceptance. This study enriches the understanding of the influence path of trust with regard to the acceptance of emerging technologies and is of great significance to relevant risk-management practices.

Keywords: epistemic trust; risk perception; genetically modified food; public acceptance; partial least squares structural equation modeling

1. Introduction

Genetically modified food (GMF) offers a significant technological advance in modern agriculture as well as enormous social and economic benefits [1]. Like any other new food technology in history, the safety of GMF has been a source of anxiety, uncertainty, controversy, and low acceptance since GMF entered the market. Previous studies have shown that consumers from Japan, the European Union (EU), and the United States (US) maintain low acceptance of GMF [2–10]. In this regard, China is no exception [11]. A survey by Cui and Shoemaker (2018) showed that the percentage of the Chinese public adverse to GMF is as high as 41.4% [12]. The commercialization of GMF as well as the decision-making of stakeholders related to food industries (e.g., governmental policymakers, farmers, and agro-biotechnology enterprises) strongly depends on its public acceptance [13–15]. Given the importance of predicting public acceptance of GMF, much scholarly attention has been paid to explore the factors that affect the public acceptance of GMF [16–22].

Among these factors, scholars are most interested in the following three: perceived risks, perceived benefits, and trust [13,17]. Siegrist (2000, 1999) proposed a causal model to explain the acceptance of gene technology, which identified perceived benefits, perceived risks, and trust as the three most important factors to affect public acceptance. Moreover, the perceived benefits and perceived risks directly influence acceptance, while trust imposes an indirect influence on acceptance through perceived risks and perceived benefits [23,24]. This model has been accepted as the basic model for the study of the acceptability of emerging technologies and is widely used in several technical fields.

Trust in the casual model of public acceptance mostly refers to social trust [25]. Social rust is a psychological state, which comprises the intention to accept vulnerability based on positive expectations of the intentions or behavior of another [26,27]. The object of social trust is trust in people, organizations, and institutions. Trust is a multi-type concept. Except social trust, epistemic trust is also one kind of trust that has an important impact on perceived risks. Epistemic trust refers to people's trust in scientific knowledge behind the technology of concern [28]. Some studies have shown that cognitive trust is an important factor in perceived risk, which is more negatively correlated with perceived risk than social trust [29]. However, with the exception of some recent studies, most causal models of public acceptance rarely consider epistemic trust. For example, Hakim et al. (2020) did not explicitly mention the concept of epistemic trust but included the content of epistemic trust in the measurement items of social trust [18].

In addition, social trust is also a multi-type concept. According to the types of trustees, some scholars divided social trust into trust in public organizations (e.g., government regulators, public research institutions) and trust in industrial organizations (e.g., farmers and agro-biotechnology enterprises) [30]. Several studies have found that these two types of social trust have different antecedents. The level of trust in public organizations depends on their abilities and competence, and the level of trust in industrial organizations depends on their intentions, honesty, and integrity [31,32]. At the same time, some studies found that public trust in these two types of trustees differ: people have more trust in public organizations than in industrial organizations [33]. Therefore, it is necessary to divide the social trust into trust in industrial organizations and trust in public organizations; then, the impact of these two types of social trust on public acceptance of GMF can be appropriately explored.

This study complements previous studies in two aspects: first, the concept of epistemic trust is introduced as an indirect factor that affects public acceptance; second, different from most previous studies, which, as outlined, regarded trust in industrial organizations and trust in public organizations as a single construct, this study treats both types of trust as two different variables.

All in all, some studies have found that epistemic trust is an important factor affecting the public risk perception; trust in public organizations and trust in industrial organizations should be treated as two different variables. By integrating epistemic trust, trust in public organizations, and trust in industrial organizations into the causal model, the impact of trust on public acceptance of GMF can be appropriately explored. However, such work has not been conducted to date. As such, this study is aimed at integrating epistemic trust, trust in public organizations, and trust in industrial organizations into one model and analyzing their impacts on public acceptance of GMF.

2. Research Hypotheses and Framework

Public acceptance of GMF (ACC) is defined as the willingness of the public to buy and their intention to use GMF [34,35]. As technical barriers disappear, a critical factor for promoting the deployment of GMF is whether people will be willing to buy and use the resulting products and enjoy the benefits of this technology [36,37].

The role ACC plays in the implementation of food technology induces a number of important research questions for social scientists, such as "which factors determine whether a particular food technology will be accepted or rejected?" A wide range of social–psychological factors influencing ACC has already been explored. Among these, three factors (social trust, perceived benefits, and perceived risks) have attracted the most scholarly attention [17,38]. To explain ACC, Siegrist (2000, 1999) proposed a causal model for the relationship among these three factors [23,24]. In that causal model, Siegrist argued that acceptance of this new technology was determined by both perceived risks and perceived benefits and that social trust exerted a strong indirect influence on acceptance through perceived risks and benefits.

This causal model has been widely used to explain public acceptance in a variety of technological domains, such as gene technology [18,39–41], financial technology [42,43], nanotechnology [44–49], renewable energy [32,50–52], unmanned aircraft [53], and automated driving technology [54,55]. The present study is also based on Siegrist's causal model.

The present study proposed a research framework to systematically examine the relationship among these various types of trust, perceived risks/benefits, and public acceptance of GMF. Figure 1 illustrates the proposed framework.

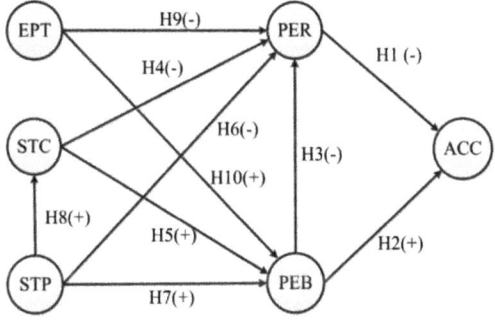

Note: ACC = Public acceptance; PEB = Perceived benefits; PER = Perceived risks; STC = Trust in industrial organizations; STP = Trust in public organizations; EPT = Epistemic trust.

Figure 1. The concept model.

2.1. Perceived Risks and Benefits

Perceived risk is an individual's impression or interpretation of the uncertainty and potential negative consequences related to an object that is perceived as a threat [56,57]. Different people will interpret the same objective facts differently and thus form different subjective cognition. It has been shown that because of the discrepancy and biases in individual cognition, not only the individuals but also the perceived risks that have been assessed by experts can differ widely [58]. Moreover, for the same risk, different individuals will have completely different perceived outcomes. Perceived benefit is an individual's perception of the benefits a certain technology or product can provide [59]. Benefits are what individuals pursue when they accept a certain technology to buy a certain product, which are thus reflections of the value these individuals want to obtain [60].

In the case of GMF, perceived risks include unknown long-term effects, side effects on human health, and both environmental and social problems [61–63]. Perceived benefits revolve around environmental issues, especially in relation to the reduction of energy and chemical inputs, high yields and diversity, lower food prices, and longer shelf life [64,65].

In general, food products have been regarded as low-involvement purchases that require only limited decision-making [66]. Perceived risks have no explanatory power unless they exceed a specific threshold [67]. Most surveys showed that the risk perceptions of the public toward GMF are high across the world [11,68–73]. In the context of GMF, perceived risks may be a key factor that determines ACC as perceived benefits [16,74,75]. Most studies and reviews have concluded that perceived benefits positively influence the acceptance of GMF. In contrast, perceived risks are considered to impose negative impacts. There have been good reviews on the relationship among perceived risks, perceived benefits, and GMF acceptance; please refer to Frewer, Lynn J., et al. (2013), Bearth A. and M. Siegrist (2016), and Machado Nardi, V.A., et al. (2020) [13,19,34].

Based on the above, the following related hypotheses are proposed:

Hypothesis H1 (H1). *Public's perceived risks of GMF will negatively affect their ACC.*

Hypothesis H2 (H2). *Public's perceived benefits of GMF will positively affect their ACC.*

Most research suggested that risk and benefit perceptions were not independent but rather inversely related [76,77]. This suggests that people do not judge risks and benefits independently, as is done in scientific risk–benefit appraisals, but rather they intuitively weigh risks and benefits against each other. When the risks people thus perceive are high, they perceive that the benefits that could be obtained are low, and vice visa. Following Siegrist (1999), this further proposes that perceived benefits influence perceived risks [24]. The public has little capacity and knowledge to properly evaluate the risks associated with GMF; however, its benefits are tangible and concrete, and people consequently are more experienced about the associated benefits [39,78]. Therefore, for normal people, it is much easier to assess the benefits associated with GMF than to assess its risks. Attributing relatively high benefits and high risks to GMF would produce cognitive dissonance. It would not be surprising if altering the level of perceived risks reduced this dissonance. Following this argument, it is more plausible that perceived benefits influence perceived risks than the opposite.

Hypothesis H3 (H3). *Public's perceived benefits of GMF will negatively affect their perceived risks.*

2.2. Social Trust

Trust is a psychological state, which comprises the intention to accept vulnerability based on positive expectations of the intentions or behavior of another [26]. In this definition, the object is trust in people, organizations, and institutions. This type of trust is also referred to as social trust [25,27,79].

Most people do not possess elaborated knowledge about GMF [20,80,81]. One way to cope with this lack of knowledge and capacities is to rely on others to evaluate and manage an associated hazard. Relevant actors are the producers of GMF, regulating organizations (e.g., governmental organizations), research institutions working in the field of GMF, and independent non-governmental organizations [82]. Therefore, social trust plays a dominant role in such circumstances. Research in the domain of GMF showed that people who trust responsible actors attributed more benefits and fewer risks to GMF. Thus, social trust indirectly impacts the acceptance of GMF [37,83,84].

Social trust is a multi-type construct. Peters, Covello, and McCallum (1997) divided social trust into trust in the industry, trust in the government, and trust in citizen groups [30]. They showed that the trust in the industry was related to public perceptions of concern and care on the part of this industry (e.g., the trustee's intentions, honesty, and integrity). The trust in the government was related to perceptions of commitment and perceptions of knowledge and expertise (e.g., trustee's abilities and competence). The trust in citizen groups was related to perceptions of knowledge and expertise (e.g., trustee's abilities and competence). Maeda and Miyahara (2003) conducted a similar study in Japan. They obtained the same results about trust in government and industry but not for citizen groups because the social positions of citizen groups are not yet stable in Japan [85]. Thus, it can be seen that different types of social trust have different antecedents. The antecedents of trust in public organizations lie in the trustee's abilities and competence, and the antecedents of trust in industrial organizations lie in the trustee's intentions, honesty, and integrity. Additionally, Lang and Hallman

(2005) and Terwel et al. (2009) found that the trust level of the public in these different organizations is also different. Generally, the trust level of public organizations is higher than that of industrial organizations [33,86]. Finally, Maeda and Miyahara (2003) found that the trusts in both government and industry were negatively related to risk perception [85].

Based on these studies, each type of social trust has different antecedents, and the public assigns different levels to every type of trust. Therefore, it is essential to distinguish between these various types of social trust and divide them into two differential constructs. In this way, we can have a deeper understanding of the influence mechanism of social trust on public acceptance of GMF.

In China, the social positions of citizen groups are not yet stable because their social positions have only recently started to be established. Following Maeda and Miyahara (2003), this study inferred that citizen groups are not well trusted by the people in China [85]. Consequently, citizen groups are not seen as relevant agents in the domain of GMF and were not included in the investigation. This study distinguished between trust in the industrial organizations which form the industry and trust in public organizations. Since previous studies showed that social trust, as one single construct, exerts significant influences on the perceived benefits and the perceived risks, it is reasonable to assume that both types of social trust might influence perceived benefits and perceived risks in the same way.

However, these two types of social trust are not independent. The responsibility of public institutions is to supervise the effective implementation of relevant risk policies and regulations by industrial organizations. López-Navarro, Llorens-Monzonís, and Tortosa-Edo (2013) argued that the more effective public institutions perform their supervision responsibilities, the higher the public's confidence in the industrial organizations' compliance with relevant risk control measures will be [14]. Consequently, trust in public organizations will directly and positively impact the trust in industrial organizations. In fact, evidence supports this argument.

Following these arguments, the following set of hypotheses was developed:

Hypothesis H4 (H4). *Higher trust in public organizations will decrease the perceived risks of GMF.*

Hypothesis H5 (H5). *Higher trust in public organizations will increase the perceived benefits of GMF.*

Hypothesis H6 (H6). *Higher trust in industrial organizations will decrease the perceived risks of GMF.*

Hypothesis H7 (H7). *Higher trust in industrial organizations will increase the perceived benefits of GMF.*

Hypothesis H8 (H8). *Trust in public organizations will directly and positively influence trust in industrial organizations.*

2.3. Epistemic Trust

In her study of the Storuman (Sweden) referendum on siting a local high-level nuclear waste repository, Drottz-Sjöberg (1996) found that even though the social trust may exist, the public may still reject a siting proposal. People may well trust the technical expertise of an industry or an agency in the area of technology of concern, but they may still reject the technology [87]. It is clear that this kind of rejection could not be explained by lower social trust. Such a contradiction is common in society. Sjöberg (2001, 1999) argued that the reason for such contradictions is that people distrust the sufficient development of the scientific basis of the technology of concern, assuming that current scientific knowledge has not completely assessed the (negative) effects of the technology [28,88].

Sjöberg (2001) thus introduced the concept of epistemic trust to represent people's trust in scientific knowledge behind the technology of concern [28]. Additionally, research showed that social trust is fairly marginal when it comes to account for perceived risks [89,90]. Follow-up work supported the notion that epistemic risk is an important factor for perceived risks, which was even more strongly negatively related to perceived risks than social trust [25,29,52,91–96].

Based on these findings, the following hypotheses were proposed:

Hypothesis H9 (H9). *Epistemic trust will negatively affect perceived risks.*

Hypothesis H10 (H10). *Epistemic trust will positively affect perceived benefits.*

3. Methods

3.1. Sample

Data were collected through self-reported, structured questionnaires. The questionnaire was developed in Chinese and was submitted to a panel of five experts at one of the key universities in Central China for content validity evaluation. Of these five experts, two work at the Department of Biology and three at the School of Public Management. The panel approved both the issue list and question format and suggested revisions to clarify questions so that the general public could fully understand the questions asked and answer them. Before the formal survey, a pilot test was conducted. In summary, 50 randomly selected individual participants (representing the public, and including both 20 undergraduates and 30 ordinary people) were interviewed individually. During the test, respondents were asked whether they could clearly understand the questions and felt comfortable answering them. According to their feedback, changes were implemented with regard to wording, expressions, and grammar to improve the questionnaire's clarity, accuracy, flow, and validity.

The questionnaire contained four parts: The first section was the screening question "Have you heard of genetically modified food?" The respondent need not continue to fill in the questionnaire if his or her answer was "no". The second section asked for socio-demographic information including gender, age, educational background, and income. The third section focused on the public's acceptance of GMF. The last part inquired about perceived risks/benefits level with regard to GMF, social trust in different objects, and epistemic trust.

The survey followed a stratified sampling. First, to account for geographical differences and to maximize representativeness, we choose eight provinces from the east (Zhejiang), south (Guangdong), west (Sichuan, Xizang, and Xinjiang), north (Hebei), northeast (Jilin), and middle (Hubei) regions in China. Two higher-income and another two lower-income counties were randomly selected in each province, resulting in 32 counties. Next, 4–6 city communities or villages were randomly selected from each county, resulting in 150 city communities or villages. Finally, 7–10 households were randomly approached in each of the city communities or villages, resulting in a total sample of 1200 observations. In June 2019, through public recruitment, 100 university students were recruited as interviewers at Central China Normal University. The home addresses of the university students were located in the 32 counties selected above; there are 3–4 interviewers in each county. Face-to-face interviews were conducted by university students during July and September 2019.

A total of 1200 paper-based questionnaires were distributed. Finally, 1168 paper-based questionnaires were thus collected, resulting in 1091 valid questionnaires after eliminating those with clerical errors or contradictions; the effective questionnaire recovery rate reached 93.41%.

3.2. Measures

The measurement scale used in this study contained six constructs and twenty-two items, which are based on several scales in relevant studies (see Table 1 for specific relevant studies) that offer high reliability and validity. Peculiarities of the Chinese language and culture were considered during the translation. A minor modification in the wording was made to suit Chinese peculiarities. The subjects were asked to indicate their agreement or disagreement with the statements provided, using a seven-point Likert scale. Table 1 provides detailed scale items for the constructed variables.

Table 1. Measures used in the study.

Construct	Items	Source
Public acceptance (ACC)	(ACC1) Would you like to buy genetically modified food?	[23,24,97]
	(ACC2) Would you like to buy this kind of food if the product trademark indicates that it contains genetically modified ingredients?	
	(ACC3) Whenever possible I avoid buying GMF (reversed scoring).	
	(ACC4) Compared with ordinary food, genetically modified food has a longer shelf life. Would you choose to buy because of this point?	
Perceived benefits (PEB)	(PEB1) Overall, GM food technology is useful for society.	[96,98]
	(PEB2) Transgenic technology can increase crop yields and feed more people.	
	(PEB3) GMF creates a higher quality of life; it is a great technological advancement.	
	(PEB4) Genetically modified foods will eventually be accepted by the majority of people.	
Perceived risks (PER)	(PER1) Overall, GMF can be dangerous to people.	[37,96,98,99]
	(PER2) Eating genetically modified food will lead to infertility.	
	(PER3) Eating genetically modified food will change the genes of us or future generations.	
	(PER4) The production of genetically modified food will destroy the diversity of animals and plants.	
	(PER5) Planting genetically modified crops will have a negative impact on the environment.	
Trust in industrial organizations (STC)	(STC1) food corporation.	[39,100]
	(STC2) agricultural corporation.	
	(STC3) pharmaceutical corporation.	
Trust in public organizations (STP)	(STP1) National Food Administration.	[39,96]
	(STP2) public research institution in the domain of GMF.	
	(STP3) National Institute of Public Health.	
Epistemic trust (EPT)	(EPT1) There could be negative side effects of GMF unknown for scientific knowledge today.	[94,96]
	(EPT2) Scientific knowledge about GMF is probably still incomplete	
	(EPT3) Researchers behind GMF technology are hardly aware of all consequences of what they create.	

To assess ACC, a 5-item measure was used that was developed by Siegrist (1999, 2000) and Zhang (2017) and represented people's willingness to buy GMF under different specified circumstances [23,24,97]. The first two items were adapted from Zhang (2017), and the remaining three items were adapted from Michael Siegrist (1999, 2000). Examples of items are "Whenever possible I avoid buying GMF" (1 = strongly disagree; 7 = strongly agree) (reverse-coded) and "Would you like to buy genetically modified food?" (1 = strongly unwilling; 7 = strongly willing).

To assess the perceived benefits of GMF, the 4-item measure was used that was developed by Sjöberg (2005) and Ghoochani et al. (2016) [96,98]. The items therein reflect the social and environmental benefits of GMF that are typically mentioned by experts and news media. Items that represent the economic benefits of GMF (e.g., lower price, reduction of production cost, and increased profit) were not included, because previous studies found that most of the public assumed that these economic benefits were only obtained by the corporations in the domain of GMF [96]. An example of these items is "Transgenic technology can increase crop yields and feed more people." (1 = strongly disagree; 7 = strongly agree).

To assess the perceived risks of GMF, respondents indicated their agreement with the 5-items developed by Sjöberg (2005), Chen M.-F. (2008), Ghoochani et al. (2016), and Zhang (2019) [37,96,98,99]. Two items reflect the possible harm of GMF to human health, and the other two items reflect the possible harm of GMF to the environment. Examples of items are "Eating genetically modified food will lead to infertility." and "Planting genetically modified crops will have a negative impact on the environment." (1 = strongly disagree; 7 = strongly agree).

Trust in industrial organizations: Although previous studies have shown that social trust contains multiple components, Lang and Hallman (2005) showed that these components were highly correlated and would converge on a common factor [86]. Therefore, the public's social trust in different objects can be measured in a specific holistic way. Based on this argument, the trust in industrial organizations was measured via the trust in various industrial organizations [39,100]. Participants were asked, "How much trust do you have in the following institutions: (1) food corporations, (2) agricultural corporations, (3) pharmaceutical corporations?" Participants had to indicate their level of trust on a 7-point-scale, ranging from no trust at all to a very high level of trust (1 = not at all; 7 = very much).

Trust in public organizations was measured via trust in various public organizations [39,96]. Participants were asked, "How much trust do you have in the following institutions: (1) National Food Administration, (2) Public research institutions in the domain of GMF, (3) National Institute of Public Health?" Participants had to indicate their level of trust on a 7-point-scale, ranging from no trust at all to a very high level of trust (1 = not at all; 7 = very much).

To measure epistemic trust, respondents indicated their agreement with the three items that were adopted from Sjöberg (2005) and that have been used elsewhere [94,96]. An example of such items is "There could be negative side effects of GMF unknown for scientific knowledge today" (1 = strongly disagree; 7 = strongly agree).

3.3. Analysis Method

Descriptive statistics and exploratory factor analysis of all questionnaire items were performed in a preliminary study by IBM SPSS Statistics (IBM, Armonk, NY, USA). In contrast to covariance-based structural equation methods (CB-SEM), partial least squares structural equation modeling (PLS-SEM) is the appropriate analytical tool in this case because it imposes minimal demands on measurement scales, sample size, and residual distributions [101]. PLS-SEM was used to test the reliability and validity of both the measurement model and the structural model. Smart PLS version 3.2.4 [102] was used to run the PLS–SEM analysis. A bootstrapping procedure of 5000 resamples was used to generate t-statistics and standard errors [103].

The process of evaluation of the results of the PLS-SEM involves two steps. In step 1, the assessment of the measurement model is conducted. When measurement quality is confirmed, the structural model evaluation is conducted in step 2 [104].

For the assessment of the measurement model, we start by examining the indicator loadings. Loadings above 0.70 indicate that the construct explains more than 50% of the indicator's variance, demonstrating that the indicator exhibits a satisfactory degree of reliability. The constructs' internal consistency reliability was assessed. For Cronbach's alpha (α), higher values indicate higher levels of internal consistency reliability. Results between 0.70 and 0.95 represent "satisfactory to good" reliability levels [104]. Composite reliability (CR) measures internal consistency reliability that assumes the same thresholds. Results between 0.70 and 0.95 represent "satisfactory to good" reliability levels [104].

Next, the convergent validity was calculated, which is the extent to which a construct converges in its indicators by explaining the items' variance. Convergent validity is assessed by the average variance extracted (AVE) across all items associated with a particular construct and is also referred to as communality. An acceptable threshold for the AVE is 0.50 or higher. This level or higher indicates that, on average, the construct explains (more than) 50% of the variance of its items [104].

The last stage is to assess discriminant validity. This analysis reveals to which extent a construct is empirically distinct from other constructs both in terms of how much it correlates with other constructs and how distinctly the indicators represent only this single construct. Discriminant validity assessment in PLS-SEM involves analyzing Henseler et al.'s (2015) heterotrait–monotrait ratio (HTMT) of correlations [105]. The suggested threshold is a value of 0.85 when the path model included constructs that are conceptually very similar.

For the assessment of the structural model, we start by testing the proposed research hypothesis about the causal relationship between latent variables by evaluating the significance of the path coefficients. A path coefficient is regarded as significant if the p-value is below the pre-defined α-level.

Next, for the significant path coefficients, it makes sense to quantify how substantial they are, which can be accomplished by assessing their effect size f^2. f^2 values above 0.35, 0.15, and 0.02 can be regarded as strong, moderate, and weak, respectively [106].

Finally, the multicollinearity of the structural model is examined. The index used is the variance inflation factor (VIF). If VIF is less than 5, it can be considered that there is no serious multicollinearity problem in the structural model [104].

4. Results

4.1. Descriptive Analysis

A total of 1091 individuals with a mean age (standard deviation) of 32.93 (14.31) years were enrolled in this study. The sample did not originate from strict random sampling, and therefore, the representativeness of the sample had to be evaluated. To do so, a χ^2 test was applied to ensure that the sample in this study is representative of the entire population. Table 2 presents the characteristics of the sample and the results of the χ^2 test, which indicate that the sample could represent the Chinese population roughly ($p \geq 0.05$).

Table 2. Descriptive statistics of the sample data.

Characteristic	Classification	Number	Sample (%)	Population (%) *	χ^2 Test (p-Value)
Gender	Male	483	44.3	51.2	0.982
	Female	608	55.7	48.8	(0.322)
Age	15–29 years old and below	523	47.9	42.9	0.902
	30–50 years old	447	41.0	42.3	(0.637)
	51 years old and above	121	11.1	14.8	
Type of Habitat	Rural inhabitant	585	53.6	55.9	0.081
	Urban inhabitant	506	46.4	44.1	(0.776)
Education background	Primary education	183	16.8	27.7	
	Junior high school	427	39.1	40.6	
	High school (including technical secondary school)	254	23.3	17.5	4.744 (0.192)
	College degree and above (including junior College)	227	20.8	14.2	
Monthly income (Chinese Yuan)	<3000	843	77.3%	No available	
	3001–5000	204	18.7%	No available	
	>5001	44	4.0%	No available	

* Source: http://www.stats.gov.cn/tjsj/zxfb/201604/t20160420_1346151.html.

4.2. Assessment of Measurement Model

Cronbach's alpha (α) and composite reliability (CR) were above 0.70 and each AVE (Average Variance Extracted) was above 0.50 (see Table 3), indicating that the measurements were reliable and that the latent construct can account for at least 50% of the variance within items. As shown in Table 3, the loadings are within an acceptable range and the t-values indicate that they are significant at the 0.001 level.

Table 3. Confirmatory factor analysis results.

Construct	Mean(SD)	Item	Mean	SD	Loading	P	α	CR	AVE
ACC	3.682(1.481)	ACC1	3.432	2.071	0.827	0.000	0.804	0.872	0.640
		ACC2	3.372	1.631	0.840	0.000			
		ACC3	4.813	1.642	0.800	0.000			
		ACC4	3.112	2.142	0.701	0.000			
EPT	2.852(1.161)	EPT1	2.531	1.379	0.801	0.000	0.777	0.857	0.668
		EPT2	2.742	1.382	0.773	0.000			
		EPT3	3.301	1.421	0.874	0.000			
PEB	4.479(1.232)	PEB1	4.711	1.501	0.858	0.000	0.816	0.879	0.645
		PEB2	4.751	1.558	0.768	0.000			
		PEB3	4.282	1.589	0.853	0.000			
		PEB4	4.169	1.519	0.725	0.000			
PER	3.887(1.129)	PER1	3.801	1.561	0.820	0.000	0.802	0.862	0.558
		PER2	3.682	1.468	0.794	0.000			
		PER3	3.551	1.659	0.761	0.000			
		PER4	4.151	1.492	0.711	0.000			
		PER5	4.282	1.371	0.634	0.000			
STC	4.078(1.292)	STC1	3.850	1.451	0.864	0.000	0.884	0.928	0.811
		STC2	4.253	1.401	0.921	0.000			
		STC3	4.161	1.471	0.916	0.000			
STP	5.258(1.191)	STP1	5.661	1.382	0.800	0.000	0.765	0.864	0.680
		STP2	5.162	1.471	0.822	0.000			
		STP3	4.961	1.460	0.850	0.000			

Note: ACC =Public acceptance; EPT = Epistemic trust; PEB = Perceived benefits; PER = Perceived risks; STC = Trust in industrial organizations; STP = Trust in public organizations.

The discriminant validity of the constructs was evaluated using the approaches recommended by the heterotrait–monotrait ratio (HTMT) of correlations [105]. If the HTMT is significantly smaller than 0.85, this is evidence of sufficient discriminant validity. The results in Table 4 suggest that all constructs had acceptable discriminant validity.

Table 4. Discriminant validity (heterotrait–monotrait ratio (HTMT)).

	ACC	EPT	PEB	PER	STC	STP
ACC						
EPT	0.239					
PEB	0.668	0.154				
PER	0.755	0.436	0.466			
STC	0.316	0.120	0.270	0.183		
STP	0.305	0.326	0.422	0.137	0.694	

Note: ACC =Public acceptance; PEB = Perceived benefits; PER = Perceived risks; STC = Trust in industrial organizations; STP = Trust in public organizations; EPT = Epistemic trust.

4.3. Common Method Bias

All data were collected by using the discussed survey method; therefore, common method bias may affect the validity of this research.

First, the data set was assessed using Harman's one-factor test to identify any potential common method biases [107]. The danger of common method bias is high if a single factor accounts for more than 50% of the variance [108]. Evidence of common method bias exists when a general construct accounts for the majority of the covariance among all constructs. A principal component factor analysis was performed and the results excluded the potential threat of common methods bias. The first (and largest) factor accounted for 27.930% and none of the general factors accounted for more than 50% of the variance, indicating that common method bias was not a serious problem in the data set.

Second, following Liang et al. (2007), the PLS model included a common method factor whose indicators included all principal constructs' indicators [109]. Each calculated indicator's variances could be substantively explained by the principal construct and by the method. The results demonstrate that the average substantively explained variance of the indicators was 0.665, while the average method-based variance was 0.015. The ratio of substantive variance to method-based variance is 44:1. In addition, all method-based factor loadings are non-significant. Given the small magnitude and insignificance of method-based variance, according to Liang et al. (2007), this indicated that the method is unlikely to be a serious concern for this study.

4.4. Assessment of Structural Model

Model fit was evaluated by examining the goodness of fit (GoF) [110] and the standardized root mean square residual (SRMR) [111]. GoF was 0.475, which exceeded the cut-off value of 0.36 for a large effect size [110]. SRMR evaluates the discrepancy between an observed correlation matrix and a predicted correlation matrix. The calculated SRMR was 0.039, which remained below the recommended threshold of 0.08 [111]. Thus, the PLS path model achieved an appropriate overall fit.

Figure 2 and Table 5 presents the estimates obtained via PLS analysis. R^2 indicates the amount of variance explained by a model [112]. To evaluate the full model, R^2 values were calculated for ACC. The R^2 value of 0.521 indicated that the model explains a substantial amount of variance for ACC.

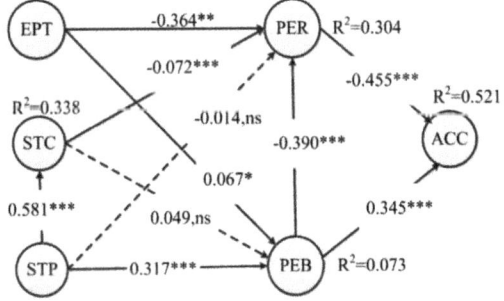

Note: ACC = Public acceptance; PEB = Perceived benefits; PER = Perceived risks; STC = Trust in industrial organizations; STP = Trust in public organizations; EPT = Epistemic trust.

* $p < 0.05$; ** $p < 0.01$; *** $p < 0.001$; ns, not significant.

Figure 2. Result of partial least squares (PLS) analysis for structural model.

Table 5. Causal relationships.

Path	Path Coefficients	Effect Size (Cohen's f^2)	t-Value	p Values	Hypothesis Check
PER -> ACC	−0.455	0.303(medium -large)	22.473	0.000	H1 (Supported)
PEB -> ACC	0.345	0.196(medium)	15.260	0.000	H2 (Supported)
PEB -> PER	−0.390	0.195(medium)	13.463	0.000	H3 (Supported)
STC -> PER	−0.072	0.006(small)	2.147	0.032	H4 (Supported)
STC -> PEB	0.049	0.003(small)	1.303	0.193	H5 (Not supported)
STP -> PEB	0.317	0.073(small–medium)	8.454	0.000	H6 (Supported)
STP -> PER	−0.014	0.001(small)	0.410	0.682	H7 (Not supported)
STP -> STC	0.581	0.513(large)	26.571	0.000	H8 (Supported)
EPT -> PER	−0.364	0.181(medium)	12.917	0.000	H9 (Supported)
EPT -> PEB	0.067	0.006(small)	1.820	0.069	H10 (Supported)

Note: ACC =Public acceptance; PEB = Perceived benefits; PER = Perceived risks; STC = Trust in industrial organizations; STP = Trust in public organizations; EPT = Epistemic trust.

Perceived risks demonstrated a direct and statistically significant negative relationship with ACC ($\beta = -0.455$, $p < 0.001$). Individuals who perceived more risks were less likely to accept GMF, thus supporting Hypothesis 1.

Perceived benefits demonstrated a direct and statistically significant positive relationship with ACC ($\beta = 0.345$, $p < 0.001$). Individuals who perceived more benefits were more likely to acceptance of GMF, thus supporting Hypothesis 2.

As shown in Table 4, perceived risks ($f^2 = 0.303$) exerted a greater influence than perceived benefits ($f^2 = 0.196$) for affecting public acceptance of GMF.

Perceived benefits demonstrated a direct and statistically significant negative relationship with perceived risks ($\beta = -0.390$, $p < 0.001$). Individuals who perceived more benefits were more likely to perceive fewer risks, thus supporting Hypothesis 3.

Higher trust in industrial organizations demonstrated a direct and statistically significant negative relationship with perceived risks (PER) ($\beta = -0.072$, $p < 0.05$). The more people trusted industrial organizations, the fewer their perceived risks, thus supporting Hypothesis 4.

Higher trust in industrial organizations did not demonstrate a direct, statistically significant relationship with perceived benefits, thus Hypothesis 5 was not supported. In this sample, individuals with high trust in an industrial organization were not likely to perceive more benefits.

With regard to Hypothesis 6, Figure 2 shows that the higher trust in public organizations → perceived risks link was not significant, thus failing to confirm that people's trust in public organizations affects their risk perception.

As shown in Figure 2, the positive higher trust in public organizations → perceived benefits link was significant ($\beta = 0.317$, $p < 0.001$), thus supporting Hypotheses 7. Individuals with high trust in public organizations were likely to perceive more benefits.

With regard to Hypothesis 8, Figure 2 shows that the higher trust in public organizations → higher trust in industrial organizations link was significant ($\beta = 0.581$, $p < 0.001$). The more people trust public organizations, the more they will trust industrial organizations.

Figure 2 also shows that the negative epistemic trust → perceived risks link was significant ($\beta = -0.364$, $p < 0.001$) and the positive epistemic trust → perceived benefits link was weakly significant ($\beta = 0.067$, $p = 0.069$), but it was only significant at $p = 0.10$, hence, supporting Hypotheses 9 and 10. Individuals with high trust in the science behind GMF were likely to perceive more benefits and fewer risks.

Trust in public organization ($f^2 = 0.073$) had a stronger influence than epistemic trust ($f^2 = 0.006$) on explaining perceived benefits. The impact of trust in the industrial organization on perceived benefits was small ($f^2 = 0.003$).

The effects of epistemic trust and perceived benefits had an influence on explaining perceived risks that were similar ($f^2 = 0.181$ and 0.195, respectively). Trust in industrial organizations on perceived risks and the impact of higher trust in public organizations were similar ($f^2 = 0.006$ and 0.001, respectively).

In tests of multicollinearity, the variance inflation factor (VIF) values were calculated for all constructs. All VIF values remained well below the acceptable threshold of 5.0 (ranging from 1.000 to 1.707), as shown in Table 6 [113].

Table 6. Variance inflation factors (VIFs) of the constructs.

	ACC	PEB	PER	STC
EPT		1.057	1.062	
PEB	1.271		1.133	
PER	1.433			
STC		1.541	1.543	
STP		1.593	1.707	1.000

Note: ACC = Public acceptance; PEB = Perceived benefits; PER = Perceived risks; STC = Trust in industrial organizations; STP = Trust in public organizations; EPT = Epistemic trust.

5. Discussion

5.1. Theoretical Implications

By integrating social trust [23,24] and epistemic trust [25,28,114] in risk perception research, this study proposes an extended model to explain GMF acceptance. The model specifies the relationship among social trust, epistemic trust, perceived risks, perceived benefits, and GMF acceptance. The model was tested with survey data of China. This study yielded three major findings: First, epistemic trust is an important antecedent to perceived risks and perceived benefits and exerts a significant indirect effect on GMF acceptance. Secondly, higher trust in industrial organizations exerts a negative impact on perceived risks, and higher trust in public organizations exerts a positive impact on perceived benefits. Therefore, higher trust in industrial organizations and higher trust in public organizations utilize different influence paths toward GMF acceptance. Thirdly, in contrast to common opinion, higher trust in industrial organizations did not exert a significant direct effect on perceived benefits, and higher trust in public organizations did not exert a significant direct effect on perceived risks. This study enriches the knowledge on the influence path of trust on the acceptance of emerging technology and has significance for risk management practice.

Consistent with prior research, these findings suggest that perceived risks and perceived benefits are two important factors that influence GMF acceptance. By demonstrating that perceived benefits have a statistically significant, negative relationship with perceived risks, this study supported that risk and benefit perceptions are not independent but rather inversely related [76,77].

More importantly, consistent with Sjöberg [25,28], the findings of the present study illustrate that epistemic trust is an important factor in GMF acceptance by exerting a direct positive effect on perceived benefits and a negative effect on perceived risks. Given that research has identified epistemic trust as an important antecedent to perceived risks and perceived benefits, future research should not omit this construct.

With regard to social trust, these findings also suggest that it is important to distinguish between trust in industrial organizations and trust in public organizations. When both types of trust are treated jointly in the same model, differences were found with respect to the GMF acceptance relationship, depending on the type of trust. Trust in industrial organizations in the domain of GMF exerts a negative impact on perceived risks, and trust in public organizations exerts a positive impact on perceived benefits. In contrast to the hypothesized relationships, higher trust in industrial organizations did not exert a significant direct effect on perceived benefits, and higher trust in public organizations did not exert a significant direct effect on perceived risks. On the one hand, these findings confirm that it is necessary to distinguish between higher trust in industrial organizations and higher trust in public organizations when operationalizing the social trust measurement. Furthermore, it is important to consider both types of trust separately as two different constructs. On the other hand, the results show that the influence paths of both types of trust on the GMF acceptance differ.

These findings are consistent with the results of a number of recent studies. When they distinguished between trust in companies and trust in public institutions, López-Navarro, Llorens-Monzonís, and Tortosa-Edo (2013) showed that trust in companies negatively affected citizens' health risk perception [14]. Moreover, trust in public institutions did not exert a direct and significant effect in the context of a petrochemical industrial complex. However, their study did not include the relationship between both types of trust and perceived benefits; therefore, a complete comparative analysis could not be conducted. Peters, Covello, and McCallum (1997), as well as Maeda and Miyahara (2003), showed that the component (or dimension) of trust in the government (i.e., public organizations) is a form of competency trust, while the component (or dimension) of trust in the industry (i.e., industrial organizations) is a form of goodwill trust [30,85]. In the context of nuclear power plants (NPPs) in China, Xiao, Liu, and Feldman (2017) showed that goodwill trust improves the acceptance of NPPs by decreasing the risk perception of the public [32]; however, competence trust improves the acceptance of NPPs by increasing the benefit perception. The authors showed that the associations between goodwill trust and benefit perception, as well as competence trust and risk perception, were not significant. Considering the results of Peters, Covello, and McCallum (1997) as well as Maeda and Miyahara (2003), the results of the present study are highly consistent with the results of Xiao, Liu, and Feldman (2017) [30,32,85].

Why does higher trust in industrial organizations only affect the perceived risks, while higher trust in public organizations only affects perceived benefits? The literature provides no explanation for this question. The risks of GMF are mainly related to industrial activities; therefore, industrial organizations are the first to bear the responsibility for managing the risks inherent to the industrial activity, which they developed [14]. Therefore, trust in industrial organizations is directly related to reducing the public's perception of the risks associated with GMF. At the same time, according to the loss aversion principle, most people apply asymmetric sensitivity to gains and losses, and the pain in the face of loss is perceived as far stronger than the pleasure in the face of gain [115]. For most people, the primary goal of decision-making is to avoid risks and losses. Only when risks are controlled and when safety is guaranteed, most people further consider the benefits. The duties of public organizations in the domain of GMF are associated with their regulatory activities as well as their functions of authorizing and monitoring relevant industrial activities. The component (or dimension) of trust in public organizations is a form of competency trust. When people have a high level of trust in public organizations, they assume that public organizations have the ability to perform their duties effectively. Under the premise that loss is avoided, the public will pay more attention to the relevant benefits of GMF. Therefore, trust in public organizations exerts a significant positive impact on perceived benefits.

5.2. Policy Implications

These results offer relevant implications for the practitioner. Scientific knowledge contains inherent uncertainty. In this sense, it is rational for the public to criticize and doubt scientific knowledge. However, such criticism and doubt should be based on relevant evidence and facts. In China, most people lack the scientific knowledge to understand transgene technology and biology in general [116]; therefore, it is difficult for them to make a reasonable judgment on the scientific evidence about GMF. It is easy for the lay public to distort the uncertainties of scientific knowledge behind GMF, which further reduces their willingness to accept GMF. To overcome this issue, the government can use a variety of popular science activities to improve the scientific literacy of the public, enhance their epistemic trust, and ultimately improve GMF acceptance.

The results of this study may be useful for industrial organizations in the domain of GMF in relation to their behavior. Industrial organizations ought to be concerned about the level of trust received by the public in response to all items representing higher trust in industrial organizations. All average values of the items were lower than the middle value of the scale (see Table 3). Given this fact, and considering that the component of higher trust in industrial organizations is goodwill trust, industrial organizations should pay more attention to public interests. Moreover, they should improve the transparency of their risk control information to enhance goodwill trust.

The findings for public organizations are of concern: contrary to the case of higher trust in industrial organizations, the average values of all items representing higher trust in public organizations were higher than the middle value of the scale (see Table 3). Although public trust in public organizations exceeds that in industrial organizations, the absolute level of higher trust in public organizations is low, and the average values of all items representing higher trust in public organizations remain below 5 (see Table 3). Therefore, and considering that the component of higher trust in public organizations is competence trust, public organizations need to properly execute their regulatory function with regard to the risk management of GMF. This will further enhance the public's trust in their capabilities and increase the perceived benefits in the public.

Both industrial organizations and public organizations in the domain of GMF should focus their efforts on prompting public trust, reducing perceived risks, and improving benefit perception, which will ultimately improve GMF acceptance. Generating and maintaining trust often constitutes the primary goal of industrial communication policies.

5.3. Limitations

Although the findings of this study provide meaningful implications for both researchers and practitioners, a number of limitations apply. On the one hand, this study used cross-section data on research methods and its acceptance intention took the place of actual acceptance behavior as the explained variable. While the current studies mostly used this method, considering that public acceptance of GMF is a dynamic process, future studies should consider longitudinal dynamic tracking surveys. Moreover, the GMF acceptance of the public should be compared for different periods to better reflect the changing regularity of this acceptance. On the other hand, this study focused on the influence of trust factors on perceived benefits, perceived risks, and public acceptance without considering other factors. Consequently, the explanatory power of a number of the variables remains limited, especially for perceived benefits ($R^2 = 0.073$). Future studies should expand the model by adding further important influencing factors.

Author Contributions: Conceptualization, L.H. and R.L.; methodology, L.H. and T.Z.; software, R.L.; writing—original draft preparation, L.H. and R.L.; writing—review and editing, W.Z.; supervision, L.H. All authors have read and agreed to the published version of the manuscript.

Funding: This research was funded by the National Natural Science Foundation of China (#71804056, #71932004, #71672111), Humanities and Social Sciences Research Project of the Ministry of Education of China (#18YJC630250), China Postdoctoral Science Foundation (2018M642033), and Central China Normal University research funding (#2017980039).

Conflicts of Interest: The authors declare no conflict of interest.

References

1. WHO. Frequently Asked Questions on Genetically Modified Foods. 2014. Available online: https://www.who.int/foodsafety/areas_work/food-technology/faq-geneically-modified-food/en/ (accessed on 11 December 2019).
2. Lusk, J.L.; Rozan, A. Consumer acceptance of ingenic foods. *Biotechnol. J.* **2006**, *1*, 1433–1434. [CrossRef] [PubMed]
3. Lusk, J.L.; Coble, K.H. Risk Perceptions, Risk Preference, and Acceptance of Risky Food. *Am. J. Agric. Econ.* **2005**, *87*, 393–405. [CrossRef]
4. Hudson, J.; Caplanova, A.; Novak, M. Public attitudes to GM foods. The balancing of risks and gains. *Appetite* **2015**, *92*, 303–313. [CrossRef] [PubMed]
5. Edenbrandt, A.K.; Gamborg, C.; Thorsen, B.J. Consumers' Preferences for Bread: Transgenic, Cisgenic, Organic or Pesticide-free? *J. Agric. Econ.* **2018**, *69*, 1–21. [CrossRef]

6. Edenbrandt, A.K. Demand for pesticide-free, cisgenic food? Exploring differences between consumers of organic and conventional food. *Br. Food J.* **2018**, *120*, 1666–1679. [CrossRef]
7. Delwaide, A.-C.; Nalley, L.L.; Dixon, B.L.; Danforth, D.M.; Nayga, R.M.N., Jr.; Van Loo, E.J.; Verbeke, W. Revisiting GMOs: Are There Differences in European Consumers' Acceptance and Valuation for Cisgenically vs Transgenically Bred Rice? *PLoS ONE* **2015**, *10*, e0126060. [CrossRef] [PubMed]
8. Christoph, I.B.; Bruhn, M.; Roosen, J. Knowledge, attitudes towards and acceptability of genetic modification in Germany. *Appetite* **2008**, *51*, 58–68. [CrossRef]
9. Ceccoli, S.; Hixon, W. Explaining attitudes toward genetically modified foods in the European Union. *Int. Political Sci. Rev.* **2012**, *33*, 301–319. [CrossRef]
10. Lusk, J.L.; Roosen, J.; Fox, J.A. Demand for beef from cattle administered growth hormones or fed genetically modified corn: A comparison of consumers in France, Germany, the United Kingdom, and the United States. *Am. J. Agric. Econ.* **2003**, *85*, 16–29. [CrossRef]
11. Xu, R.; Wu, Y.; Luan, J. Consumer-perceived risks of genetically modified food in China. *Appetite* **2020**, *147*, 104520. [CrossRef]
12. Cui, K.; Shoemaker, S.P. Public perception of genetically-modified (GM) food: A Nationwide Chinese Consumer Study. *NPJ Sci. Food* **2018**, *2*, 1–8. [CrossRef] [PubMed]
13. Frewer, L.J.; van der Lans, I.A.; Fischer, A.R.; Reinders, M.J.; Menozzi, D.; Zhang, X.; van den Berg, I.; Zimmermann, K.L. Public perceptions of agri-food applications of genetic modification—A systematic review and meta-analysis. *Trends Food Sci. Technol.* **2013**, *30*, 142–152. [CrossRef]
14. López-Navarro, M.A.; Llorens-Monzonís, J.; Tortosa-Edo, V. The Effect of Social Trust on Citizens' Health Risk Perception in the Context of a Petrochemical Industrial Complex. *Int. J. Environ. Res. Public Health* **2013**, *10*, 399–416. [CrossRef] [PubMed]
15. Rodríguez-Entrena, M.; Salazar-Ordóñez, M. Influence of scientific-technical literacy on consumers' behavioural intentions regarding new food. *Appetite* **2013**, *60*, 193–202. [CrossRef]
16. Frewer, L.J.; Von Bergmann, K.; Brennan, M.; Lion, R.; Meertens, R.M.; Rowe, G.; Siegrist, M.; Vereijken, C.M.J.L. Consumer response to novel agri-food technologies: Implications for predicting consumer acceptance of emerging food technologies. *Trends Food Sci. Technol.* **2011**, *22*, 442–456. [CrossRef]
17. Gupta, N.; Fischer, A.R.; Frewer, L.J. Socio-psychological determinants of public acceptance of technologies: A review. *Public Underst. Sci.* **2012**, *21*, 782–795. [CrossRef]
18. Hakim, M.P.; Zanetta, L.D.; De Oliveira, J.M.; Da Cunha, D.T. The mandatory labeling of genetically modified foods in Brazil: Consumer's knowledge, trust, and risk perception. *Food Res. Int.* **2020**, *132*, 109053. [CrossRef]
19. Nardi, V.A.M.; Teixeira, R.; Ladeira, W.J.; Santini, F.D.O. A meta-analytic review of food safety risk perception. *Food Control* **2020**, *112*, 107089. [CrossRef]
20. Guo, Q.; Yao, N.; Zhu, W. How consumers' perception and information processing affect their acceptance of genetically modified foods in China: A risk communication perspective. *Food Res. Int.* **2020**, *137*, 109518. [CrossRef]
21. Butkowski, O.K.; Baum, C.M.; Pakseresht, A.; Bröring, S.; Lagerkvist, C.J. Examining the social acceptance of genetically modified bioenergy in Germany: Labels, information valence, corporate actors, and consumer decisions. *Energy Res. Soc. Sci.* **2020**, *60*, 101308. [CrossRef]
22. Ardebili, A.T.; Rickertsen, K. Personality traits, knowledge, and consumer acceptance of genetically modified plant and animal products. *Food Qual. Prefer.* **2020**, *80*, 103825. [CrossRef]
23. Siegrist, M. The Influence of Trust and Perceptions of Risks and Benefits on the Acceptance of Gene Technology. *Risk Anal.* **2000**, *20*, 195–203. [CrossRef] [PubMed]
24. Siegrist, M. A Causal Model Explaining the Perception and Acceptance of Gene Technology. *J. Appl. Soc. Psychol.* **1999**, *29*, 2093–2106. [CrossRef]
25. Sjöberg, L. Antagonism, Trust and Perceived Risk. *Risk Manag.* **2008**, *10*, 32–55. [CrossRef]
26. Rousseau, D.M.; Sitkin, S.B.; Burt, R.S.; Camerer, C. Not So Different After All–A Cross-Discipline View of Trust. *Academy Manag. Rev.* **1998**, *23*, 393–404. [CrossRef]
27. Eiser, J.R.; Miles, S.; Frewer, L.J. Trust, Perceived Risk, and Attitudes Toward food technologies. *J. Appl. Soc. Psychol.* **2002**, *32*, 2423–2433. [CrossRef]
28. Sjöberg, L. Limits of Knowledge and the Limited Importance of Trust. *Risk Anal.* **2001**, *21*, 189–198. [CrossRef]
29. Sjöberg, L.; Herber, M.W. Too much trust in (social) trust? The importance of epistemic concerns and perceived antagonism. *Int. J. Glob. Environ. Issues* **2008**, *8*, 30–44. [CrossRef]

30. Peters, R.G.; Covello, V.T.; McCallum, D.B. The Determinants of Trust and Credibility in Environmental Risk Communication: An Empirical Study. *Risk Anal.* **1997**, *17*, 43–54. [CrossRef]
31. Deljoo, A.; Van Engers, T.; Gommans, L.; De Laat, C. The Impact of Competence and Benevolence in a Computational Model of Trust. In *International Federation for Information Processing 2018*; Gal-Oz, N., Lewis, P.R., Eds.; Springer: Berlin/Heidelberg, Germany, 2018; pp. 45–57.
32. Xiao, Q.; Liu, H.; Feldman, M.W. How does trust affect acceptance of a nuclear power plant (NPP): A survey among people living with Qinshan NPP in China. *PLoS ONE* **2017**, *12*, e0187941. [CrossRef] [PubMed]
33. Terwel, B.W.; Harinck, F.; Ellemers, N.; Daamen, D.D.L. Competence-based and integrity-based trust as predictors of acceptance of carbon dioxide capture and storage (CCS). *Risk Anal.* **2009**, *29*, 1129–1140. [CrossRef] [PubMed]
34. Bearth, A.; Siegrist, M. Are risk or benefit perceptions more important for public acceptance of innovative food technologies: A meta-analysis. *Trends Food Sci. Technol.* **2016**, *49*, 14–23. [CrossRef]
35. Adell, E.; Varhelyi, A.; Nilsson, L. The Definition of Acceptance and Acceptability: Theory, measurement and optimisation. In *Driver Acceptance of New Technology*; Reagan, M.A., Horberry, T., Stevens, A., Eds.; CRC Press: Boca Raton, FL, USA, 2014; pp. 11–21.
36. Chen, Y.; Chang, C. Enhance green purchase intentions. *Manag. Decis.* **2012**, *50*, 502–520. [CrossRef]
37. Chen, M.-F. An integrated research framework to understand consumer attitudes and purchase intentions toward genetically modified foods. *Br. Food J.* **2008**, *110*, 559–579. [CrossRef]
38. Huijts, N.M.A.; Molin, E.J.E.; Steg, L. Psychological factors influencing sustainable energy technology acceptance: A review-based comprehensive framework. *Renew. Sustain. Energy Rev.* **2012**, *16*, 525–531. [CrossRef]
39. Connor, M.; Siegrist, M. Factors Influencing People's Acceptance of Gene Technology: The Role of Knowledge, Health Expectations, Naturalness, and Social Trust. *Sci. Commun.* **2010**, *32*, 514–538. [CrossRef]
40. Zhang, Y.; Jing, L.; Bai, Q.; Shao, W.; Feng, Y.; Yin, S.; Zhang, M. Application of an integrated framework to examine Chinese consumers' purchase intention toward genetically modified food. *Food Qual. Prefer.* **2018**, *65*, 118–128. [CrossRef]
41. Hall, C.R. Genetically Modified Food and Crops: Perceptions of Risks. Ph.D. Thesis, The University of Edinburgh, Edinburgh, UK, May 2010.
42. Hu, Z.; Ding, S.; Li, S.; Chen, L.; Yang, S. Adoption Intention of Fintech Services for Bank Users: An Empirical Examination with an Extended Technology Acceptance Model. *Symmetry* **2019**, *11*, 340. [CrossRef]
43. Martins, C.; Oliveira, T.; Popovič, A. Understanding the Internet banking adoption: A unified theory of acceptance and use of technology and perceived risk application. *Int. J. Inf. Manag.* **2014**, *34*, 1–13. [CrossRef]
44. Kamarulzaman, N.A.; Lee, K.E.; Siow, K.S.; Mokhtar, M. Public benefit and risk perceptions of nanotechnology development: Psychological and sociological aspects. *Technol. Soc.* **2020**, *62*, 101329. [CrossRef]
45. Joubert, I.A.; Geppert, M.; Ess, S.; Nestelbacher, R.; Gadermaier, G.; Duschl, A.; Bathke, A.C.; Himly, M. Public perception and knowledge on nanotechnology: A study based on a citizen science approach. *NanoImpact* **2020**, *17*, 100201. [CrossRef]
46. Ho, S.S.; Scheufele, D.A.; Corley, E.A. Factors influencing public risk-benefit considerations of nanotechnology: Assessing the effects of mass media, interpersonal communication, and elaborative processing. *Public Underst. Sci.* **2013**, *22*, 606–623. [CrossRef] [PubMed]
47. Capon, A.; A Gillespie, J.; Rolfe, M.; Smith, W. Perceptions of risk from nanotechnologies and trust in stakeholders: A cross sectional study of public, academic, government and business attitudes. *BMC Public Health* **2015**, *15*, 424–436. [CrossRef]
48. Kim, J.; Yeo, S.K.; Brossard, D.; Scheufele, D.A.; Xenos, M.A. Disentangling the Influence of Value Predispositions and Risk/Benefit Perceptions on Support for Nanotechnology Among the American Public. *Risk Anal.* **2014**, *34*, 965–980. [CrossRef] [PubMed]
49. Siegrist, M.; Keller, C. Labeling of Nanotechnology Consumer Products Can Influence Risk and Benefit Perceptions. *Risk Anal.* **2011**, *31*, 1762–1769. [CrossRef]
50. Yasmin, N.; Grundmann, P. Pre- and Post-Adoption Beliefs about the Diffusion and Continuation of Biogas-Based Cooking Fuel Technology in Pakistan. *Energies* **2019**, *12*, 3184. [CrossRef]
51. Ho, J.-C.; Kao, S.-F.; Wang, J.-D.; Su, C.-T.; Lee, C.-T.P.; Chen, R.-Y.; Chang, H.-L.; Ieong, M.C.F.; Chang, P.W. Risk perception, trust, and factors related to a planned new nuclear power plant in Taiwan after the 2011 Fukushima disaster. *J. Radiol. Prot.* **2013**, *33*, 773–789. [CrossRef]

52. Sjöberg, L.; Drottz-Sjoberg, B.-M. Public risk perception of nuclear waste. *Int. J. Risk Assess. Manag.* **2009**, *11*, 248–280. [CrossRef]
53. Clothier, R.; Greer, D.A.; Greer, D.G.; Mehta, A.M. Risk Perception and The Public Acceptance of Drones. *Risk Anal.* **2015**, *35*, 1167–1183. [CrossRef]
54. Liu, P.; Yang, R.; Xu, Z. Public Acceptance of Fully Automated Driving: Effects of Social Trust and Risk/Benefit Perceptions. *Risk Anal.* **2018**, *39*, 326–341. [CrossRef]
55. Zhang, T.; Tao, D.; Qu, X.; Zhang, X.; Lin, R.; Zhang, W. The roles of initial trust and perceived risk in public's acceptance of automated vehicles. *Transp. Res. Part C Emerg. Technol.* **2019**, *98*, 207–220. [CrossRef]
56. Mitchell, V.-W. Consumer Perceived Risk: Conceptualizations and Models. *Eur. J. Mark.* **1999**, *33*, 163–195. [CrossRef]
57. Renn, O.; Benighaus, C. Perception of technological risk: Insights from research and lessons for risk communication and management. *J. Risk Res.* **2013**, *16*, 293–313. [CrossRef]
58. Slovic, P. Perception of risk. *Science* **1987**, *236*, 280–285. [CrossRef] [PubMed]
59. Puth, G.; Mostert, P.; Ewing, M.T. Consumer perceptions of mentioned product and brand attributes in magazine advertising. *J. Prod. Brand Manag.* **1999**, *8*, 38–50. [CrossRef]
60. Kotler, P. *Marketing Management: Analysis, Planning, Implementation, and Control*, 9th ed.; Prentice Hall: Upper Saddle River, NJ, USA, 1999.
61. Margulis, C. The Hazards of Genetically Engineered Foods. *Environ. Health Perspect.* **2006**, *114*, A146–A147. [CrossRef]
62. Séralini, G.-E.; Cellier, D.; De Vendômois, J.S. New Analysis of a Rat Feeding Study with a Genetically Modified Maize Reveals Signs of Hepatorenal Toxicity. *Arch. Environ. Contam. Toxicol.* **2007**, *52*, 596–602. [CrossRef]
63. Zawide, F.; Birke, W. Emerging Risks of Genetically Modified Foods. *EC Nutr.* **2017**, *8*, 233–236. [CrossRef]
64. Amin, L.; Hamdan, F.; Hashim, R.; Samani, M.C.; Anuar, N.; Zainol, Z.A.; Jusoff, K. Risks and benefits of genetically modified foods. *Afr. J. Biotechnol.* **2011**, *10*, 12481–12485.
65. Knight, J.G.; Gao, H. Chinese gatekeeper perceptions of genetically modified food. *Br. Food J.* **2009**, *111*, 56–69. [CrossRef]
66. Blackwell, R.F.; Miniard, P.W.; Engel, J.F. *Consumer Behavior*, 9th ed.; Harcourt Collage Publishers: New York, NY, USA, 2001.
67. Dowling, G.R.; Staelin, R. A Model of Perceived Risk and Intended Risk-handling Activity. *J. Consum. Res.* **1994**, *21*, 119–134. [CrossRef]
68. Sajiwani, J.W.A.; Rathnayaka, R.M.U.S.K. Consumer Perception on Genetically Modified Food in Sri Lanka. *Adv. Res.* **2014**, *2*, 846–855. [CrossRef]
69. Lü, L.; Chen, H. Chinese Publics Risk Perceptions of Genetically Modified Food: From the 1990s to 2015. *Sci. Technol. Soc.* **2016**, *21*, 110–128. [CrossRef]
70. Animashaun, J.O. *Consumers' Evaluation of Genetically Modified (GM) Food: A Meta-Review and Implications for Policy Regulation in Africa*; African Association of Agricultural Economists (AAAE): Nairobi, Kenya, 2019.
71. Marques, M.D.; Critchley, C.R.; Walshe, J. Attitudes to genetically modified food over time: How trust in organizations and the media cycle predict support. *Public Underst. Sci.* **2015**, *24*, 601–618. [CrossRef] [PubMed]
72. Buah, J.N. Public Perception of Genetically Modified Food in Ghana. *Am. J. Food Technol.* **2011**, *6*, 541–554. [CrossRef]
73. Augoustinos, M.; Crabb, S.; Shepherd, R. Genetically modified food in the news: Media representations of the GM debate in the UK. *Public Underst. Sci.* **2010**, *19*, 98–114. [CrossRef]
74. Prati, G.; Pietrantoni, L.; Zani, B. The prediction of intention to consume genetically modified food: Test of an integrated psychosocial model. *Food Qual. Prefer.* **2012**, *25*, 163–170. [CrossRef]
75. Pham, N.; Mandel, N. What Influences Consumer Evaluation of Genetically Modified Foods? *J. Public Policy Mark.* **2019**, *38*, 263–279. [CrossRef]
76. AlHakami, A.S.; Slovic, P. A psychological study of the inverse relationship between perceived risk and perceived benefit. *Risk Anal.* **1994**, *14*, 1085–1096. [CrossRef]
77. Finucane, M.L.; Alhakami, A.; Slovic, P.; Johnson, S.M. The Affect Heuristic in Judgments of Risks and Benefits. *J. Behav. Decis. Mak.* **2000**, *13*, 1–17. [CrossRef]
78. Huang, J.; Qiu, H.; Bai, J.; Pray, C. Awareness, acceptance of and willingness to buy genetically modified foods in Urban China. *Appetite* **2006**, *46*, 144–151. [CrossRef]

79. Eiser, J.R.; Donovan, A.; Sparks, R.S.J. Risk Perceptions and Trust Following the 2010 and 2011 Icelandic Volcanic Ash Crises. *Risk Anal.* **2015**, *35*, 332–343. [CrossRef] [PubMed]
80. Zhu, X.; Xie, X. Effects of Knowledge on Attitude Formation and Change toward Genetically Modified Foods. *Risk Anal.* **2015**, *35*, 790–810. [CrossRef] [PubMed]
81. Klerck, D.; Sweeney, J.C. The effect of knowledge types on consumer-perceived risk and adoption of genetically modified foods. *Psychol. Mark.* **2007**, *24*, 171–193. [CrossRef]
82. Visschers, V.H.M.; Siegrist, M. Differences in Risk Perception between Hazards and Between Individuals. In *Psychological Perspectives on Risk and Risk Analysis: Theory, Models, and Applications*; Raue, M., Lerme, E., Streicher, B., Eds.; Springer: Berlin/Heidelberg, Germany, 2018; pp. 63–80.
83. Frewer, L.J.; Scholderer, J.; Bredahl, L. Communicating about the Risks and Benefits of Genetically Modified Foods: The Mediating Role of Trust. *Risk Anal.* **2003**, *23*, 1117–1133. [CrossRef]
84. Chen, M.F. Consumer trust in food safety–a multidisciplinary approach and empirical evidence from Taiwan. *Risk Anal.* **2008**, *28*, 1553–1569. [CrossRef]
85. Maeda, Y.; Miyahara, M. Determinants of Trust in Industry, Government, and Citizen's Groups in Japan. *Risk Anal.* **2003**, *23*, 303–310. [CrossRef] [PubMed]
86. Lang, J.T.; Hallman, W.K. Who does the public trust? The case of genetically modified food in the United States. *Risk Anal.* **2005**, *25*, 1241–1252. [CrossRef]
87. Drottz-Sjöberg, B.M. *Stämningar i Storuman efter Folkomröstningen om ett Djupförvar [Sentiments in Storuman after the Referendum on a Deep Level Repository]*; SKB: Stockholm, Sweden, 1996.
88. Sjöberg, L. Risk Perception by the Public and by Experts: A Dilemma in Risk Management. *Res. Hum. Ecol.* **1999**, *6*, 1–9.
89. Sjöberg, L. Attitudes toward technology and risk: Going beyond what is immediately given. *Policy Sci.* **2002**, *35*, 379–400. [CrossRef]
90. Sjöberg, L. Policy Implications of Risk Perception Research: A Case of the Emperor's New Clothes? *Risk Manag.* **2002**, *4*, 11–20. [CrossRef]
91. Drottz-Sjöberg, B.-M. Perceptions of Nuclear Wastes across Extreme Time Perspectives. *Risk Hazards Crisis Public Policy* **2010**, *1*, 231–253. [CrossRef]
92. Sjöberg, L.; Drottz-Sjöberg, B.-M. Attitudes toward nuclear waste and siting policy:expert and the public. In *Nuclear Waste Research: Siting, Technology and Treatment*; Lattefer, A.P., Ed.; Nova Science Publishers, Inc.: Hauppauge, NY, USA, 2008; p. 28.
93. Sjoberg, L.; Engelberg, E. Risk perception and movies: A study of availability as a factor in risk perception. *Risk Anal.* **2010**, *30*, 95–106. [CrossRef]
94. Sjöberg, L. Genetically Modified Food in The Eyes of the Public and Experts. *Risk Manag.* **2008**, *10*, 168–193. [CrossRef]
95. Sjöberg, L. As Time Goes By: The Beginnings of Social and Behavioural Science Risk Research. *J. Risk Res.* **2006**, *9*, 601–604. [CrossRef]
96. Sjöberg, L. *Gene Technology in the Eyes of the Public and Experts: Moral Opinions, Attitudes and Risk Perception*; SSE/EFI Working Paper Series in Business Administration; Stockholm School of Economics: Stockholm, Sweden, May 2005.
97. Zhang, W. Study on the Consumption Behavior for Genetically Modified Food. Ph.D. Thesis, Northwest A & F University, Xian, China, May 2017.
98. Ghoochani, O.M.; Ghanian, M.; Baradaran, M.; Alimirzaei, E.; Azadi, H. Behavioral intentions toward genetically modified crops in Southwest Iran: A multi-stakeholder analysis. *Environ. Dev. Sustain.* **2016**, *20*, 233–253. [CrossRef]
99. Zhang, W.; Xue, J.; Folmer, H.; Hussain, K. Perceived Risk of Genetically Modified Foods among Residents in Xi'an, China: A Structural Equation Modeling Approach. *Int. J. Environ. Res. Public Health* **2019**, *16*, 574. [CrossRef]
100. Chen, M.-F.; Li, H.-L. The consumer's attitude toward genetically modified foods in Taiwan. *Food Qual. Prefer.* **2007**, *18*, 662–674. [CrossRef]
101. Chin, W.; Marcolin, B.; Newsted, P. A partial least squares latent variable modeling app roach for measuring interaction effects: Results from a Monte Carlo simulation study and voice mail emotion/adoption study. In Proceedings of the 15th International Conference on Information Systems, Cleveland, OH, USA, 16–18 December 1996; pp. 21–41.

102. Ringle, C.M.; Wende, S.; Becker, J.-M. "SmartPLS 3.". Boenningstedt: SmartPLS GmbH. 2015. Available online: http://www.smartpls.com (accessed on 11 March 2016).
103. Chin, W.W. The partial least squares approach for structural equation modeling. In *Modern Methods for Business Research*; Marcoulides, G.A., Ed.; Lawrence Erlbaum Associates: Mahwah, NJ, USA, 1998; pp. 295–336.
104. Hair, J.F., Jr.; Hult, G.T.M.; Ringle, C.; Sarstedt, M. *A Primer on Partial Least Squares StructuralEquation Modeling (PLS-SEM)*, 2nd ed.; SAGE Publications, Inc.: Thousand Oaks, CA, USA, 2017.
105. Henseler, J.; Ringle, C.M.; Sarstedt, M. A new criterion for assessing discriminant validity in variance-based structural equation modeling. *J. Acad. Mark. Sci.* **2015**, *43*, 115–135. [CrossRef]
106. Cohen, J. *Statistical Power Analysis for the Behavioral Sciences*; Lawrence Erlbaum: Mahwah, NJ, USA, 1988.
107. Podsakoff, P.M.; MacKenzie, S.B.; Lee, J.Y.; Podsakoff, N.P. Common Method Biases in Behavioral Research: A Critical Review of the Literature and Recommended Remedies. *J. Appl. Psychol.* **2003**, *88*, 879–903. [CrossRef]
108. Harman, H.H. *Modern Factor Analysis*; University of Chicago Press: Chicago, IL, USA, 1976.
109. Liang, H.; Saraf, N.; Hu, Q.; Xue, Y. Assimilation of Enterprise Systems: The Effect of Institutional Pressures and the Mediating Role of Top Management. *MIS Q.* **2007**, *31*, 59–87. [CrossRef]
110. Tenenhaus, M.; Vinzi, V.E.; Chatelin, Y.-M.; Lauro, C. PLS path modeling. *Comput. Stat. Data Anal* **2005**, *48*, 159–205. [CrossRef]
111. Hu, L.; Bentler, P.M. Cutoff criteria for fit indexes in covariance structure analysis: Conventional criteria versus new alternatives. *Struct. Equ. Model. A Multidiscip. J.* **1999**, *6*, 1–55. [CrossRef]
112. Barclay, D.; Thompson, R.; Higgins, C. The Partial Least Squares (PLS) Approach to Causal Modeling: Personal Computer Adoption and Use as an Illustration. *Technol. Stud.* **1995**, *2*, 285–309.
113. Neter, J.; Wasserman, W.; Kutner, M.H. *Applied Linear Statistical Models*; Irwin Inc.: Boston, MA, USA, 1990.
114. Siegrist, M.; Gutscher, H.; Earle, T.C. Perception of risk: The influence of general trust, and general confidence. *J. Risk Res.* **2006**, *8*, 145–156. [CrossRef]
115. Thaler, R.H.; Tversky, A.; Kahneman, D.; Schwartz, A. The Effect of Myopia and Loss Aversion on Risk Taking: An Experimental Test. *Q. J. Econ.* **1997**, *112*, 647–661. [CrossRef]
116. Zhang, X.M. GM Food: A Study of Chinese Public's Recognition and Attitude. *J. Anhui Agric. Sci.* **2014**, *42*, 6783–6786.

Publisher's Note: MDPI stays neutral with regard to jurisdictional claims in published maps and institutional affiliations.

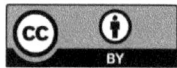

© 2020 by the authors. Licensee MDPI, Basel, Switzerland. This article is an open access article distributed under the terms and conditions of the Creative Commons Attribution (CC BY) license (http://creativecommons.org/licenses/by/4.0/).

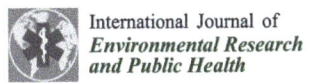

Article

Effects of a Community-Based Pilot Intervention on Home Food Availability among U.S. Households

Rachel A. Cassinat [1], Meg Bruening [1], Noe C. Crespo [2], Mónica Gutiérrez [1], Adrian Chavez [1], Frank Ray [3] and Sonia Vega-López [1,4,*]

1. College of Health Solutions, Arizona State University, 550 North 3rd Street, Phoenix, AZ 85004, USA; rachel.cassinat@gmail.com (R.A.C.); meg.bruening@asu.edu (M.B.); moni.gutierrez@asu.edu (M.G.); drachavez31@gmail.com (A.C.)
2. School of Public Health, San Diego State University, 9245 Sky Park Ct. Suite 224, San Diego, CA 92123, USA; ncrespo@sdsu.edu
3. City of Phoenix, Parks and Recreation Department, 212 E. Alta Vista Rd., Phoenix, AZ 85402, USA; frank.ray@phoenix.gov
4. Southwest Interdisciplinary Research Center, Arizona State University, 201 N. Central Ave, Room 3346, Phoenix, AZ 85004, USA
* Correspondence: sonia.vega.lopez@asu.edu; Tel.: +1-60-2496-3350

Received: 3 October 2020; Accepted: 9 November 2020; Published: 11 November 2020

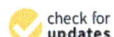

Abstract: The purpose of this study was to assess the effects of a pilot community-based behavioral intervention on the home food environment in U.S. households. Parents (21 females, 2 males; age = 36 ± 5.5 years; 78% Hispanic) of elementary school-aged children attended a 10-week dietary improvement behavioral intervention targeting an increase in fruit and vegetable consumption and a reduction in sugar intake. Home food availability of fruit, vegetables, and sugar-laden foods and beverages were assessed before and after the intervention using a modified version of the Home Food Inventory. Relative to baseline, the intervention resulted in significant increases in fruit availability (7.7 ± 3.2 items vs. 9.4 ± 3.1 items; $p = 0.004$) and low sugar cereal (2.3 ± 1.4 types vs. 2.7 ± 1.4 types; $p = 0.033$). There was a significant reduction in sugar-sweetened beverage availability (3.2 ± 1.9 types vs. 1.7 ± 1.3 types; $p = 0.004$). There was a significant increase in the number of households with accessible ready-to-eat vegetables and fruit, and a significant reduction in available prepared desserts, and candy ($p < 0.01$). There were no significant changes in the availability of vegetables and sugar-laden cereals. The current intervention resulted in positive changes in the home food environment. Further research to confirm these results in a randomized controlled trial is warranted.

Keywords: community-based intervention; diet; home food availability; home food environment; sugar sweetened beverages; fruit and vegetable intake

1. Introduction

Poor dietary quality, roughly described as low adherence to dietary recommendations [1], plays a role in the development of obesity and chronic diseases [2,3]. While fresh fruit and vegetables aid in the prevention of cardiometabolic diseases [2], sugar intake can trigger weight gain and may play a catalytic role in obesity and chronic disease development [3]. Individuals from ethnically-diverse communities, susceptible to disparities in chronic diseases, often have limited access to fresh fruit and vegetables, and have a greater consumption of sugar-laden foods [3,4].

Hispanics are the largest and fastest growing ethnic minority group in the U.S. [5,6]. Hispanics are a population of concern because of their greater prevalence of chronic disease risk factors such as abdominal obesity, dyslipidemias, and insulin resistance, relative to non-Hispanic Whites and

Blacks [7–14]. It has also been reported that Hispanics have a lower overall dietary quality than non-Hispanic Whites [15], further contributing to chronic disease risk. Poor dietary quality is of particular concern among Hispanic youth, as it has been documented that fewer than 10% of Mexican American youths adhere to dietary recommendations regarding fruit and vegetables, fish, whole grains, or sodium intake, and fewer than 35% adhere to sugar-sweetened beverage recommendations [16]. When considering these five components combined, 79–85% of Mexican Americans 5 to 19 years of age had a poor diet score [16]. Given the importance of nutrition for chronic disease prevention, more research is needed to promote healthier dietary intake among this vulnerable population.

Evidence suggests that interventions which target parents and focus on behavioral change from a family context can improve the parents' behavior while also improving the behavior of the children in the family, particularly prior to adolescence when parents are still the primary influence on dietary behavior [17–19]. This approach has been shown to have positive effects on parent cardiovascular risk factors, parent weight, child weight, and parent- and child-reported eating behaviors [20–25]. Conceptually, this approach relies on helping the parents to develop skills related to eating and parenting while encouraging them to model these behaviors, promote healthy behavioral choices in their children and reinforce them, and make changes in the home food environment (HFE) [26]. This intervention approach has the potential to simultaneously affect change at the personal (individual), interpersonal (family) and environmental (home) levels. Currently, there is a lack of evidence to support the use of this model in underserved populations for whom need for behavior change may be greatest [20].

The HFE is a multifactorial concept that comprises the dietary choices available and accessible within a household, as well as the choices around mealtimes that may influence food intake by family members (e.g., media exposure, how meals are served) [27]. The HFE has been suggested as the most influential environmental factor on a child's dietary intake [28]. Particularly related to dietary choices, two relevant HFE dimensions are home food availability (i.e., the presence or absence of specific foods in the home) and food accessibility (i.e., whether foods are visible and readily obtainable, and therefore more likely to be consumed) [29]. Although it has been suggested that the HFE has a localized and direct impact on food choice and diet quality [30–32], the focus of dietary interventions on environmental influences on dietary quality at the family or household level has been limited [26,33]. Behavioral interventions that target the HFE have resulted in significant decreases in energy-dense foods and beverages, and an increase in the amount of fruit and vegetables in the home [34,35]. However, those focusing on ethnically-diverse populations are scarce, and have mainly focused on African-Americans [35]. Therefore, there is a need to assess whether interventions aimed at influencing the HFE are also beneficial in primarily Hispanic populations.

Several HFE measurement tools [29,36–38], including a version adapted for low-income Spanish and Somali-speaking households [39], have been validated. However, existing literature involving assessment of the HFE has mostly relied on self-reported data. Studies in which HFE assessment takes place using open inventories (i.e., home visits where home food information is recorded by research staff rather than relying on self-reported data), are scarce [40]. Moreover, open inventories have not been used to assess the efficacy of a behavior change intervention. Therefore, this quasi-experimental pilot study used open inventories to assess the effects of a community-based dietary behavior change intervention delivered to parents of school-aged children on their HFE. Such an assessment is important as it allows for an objective evaluation of whether a behavioral intervention can influence household-level factors that directly influence dietary intake.

2. Materials and Methods

2.1. Participants

One adult parent (≥18 years) and one 6–11-year-old child from the same household were enrolled in a 10-week quasi-experimental dietary behavior change pilot intervention delivered concurrently at an inner-city elementary school and a community center in Phoenix, AZ. The study team did not have a say as to which parent within a household enrolled in the study. Parent participation depended on willingness and availability to take part of the intervention sessions. Enrolled parents participated in the behavioral intervention described below, while their children took part in concurrent physical activity sessions that did not include information about the HFE. For the purposes of the current analysis, we only included data from the parent participants given that they were the ones consenting to the home data collection procedures to assess the HFE (see below).

Participants were recruited through the use of flyers distributed at both locations, referrals from prior participants, and word of mouth. Exclusion criteria (for both, parents or children) were: (a) medical conditions requiring a specialized diet (e.g., food allergy, phenylketonuria); (b) participation in a separate diet modification program; (c) fruit and vegetable intake ≥5 servings/day; (d) inability to attend sessions; and (e) pregnancy. The questions used in the screening process to verify participant eligibility are available in Supplementary Material 1. Although the original intent was to exclusively enroll Hispanic families, all interested families were admitted to the study regardless of ethnicity, per request of our community partners where the intervention was delivered. Nevertheless, both locations were located in an area with a large Hispanic population (63%) [41], and most enrolled participants were Hispanic (see results). Sessions at the community center were conducted in Spanish to accommodate the high percentage of Hispanic participants; sessions at the school were delivered in English. For the current report, parent participants had to consent to a home visit for assessment of the HFE. Out of 34 participating families, 27 consented for baseline home visits (19 attending the program at the community center and 8 attending at the elementary school), and 23 completed post-intervention follow-up visits and were included in the present analysis. All participants provided written informed consent both for program participation and the home visits. This study was approved by the Institutional Review Board at Arizona State University (IRB#STUDY00000427 and IRB # STUDY00000267).

2.2. Intervention

The 10-week group-based program was delivered once weekly at the inner-city school (90 min/session) and twice weekly at the community center (45 min/session) and included a variety of behavioral modification techniques demonstrated to promote dietary behavior change, particularly targeting an increase in fruit and vegetable consumption and a reduction in sugar intake. A variety of behavioral modification techniques grounded in principles from social-cognitive theory [42] and operant conditioning [43] were used, with particular emphasis on goal-setting, generating social support, skill practice, and habitual self-monitoring [44]. These techniques were combined with nutrition education focused on maintaining a healthy diet and keeping healthy foods in the home. The curriculum had a module specifically dedicated to discussing improvements in the HFE which reviewed home food availability and the selection of healthier options at the store. Moreover, the intervention emphasized HFE improvements as part of the behavioral strategies promoted throughout multiple sessions. The curriculum content and corresponding activities were consistent at both study sites. Table 1 includes a list of the intervention topics and a brief description of their content. The main diet improvement targets were increasing the availability and intake of fruit and vegetables and reducing the availability and intake of sugar-containing foods and beverages. No interventions took place in the homes of participants during HFE data collection.

Table 1. Outline of Intervention Topics.

Module	Topic(s)	Content
1	Introduction/Chronic disease risk reduction	Description of the program. Discussion about common chronic diseases related to lifestyle.
2	Overview of a healthy diet/Meal planning	Introduction of basic nutrition concepts related to dietary guidance. Recommendations for the preparation of a weekly meal plan and grocery list as a way to incorporate dietary guidance in the family meals and increase fruit/vegetable availability in the home.
3	Fats and sugars/Reading food labels	Discussion about the role of dietary fat and sugar in chronic disease risk. Review of the key items on the nutrition facts panel and examples of how to use them for making food choices.
4	Recipe modification/Portion control	Discussion of ways to modify recipes to reduce sugar and fat content and increase fruit/vegetable consumption. Review of standard portion sizes for commonly consumed foods.
5	Benefits of physical activity/Healthy foods on a budget	Discussion of the importance of physical activity as a way to reduce chronic disease risk. Discussion of strategies to purchase less expensive foods without compromising dietary quality.
6	Healthy home food environment/Smart shopping	Discussion of the importance of the home environment for making smart diet choices and for providing healthy foods for the family, and the benefits of having healthy options as the more easily accessible foods for children. Strategies for improving the home food environment by selecting healthier food options when shopping.
7	Involving the family/Family mealtime	Discussion of the importance of involving children and other family members in healthy food selection and preparation. Discussion of the importance of having meals as a family.
8	Why we eat: hunger vs. nourishment	Discussion of the difference between high-calorie and high-nutrient foods.
9	Physical activity and sedentary behaviors	Discussion of the role of physical activity and sedentary behaviors on health.
10	Final review and graduation	Question and answer session. Potluck to celebrate the end of the program.

2.3. Measures

Data were collected in the households of participating families at baseline (after screening and consenting but before the start of intervention sessions) and within four weeks after completion of the intervention. Parent participants completed a survey to gather information on gender, age, income, number of people living in the household, employment status, education level, ethnicity, and if a household received any public food assistance (i.e., Women, Infants & Children [WIC], Supplemental Nutrition Assistance Program [SNAP]). HFE was assessed by trained research assistants using a modified version of the Home Food Inventory [29]. This tool captures the presence or absence of specific foods found in the main storage areas (i.e., home food availability), and whether foods are visible and readily obtainable on kitchen surfaces or without moving other items around in the refrigerator (i.e., kitchen and refrigerator accessibility, respectively). The inventory was modified by only including food categories within the main study outcomes of interest (fruits, vegetables, sugar-laden foods and beverages, and sugar-free beverages), and was culturally adapted to include foods commonly consumed by Hispanic individuals (e.g., pan dulce, aguas frescas). A section devoted to inventorying dry breakfast cereal was added. Dry cereal was categorized based on 2014 Arizona WIC guidelines as WIC-approved (low-sugar; no more than 6 grams of sugar per 1-ounce serving) or as sugar-laden (more than 6 grams of sugar per 1-ounce serving), regardless of fiber content [45]. Table 2 displays a list of the food items included in the modified inventory and used for the present analysis. The full instrument used for this study is available in Supplementary Material 2.

Table 2. Food items included in the modified Home Food Inventory.

Food Category	Items Included
Fruits and Vegetables	
Fruits	Apples, apple sauce, apricots, avocado, bananas, blueberries, cranberries, dates, grapes, grapefruit, kiwi, lemons or limes, mango, melon, mixed fruit/fruit cocktail, nectarines, oranges, pears, peaches, pineapple, plums, prunes, raisins, raspberries, strawberries, tangerines/clementines
Vegetables	Asparagus, beets, bell peppers, broccoli, cabbage, cauliflower, carrots, celery, corn, cucumbers, green beans, lettuce, mushrooms, peas, potatoes, spinach/other greens, squash
Sugar-containing products	
Beverages	Soda, prepared iced teas and lemonades, sports drinks, fruit drinks, flavored milks, aguas frescas, energy drinks, 100% fruit juice
Prepared desserts	Cookies, cakes/cupcakes, muffins, brownies, other snack cakes, pastries/sweet rolls/donuts, flan, pan dulce, ice cream, pudding/jello
Candy	Chocolate, hard candy, gummy candy varieties, fruit rollups/fruit snacks or other fruit-based candy, chewy candy
Dry breakfast cereal	WIC-approved low sugar, sugar-laden breakfast cereal
Sugar-free alternatives	
Beverages	Diet soda, diet iced tea, water

2.4. Analysis

Statistical analyses were conducted using IBM SPSS Statistics, version 21.0 (SPSS Inc., Chicago, IL, USA). All continuous variables are presented in text and tables as mean ± standard deviation (Mean ± SD) or frequency where appropriate. Data were summarized using descriptive statistics to capture the baseline characteristics of participants. Food availability values reported indicate the number (count) of different items present in a household at baseline or follow-up, and the difference between the two time points. Kitchen or refrigerator accessibility data represent the number of households that had each item being accessible (i.e., readily obtainable without moving other food items) at baseline or follow-up. Changes in home food availability were compared using a paired samples *t*-test for normally distributed variables (fruits and vegetables) or a Wilcoxon Signed Rank test for all other variables which were not normally distributed and/or could not be transformed (sugar-sweetened beverages, prepared desserts, candy, sugar-laden cereal, and high fiber/low sugar cereal). Vegetables were analyzed separately to include and exclude potatoes. Sugar-containing beverages, diet-beverages, and water were counted separately. Changes in kitchen and refrigerator accessibility are reported as the number of households that had those items readily obtainable, and were compared using a McNemar Test using the Quick Calcs calculator [46].

3. Results

3.1. Participant Sociodemographic Characteristics and Program Attendance

The mean age was 36.0 ± 5.5 years with an average household size of 2.4 ± 1.0 adults and 2.7 ± 1.1 children. The majority of participants were female ($n = 21$; 91%) and identified themselves as Hispanic ($n = 18$; 78%). Other participants self-identified as African-American ($n = 1$), Native American ($n = 1$), Caucasian ($n = 2$) and Somali ($n = 1$). Overall, the level of education was high school or lower for 52% of participants; 22% of participants were college graduates. Fewer than half of the participants reported working either full-time (22%) or part-time (17%); 39% of participants reported being homemakers. About 61% of households had an income less than USD 2000/month, and 39% of households reported to be receiving public food assistance. Participants' mean attendance was 7.7 ± 1.2 sessions.

3.2. Changes in Food Availability

Changes in the number of available food items per household from baseline to follow-up are depicted in Table 3. There was a significant increase in the availability of fruit (1.7 items; $p = 0.004$)

but not vegetables ($p = 0.111$), and significant reductions in sugar-sweetened beverages (−1.5 items; $p = 0.004$), available prepared desserts (−1.3 items; $p = 0.005$) and available types of candy (−1.4 items; $p < 0.001$). There were no significant differences in sugar-laden dry cereal availability ($p = 0.090$), but low-sugar cereal significantly increased (0.4 items; $p = 0.033$).

Table 3. Changes in home availability of food items from baseline to post-intervention [1].

Food Group	Baseline	Follow-up	Difference	p Value
		items		
Fruit	7.7 (3.2)	9.4 (3.1)	1.7	**0.004**
Vegetables (excluding potatoes)	8.7 (2.9)	9.5 (2.8)	0.8	0.111
Sugar-sweetened beverages	3.2 (1.9)	1.7 (1.3)	−1.5	**0.004**
Prepared desserts	3.0 (2.0)	1.7 (1.3)	−1.3	**0.005**
Candy	2.0 (1.7)	0.6 (0.7)	−1.4	**<0.001**
Sugar-laden cereal	2.4 (2.1)	1.8 (1.5)	−0.6	0.090
High fiber/low sugar cereal	2.3 (1.4)	2.7 (1.4)	0.4	**0.033**

[1] Values are presented as Mean (SD) and represent the number of items within each category present in the household ($n = 23$). Mean values were compared using a paired samples t-test for normally distributed variables (fruit and vegetables), or a Wilcoxon Signed rank test for all other variables. Emboldened p values indicate statistical significance.

3.3. Changes in Kitchen and Refrigerator Food Accessibility

There were no changes in the number of households with readily accessible fresh fruit or vegetables, dry cereal, regular soda, candy, or prepared desserts within the kitchen (Table 4). At baseline, chocolate and strawberry flavored milk were accessible in seven and three households, respectively; those products were not accessible at follow-up ($p = 0.023$ for chocolate flavored milk; n.s. for strawberry flavored milk). Changes in refrigerator accessibility of beverages included significant increases in 100% fruit juice (+14 households; $p = 0.001$) and bottled/contained water (+13 households; $p < 0.001$), a non-significant reduction in fruit drinks and sports drinks (−7 households; $p = 0.065$), and no changes in regular or diet soda ($p = 0.453$ and $p = 0.480$, respectively). There were significant increases in refrigerator-accessible ready-to-eat fruits (+9 households; $p = 0.022$) and vegetables (+11 households; $p = 0.007$).

Table 4. Changes in kitchen and refrigerator accessibility from baseline to follow-up [1].

Food Item	Pre	Post	Difference	p Value
		households		
Kitchen accessibility				
Fresh fruit	19	22	3	0.250
Fresh vegetables	5	6	1	1.000
Dry cereal	11	8	−3	0.375
Regular soda pop	3	2	−1	1.000
Candy	5	3	−2	0.688
Regular prepared desserts [2]	3	7	4	0.289
Refrigerator accessibility				
Flavored milk (chocolate)	7	0	−7	**0.023**
Flavored milk (strawberry)	3	0	−3	0.248
100% fruit juice	3	17	14	**0.001**
Fruit drinks/sports drinks	13	6	−7	0.065
Regular soda pop	9	6	−3	0.453
Diet soda pop	2	0	−2	0.480
Bottled/contained water	9	22	13	**<0.001**
Fresh ready-to-eat vegetables	8	19	11	**0.007**
Fresh ready-to-eat fruit	8	17	9	**0.022**

[1] Values represent the frequency of households in which each item was accessible in the kitchen or refrigerator ($n = 23$). The frequency of households having an item accessible in the kitchen or refrigerator was compared using a McNemar Test. Emboldened p values indicate statistical significance; [2] Accessible regular prepared desserts included cookies, cakes, cupcakes, and muffins. Emboldened p values indicate statistical significance.

4. Discussion

Given that the HFE is a key influence on food choice and diet quality [30–32], effective intervention strategies to increase the intake of fruits and vegetables among children include those that target potential environmental determinants of intake, such as the availability and accessibility of these items in the household [47]. This is particularly important among Hispanic families, given their lower compliance with dietary guidance [16]. The current pilot study findings pose the possibility for community-based programs to improve diet quality by increasing home availability of fruits and WIC-approved cereal, while decreasing sugar-containing products. The intervention used for the current study emphasized HFE improvements as part of the behavioral strategies promoted throughout the program, particularly focusing on encouraging fruit and vegetable intake and reduced consumption of sugar-containing foods and beverages. Furthermore, the intervention had a session dedicated to discussing HFE improvements, including specific strategies to increase the home availability of fruit and vegetables, and the replacement of sugar-containing foods with more healthy options.

In this study, intervention participation resulted in increased home availability of fruit but not vegetables. Other interventions relying on self-reported data have also documented increased home availability of fruit or vegetables in households with children [26,35,48], with greater changes in fruit availability than vegetable availability [35]. Parents may be more likely to increase availability of fruit, as those tend to be more acceptable among children than vegetables, and do not require additional preparation (e.g., cooking) for consumption. Home environmental triggers may not impact fruit and vegetable consumption in comparable ways. Evidence suggests that placing a fruit bowl on the table may prompt increased fruit intake, while other factors such as culture-specific eating patterns practiced in the home may determine the amount of vegetables consumed at meal times [27]. This represents an opportunity to integrate more activities that focus on food preparation and cooking skills aimed at including more vegetables in meals in future interventions.

Although the current study did not compare dietary intake data to the observed changes in the HFE, previous research suggests that home food availability and accessibility play a role in consumption behaviors, food preferences, dietary quality, and weight status [30,32,48,49]. Homes with more fruits and vegetables available have been described as being overall more motivating and supportive for both adult and child fruit and vegetable intake when compared to homes with low fruit and vegetable availability [26,50]. This suggests the importance of combining parental encouragement for children to eat fruits and vegetables while also providing a home environment to encourage this behavior.

The current intervention resulted in lower home availability of sugar-sweetened beverages, prepared desserts, and candy. Home availability of sugar-containing foods and beverages has been reported to impact sugar intake and health outcomes [48,51]. However, a systematic review of studies assessing correlates or determinants of sugar-sweetened beverage consumption concluded that the evidence associating intake with home availability is equivocal [52]. Nevertheless, some interventions resulting in a lower home availability of sugar-containing foods have also reported reduced sugar intake [53]. Given the disparities in diet quality observed among underrepresented populations [54], strategies that reduce the availability of sugar-laden foods in the household may be good approaches to reduce overall sugar intake and improve diet quality. Replication studies are needed in order to compare results by differences in household racial and ethnic make-up.

Whereas this study is novel and adds to the literature on the HFE, several potential strengths and limitations deserve mention. A major strength of the current study is that it assessed the HFE through open inventories conducted by research staff during home visits instead of self-reported data, to avoid recall and social-desirability biases [40]. However, social desirability bias could not be completely eliminated given that home visits were scheduled, and study participants could have altered or hidden food items and beverages in the home on observation day. Open inventories have not been used to assess the efficacy of a behavior change intervention. Though this study attempted to evaluate a potential causal relationship between the intervention and the HFE through the availability and accessibility of fruits, vegetables, and sugar-sweetened products, the quasi-experimental design of this pilot study prohibits us from drawing causal conclusions. Household characteristics (e.g., household size, physical layout of dining and kitchen areas, cultural practices) may also contribute to availability and consumption behaviors. However, the study was strengthened by precautions to limit additional influence on the HFE of participants, particularly through our efforts to reduce or eliminate social desirability bias by collecting data through open inventories. Research assistants were extensively trained in the use of the Home Food Inventory, but HFE data were not collected in duplicate due to budgetary constraints. The lack of inter-rater reliability data is a methodological limitation of the study. Only study participants who consented to the home visit were included in this analysis, therefore the study sample may not be representative of the general population. Moreover, although the original intent was to exclusively enroll Hispanic families in the study, participation of parents from other ethnic groups limits the generalizability of findings to the overall Hispanic population. Parent participant enrollment was based on their willingness and availability to attend sessions, rather than their involvement in food procurement for the household. Focusing on the caregiver with the primary responsibility on food purchasing and preparation may lead to a greater impact of future interventions. The current analysis did not control for additional factors that may have affected findings, including seasonality, holidays, household socioeconomic status, dietary restrictions from other family members not enrolled in the study, and parental education. Though several culturally-relevant items were added to the home food inventory prior to the start of the intervention, other popular items were not included (e.g., papaya, jicama, radish). The analysis was limited to assessing food availability and accessibility and did not confirm whether observed changes actually resulted in modified food intake. Feasibly data regarding intervention implementation were not collected. Future work should collect feasibility data in order to inform large scale implementation efforts. Finally, the study tool used to assess home food availability was not quantitative (i.e., it captures variety but not amount of food items maintained at home); this is a limitation for many validated inventory tools, including a tool comparably designed to measure household food availability among low-income Mexican families [55].

5. Conclusions

Results suggest that the current intervention resulted in favorable changes in the HFE among a sample of primarily Hispanic participants. Existing health education programs could benefit from focusing on modifying the HFE to promote healthier eating behaviors of families, and health behavior change interventions focused on modifying the HFE could utilize home visits as an additional feasible measure of program efficacy. In addition to focusing on how to improve the HFE, programs should also include strategies for navigating the food environment outside of the home. Future research should explore the relationship between HFE and intake, dietary quality, and weight, incorporate more food preparation activities aimed at including vegetables in family meals, and add strategies for sustaining intervention effects after the intervention is completed.

Supplementary Materials: The following are available online at http://www.mdpi.com/1660-4601/17/22/8327/s1.

Author Contributions: Conceptualization, R.A.C., M.B., N.C.C. and S.V.-L.; methodology, R.A.C., M.B., A.C. and S.V.-L.; formal analysis, R.A.C.; resources, N.C.C., F.R. and S.V.-L.; writing—original draft preparation, R.A.C.; writing—review and editing, R.A.C., M.B. and S.V.-L.; supervision, S.V.-L.; project administration, M.G. and A.C. All authors have read and agreed to the published version of the manuscript.

Funding: This research received no external funding.

Acknowledgments: The authors want to thank study participants for their contributions to this study, and staff members of the South Mountain Community Center for their support in carrying out this project.

Conflicts of Interest: The authors declare no conflict of interest.

References

1. Wirt, A.; Collins, C.E. Diet quality—What is it and does it matter? *Public Health Nutr.* **2009**, *12*, 2473–2492. [CrossRef] [PubMed]

2. Joshipura, K.J.; Hu, F.B.; Manson, J.E.; Stampfer, M.J.; Rimm, E.B.; Speizer, F.E.; Colditz, G.; Ascherio, A.; Rosner, B.; Spiegelman, D.; et al. The effect of fruit and vegetable intake on risk for coronary heart disease. *Ann. Intern. Med.* **2001**, *134*, 1106–1114. [CrossRef] [PubMed]
3. Johnson, R.J.; Segal, M.S.; Sautin, Y.; Nakagawa, T.; Feig, D.I.; Kang, D.H.; Gersch, M.S.; Benner, S.; Sanchez-Lozada, L.G. Potential role of sugar (fructose) in the epidemic of hypertension, obesity and the metabolic syndrome, diabetes, kidney disease, and cardiovascular disease. *Am. J. Clin. Nutr.* **2007**, *86*, 899–906. [PubMed]
4. Hosler, A.S.; Rajulu, D.T.; Fredrick, B.L.; Ronsani, A.E. Assessing retail fruit and vegetable availability in urban and rural underserved communities. *Prev. Chronic Dis.* **2008**, *54*. Available online: http://www.cdc.gov/pcd/issues/2008/oct/07_0169.htm (accessed on 17 April 2017).
5. Population Division—US, Census Bureau. *Table 6. Percent of the Projected Population by Race and Hispanic Origin for the United States: 2010 to 2050 (NP2008-T6)*; Census Bureau: Washington, DC, USA, 2008.
6. Colby, S.L.; Ortman, J.M. *Projections of the Size and Composition of the U.S. Population: 2014 to 2060*; Bureau, Ed.; U.S. Census: Washington, DC, USA, 2014; pp. 25–1143.
7. Kurian, A.; Cardarelli, K. Racial and ethnic differences in cardiovascular disease risk factors: A systematic review. *Ethn. Dis.* **2007**, *17*, 143–152.
8. Centers for Disease Control and Prevention. *National Diabetes Fact Sheet: National Estimates and General Information on Diabetes and Prediabetes in the United States, 2011*; U.S. Department of Health and Human Services, Centers for Disease Control and Prevention: Atlanta, GA, USA, 2011.
9. Pan, L.; Galuska, D.A.; Sherry, B.; Hunter, A.S.; Rutledge, G.E.; Dietz, W.H.; Balluz, L.S. Differences in Prevalence of Obesity among Black, White and Hispanic Adults—United States, 2006–2008. In *Morbidity and Mortality Weekly Reports*; Centers for Disease Control and Prevention, U.S. Department of Health and Human Services: Atlanta, GA, USA, 2009; Volume 58, pp. 740–744.
10. Wang, Y.; Beydoun, M.A. The obesity epidemic in the United States. Gender, age, socioeconomic, racial/ethnic, and geographic characteristics: A systematic review and meta-regression analysis. *Epidemiol. Rev.* **2007**, *29*, 6–28. [CrossRef]
11. Beckles, G.L.; Zhu, J.; Moonesinghe, R. Diabetes—United States, 2004 and 2008. In *MMWR Morbidity and Mortality Weekly Reports*; U.S. Department of Health and Human Services, Centers for Disease Control and Prevention: Atlanta, GA, USA, 2011; Volume 60, pp. 90–93.
12. Daviglus, M.L.; Talavera, G.A.; Avilés-Santa, M.L.; Allison, M.; Cai, J.; Cirqui, M.H.; Gellman, M.; Giachello, A.L.; Gouskova, N.; Kaplan, R.C.; et al. Prevalence of major cardiovascular risk factors and cardiovascular diseases among hispanic/latino individuals of diverse backgrounds in the united states. *JAMA* **2012**, *308*, 1775–1784. [CrossRef]
13. Ford, E.S.; Giles, W.H.; Dietz, W.H. Prevalence of the metabolic syndrome among US adults: Findings from the Third National Health and Nutrition Examination Survey. *JAMA* **2002**, *287*, 356–359. [CrossRef]
14. Ong, K.L.; Cheung, B.M.Y.; Wong, L.Y.F.; Wat, N.M.S.; Tan, K.C.B.; Lam, K.S.L. Prevalence, treatment, and control of diagnosed diabetes in the U.S. National Health and Nutrition Examination Survey 1999–2004. *Ann. Epidemiol.* **2008**, *18*, 222–229. [CrossRef]
15. Gao, S.K.; Beresford, S.A.; Frank, L.L.; Schreiner, P.J.; Burke, G.L.; Fitzpatrick, A.L. Modifications to the Healthy Eating Index and its ability to predict obesity: The Multi-Ethnic Study of Atherosclerosis. *Am. J. Clin. Nutr.* **2008**, *88*, 64–69. [CrossRef]
16. Steinberger, J.; Daniels, S.R.; Hagberg, N.; Isasi, C.R.; Kelly, A.S.; Lloyd-Jones, D.; Pate, R.R.; Pratt, C.; Shay, C.M.; Towbin, J.A.; et al. Cardiovascular Health Promotion in Children: Challenges and Opportunities for 2020 and Beyond: A Scientific Statement From the American Heart Association. *Circulation* **2016**, *134*, e236–e255. [CrossRef] [PubMed]
17. Salvy, S.J.; Elmo, A.; Nitecki, L.A.; Kluczynski, M.A.; Roemmich, J.N. Influence of parents and friends on children's and adolescents' food intake and food selection. *Am. J. Clin. Nutr.* **2011**, *93*, 87–92. [CrossRef] [PubMed]
18. Anzman, S.L.; Rollins, B.Y.; Birch, L.L. Parental influence on children's early eating environments and obesity risk: Implications for prevention. *Int. J. Obes.* **2010**, *34*, 1116–1124. [CrossRef] [PubMed]
19. Gross, S.M.; Pollock, E.D.; Braun, B. Family influence: Key to fruit and vegetable consumption among fourth- and fifth-grade students. *J. Nutr. Educ. Behav.* **2010**, *42*, 235–241. [CrossRef]

20. Artinian, N.T.; Fletcher, G.F.; Mozaffarian, D.; Kris-Etherton, P.; Van Horn, L.; Lichtenstein, A.H.; Kumanyika, S.; Kraus, W.E.; Fleg, J.L.; Redeker, N.S.; et al. Interventions to promote physical activity and dietary lifestyle changes for cardiovascular risk factor reduction in adults: A scientific statement from the American Heart Association. *Circulation* **2010**, *122*, 406–441. [CrossRef]
21. Faith, M.S.; Van Horn, L.; Appel, L.J.; Burke, L.E.; Carson, J.A.; Franch, H.A.; Jakicic, J.M.; Kral, T.V.; Odoms-Young, A.; Wansink, B.; et al. Evaluating parents and adult caregivers as "agents of change" for treating obese children: Evidence for parent behavior change strategies and research gaps: A scientific statement from the American Heart Association. *Circulation* **2012**, *125*, 1186–1207. [CrossRef]
22. Epstein, L.H.; Gordy, C.C.; Raynor, H.A.; Beddome, M.; Kilanowski, C.K.; Paluch, R. Increasing Fruit and Vegetable Intake and Decreasing Fat and Sugar Intake in Families at Risk for Childhood Obesity. *Obesity* **2001**, *9*, 171–178. [CrossRef]
23. Golan, M.; Kaufman, V.; Shahar, D.R. Childhood obesity treatment: Targeting parents exclusively v. parents and children. *Br. J. Nutr.* **2006**, *95*, 1008–1015. [CrossRef]
24. Golan, M.; Crow, S. Targeting Parents Exclusively in the Treatment of Childhood Obesity: Long-Term Results[ast]. *Obesity* **2004**, *12*, 357–361. [CrossRef]
25. West, F.; Sanders, M.R.; Cleghorn, G.J.; Davies, P.S. Randomised clinical trial of a family-based lifestyle intervention for childhood obesity involving parents as the exclusive agents of change. *Behav. Res. Ther.* **2010**, *48*, 1170–1179. [CrossRef]
26. Heim, S.; Bauer, K.W.; Stang, J.; Ireland, M. Can a community-based intervention improve the home food environment? parental perspectives of the influence of the delicious and nutritious garden. *J. Nutr. Educ. Behav.* **2011**, *43*, 130–134. [CrossRef] [PubMed]
27. Kamphuis, C.B.; Giskes, K.; de Bruijn, G.J.; Wendel-Vos, W.; Brug, J.; van Lenthe, F.J. Environmental determinants of fruit and vegetable consumption among adults: A systematic review. *Br. J. Nutr.* **2006**, *96*, 620–635. [PubMed]
28. Birch, L.L.; Fisher, J.O. Development of eating behaviors among children and adolescents. *Pediatrics* **1998**, *101*, 539–549. [PubMed]
29. Fulkerson, J.A.; Nelson, M.C.; Lytle, L.; Moe, S.; Heitzler, C.; Pasch, K.E. The validation of a home food inventory. *Int. J. Behav. Nutr. Phys. Act.* **2008**, *5*, 55. [CrossRef]
30. Ding, D.; Sallis, J.F.; Norman, G.J.; Saelens, B.E.; Harris, S.K.; Kerr, J.; Rosenberg, D.; Durant, N.; Glanz, K. Community food environment, home food environment, and fruit and vegetable intake of children and adolescents. *J. Nutr. Educ. Behav.* **2012**, *44*, 634–638. [CrossRef]
31. Wyse, R.; Campbell, E.; Nathan, N.; Wolfenden, L. Associations between characteristics of the home food environment and fruit and vegetable intake in preschool children: A cross-sectional study. *BMC Public Health* **2011**, *11*, 938. [CrossRef]
32. Couch, S.C.; Glanz, K.; Zhou, C.; Sallis, J.F.; Saelens, B.E. Home food environment in relation to children's diet quality and weight status. *J. Acad. Nutr. Diet.* **2014**, *114*, 1569–1579. [CrossRef]
33. Black, A.P.; D'Onise, K.; McDermott, R.; Vally, H.; O'Dea, K. How effective are family-based and institutional nutrition interventions in improving children's diet and health? A systematic review. *BMC Public Health* **2017**, *17*, 818. [CrossRef]
34. Stark, L.J.; Spear, S.; Boles, R.; Kuhl, E.; Ratcliff, M.; Scharf, C.; Bolling, C.; Rausch, J. A pilot randomized controlled trial of a clinic and home-based behavioral intervention to decrease obesity in preschoolers. *Obesity* **2011**, *19*, 134–141. [CrossRef]
35. Baranowski, T.; Baranowski, J.; Cullen, K.W.; de Moor, C.; Rittenberry, L.; Hebert, D.; Jones, L. 5 a day Achievement Badge for African-American Boy Scouts: Pilot outcome results. *Prev. Med.* **2002**, *34*, 353–363. [CrossRef]
36. Marsh, T.; Cullen, K.W.; Baranowski, T. Validation of a fruit, juice, and vegetable availability questionnaire. *J. Nutr. Educ. Behav.* **2003**, *35*, 93–97. [CrossRef]
37. Miller, P.E.; Mitchell, D.C.; Harala, P.L.; Pettit, J.M.; Smiciklas-Wright, H.; Hartman, T.J. Development and evaluation of a method for calculating the Healthy Eating Index-2005 using the Nutrition Data System for Research. *Public Health Nutr.* **2011**, *14*, 306–313. [CrossRef] [PubMed]
38. Iwaoka, F.; Yoshiike, N.; Date, C.; Shimada, T.; Tanaka, H. A validation study on a method to estimate nutrient intake by family members through a household-based food-weighing survey. *J. Nutr. Sci. Vitam.* **2001**, *47*, 222–227. [CrossRef] [PubMed]

39. Hearst, M.O.; Fulkerson, J.A.; Parke, M.; Martin, L. Validation of a home food inventory among low-income Spanish- and Somali-speaking families. *Public Health Nutr.* **2013**, *16*, 1151–1158. [CrossRef] [PubMed]
40. Bryant, M.; Stevens, J. Measurement of food availability in the home. *Nutr. Rev.* **2006**, *64*, 67–76. [CrossRef]
41. U.S. Census Bureau. *Annual Estimates of the Resident Population by Sex, Age, Race and Hispanic Origin for the United States and States: April 1, 2010 to July 1, 2018*; U.S. Department of Commerce: Suitland, MD, USA, 2018.
42. Bandura, A. *Social Foundations of Thougth and Action: A Social Cognitive Theory*; Prentice-Hall: Englewood Cliffs, NJ, USA, 1986.
43. Skinner, B.F. Operant-Behavior. *Am. Psychol.* **1963**, *18*, 503–515. [CrossRef]
44. Michie, S.; Abraham, C.; Whittington, C.; McAteer, J.; Gupta, S. Effective techniques in healthy eating and physical activity interventions: A meta-regression. *Health Psychol.* **2009**, *28*, 690–701. [CrossRef]
45. Arizona Department of Health Services. Arizona Women, Infants & Children (WIC) Program Food List. Available online: http://azdhs.gov/azwic/food-pack.htm (accessed on 1 October 2013).
46. GraphPad. Quick Calcs McNemar's Test to Analyze a Matched Case-Control Study. Available online: https://www.graphpad.com/quickcalcs/mcNemar1/ (accessed on 6 November 2020).
47. Blanchette, L.; Brug, J. Determinants of fruit and vegetable consumption among 6-12-year-old children and effective interventions to increase consumption. *J. Hum. Nutr. Diet.* **2005**, *18*, 431–443. [CrossRef]
48. Wang, L.; Dalton, W.T.; Schetzina, K.E.; Fulton-Robinson, H.; Holt, N.; Ho, A.L.; Tudiver, F.; Wu, T. Home food environment, dietary intake, and weight among overweight and obese children in Southern Appalachia. *South. Med J.* **2013**, *106*, 550–557. [CrossRef]
49. Cullen, K.W.; Baranowski, T.; Owens, E.; Marsh, T.; Rittenberry, L.; de Moor, C. Availability, accessibility, and preferences for fruit, 100% fruit juice, and vegetables influence children's dietary behavior. *Health Educ. Behav.* **2003**, *30*, 615–626. [CrossRef]
50. Kratt, P.; Reynolds, K.; Shewchuk, R. The role of availability as a moderator of family fruit and vegetable consumption. *Health Educ. Behav.* **2000**, *27*, 471–482. [CrossRef] [PubMed]
51. van Ansem, W.J.; van Lenthe, F.J.; Schrijvers, C.T.; Rodenburg, G.; van de Mheen, D. Socio-economic inequalities in children's snack consumption and sugar-sweetened beverage consumption: The contribution of home environmental factors. *Br. J. Nutr.* **2014**, *112*, 467–476. [CrossRef] [PubMed]
52. Mazarello Paes, V.; Hesketh, K.; O'Malley, C.; Moore, H.; Summerbell, C.; Griffin, S.; van Sluijs, E.M.; Ong, K.K.; Lakshman, R. Determinants of sugar-sweetened beverage consumption in young children: A systematic review. *Obes. Rev.* **2015**, *16*, 903–913. [CrossRef] [PubMed]
53. Ezendam, N.P.; Evans, A.E.; Stigler, M.H.; Brug, J.; Oenema, A. Cognitive and home environmental predictors of change in sugar-sweetened beverage consumption among adolescents. *Br. J. Nutr.* **2010**, *103*, 768–774. [CrossRef] [PubMed]
54. Satia, J.A. Diet-Related Disparities: Understanding the Problem and Accelerating Solutions. *J. Am. Diet. Assoc.* **2009**, *109*, 610–615. [CrossRef]
55. Sharkey, J.R.; Dean, W.R.; St John, J.A.; Huber, J.C., Jr. Using direct observations on multiple occasions to measure household food availability among low-income Mexicano residents in Texas colonias. *BMC Public Health* **2010**, *10*, 445. [CrossRef]

Publisher's Note: MDPI stays neutral with regard to jurisdictional claims in published maps and institutional affiliations.

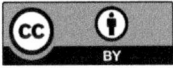

© 2020 by the authors. Licensee MDPI, Basel, Switzerland. This article is an open access article distributed under the terms and conditions of the Creative Commons Attribution (CC BY) license (http://creativecommons.org/licenses/by/4.0/).

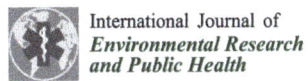

Article

Outcomes of Culturally Tailored Dietary Intervention in the North African and Bangladeshi Diabetic Patients in Italy

Laura Piombo [1,*], Gianluca Nicolella [1], Giulia Barbarossa [1], Claudio Tubili [2], Mayme Mary Pandolfo [2], Miriam Castaldo [1], Gianfranco Costanzo [1], Concetta Mirisola [1] and Andrea Cavani [1]

[1] National Institute for Health, Migration and Poverty (INMP/NIHMP), 00153 Rome, Italy; gianluca.nicolella@inmp.it (G.N.); giulia.barbarossa@inmp.it (G.B.); miriam.castaldo@inmp.it (M.C.); gianfranco.costanzo@inmp.it (G.C.); concetta.mirisola@inmp.it (C.M.); andrea.cavani@inmp.it (A.C.)

[2] Diabetes Unit, San Camillo-Forlanini Hospital, 00152 Rome, Italy; ctubili@scamilloforlanini.rm.it (C.T.); mmpandolfo@gmail.com (M.M.P.)

* Correspondence: laura.piombo@inmp.it

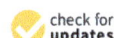

Received: 16 October 2020; Accepted: 29 November 2020; Published: 1 December 2020

Abstract: Immigrants show higher adjusted diabetes prevalence than Italians, especially among South-East Asians followed by North and Sub-Saharan Africans. Diabetes progression is influenced by food behaviors, and diet control is a critical aspect in disease management. Food habits have many cultural and symbolic implications. Guidelines recommend that every patient should receive appropriate self-management education according to cultural and socioeconomic characteristics. This study aims to test whether a customized diet and transcultural mediator's support can improve immigrants' food habits. A pre-post quali-quantitative study was conducted among 20–79-year-old Bangladeshi and North African diabetic immigrants. The INMP transcultural mediator, an expert in the social and health care field, actively participates in clinical activity by decoding linguistic and cultural needs expressed by the foreigner patient. Five culturally tailored dietary profiles were designed according to international diabetes guidelines and adjusted to traditional food habits. Data were collected with two different semi-structured questionnaires. Changes in food consumption were assessed through McNemar's test, while paired Wilcoxon Signed-Rank test was used to analyze pre and post intervention. Fifty-five patients were enrolled. At follow-up, cereals, meat, and potatoes intake significantly improved, and the number of adequate dietary habits for each patient increased significantly. Transcultural mediator support was 90% positively evaluated. Adherence to dietary control is favorably influenced by a transcultural intervention, which is based on clinical and socio-cultural criteria, in compliance with patient's lifestyles.

Keywords: migrants; diabetes; food habits; culturally tailored diet; transcultural mediator

1. Introduction

In 2019, the global international migrant population was around 272 million. International migrants in Europe were about 82 million and in Italy around 6 million, representing 10% of the whole Italian population [1]. The literature indicates a greater self-reported change in diet associated with deterioration in health with increasing length of stay [2]. Low education level, lack of employment, and negative self-perceived economic resources were conditions associated with the risk of hospitalization, longer hospital stay, and greater recourse to urgent hospitalization [3].

The increased migratory phenomenon created new challenges for health systems, which have to adapt to the needs of a multicultural society. World Health Organization (WHO) underlines the necessity of choosing adequate care models respectful of the patient's culture [4]. Migrants appear more subject to communicable diseases (CDs), due to disease patterns in their origin countries, poor living conditions, precarious employment, and traumatic migratory experience [5]. However, non-communicable diseases (NCDs) are increasing among long-term resident migrants [6]. The "healthy migrant effect" tends to disappear over time. Unemployment increases and lower income also makes access to medical care more difficult, particularly among the most fragile population groups, including migrants [7]. Adult male immigrants are at higher risk of experiencing avoidable hospitalization for diabetes than Italians, with differences by area of origin, suggesting that they may experience lower access to and lower quality of primary care for diabetes [8].

Type 2 diabetes is one of the most widespread NCDs. It represents a major health burden worldwide and its incidence is increasing at an alarming rate. In Italy, immigrants show a higher adjusted diabetes prevalence than Italians [9]. Moreover, different prevalence rates exist across ethnic groups, with the highest among South-East Asians followed by North and Sub-Saharan Africans [10,11].

Diabetes progression is influenced by food behaviors, and diet control is one of the most critical aspects of disease management [12–14]. Food habits have many cultural and symbolic implications [15]. Indeed, migrants tend to maintain their traditional food habits, despite their negative impact on health. Food Balance Sheet indicate 2596 kcal/capita/day available in Bangladesh (data from FAOSTAT). The staple foods are rice and tubers and pulses (lentils) and are widely consumed. Intake of vegetables, fruit, meat, and fish is low. In North-African countries, food intake is, on average, 3300 kcal/capita/day. Staple foods are cereals (wheat, rice, corn, or barley) and pulses (chickpeas), and sugar and sweeteners are widely consumed. Intakes of vegetables, fruit (dates), and foods of animal origin is medium. The consumption of pork and alcohol is absent in all countries due to religious prohibitions.

The proposal of non-culturally tailored diets for diabetes control usually fails [16]. Therefore, strict adherence to traditional food, together with different language and religious beliefs, have been identified as an informal barrier to access to healthcare [17–19].

Studies have demonstrated that culturally tailored diabetes educational interventions are effective for improving glycemic control among ethnic minorities [20–23]. It was also observed that the more distant the recommended diet is from the actual habits of the patients, the more difficult it is to promote a good adherence to the nutritional therapy [24]. Guidelines recommend that every diabetic patient should receive appropriate self-management education according to specific cultural, socioeconomic, and literacy characteristics [20,25]. Cultural background influences the ability to adhere to indications for healthy eating habits among ethnic groups [26]. Nevertheless, the role of a customized diet according to immigrant culture in diabetes self-efficacy has not been highlighted in practice. The purpose of this study is to test if a culturally tailored intervention, based on customized diet and transcultural mediator's support, can improve diabetic immigrants' food habits.

2. Materials and Methods

A pre-post quali-quantitative study was conducted at the National Institute for Health, Migration, and Poverty (INMP-Italy) outpatient clinic. The typical target of INMP are Italian and migrant disadvantaged people, refugees, asylum seekers, homeless people, victims of prostitution trade, unaccompanied minors, women with female genital mutilations, and victims of torture. Patients usually are unemployed or have casual and part-time work. Their level of education is medium-low. They often are undocumented, and cannot be registered within the Italian National Health Service. Between January 2017 and April 2018, 20–79-year-old first-generation migrants from Bangladesh, Maghreb (Tunisia, Morocco, Algeria) and Egypt were opportunistically recruited and screened for diabetes. Screening was offered to every adult patient accessing INMP outpatient clinic for an internal medicine examination and coming from the above-mentioned geographical areas. Only diabetic migrants were enrolled after written informed consent. The study was conducted in accordance with the Declaration of Helsinki, and the protocol was approved by the Ethics Committee of Ethics Committee of Istituto Superiore di Sanità (Italian higher institute for Health—PRE 565/16). Exclusion criteria included normoglycemic patients, not neo-diagnosed ones, people regularly followed elsewhere, or who declined to participate to the study.

Two different semi-structured questionnaires were designed by the nutritionist. The baseline questionnaire, with 25 items (7 open), aimed at investigating socio-demographic characteristics, food habits, food choice determinants, barriers in dietary management, and contained a simplified food frequency questionnaire (FFQ) [27,28]. The follow-up questionnaire included the FFQ and additional 16 items (7 open) aimed at analyzing customer satisfaction, adherence to diet and the recommended activity levels. Customer's satisfaction for perceived health conditions and the multidisciplinary care received, adherence to the diet (referred), recommended level of physical activity (referred), and usefulness of transcultural mediation were evaluated using a Likert scale ranging from (1) 'very low' to (5) 'very high'.

Anthropological support was critical for including socio-cultural and migration-focused items. In particular, the anthropologist contributed to design the baseline questionnaire aimed at identifying the salient stages of the migratory path and related main breaking points that may have affected eating habits. The anthropologist's support was also important to contextualize the social environment of the patients and highlight potential barriers to diet adherence (e.g., domestic overcrowding, loss of family ties, social hierarchy and roles, different meanings of the reasons for migration). This information was critical for the nutritionist to conduct an in-depth interview. The questionnaires were previously tested on a number of pre-diabetic patients who helped to circumscribe the list of customized questions, then included in the final questionnaire.

The multidisciplinary team included a nutritionist, a diabetologist, a medical anthropologist, medical dietitians, nurses, and three transcultural mediators (two Bangladeshi and one Arabic). The INMP transcultural mediator is an expert in the social and healthcare field who actively participates in routine clinic activity by decoding linguistic and cultural codes in the relationship between the foreign patient and Italian health professionals. In this project, transcultural mediators were also skilled on diabetes management to best contribute to a culturally oriented care model for foreign diabetic patients. Five culturally tailored dietary profiles were developed by the nutritionist supported by the diabetologist. Each one followed the international diabetes guidelines and was adjusted according to traditional food habits, as reported by the literature [29]. Based on a conventional diet for diabetic patients, profiles were designed according to traditional dishes, typical spices, and cooking techniques, giving preference to food preparations suitable for diabetic patients. In particular, the main cereals chosen for Bangladeshi and Egyptian diet were rice and wheat or derivatives such as *ruti* for Bangladesh or bread for Egypt. The main cereal used for Maghreb countries was wheat or derivatives such as bread, couscous, or pasta. For each profile, alternative menus were provided. Transcultural mediators contributed to creating a more suitable dietary profile suggesting national dishes and food, respectful of religious restrictions. Table 1 shows an extract of 2 out of 5 profiles created (only main meals/not during Ramadan).

A diet plan was prepared by the nutritionist according to the patient's culture of origin as described above. At baseline (T_0), patients were recruited by the diabetologist according to their age and country of origin. Diabetic patients were enrolled and interviewed by the nutritionist. Information collected with baseline questionnaire (pre-questionnaire) allowed to customize each dietary profile according to patients' lifestyle and social determinants of health, such as purchasing power, ease of consumption, and family habits. Together with the culturally tailored dietary, patients also received nutritional counseling using translated iconographic material (seasonal fruit and vegetable calendar). Patients who completed the baseline questionnaire were sent to the San Camillo-Forlanini Hospital Diabetic Center of Rome, where the dietitian finally planned a balanced intake diet. Customized diets were available both in Arabic or Bangladeshi and Italian. The administration of the 6-month-follow-up questionnaire (post- questionnaire) completed the intervention. Transcultural mediators actively participated to each setting. Figure 1 presents the study workflow.

Table 1. Culturally tailored dietary profiles for North African and Bangladeshi diabetic patients: Two main meals extract.

Main Meal	Bangladesh	Egypt
Breakfast	Salty Tea/coffee (sugar free) with *ruti* and boiled *shak* vegetable (no peas or potatoes)	Sweety Light yogurt and sugar free tea with biscuits
Lunch	A meal of parboiled/brown rice and salad as aperitif Rice with *dhal* or Rice with meat/fish curry or Rice with *shobji* and eggs or Rice with *shak*	A meal of parboiled/brown rice *Koshari* and vegetables or *Sayydaiah* and rice with vegetables or *Melokhia* with meat and rice
Dinner	*Ruti* with *shobji* (no potatoes) and light yogurt or Fish *rui/tengra/rupchada* with turmeric and *ruti* or ½ *ruti* with *aloo* or *Ruti* with *dhal*	Couscous with chickpeas/fish/meat and vegetables or Pasta with vegetables/meat/fish sauce and salad

ruti: Flat-bread made with millet flour, barley, wheat (without yeast); *shak*: Broad leafy vegetables (beet, spinach, chicory); *shobji*: Vegetables (zucchini, tomatoes, cauliflower, cabbage, onion, green beans, pepper, pumpkin); *salad*: Salad of lettuce, tomatoes, cucumber, onion with coriander; *dhal*: Lentils (cream); *rui*: River fish (*Labeorohita*); *tengra*: River fish (*Mystustengara*); *rupchada*: Sea fish (*Pampuschinensis*); *aloo*: Potatoes; *koshari*: A rice with pulses dish (lentils or chickpeas); *sayydaiah*: A fish dish; *melokhia*: A spinach soup.

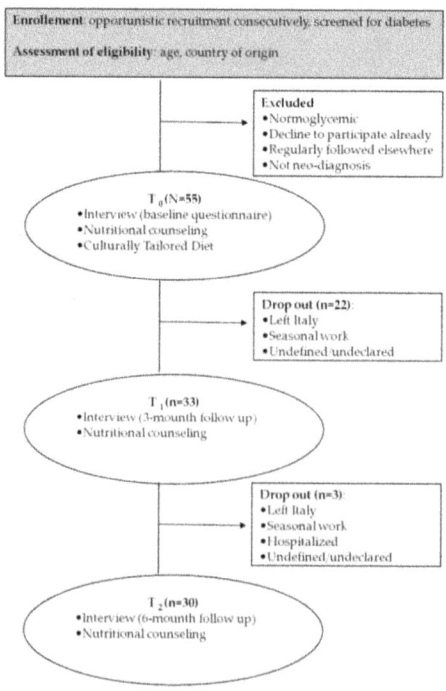

Figure 1. Workflow of the transcultural intervention design.

The questionnaires were administered by the nutritionist supported by the transcultural mediator, at the baseline, and at the follow-up (after 3 and 6 months). Each T_0 interview took about 45–50 min and each T_{1-2} one 30–40 min in a comfortable environment. Information collected with FFQ was used to classify dietary habits.

Level of food consumption was dichotomously categorized ('adequate' or 'non adequate') according to diabetes guidelines [30]. Changes in food consumption were assessed through McNemar's test, while paired Wilcoxon Signed-Rank test was used to analyze pre- and post-intervention differences in food habits of each patient. Only differences with $p < 0.05$ were considered statistically significant.

Statistical analyses were conducted in R software (version 3.5.1; R Foundation for Statistical Computing, Vienna, Austria) [31]. Post-hoc power analysis was done by using G*Power (version 3.1.9.7; Universitat, Kiel, Germany) [32]. The incisiveness of the culturally tailored intervention was assessed using a constant comparative method (CCM).

3. Results

Fifty-five patients were enrolled. Table 2 describes patients' socio-demographic characteristics, while Table 3 presents principal food choices and main barriers encountered in dietary management. Most participants were males, Bangladeshi, and living in rented accommodation with family or compatriots. Many of the interviewed were satisfied with their food habits and the majority reported to follow a typical or like-typical diet from the origin country, according to 'their taste' or because of 'no real free choice', especially those who did not live alone, or for scarce personal finances. Generic inadequate food intake and excessive sugar consumption were identified as the worst dietary habits.

Table 2. Socio-demographic characteristics of patients ($n = 55$).

Characteristic	M (Range)	n	%
Sex (n, %)			
Male		49	89
Female		6	11
Age, y (M, range)	44.3 (22–65)		
≤29		3	5
30-39		14	25
40-49		20	36
≥50		18	34
Origin (n, %)			
Bangladesh		37	67
Morocco		10	18
Algeria		2	4
Tunisia		1	2
Egypt		5	9
Religion (n, %)			
Muslim		53	96
Hinduism		2	4
Qualification (n, %)			
Not schooled		7	13
Junior high school diploma		28	51
High school diploma		11	20
Degree and beyond		9	16
Area of origin (n, %)			
Rural area		21	56
Urban area		24	44
Living in Italy, y (M, range)	11.4 (0–41)		

Table 2. Cont.

Characteristic	M (Range)	n	%
Accommodation (n, %)			
House rent with family or compatriots		36	66
As guest		9	16
Migrants helter		5	9
Homeless		4	7
Own house		1	2
Juridical status (n, %)			
Irregular		26	47
Regular		29	53
Work (n, %)			
Unemployed		16	29
Employed		39	71

Table 3. Food habits, barriers, and motivations in dietary management of patients ($N = 55$).

Items	Categories	n	%
Degree of satisfaction with the diet [1]	1	6	11
	2	4	7
	3	17	31
	4	12	22
	5	16	29
How much diet have changed after arriving in Italy [2]	1	9	16
	2	9	16
	3	14	26
	4	10	18
	5	13	24
Kind of diet followed in Italy	Only or mainly typical of own country	40	73
	Only or mainly Italian	15	27
Principal reasons	«I prefer it»	31	56
	«I have no choice»	20	36
	«People who cook for me prefer it»	2	4
	«It's cheaper»	1	2
	«Other»	1	2
Most common bad dietary habits	«I don't know»	32	57
	«I eat badly (qualitatively)»	11	20
	«I eat too many sweets»	7	13
	«I often eat out of meals»	2	4
	«I eat too much»	1	2
	«Other»	2	4
What the patient eats depends on...	«My personal taste»	27	49
	«What I find ready to eat»	13	24
	«Taste of people I live with»	11	20
	«How much money I can spend»	3	5
	«What is given to me (food parcels, gifts)»	1	2
Principal difficulties in management of food behaviors	«Eating well is expensive»	11	20
	«I don't have any difficulties»	21	38
	«I have no choice»	7	13
	«Laziness or lack of time»	4	7
	«I always have stomachache»	2	4
	«Respect for religious prescriptions»	1	2
	«Fear of forgetting the origins»	1	2
	«Other»	8	14

[1] from 1 'very bad' to 5 'excellent'. [2] from 1 'not at all' to 5 'completely'.

Thirty patients completed the follow up. Four out of the 25 dropouts were caused by returning to their origin country, three patients had a seasonal work far from the outpatient clinic, and one was hospitalized, whereas we do not have information about the remaining 17 dropouts. No particular socio-demographic differences were found between this group and the rest of the patients.

Patients' food habits improved at six-month follow-up. As shown in Table 4, the number of patients with adequate consumption increased in almost all food categories. Significant changes were reported for cereals and derivatives ($p = 0.04$), meat ($p = 0.02$) and potatoes ($p = 0.03$). Furthermore, the number per patient of food categories in which adequate consumption was reached in adequate dietary habits significantly improved ($p < 0.001$). The power of Wilcoxon Signed-Rank test ($1-\beta$) turned out to be as high as 0.99 at the effect size of 1.25, $\alpha = 0.05$, and the given sample size. For changes in food consumption assessed through McNemar's test, when the significance level was set at 0.05, post hoc power analysis results of cereals and derivates, meat, and potatoes were 0.60, 0.94, and 0.77, respectively.

Table 4. Food frequency before and after six months ($n = 30$).

Food Categories	Patients with Adequate Consumption n (%)		
	Before	After	Δ
Daily			
Meals (4–5)	7 (23.3)	13 (43.3)	+6 (+20.0)
Fruit and vegetable (3–5)	5 (16.7)	10 (33.3)	+5 (+16.6)
Cereals and derivatives (3)	7 (23.3)	14 (46.7)	+7 (+23.4) [1]
Milk and yogurt (1–2)	15 (50.0)	18 (60.0)	+3 (+10.0)
Weekly			
Meat (2–3)	3 (10.0)	12 (40.0)	+9 (+30.0) [1]
Legumes (≥ 2)	24 (80.0)	26 (86.7)	+2 (+6.7)
Fish (≥ 2)	26 (86.7)	27 (90.0)	+1 (+3.3)
Potatoes (≤ 2)	19 (63.3)	27 (90.0)	+8 (+26.7) [1]
Cheese (≤ 2)	24 (80.0)	27 (90.0)	+3 (+10.0)
Monthly (rare)			
Snack	22 (73.3)	21 (70.0)	−1 (−3.3)
Alcohol drinks	30 (100)	29 (96.7)	−1 (−3.3)
Soft drinks	16 (53.3)	18 (60.0)	+2 (+6.7)
Nr of adequate dietary habits per patient (median)	7	8	+1 [2]

[1] Statistically significant changes assessed by one-tail McNemar's test $p < 0.05$. [2] Statistically significant changes assessed by Wilcoxon Signed-Rank test $p < 0.05$.

With regard to patients' feedback, 93% reported a positive life change after nutrition recommendations. Customer satisfaction was generally high, both regarding perceived health conditions (average score = 3.7) and the multidisciplinary care received (average score = 4.9). Compliance to diet (average score = 3.3) and to recommended level of physical activity (average score = 3.9) was moderately good. Support from transcultural mediators was positively evaluated by 90% with an average score of 4.6. The main comments from the patients were: *'To better understand what my illness consists of'*, *'In order to communicate better with my doctor'*, *'For clearer information on how/when to visit'*, *'To better understand the dietary indications or how take medicine'*, *'I didn't feel alone'*, *'They accompanied me to the doctor'*, *'Finding a person from your country who explains in your language is a fact that makes you feel comfortable, you feel welcomed'*.

4. Discussion

The intervention had a significantly positive effect on patients' eating habits, a critical step for the management of diabetic patients. At the six-month follow-up, improvement in dietary habits and diabetes management was achieved. Positive effects were reported for almost all considered food categories. The best results were observed for meat, potatoes, and cereals and derivatives.

Initially, their intakes were really high due to cultural food habits. Excessive daily cereal intake decreased in favor of wholegrain foods. The suitable intake of fruit and vegetables increased, as well as appropriate number of daily meals. On the contrary, snacks and soft drinks consumption were still high mainly among Bangladeshis and Moroccans. They represent typical comfort foods and a risk factor for diabetes and cardiovascular disease [33], difficult to reduce because of their gratifying power. Dietary habits in affluent countries are characterized by high sugar and carbohydrate consumption and this seems to be related to high total and cardiovascular mortality [33]. The literature indicates a greater self-reported change in diet being associated with worsening health conditions at increasing immigrants' length of stay [2,34].

At baseline, food habits of patients included in the study were unhealthy, and there was urgent need to implement nutritional interventions to improve their health status. The aim of this study was to assess how the culturally tailored intervention, based on a customized diet and transcultural mediator's support, affects dietary changes. Our study confirmed that migrants maintain their country's food habits for multiple reasons, but it underlines that it is also possible to direct the diet towards healthy paths by leveraging cultural aspects. However, in our study, we were not able to confirm a significant relationship between the ease of adapting to a healthier diet and the immigrants' length of stay in Italy. Cohabitation with only one cooker and economic constraints play a decisive negative influence on diet. Additionally, food choices are affected by low or absent purchasing power. Above all, in low- and middle-income patients, the use of mobile phones may be useful [35], and at the same time a technological effort is needed to protect the data collected in the design process of personalized nutritional therapies [36]. Other intervention strategies for eating behavior improvement emphasize the involvement of social and health workers of the same language in the case of Arabic patients [37]. However, strong adherence to culturally oriented diet and to religious prescriptions often puts diabetes self-management in the background when patients are not correctly informed [38]. According to Bailey et al. [39], identifying food choices determinants is essential for achieving good adherence to diet and reduce dropouts. Using traditional food to design appropriate dietary profiles has been the key to overcome cultural barriers [40]. Nutritional counseling and the choice of personalized diets have been oriented towards the eating habits of the countries of origin, promoting the healthiest ones (e.g., fish and legumes for Bangladesh, unique dishes for North Africa). The limiting factors and the barriers to access to correct lifestyles have been contextualized with the specific social determinants of the person's health: Economic availability, time to devote to buying and preparing dishes, place of consumption of main meals, and responsible of daily nutrition. Particular attention was paid to the most dangerous categories of foods for a diabetic patient, rich in starch, correcting the excess consumption of meat. Patients' culture and lifestyle were respected. Adapting diets to people's cultural background can help reinforce the impact of dietary interventions. In our study, the cultural aspects of the intervention were stressed. Alongside with a culturally tailored diet, transcultural mediators were central for the success of the intervention. As evidenced by the words of the interviewees, they were fundamental to establish a 'pact with the patient' and support the process under both linguistic and logistic aspects. Many patients have highlighted how the mediator is 'listening', 'in tune with', activating a deeper feeling. The mediator physically accompanying the patient represented a sort of 'protective network', providing the patient with both critical orientation to services and psychological support.

To our knowledge there are no studies investigating the efficacy of a culturally tailored diet administered with the support of a transcultural mediator. Nevertheless, there are increasing indications that personalized dietary advice is more effective than generic nutritional information provided to consumers. Advices can be personalized in different ways: Personal preferences, self-formulated goals, eating habits, health status, or DNA profile [41,42]. Interventions of personalized medicine are also designed on the basis of behavior and social determinants such as personal and family history, cultural background, and personal beliefs and preferences [43].

Our study limitations include the lack of sex balance. Migration from Bangladesh to Italy is predominantly male and low participation of women in the sample was consistent with migratory flows. Many studies highlight the inequalities in the quality of healthcare access to specialized care and inappropriateness, due to migrant status and gender [44–46]. Difficulties were recorded to recruit women, notwithstanding the involvement of migrant reception centers and the organization of 'awareness days' in aggregation places. The role of gender differences in food supply should be investigated to understand if it can influence adherence to nutritional treatment. Due to the limited number of patients engaged, it was not possible to make any comparisons between countries of origin, nor provide clear-cut conclusion on the entire migrant population in Italy. Furthermore, although a 12-month follow-up could have been useful to confirm the improvement in eating habits, a longer follow-up was not feasible, given the characteristic mobility of the population recruited in the study. A strength of this study is that in-depth interviews allowed to get useful elements to better direct the patient towards healthier food habits, forms of cooking and preparation of the recipes, in respect of their culture and lifestyle.

5. Conclusions

This study underlines the importance to preventively evaluate the feasibility of nutritional therapy according to patient's lifestyle and to analyze the difficulties actually perceived by patients in accessing and continuing care [47,48]. In order to develop appropriate nutritional interventions for diabetes care, it has been critical to first manage formal barriers, such as legal restrictions and low-income lifestyle, evaluating patient's working hours, distance from the medical center, and returns for main meals in the reception centers.

Nutritional interventions based on both clinic and socio-cultural criteria and on the support of transcultural mediator are functional for improving diabetic immigrant's compliance to the therapy and healthier food habits.

Author Contributions: Conceptualization, L.P., G.B., M.C., and A.C.; methodology, L.P. and A.C.; formal analysis, G.N. and L.P.; investigation, L.P., G.B., C.T., and M.M.P.; data curation, L.P. and G.N.; writing—original draft preparation, L.P., G.N., and A.C.; writing—review and editing, L.P., G.N., G.B., C.T., M.M.P., M.C., G.C., C.M., and A.C.; supervision, A.C.; funding acquisition, C.M. and G.C. All authors have read and agreed to the published version of the manuscript.

Funding: This research was carried out under a project financed by Italian Ministry of Health (Cod. MINSAL-2016_002–CUP J82I15000870005).

Acknowledgments: The authors would like to acknowledge and thank transcultural mediators Papia Aktar, Moez Chamkhi, Kabir Md Rifat for their precious support in the study, Chiara Moncada for her help in bibliography, Cecilia Fazioli for critical revision of the English language and the San Camillo-Forlanini Hospital Diabetic Center staff.

Conflicts of Interest: The authors declare no conflict of interest. The funders had no role in the design of the study; in the collection, analyses, or interpretation of data; in the writing of the manuscript, or in the decision to publish the results.

References

1. McAuliffe, M.; Khadria, B. (Eds.) *World Migration Report 2020*; International Organization for Migration: Geneva, Switzerland, 2019; ISBN 978-92-9068-789-4.
2. Lee, S.; O'Neill, A.H.; Ihara, E.S.; Chae, D.H. Change in self-reported health status among immigrants in the United States: Associations with measures of acculturation. *PLoS ONE* **2013**, *8*, e76494. [CrossRef] [PubMed]
3. Petrelli, A.; Di Napoli, A.; Demuru, E.; Ventura, M.; Gnavi, R.; Di Minco, L.; Tamburini, C.; Mirisola, C.; Sebastiani, G. Socioeconomic and citizenship inequalities in hospitalisation of the adult population in Italy. *PLoS ONE* **2020**, *15*, e0231564. [CrossRef]
4. Rechel, B. (Ed.) *Migration and Health in EUROPEAN Union*; European Observatory on Health Systems and Policies Series; McGraw Hill/Open University Press: Maidenhead, UK, 2011; ISBN 978-0-335-24567-3.
5. Gushulak, B.; Weekers, J.; MacPherson, D. Migrants and emerging public health issues in a globalized world: Threats, risks and challenges, an evidence-based framework. *Emerg. Health Threat. J.* **2010**, *2*. [CrossRef]

6. Commodore-Mensah, Y.; Selvin, E.; Aboagye, J.; Turkson-Ocran, R.-A.; Li, X.; Himmelfarb, C.D.; Ahima, R.S.; Cooper, L.A. Hypertension, overweight/obesity, and diabetes among immigrants in the United States: An analysis of the 2010–2016 National Health Interview Survey. *BMC Public Health* **2018**, *18*, 773. [CrossRef]
7. Petrelli, A.; Di Napoli, A.; Perez, M.; Gargiulo, L. The health status of the immigrant population in Italy: Evidence from multipurpose surveys of the Italian National Institute of Statistics (Istat). *Epidemiol. Prev.* **2017**, *41*, 11–17. [CrossRef] [PubMed]
8. Dalla Zuanna, T.; Cacciani, L.; Barbieri, G.; Ferracin, E.; Zengarini, N.; Di Girolamo, C.; Caranci, N.; Petrelli, A.; Marino, C.; Agabiti, N.; et al. Avoidable hospitalisation for diabetes mellitus among immigrants and natives: Results from the Italian Network for Longitudinal Metropolitan Studies. *Nutr. Metab. Cardiovasc. Dis.* **2020**, *30*, 1535–1543. [CrossRef] [PubMed]
9. Marzona, I.; Avanzini, F.; Tettamanti, M.; Vannini, T.; Fortino, I.; Bortolotti, A.; Merlino, L.; Genovese, S.; Roncaglioni, M.C. Prevalence and management of diabetes in immigrants resident in the Lombardy Region: The importance of ethnicity and duration of stay. *Acta Diabetol.* **2018**, *55*, 355–362. [CrossRef] [PubMed]
10. Fedeli, U.; Casotto, V.; Ferroni, E.; Saugo, M.; Targher, G.; Zoppini, G. Prevalence of diabetes across different immigrant groups in North-eastern Italy. *Nutr. Metab. Cardiovasc. Dis.* **2015**, *25*, 924–930. [CrossRef]
11. Jabbar, A.; Abdallah, K.; Hassoun, A.; Malek, R.; Senyucel, C.; Spaepen, E.; Treuer, T.; Bhattacharya, I. Patterns and trends in insulin initiation and intensification among patients with Type 2 diabetes mellitus in the Middle East and North Africa region. *Diabetes Res. Clin. Pract.* **2019**, *149*, 18–26. [CrossRef]
12. Abdulah, D.M.; Hassan, A.B.; Saadi, F.S.; Mohammed, A.H. Impacts of self-management education on glycaemic control in patients with type 2 diabetes mellitus. *Diabetes Metab. Syndr. Clin. Res. Rev.* **2018**, *12*, 969–975. [CrossRef]
13. Ley, S.H.; Hamdy, O.; Mohan, V.; Hu, F.B. Prevention and management of type 2 diabetes: Dietary components and nutritional strategies. *Lancet* **2014**, *383*, 1999–2007. [CrossRef]
14. Pan, B.; Wu, Y.; Yang, Q.; Ge, L.; Gao, C.; Xun, Y.; Tian, J.; Ding, G. The impact of major dietary patterns on glycemic control, cardiovascular risk factors, and weight loss in patients with type 2 diabetes: A network meta-analysis. *J. Evid. Based Med.* **2019**, *12*, 29–39. [CrossRef] [PubMed]
15. Mora, N.; Golden, S.H. Understanding Cultural Influences on Dietary Habits in Asian, Middle Eastern, and Latino Patients with Type 2 Diabetes: A Review of Current Literature and Future Directions. *Curr. Diab Rep.* **2017**, *17*, 126. [CrossRef] [PubMed]
16. Vanstone, M.; Giacomini, M.; Smith, A.; Brundisini, F.; DeJean, D.; Winsor, S. How diet modification challenges are magnified in vulnerable or marginalized people with diabetes and heart disease: A systematic review and qualitative meta-synthesis. *Ont. Health Technol. Assess. Ser.* **2013**, *13*, 1–40.
17. Chambre, C.; Gbedo, C.; Kouacou, N.; Fysekidis, M.; Reach, G.; Le Clesiau, H.; Bihan, H. Migrant adults with diabetes in France: Influence of family migration. *J. Clin. Transl. Endocrinol.* **2017**, *7*, 28–32. [CrossRef]
18. Smith-Miller, C.A.; Berry, D.C.; Miller, C.T. Diabetes affects everything: Type 2 diabetes self-management among Spanish-speaking hispanic immigrants. *Res. Nurs. Health* **2017**, *40*, 541–554. [CrossRef]
19. Zeh, P.; Sandhu, H.K.; Cannaby, A.M.; Sturt, J.A. Cultural barriers impeding ethnic minority groups from accessing effective diabetes care services: A systematic review of observational studies. *Divers. Equal. Health Care* **2014**, *11*. [CrossRef]
20. Association, A.D. 4. Lifestyle Management: Standards of Medical Care in Diabetes—2018. *Diabetes Care* **2018**, *41*, S38–S50. [CrossRef]
21. Islam, N.S.; Wyatt, L.C.; Taher, M.D.; Riley, L.; Tandon, S.D.; Tanner, M.; Mukherji, B.R.; Trinh-Shevrin, C. A Culturally Tailored Community Health Worker Intervention Leads to Improvement in Patient-Centered Outcomes for Immigrant Patients With Type 2 Diabetes. *Clin. Diabetes* **2018**, *36*, 100–111. [CrossRef]
22. Lagisetty, P.A.; Priyadarshini, S.; Terrell, S.; Hamati, M.; Landgraf, J.; Chopra, V.; Heisler, M. Culturally Targeted Strategies for Diabetes Prevention in Minority Population: A Systematic Review and Framework. *Diabetes Educ.* **2017**, *43*, 54–77. [CrossRef]
23. Nam, S.; Janson, S.L.; Stotts, N.A.; Chesla, C.; Kroon, L. Effect of Culturally Tailored Diabetes Education in Ethnic Minorities With Type 2 Diabetes: A Meta-analysis. *J. Cardiovasc. Nurs.* **2012**, *27*, 505–518. [CrossRef]
24. Jaworski, M.; Panczyk, M.; Cedro, M.; Kucharska, A. Adherence to dietary recommendations in diabetes mellitus: Disease acceptance as a potential mediator. *Patient Prefer. Adherence* **2018**, *12*, 163–174. [CrossRef]
25. Franz, M.J.; MacLeod, J.; Evert, A.; Brown, C.; Gradwell, E.; Handu, D.; Reppert, A.; Robinson, M. Academy of Nutrition and Dietetics Nutrition Practice Guideline for Type 1 and Type 2 Diabetes in Adults: Systematic

Review of Evidence for Medical Nutrition Therapy Effectiveness and Recommendations for Integration into the Nutrition Care Process. *J. Acad. Nutr. Diet.* **2017**, *117*, 1659–1679. [CrossRef] [PubMed]
26. Li, S.; van Halen, C.; van Baaren, R.B.; Müller, B.C.N. Self-Persuasion Increases Healthy Eating Intention Depending on Cultural Background. *Int. J. Environ. Res. Public Health* **2020**, *17*, 3405. [CrossRef]
27. Cunha, L.M.; Cabral, D.; Moura, A.P.; de Almeida, M.D.V. Application of the Food Choice Questionnaire across cultures: Systematic review of cross-cultural and single country studies. *Food Qual. Prefer.* **2018**, *64*, 21–36. [CrossRef]
28. Gibson, R.S. *Principles of Nutritional Assessment*; Oxford University Press: New York, NY, USA, 2005; ISBN 978-0-19-517169-3.
29. FAOSTAT. Available online: http://www.fao.org/faostat/en/#data/FBS/report (accessed on 21 January 2017).
30. Association, A.D. Standards of Medical Care in Diabetes—2016: Summary of Revisions. *Diabetes Care* **2016**, *39*, S4–S5. [CrossRef]
31. R Core Team. *R: A Language and Environment for Statistical Computing*; R Foundation for Statistical Computing: Vienna, Austria, 2018.
32. Faul, F.; Erdfelder, E.; Lang, A.-G.; Buchner, A. G*Power 3: A flexible statistical power analysis program for the social, behavioral, and biomedical sciences. *Behav. Res. Methods* **2007**, *39*, 175–191. [CrossRef] [PubMed]
33. Dehghan, M.; Mente, A.; Zhang, X.; Swaminathan, S.; Li, W.; Mohan, V.; Iqbal, R.; Kumar, R.; Wentzel-Viljoen, E.; Rosengren, A.; et al. Associations of fats and carbohydrate intake with cardiovascular disease and mortality in 18 countries from five continents (PURE): A prospective cohort study. *Lancet* **2017**, *390*, 2050–2062. [CrossRef]
34. Gilbert, P.A.; Khokhar, S. Changing dietary habits of ethnic groups in Europe and implications for health Affiliations. *Nutr. Rev.* **2008**, *66*, 203–215. [CrossRef]
35. Abaza, H.; Marschollek, M. SMS education for the promotion of diabetes self-management in low & middle income countries: A pilot randomized controlled trial in Egypt. *BMC Public Health* **2017**, *17*, 962. [CrossRef]
36. Stewart-Knox, B.; Rankin, A.; Kuznesof, S.; Poínhos, R.; de Almeida, M.D.V.; Fischer, A.; Frewer, L.J. Promoting healthy dietary behaviour through personalised nutrition: Technology push or technology pull? *Proc. Nutr. Soc.* **2015**, *74*, 171–176. [CrossRef]
37. Alzubaidi, H.; Namara, K.M.; Browning, C. Time to question diabetes self-management support for Arabic-speaking migrants: Exploring a new model of care. *Diabet. Med.* **2017**, *34*, 348–355. [CrossRef]
38. Abuelmagd, W.; Håkonsen, H.; Mahmood, K.Q.-A.; Taghizadeh, N.; Toverud, E.-L. Living with Diabetes: Personal Interviews with Pakistani Women in Norway. *J. Immigr. Minority Health* **2018**, *20*, 848–853. [CrossRef] [PubMed]
39. Bailey, C.; Garg, V.; Kapoor, D.; Wasser, H.; Prabhakaran, D.; Jaacks, L.M. Food Choice Drivers in the Context of the Nutrition Transition in Delhi, India. *J. Nutr. Educ. Behav.* **2018**, *50*, 675–686. [CrossRef] [PubMed]
40. Kohinor, M.J.E.; Stronks, K.; Nicolaou, M.; Haafkens, J.A. Considerations affecting dietary behaviour of immigrants with type 2 diabetes: A qualitative study among Surinamese in the Netherlands. *Ethn. Health* **2011**, *16*, 245–258. [CrossRef] [PubMed]
41. Reinders, M.J.; Bouwman, E.P.; van den Puttelaar, J.; Verain, M.C.D. Consumer acceptance of personalised nutrition: The role of ambivalent feelings and eating context. *PLoS ONE* **2020**, *15*, e0231342. [CrossRef] [PubMed]
42. Celis-Morales, C.; Livingstone, K.M.; Marsaux, C.F.; Macready, A.L.; Fallaize, R.; O'Donovan, C.B.; Woolhead, C.; Forster, H.; Walsh, M.C.; Navas-Carretero, S.; et al. Effect of personalized nutrition on health-related behaviour change: Evidence from the Food4Me European randomized controlled trial. *Int. J. Epidemiol.* **2017**, *46*, 578–588. [CrossRef]
43. Bush, C.L.; Blumberg, J.B.; El-Sohemy, A.; Minich, D.M.; Ordovás, J.M.; Reed, D.G.; Behm, V.A.Y. Toward the Definition of Personalized Nutrition: A Proposal by The American Nutrition Association. *J. Am. Coll. Nutr.* **2020**, *39*, 5–15. [CrossRef]
44. Malmusi, D.; Borrella, C.; Benach, J. Migration-related health inequalities: Showing the complex interactions between gender, social class and place of origin. *Soc. Sci. Med.* **2010**, *71*, 1610–1619. [CrossRef]
45. de Waure, C.; Bruno, S.; Furia, G.; Di Sciullo, L.; Carovillano, S.; Specchia, M.L.; Geraci, S.; Ricciardi, W. Health inequalities: An analysis of hospitalizations with respect to migrant status, gender and geographical area. *BMC Int. Health Hum. Rights* **2015**, *15*, 2. [CrossRef]

46. Gkiouleka, A.; Huijts, T. Intersectional migration-related health inequalities in Europe: Exploring the role of migrant generation, occupational status & gender. *Soc. Sci. Med.* **2020**, *17*, 113218. [CrossRef]
47. Sugerman, S.; Backman, D.; Foerster, S.B.; Ghirardelli, A.; Linares, A.; Fong, A. Using an Opinion Poll to Build an Obesity-Prevention Social Marketing Campaign for Low-Income Asian and Hispanic Immigrants: Report of Findings. *J. Nutr. Educ. Behav.* **2011**, *43*, S53–S66. [CrossRef] [PubMed]
48. Metwally, A.M.; Soliman, M.; Abdelmohsen, A.M.; Kandeel, W.A.; Saber, M.; Elmosalami, D.M.; Asem, N.; Fathy, A.M. Effect of Counteracting Lifestyle Barriers through Health Education in Egyptian Type 2 Diabetic Patients. *Open Access. Maced J. Med. Sci.* **2019**, *7*, 2886–2894. [CrossRef] [PubMed]

Publisher's Note: MDPI stays neutral with regard to jurisdictional claims in published maps and institutional affiliations.

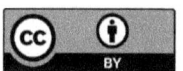

© 2020 by the authors. Licensee MDPI, Basel, Switzerland. This article is an open access article distributed under the terms and conditions of the Creative Commons Attribution (CC BY) license (http://creativecommons.org/licenses/by/4.0/).

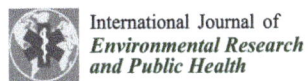 International Journal of
Environmental Research and Public Health

Article

Exploring Effective Sensory Experience in the Environmental Design of Sustainable Cafés

Yen-Cheng Chen [1] and Hsiang-Chun Lin [2,3,*]

1 Department of Applied Science of Living, Chinese Culture University, Taipei City 111, Taiwan; cyc4@g.pccu.edu.tw
2 Department of Hotel Management, Jin Wen University of Science & Technology, New Taipei City 231, Taiwan
3 Department of Geography, National Taiwan Normal University, Taipei City 106, Taiwan
* Correspondence: shiajune@just.edu.tw

Received: 10 October 2020; Accepted: 9 November 2020; Published: 2 December 2020

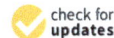

Abstract: The aim of this study was to explore and construct spatial indicators suitable for green café ambience. The indicators were further empirically verified. A three-round questionnaire survey, based on the Delphi method, was conducted with 15 experts, including university professors (food and beverage services management and interior environmental design), café operators, and personnel from government agencies. Data were collected, and the results on the characteristics of the repeated feedback from the experts were convergent. Thirty-six indicators suitable for the design of green café ambience were extracted, of which 17 were verified by actual cafés as highly operable. The five-sense indicators of sustainable green ambience design obtained in this study can facilitate positive customer experiences and enhance the appeal of maintaining sustainable green trends for cafés. These indicators can also provide references for café operators in business planning and green café ambience design.

Keywords: café; green ambience; Delphi method; indicator design

1. Introduction

In recent years, the issue of green sustainability has been attributed increasingly more importance around the world, and the concept of green consumption is trending. The question of how to apply this concept to the food and beverage service industry to reduce its adverse environmental impact is becoming important in the catering industry [1–3]. According to Chiang [4], in Taiwan, cafés have flourished in the streets and alleys of cities in recent years, providing quality dining spaces, food service, and situational experiences and becoming one of the fast-growing food and beverage industry sectors as well as an important part of the social life of locals. Consumers go to cafés not just to drink coffee but also to enjoy their ambience [5].

When consumers choose a restaurant, environmental factors affect their choice [1,3,6]. Influenced by the awareness of green sustainability, consumers have realized that green spaces function as ecological environments, and the introduction of a green theme can attract customers and thus create economic value [7]. Previous studies have also pointed out that café operators need to react quickly to new trends in coffee consumption and be able to provide new experiences to consumers [8]. Usually, the creation of an appropriate environment and ambience can benefit the sale of food and beverage products, provide positive sensory stimuli to consumers, and produce a unique style for the store that attracts consumers and strengthens their loyalty [9–11]. According to Kim and Jang [12], café managers need to foster a relationship between consumers and such venues so that consumers form a sense of place attachment. However, in the design of cafés in Taipei, Taiwan, in the past, only the visual sense has been paid attention to, while consumers' overall comprehensive feeling based on the information they receive through their 5 senses (touch, sight, hearing, smell, and taste) and then assess this information via the brain has been overlooked. Therefore, the innovation and contribution of this study stem from its evaluation of green sustainability-themed ambience indicators in 5 dimensions, which supports the more comprehensive design of the necessary ambience for sustainable green cafés.

Since the Industrial Revolution in the eighteenth century, industrialization has caused serious environmental damage, and environmental protection and sustainable management have become global issues. To maintain economic growth while mitigating environmental damage, many governments have been actively promoting sustainable green industries, to which the hospitality and food services industries belong [1,3]. Xu and Jeong [13] found that most environmental protection actions in the past have focused on environmental problems caused by the manufacturing industry and that, more recently, as consumer environmental awareness has improved, people have gradually realized that the hospitality and tourism industries also exert an impact on the environment. The food and beverage services industry is an important part of the tourism industry, consuming a significant proportion of resources used by the tourism system as a whole [2]. However, while the issue of green sustainability has begun to receive attention in the food and beverage industry, sustainable environmental design for cafés in Taiwan has rarely been addressed in depth, indicating a research gap. Thus, in this study, we wanted to answer the following questions: (1) What are the important indicators in the analysis of options for the ambience design of sustainable café in Taiwan? (2) What are indicators that can be used in analysing options that can be implemented in cafés?

Therefore, in this study, based on the basic principles of the Green Restaurant Association (GRA), we examined the development of green restaurants and the potential development patterns of green cafés and their integration of different aspects of ambience; based on the 5 dimensions of ambience proposed in a previous study [14], we investigated and constructed 5 system dimensions, i.e., auditory ambience, visual ambience, tactile ambience, olfactory ambience, and taste ambience, according to selection criteria with respect to balance, feasibility, operability, independence, and systematicity to construct an index system for the evaluation of green café ambience design that is of practical significance to the coffee and beverage services industry and consumers. Therefore, the objectives of this study were as follows:

1. To investigate and construct the indicators that are important to and suitable for green café ambience design
2. To empirically analyse indicators with high operability that are suitable for green café ambience design.

2. Literature Review

2.1. Green Food and Beverage Industry

In the late 1990s, due to environmental pollution, countries began to attach importance to environmental protection and sustainable development [3]. Compared with the concept of general environmental protection, green environmental protection started late in the catering industry, but because the catering industry is prone to a plethora of resource waste and pollution issues, the concept of "green restaurants" emerged in response to the call for green environmental protection [15,16].

The term "green" has become a synonym for pollution abolishment and environment protection, signifying health and sustainability [3]. The essence of green restaurants is to protect the global environment and create an environmentally sustainable catering industry in a way that reduces adverse impacts on the environment while providing products and services to meet people's needs and improve their quality of life [2]. The international environmental protection movement that has developed since the 1970s has re-examined the environmental damage caused by rapid economic development after the Industrial Revolution and has prompted people to pay increasingly more attention to the idea of environmental protection. The state, enterprises, and citizens can contribute to the sustainable development of the environment, and "eating and drinking", the most common behaviour in daily life, could be the most feasible way to promote the concept of a green diet [1,15].

The GRA was established in 1990; their mission is to help the catering industry become an environmentally sustainable business while promoting energy conservation. An increasing number of restaurants are designing suitable plans for environmental protection measures. For example, food material procurement, tableware material, recycled paper use, waste processing, water resource use, etc., have become important aspects in the design of green restaurants. In 1995, the GRA issued a green restaurant standard that includes 7 items, i.e., saving water, reducing waste, using sustainable furniture and building materials, using sustainable food materials, saving energy, reducing the use of disposable products, and reducing the use of chemical products and pollutants, and they advocated for the annual education of employees regarding environmental protection [17].

2.2. Ambience

With economic growth and social structural transformation, people's requirements for quality of life are increasing day by day, which is reflected, in particular, in the transition from dining solely for the purpose of having a meal to dining with a focus on the food itself and the restaurant environment, which are aspects that are becoming increasingly emphasized [18]. Baker et al. [19] suggest that consumers' sentiment is often related to consumption ambience; the design and creation of ambience can create a favourable consumption situation for an establishment, fostering positive consumer emotions [20]. Liu and Jang [21] also note the significant impact of ambience on customer emotions. Clearly, consumer demand for catering quality no longer concerns only dining but also concerns eating well, so the physical environment of the restaurant and dining ambience affect their consumption mood, which is closely associated with ambience. Schmitt [14] argue that the creation of ambience can affect consumers' perceptions of products. In a literature review, Turley and Milliman [22] note that environmental factors such as lighting, music, temperature, smell, interior design, and tableware placement are important for creating ambience in a restaurant. Therefore, providing a good environment can enhance consumers' consumption experience, making them happy.

When cafés flourish, this indicates that the consumer population is also expanding. Current consumers have developed different coffee consumption patterns from those of past consumers. Previously, people went to cafés for social, leisure, and dining purposes, but now, they want to relax and relieve stress at cafés [23,24]. With this transformation, when choosing a café, consumers pay attention not just to internal factors, such as products and services, but also to external factors, such as the ambience of the café itself [25]. The experience created by ambience in a café and the design and creation of ambience have become the main factors that attract consumers and influence their consumption behaviours [26]. Schmitt [14] note that the development of sentiment is most intense during consumption, for which the consumption ambience is the most important; consumers construct their perceptions of the world through the 5 senses, i.e., touch, sight, hearing, smell, and taste, which enable customers to have good consumption experiences, deepening their positive impressions while increasing their return rate. Therefore, multi-sense designs have become a trend for stores to increase consumer appeal [9,15,27,28].

2.3. Ambience Creation and Sensory Experience

Chen et al. [6] show that proper ambience creation and sensory experience have positive impacts on consumer emotions. The design of a restaurant's environment and ambience can enable consumers to generate more consumption desires and specific attitudes and behavioural responses [29]; thus, restaurant managers should improve service quality and adopt marketing strategies that meet the needs of the restaurant to improve consumer satisfaction [30]. Turley and Milliman [22] also indicate that a restaurant's ambience can positively affect consumer satisfaction with meals.

Furthermore, Leena [31] argue that in addition to providing meals, to increase competitiveness, the catering industry needs to provide consumers with a comfortable dining environment. Importantly, the design of a restaurant's ambience affects consumer satisfaction and behaviour [32]. To improve consumer satisfaction, food and beverage service providers must understand and design the appropriate ambience for their establishments to improve consumers' positive emotions, which in turn will affect an establishment's market competitiveness. Moreover, Rhee et al. [29] show that the design of a restaurant's ambience enables consumers to have higher consumer sentiment and specific attitudes and behavioural responses. Hamlin [33] also note that sensory designs have great impacts on consumers and that emotions can play a key role for many consumers. Consumers are paying an increasing amount of attention to an establishment's ambience when they make patronage choices because the ambience affects their emotions [34].

Therefore, sensory stimulation-focused ambience designs can trigger consumers' consumption sentiment, enhance their purchase intention, and lengthen their time spent in an establishment; ambience design for different consumer groups can have a key impact, the degree of which should not be underestimated [23,35]. In summary, environmental issues have become the focus of attention in various countries. If we can introduce the concept of green restaurants to Taiwan, it will be feasible to apply this concept in cafés through the creation of a five-sense ambience experience so that consumers' green and sustainable ambience experience is taken into account in the design of green and environmentally friendly cafés and so that their consumption experience and overall image of the café are enhanced

3. Materials and Methods

Based on the Delphi method, we collected and analysed data, determined the indicators, and constructed a research framework according to the aforementioned research motivation, objectives, and literature review; the details of those processes are described below.

3.1. Indicator Selection

In this research, we drew on the green restaurant standard proposed by the GRA; the five-sense experience proposed by Schmitt [14], Bitner [36] and Kotler [37]; and the guidance on choice criteria that take into account balance, feasibility, operability, independence and systematic aspects recommended by Dalkey and Helmer [38] on the basis of the 5 dimensions of ambience. Based on these references, we constructed 5 system dimensions: auditory ambience, visual ambience, tactile ambience, olfactory ambience, and taste ambience.

3.2. Selection of Subjects for the Delphi Method-Based Questionnaire Survey

This aim of this study was to establish criteria for the design of green ambience in cafés. Because the scope of issues is associated with the management of food and beverage services and the planning of environmental policy and infrastructure, experts from these fields were included as subjects. According to Dalkey and Helmer [38], for the Delphi method, a sample size of over 10 individuals can decrease the group-level error and thus achieve the highest reliability, which can be achieved by including 51–0 individuals in the case of a heterogeneous group. The participants of this study included college professors (catering services management and interior design), experts from government agencies responsible for overseeing catering businesses and protecting the environment, and café operators, constituting a heterogeneous group. For the rigour of the study, the number of experts recruited for this study was set at 15 (Table 1).

Table 1. Proportions of experts from different fields.

Expert Category	Food and Beverage Business Management and Interior Design	Government Agencies	Café Operator
Number of experts	5	5	5

3.3. Questionnaire Design and Distribution

Green et al. [39] demonstrated that for the Delphi method, 2 or 3 questionnaire rounds will lead to consensus, and therefore, a further increase in the number of questionnaire rounds will not affect the results because respondents will no longer change their answers to the questionnaire items. Therefore, in this study, we conducted a three-round questionnaire survey to reach a consensus among the participating experts. The questionnaire was scored using a Likert scale (very important or very easy = 5 points; important = 4 points; fair = 3 points; not so important = 2 points; not important at all = 1 point; and no opinion or cannot decide = 0 points).

After the first-round questionnaire was collected, the average score and standard deviation of each candidate indicator were calculated. For the second-round questionnaires, the scores for each candidate indicator and the average score for each candidate indicator obtained in the first-round questionnaire were included; this allowed the experts could score the indicators in the second-round questionnaire in terms of their importance and operability in reference to the answers that the others experts provided and the average score for each indicator in the previous round.

Further, as described above, based on the experts' suggestions and comments made in the first round, which were included in the second-round questionnaire, the wording of some candidate indicators was revised without changing the original meaning, and 6 new candidate indicators were added. This process resulted in the second-round questionnaire, which contained a total of 103 candidate indicators. After the second-round questionnaire was collected, the average score of the experts for each candidate indicator was calculated, which, together with the score for each candidate indicator provided by each expert, was included in the third-round questionnaire to provide information for scoring the indicators in terms of their importance and operability. This process resulted in the third-round questionnaire. Finally, after the third-round survey was completed using the formal questionnaire, stability analysis was performed on the first-round and the second-round questionnaires and the second-round and third-round questionnaires. The average score and standard deviation of each candidate indicator in the third-round questionnaire were calculated (Figure 1).

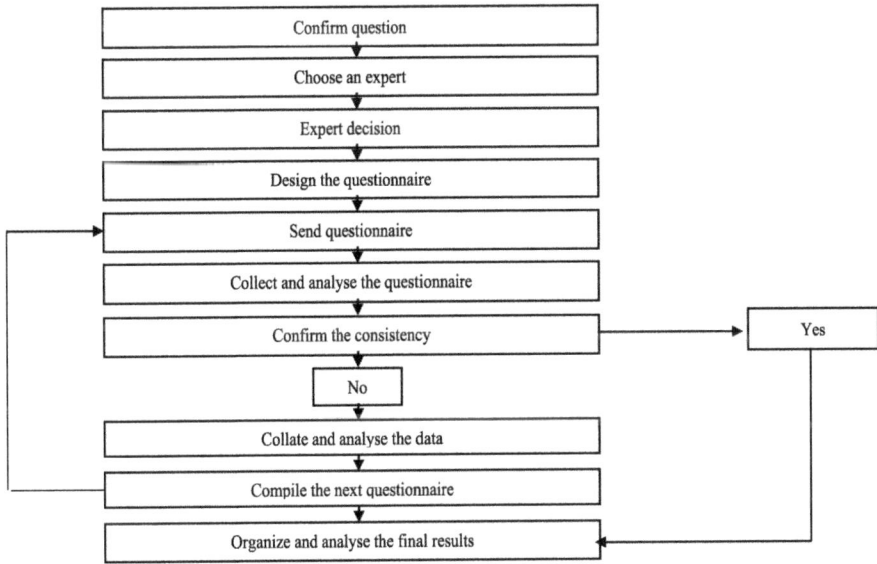

Figure 1. Delphi process.

3.4. Choice and Verification of Actual Cafés and the Design of the Verification Questionnaire for Actual Cafés

To verify the indicators of green café ambience designed in this study, after applying the Delphi method, we issued questionnaires to 10 non-chain cafés in Taipei to empirically strengthen the applicability of the findings from this study. Cafés that had more than 20 tables, sold coffee drinks and light food, were located in business areas of Taipei City, and had a unique decoration style were chosen. A total of 36 indicators of green café ambience design with high operability were analysed and verified through a questionnaire survey administered to on-site to owners or managers of 6 cafés; the questionnaires were answered anonymously and were scored using a Likert scale (very important or very easy = 5 points; important = 4 points; fair = 3 points; not so important = 2 points; not important at all = 1 point; and no opinion or cannot decide = 0 points).

3.5. Data Processing and Analysis

Based on the questionnaires issued in this study, in addition to the collation and revisions based on experts' opinions, the data for the quantitative part of the questionnaires were measured using the average score as the standard measure of the importance of the indicators. According to Linstone and Turoff [40], stability can be used to determine whether experts' opinions on questionnaire items are consistent and stable, the details of which are described below.

3.5.1. Stability Analysis

In the stability analysis, after the administration of the first-round and second-round questionnaires and the second-round and third-round questionnaires, the numbers of respondents who revised their scores for each indicator (scored based on a 5-point Likert scale, in which very important = 5 points and not important at all = 1 point) were added and then divided by 2, yielding the number of respondents who revised their opinions. This number was then divided by the number of total respondents who participated in the questionnaire survey, yielding the stability index.

3.5.2. Screening of Averages

Through the feedback component of the Delphi method, each item of the recovered questionnaire was listed, and its importance and operability were determined; furthermore, the score provided by each participating expert was provided so that others' feedback on each item could be known without the need for the experts to directly communicate with each other and so that the feedback could be used as a reference [38].

After the experts' opinions for the first-round questionnaire were integrated, the average score of each candidate indicator was calculated; then the average of each indicator for the first-round questionnaire was included in the second-round questionnaire to provide a reference for the experts when they answered the second-round questionnaire; after the second-round questionnaires were recovered, the average of each indicator was also calculated individually and included in the third-round questionnaire, and the experts' opinions were similarly revised for the third-round questionnaire. The above processes were repeated until the questionnaire results were consistently convergent when statistical analysis of the results was performed. In addition, after the third-round questionnaire survey was completed, indicators with a stability index greater than 15% were excluded through the stability analysis.

Finally, based on the overall average score, the average score for each dimension, and the importance score (of 4 points or above) obtained from the third-round questionnaire, the average selection process was performed on each of the retained indicators. Through the observation of the structure and distribution of all averages, a suitable index was chosen as the basis for the third-round screening of the indicators. The screening principle used to generate this value needed to allow a complete structure of the overall index system for green café ambience to be maintained, i.e., with at least one indicator from each dimension with a final score of 4 points or above retained in the final list of indicators based on the average importance score of the third-round questionnaire indicators (with a score of 4 or above).

3.5.3. Discussion based on the Standard Deviation

The consistency of the experts' opinions was measured using the standard deviation; the greater the standard deviation was, the higher the inconsistency on the item among the experts, and vice versa [38].

The calculation of the standard deviation was intended to examine the difference in experts' views regarding each questionnaire item. An indicator with a high and significant standard deviation value in the first-round questionnaire suggested that the experts' views on this item were still highly inconsistent, and vice versa. The calculation was performed until the third-round questionnaires were collected, and if the standard deviation value of a certain indicator was still significant, the indicator was further discussed.

4. Results

4.1. Questionnaire Distribution and Recovery

Questionnaires were distributed to experts, including scholars (food and beverage services management or environmental management), personnel from government agencies and café operators, by mail or e-mail or by on-site distribution. The three-round questionnaire survey was completed in approximately 2 months. A total of 15 questionnaires were recovered from the participants who completed the entire survey process, for a recovery rate of 100%.

4.2. Analysis of Importance Indicators

Stability analysis is mainly used to determine whether the scores of an indicator are convergent. In this study, the calculation formula for stability proposed by Linstone and Turoff [40] was used to calculate the stability index. After the third-round questionnaires were recovered, stability analysis was performed for each indicator by first measuring the stability of the score of each indicator provided by each expert in the first-round questionnaire and that in the second-round questionnaire and then performing the same stability measurement on the scores of each indicator provided by each expert in the second-round and the third-round questionnaires once the third-round questionnaires were collected. A stability index value below 15% suggested that the experts' opinions on this indicator reached a stable level and that the indicator could be included in the index system. The stability analysis results suggested that 20 indicators did not meet the stability index standard, i.e., had index values lower than 15%:

(1) 2 indicators in the auditory ambience dimension, i.e., "It is appropriate for green cafés to play audio recordings of the sound of rain" and "It is appropriate for green cafés to play violin music";

(2) 6 indicators in the visual ambience dimension, i.e., "It is appropriate for green cafés to use plastic as the main material for tables and chairs", "It is appropriate for green cafés to use candlelight", "It is appropriate for green cafés to use neon lights", "It is appropriate for green cafés to use ceiling lamps", "It is appropriate for green cafés to use ceiling fans", and "It is appropriate for green cafés to have their service staff dressed predominantly in green";

(3) 6 indicators in the tactile ambience dimension, i.e., "It is appropriate for green cafés to use dehumidifiers to keep the air dry", "It is appropriate for green cafés to use plastic utensils such as trays, cups, spoons, knives, forks, etc.", "It is appropriate for green cafés to use a plastic floor", "It is appropriate for green cafés to use plastic chairs", "It is appropriate for green cafés to use steel chairs", and "It is appropriate for green cafés to use plastic tables";

(4) 2 indicators in the olfactory ambience dimension, i.e., "It is appropriate for green cafés to have a food aroma", and "It is appropriate for green cafés to use incense"; and

(5) 4 indicators in the taste ambience dimension, i.e., "It is appropriate for green cafés to predominantly provide meat-based food", "It is appropriate for green cafés to provide fried food", "It is appropriate for green cafés to provide cured food", and "It is appropriate for green cafés to provide grilled food".

The above indicators did not meet the stability analysis criterion, meaning that experts did not reach a consensus on each of these indicators; therefore, these indicators were excluded, while the remaining candidate indicators had stability index values lower than 15%. After the above 20 candidate indicators were excluded, the remaining 83 candidate indicators were retained for the subsequent average screening stage.

The following criterion was used for the average screening: with the purpose of not disrupting the system structure, an appropriate average was chosen as the standard for the removal of candidate indicators. In this study, the candidate indicators were screened based on 3 criteria: (1) the overall average score (3.5 points); (2) the average score for each dimension (after calculation, the average scores for the dimensions were as follows: audible ambience, 3.7 points; visual ambience, 3.5 points; tactile ambience, 3.6 points; olfactory ambience, 3.2 points; and taste ambience, 3.4 points); and (3) the importance score (greater than 4 points).

The results are shown in Table 2. Ultimately, to ensure the integrity of the overall system structure and the high scores of the selected indicators, an importance score above 4 points for each dimension scored in the third-round questionnaire was used as the screening criterion for this stage.

Table 2. Comparison of the screening results for the indicators using different criteria.

Screening Criterion	No. of Remaining Indicators	Remarks
Overall average score: 3.5 points	62	"Olfactory ambience" and "taste ambience" were eliminated
Importance score: greater than 4 points	40	All dimensions showed an important score of 4 or greater
Average score for each dimension	59	"Olfactory ambience" and "taste ambience" had scores lower than the overall average score, indicating uneven levels

Therefore, we used this criterion as the basis for selecting indicators, and the system not only included indicators with high importance scores (4 points or above) but also excluded those with a stability index below 15%; however, the average importance score was lower when the indicators for all dimensions were considered. Finally, after the candidate indicators with a stability index value above 15% and an average score below 4 points were deleted, a total of 36 candidate indicators were selected.

The establishment of the above importance indicators was achieved through the following processes: after repeated feedback from the three-round expert questionnaire surveys, initial indicators with stability index values below 15% on the second- and third-round questionnaires for which the experts reached a consensus were chosen and subsequently screened based on the average for each dimension in the third-round questionnaire. Ultimately, a total of 36 indicators were selected as indicators of green café ambience: 5 auditory ambience indicators, 7 visual ambience indicators, 12 tactile ambience indicators, 4 olfactory ambience indicators, and 8 taste ambience indicators (Figure 2).

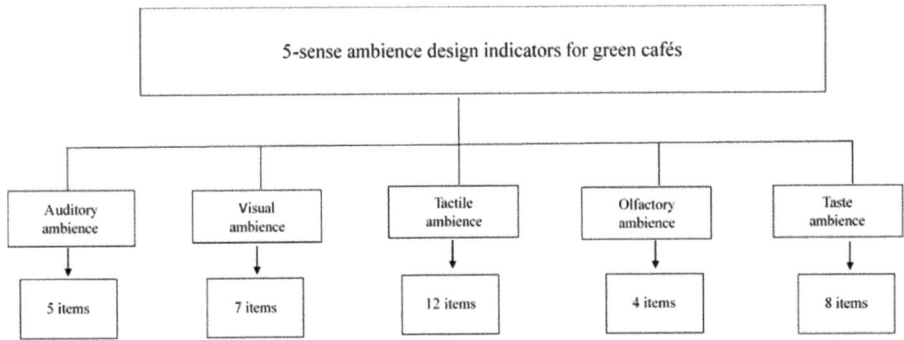

Figure 2. Indicators for green café ambience design.

4.3. Analysis of the Operability of the Indicators

In this study, the average score in the third-round questionnaire (easy, 4 points) was used as the criterion to measure the operability of the selected 36 indicators; i.e., indicators with an average value of 4 points or above were considered highly operable, as they had an operativity level of "easy" or above (Table 3).

After the experts' three-round analyses of the indicators, we chose 10 cafés to verify the selected indicators. The managers of the front and back lines and staff were asked to evaluate the indicators for the design of green café ambience; the evaluations were scored using a 5-point Likert scale, and the average scores were compared with the selected indicators to verify that these indicators could truly serve as the indicators for the design of green café ambience.

Table 3. The operability of the indicators of green café ambience design.

Operativity	System Dimension	Selected Indicators	Average Importance Score		
			Scholar	Government	Business
	Auditory ambience	A1. It is appropriate for green cafés to play audio recordings of the sound of streams	4.6	4.5	4.7
		A2. It is appropriate for green cafés to play audio recordings of the chirping sound of insects	4.4	4.5	4.3
		A3. It is appropriate for green cafés to play audio recordings of the sound of birds singing	4.1	4.5	4.3
		A4. It is appropriate for green cafés to play cello music	4.1	4.5	4.2
		A5. It is appropriate for green café service staff to greet and converse with patrons in a predominantly soft tone	4.1	4.0	4.0

Table 3. Cont.

Operativity	System Dimension	Selected Indicators	Average Importance Score		
			Scholar	Government	Business
High	Visual ambience	V1. It is appropriate to decorate green cafés predominantly in wood tones	4.7	4.5	4.5
		V2. It is appropriate to decorate green cafés predominantly with transparent glass to introduce natural light into the establishment	4.4	4.5	4.7
		V3. It is appropriate for green cafés to use tables and chairs predominantly with warm colours	4.4	5.0	4.3
		V4. It is appropriate to decorate green cafés with flowers and plants	4.7	5.0	4.7
		V5. It is appropriate to plant flowers and trees outside green cafés	5.0	5.0	4.8
		V6. It is appropriate to light green cafés predominantly with warm colours	4.4	4.0	4.8
		V7. It is appropriate for green café service staff to dress predominantly in green and earth tones	4.4	5.0	4.3
	Tactile Ambience	T1. It is appropriate for green cafés to use electric fans for air circulation in the establishment	4.6	4.5	4.3
		T2. It is appropriate for green cafés to use dehumidifiers to dry the air in the establishment	4.1	4.5	4.2
		T3. It is appropriate for green cafés to use air purifiers to freshen the air in the establishment	4.3	4.5	4.3
		T4. It is appropriate for green cafés to use air conditioners to control the temperature in the establishment	4.1	4.0	4.3
		T5. It is appropriate for green cafés to have windows to facilitate air circulation	4.9	5.0	4.8
		T6. It is appropriate for green cafés to use wooden utensils, e.g., dinner trays, plates, knives, forks, and spoons	4.3	4.5	4.5

Table 3. Cont.

Operativity	System Dimension	Selected Indicators	Average Importance Score		
			Scholar	Government	Business
		T7. It is appropriate for green cafés to use glass utensils, e.g., dinner trays, plates, knives, forks, and spoons	3.9	4.0	4.3
		T8. It is appropriate for green cafés to use wooden wall facades	4.6	4.5	4.5
		T9. It is appropriate for green cafés to use wood floors	4.3	5.0	4.3
		T10. It is appropriate for green cafés to use stone tile floors	4.4	4.5	4.2
		T11. It is appropriate for green cafés to use seats made of wood	4.4	5.0	4.3
		T12. It is appropriate for green cafés to use tables made of wood	4.4	5.0	4.7
	Olfactory ambience	O1. It is appropriate for green cafés to have a coffee aroma	5.0	4.5	5.0
		O2. It is appropriate for green cafés to have a wood aroma	4.4	4.5	4.0
		O3. It is appropriate for green cafés to have a fruit aroma	4.4	4.5	4.2
		O4. It is appropriate for green cafés to have a food aroma	4.3	4.5	4.0
	Taste Ambience	t1. It is appropriate for green cafés to provide predominantly fresh vegetables	5.0	4.5	4.8
		t2. It is appropriate for green cafés to provide predominantly bland food	4.3	4.5	4.2
		t3. It is appropriate for green cafés to provide food predominantly in its original flavour	4.7	4.5	4.6
		t4. It is appropriate for green cafés to provide predominantly light food	4.6	4.0	4.8
		t5. It is appropriate for green cafés to provide juice drinks	4.1	4.0	4.4
		t6. It is appropriate for green cafés to provide dairy drinks	4.3	4.0	4.2

Table 3. Cont.

Operativity	System Dimension	Selected Indicators	Average Importance Score		
			Scholar	Government	Business
		t7. It is appropriate for green cafés to provide predominantly freshly made coffee drinks	4.0	4.0	4.8
		t8. It is appropriate for green cafés to provide predominantly freshly made juice drinks	4.1	4.5	4.5

Last, based on the average scores of the 36 selected indicators, the average scores derived from the verification by actual café managers, and the criterion of an average value of 4 points or higher and small variation, 17 indicators with operability levels of "easy" or above that were scored in the verification were ascertained (Table 4).

Table 4. Selected indicators in this study for verification with actual cafés.

System Dimension	Indicator Content
Auditory ambience	A1. It is appropriate for green cafés to play audio recordings of the sound of streams
Visual ambience	V1. It is appropriate to decorate green cafés predominantly in wood tones
	V2. It is appropriate to decorate green cafés predominantly with transparent glass to introduce natural light into the establishment
	V3. It is appropriate for green cafés to use tables and chairs predominantly with warm colours
	V6. It is appropriate to light green cafés predominantly with warm colours
Tactile ambience	T4. It is appropriate for green cafés to use air conditioners to control the temperature in the establishment
	T6. It is appropriate for green cafés to use wooden utensils, e.g., dinner trays, plates, knives, forks, and spoons
	T9. It is appropriate for green cafés to use wood floors
	T11. It is appropriate for green cafés to use seats made of wood
	T12. It is appropriate for green cafés to use tables made of wood
Olfactory ambience	O1. It is appropriate for green cafés to have a coffee aroma
Taste ambience	t1. It is appropriate for green cafés to provide predominantly fresh vegetables
	t2. It is appropriate for green cafés to provide predominantly bland food
	t3. It is appropriate for green cafés to provide food predominantly in its original flavour
	t4. It is appropriate for green cafés to provide predominantly light food
	T7. It is appropriate for green cafés to provide predominantly freshly made coffee drinks
	T8. It is appropriate for green cafés to provide predominantly freshly made juice drinks

5. Discussion

5.1. Selected Indicators

In terms of the average operability score, 3 items, i.e., "It is appropriate to plant flowers and trees outside green cafés" in the visual ambience dimension (4.93 points), "It is appropriate for green cafés to have a coffee aroma" in the olfactory ambience dimension (4.83 points), and "It is appropriate for green cafés to provide predominantly fresh vegetables as food" in the taste ambience dimension (4.76 points), had high scores, indicating that the experts agreed that the 3 indicators are highly important for the design of green café ambience and are highly feasible.

In terms of the overall dimensions, auditory ambience (3.7 points), tactile ambience (3.6 points), and visual ambience (3.5 points) all had an average importance score above 3.5 points, indicating that these 3 dimensions are important indicators of green café ambience design.

5.2. Empirical Verification

5.2.1. Auditory Ambience Dimension

In this dimension, the item "It is appropriate for green cafés to play audio recordings of the sound of streams" showed the lowest score variation, indicating the high operability of the item in cafés, while other items, i.e., "It is appropriate for green cafés to play audio recordings of the chirping sound of insects", "It is appropriate for green cafés to play audio recordings of birds singing", "It is appropriate for green cafés to play audio recordings of the calling sound of frogs", and "It is appropriate for green cafés to play cellos music" showed high score variation. Although these items met the standard in terms of the average score, they did not attain an average score of 4 points or higher in the verification study with actual cafés, indicating that these items have low operability or would be impossible to implement.

5.2.2. Visual Ambience Dimension

In this dimension, 3 items, i.e., "It is appropriate for green cafés to predominantly use white light", "It is appropriate for green cafés to have flowers and plants", and "It is appropriate for green cafés to plant flowers and trees outside the establishment", showed high score variation and did not attain an average score of 4 points or higher in the verification study with actual cafés. Thus, these items have a low level of operability.

5.2.3. Tactile Ambience Dimension

In this dimension, 7 items failed to meet the criterion in the verification study with actual cafés: "It is appropriate for green cafés to use electric fans for air circulation in the establishment"; "It is appropriate for green cafés to use air purifiers for fresh air in the establishment"; "It is appropriate for green cafés to use glass utensils, e.g., dinner trays, plates, knives, forks, and spoons"; "It is appropriate for green cafés to have windows to facilitate air circulation"; "It is appropriate for green cafés to use wooden wall facades"; "It is appropriate for green cafés to use stone tile floors"; and "It is appropriate for green cafés to use cement floors". This finding indicates that these items have a low level of operability for implementation by cafés.

5.2.4. Olfactory Ambience Dimension

In this dimension, only 1 item, "It is appropriate for green cafés to have a coffee aroma", met the criterion in the verification study with actual cafés. Meanwhile, 3 items, i.e., "It is appropriate for green cafés to have a wood aroma", "It is appropriate for green cafés to have a fruit aroma", and "It is appropriate for green café stores to have a flower aroma", did not meet the criterion of an average score of 4 points or higher and had large differences in their average scores, indicating that these items have a low level of operability for implementation by cafés.

5.2.5. Taste Ambience Dimension

All 6 items in this dimension showed small differences in their average scores and the actual café verification results and had an average score of 4 points or higher, indicating that these items have a high level of operability for implementation by cafés.

6. Conclusions

After repeated feedback through three-round questionnaire surveys, among the 103 original indicators for the design of green café ambience, 36 indicators, including 5 indicators in the auditory ambience dimension, 7 indicators in the visual ambience dimension, 12 indicators in the tactile ambience dimension, 4 indicators in the olfactory ambience dimension and 8 indicators in the taste ambience dimension, were selected through stability analysis based on the criterion of an average importance score of 4 points or higher.

In this study, we found that because the concept of green café ambience has not yet been popularized, Taiwanese café operators would need to invest heavily in marketing to attract consumers based on ambience; therefore, it is recommended that when opening cafés, operators should take into account the capital and the regional target customer group. Based on the indicators selected by the experts in this study and the verification of the indicators with actual cafés, the items in the auditory ambience, tactile ambience, and olfactory ambience dimensions showed large variation in their scores; therefore, for the determination of green café ambience indicators in the future, items in these dimensions and the actual situation of café operations must be emphasized.

Further, when designing cafés, operators must consider the importance of ambience as experienced with all 5 senses; in the past, only visual ambience has been the focus of design [41,42], and the fact that humans receive information through 5 senses (touch, sight, hearing, smell, and taste) and assess this information with the brain to generate overall perception has not been considered [6,9,43]. The establishment of indicators of green café ambience design requires multi-party support and cooperation from academia, government, industry, and consumers, whose mutual assistance and joint efforts enable design implementation.

Limitations and Future Research Directions

Among the indicators that were not included, 2 items, i.e., "It is appropriate for green cafés to have their service staff dress predominantly in green" in the visual ambience dimension and "It is appropriate for green cafés to have unique aromas of all types of food" in the olfactory ambience dimension, had importance scores of 4 points or higher. It is recommended that these items be included when new indicators are added in the future.

In this study, in the design of the green café ambience indicators, the "conceptual" principle, which is qualitative but not representative, was established set as the main research direction in the first stage. Therefore, it is recommended that investigators further formulate indicators for "specific manoeuvrability" to establish a complete café scale to provide a tool for the industry, governmental departments, and academia to evaluate green cafés in the future and to provide guidelines for green café practices.

In the present study, due to human power and time restrictions, cafés were not distinguished based on their size and regional characteristics in the discussion. There was also no analysis of consumers. Cafés in Taiwan are diverse; therefore, in the future, different types of cafés should be differentiated in terms of their size and category for in-depth examination. Green consumption is often associated with high prices, and economic factors affect people's perceptions and quality of life, but this issue was not examined in this study. Therefore, it is recommended that in the future, price, income, and other economic factors be taken into account.

Author Contributions: Conceptualization, Y.-C.C.; Data curation, Y.-C.C.; Formal analysis, H.-C.L.; Funding acquisition, H.-C.L.; Investigation, H.-C.L.; Methodology, Y.-C.C.; Project administration, H.-C.L.; Visualization, Y.-C.C.; Writing–original draft, H.-C.L. All authors have read and agreed to the published version of the manuscript.

Funding: This research was funded by Ministry of Science and Technology, Taiwan: 109-2410-H-034-011.

Acknowledgments: The author is grateful to all those who volunteered to participate in this study. Special thanks to the data collected by Yi-Ting Chen.

Conflicts of Interest: The authors declare no conflict of interest.

References

1. Kwok, L.; Huang, Y.K. Green attributes of restaurants: Do consumers, owners, and managers think alike? *Int. J. Hosp. Manag.* **2019**, *83*, 28–32. [CrossRef]
2. Teng, Y.M.; Wu, K.S. Sustainability development in hospitality: The effect of perceived value on customers' green restaurant behavioral intention. *Sustainability* **2019**, *11*, 1987. [CrossRef]
3. Yu, Y.; Luo, M.; Zhu, D. The effect of quality attributes on visiting consumers' patronage intentions of green restaurants. *Sustainability* **2018**, *10*, 1187. [CrossRef]
4. Chiang, W.Y. Applying data mining for online CRM marketing strategy. *Br. Food J.* **2018**, *120*, 665–675. [CrossRef]
5. Filimonau, V.; Krivcova, M.; Pettit, F. An exploratory study of managerial approaches to food waste mitigation in coffee shops. *Int. J. Hosp. Manag.* **2019**, *76*, 48–57. [CrossRef]
6. Chen, Y.C.; Tsui, P.L.; Chen, H.I.; Tseng, H.L.; Lee, C.S. A dining table without food: The floral experience at ethnic fine dining restaurants. *Br. Food J.* **2019**, *122*, 1819–1832. [CrossRef]
7. Ziaabadi, M.; Malakootian, M.; Zare Mehrjerdi, M.R.; Jalaee, S.A.; Mehrabi Boshrabadi, H. How to use composite indicator and linear programming model for determine sustainable tourism. *J. Environ. Health Sci. Eng.* **2017**, *15*, 9. [CrossRef]
8. Carvalho, J.M.; Paiva, E.L.; Vieira, L.M. Quality attributes of a high specification product: Evidences from the speciality coffee business. *Br. Food J.* **2016**, *118*, 132–149. [CrossRef]
9. Chen, Y.C.; Tsui, P.L.; Lee, C.S.; Chen, G.L. Can plate colour promote appetite and joy while dining? An investigative study in Chinese fine dining restaurants. *Asia Pac. J. Mark. Logist.* **2019**, *32*, 105–116. [CrossRef]
10. Martínez-Ruiz, M.P.; Ruiz-Palomino, P.; Martinez-Canas, R.; Blázquez-Resino, J.J. Consumer satisfaction and loyalty in private-label food stores. *Br. Food J.* **2014**, *116*, 849–871. [CrossRef]
11. Song, H.; Wang, J.; Han, H. Effect of image, satisfaction, trust, love, and respect on loyalty formation for name-brand coffee shops. *Int. J. Hosp. Manag.* **2019**, *79*, 50–59. [CrossRef]
12. Kim, D.; Jang, S. Symbolic consumption in upscale cafés: Examining Korean Gen Y consumers' materialism, conformity, conspicuous tendencies, and functional qualities. *J. Hosp. Tour. Res.* **2014**, *41*, 154–179. [CrossRef]
13. Xu, Y.; Jeong, E. The effect of message framings and green practices on customers' attitudes and behavior intentions toward green restaurants. *Int. J. Contemp. Hosp. Manag.* **2019**, *31*, 2270–2296. [CrossRef]
14. Schmitt, B. Experiential marketing. *J. Mark. Manag.* **1999**, *15*, 53–67. [CrossRef]
15. Tan, B.C.; Khan, N.; Lau, T.C. Investigating the determinants of green restaurant patronage intention. *Soc. Responsib. J.* **2018**, *14*, 469–484. [CrossRef]
16. Wu, Z.; Cho, J.H. Research and practice on new technology for architectural green environment in cities. *IOP Conf. Ser. Mater. Sci. Eng.* **2018**, *317*, 012062. [CrossRef]
17. Green Restaurant Association. New Certification Standards. Available online: http://www.dinegree.com (accessed on 12 September 2015).
18. Wade, R.; Holmes, M.R.; Gibbs, C. The challenges of full-service restaurant brand internationalization: A United States/Canada perspective. *J. Foodserv. Bus. Res.* **2018**, *21*, 139–153. [CrossRef]
19. Baker, J.; Grewal, D.; Parasuraman, A. The influence of store environment on quality inferences and store image. *J. Acad. Mark. Sci.* **1994**, *22*, 328–339. [CrossRef]
20. Sirgy, M.J.; Grewal, D.; Mangleburg, T. Retail environment, self-congruity, and retail patronage. *J. Bus. Res.* **2000**, *49*, 127–138. [CrossRef]
21. Liu, Y.; Jang, S. The effects of dining atmospherics: An extended Mehrabian—Russell model. *Int. J. Hosp. Manag.* **2009**, *28*, 494–503. [CrossRef]

22. Turley, L.W.; Milliman, R.E. Atmospheric effects on shopping behavior: A review of the experimental evidence. *J. Bus. Res.* **2000**, *49*, 193–211. [CrossRef]
23. Atzori, R.; Shapoval, V.; Murphy, K.S. Measuring generation Y consumers' perceptions of green practices at Starbucks: An IPA analysis. *J. Foodserv. Bus. Res.* **2018**, *21*, 1–21. [CrossRef]
24. Kim, D.; Kim, B. An integrative view of emotion and the dedication-constraint model in the case of coffee chain retailers. *Sustainability* **2018**, *10*, 4284. [CrossRef]
25. Lim, W.M.; Jee, T.W.; Loh, K.S.; Chai, E.G.C.F. Ambience and social interaction effects on customer patronage of traditional coffeehouses: Insights from kopitiams. *J. Hosp. Mark. Manag.* **2020**, *29*, 182–201. [CrossRef]
26. Carvalho, F.M.; Spence, C. Cup colour influences consumers' expectations and experience on tasting specialty coffee. *Food Qual. Prefer.* **2019**, *75*, 157–169. [CrossRef]
27. Oh, D.; Yoo, M.; Lee, Y. A holistic view of the service experience at coffee franchises: A cross-cultural study. *Int. J. Hosp. Manag.* **2019**, *82*, 68–81. [CrossRef]
28. Tsui, P.L.; Lee, C.S.; Chen, Y.C. Building a model for the evaluation of the atmosphere of fine-dining restaurants. *J. Archit.* **2018**, *106*, 89–100.
29. Rhee, H.T.; Yang, S.B.; Kim, K. Exploring the comparative salience of restaurant attributes: A conjoint analysis approach. *Int. J. Inf. Manag.* **2016**, *36*, 1360–1370. [CrossRef]
30. Adams, C.; Doucé, L. What's in a scent? Meaning, shape, and sensorial concepts elicited by scents. *J. Sens. Stud.* **2017**, *32*, e12256. [CrossRef]
31. Leena, S.J. The Role of Perceived Value and Emotion in Determining Consumer Satisfaction and Loyalty: A Case of Asian Restaurants. Ph.D. Thesis, Oklahoma State University, Stillwater, OK, USA, 2014.
32. Heung, V.C.S.; Gu, T. Influence of restaurant atmospherics on patron satisfaction and behavioral intentions. *Int. J. Hosp. Manag.* **2012**, *31*, 1167–1177. [CrossRef]
33. Hamlin, R.P. The consumer testing of food package graphic design. *Br. Food J.* **2016**, *118*, 379–395. [CrossRef]
34. Rosenbaum, P.R. Evidence factors in observational studies. *Biometrika* **2010**, *97*, 333–345. [CrossRef]
35. Huang, H.C.; Perng, Y.H. Multi-criteria decision support system for green commercial space design. *Open House Int.* **2018**, *43*, 5–15.
36. Bitner, M.J. Servicescapes: The impact of physical surroundings on customers and employees. *J. Mark.* **1992**, *56*, 57–71. [CrossRef]
37. Kotler, P. Atmospherics as a marketing tool. *J. Retail.* **1973**, *49*, 48–64.
38. Dalkey, N.; Helmer, O. An experimental application of the DELPHI method to the use of experts. *Manag. Sci.* **1963**, *9*, 458–467. [CrossRef]
39. Green, H.; Hunter, C.; Moore, B. Assessing the environmental impact of tourism development. *Tour. Manag.* **1990**, *11*, 111–120. [CrossRef]
40. Linstone, H.A.; Turoff, M. *The Delphi Method: Techniques and Application*; Addison-Wesley: Upper Saddle River, NJ, USA, 1975.
41. Chen, Y.C.D.; Lee, C.S. Is it the staff or is it the food? How the attire of restaurant employees affects customer judgments of food quality. *Br. Food J.* **2018**, *120*, 1223–1235. [CrossRef]
42. Lindstrom, M. *Brand Sense: How to Build Powerful Brands through Touch, Taste, Smell, Sight, and Sound*; Free Press: New York, NY, USA, 2005.
43. Van Rompay, T.J.L.; Pruyn, A.T.H. When visual product features speak the same language: Effects of shape-typeface congruence on brand perception and price expectations. *J. Prod. Innov. Manag.* **2011**, *28*, 599–610. [CrossRef]

Publisher's Note: MDPI stays neutral with regard to jurisdictional claims in published maps and institutional affiliations.

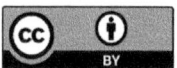

© 2020 by the authors. Licensee MDPI, Basel, Switzerland. This article is an open access article distributed under the terms and conditions of the Creative Commons Attribution (CC BY) license (http://creativecommons.org/licenses/by/4.0/).

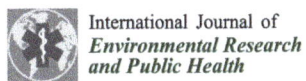

Article

Spatial-Temporal Characteristics in Grain Production and Its Influencing Factors in the Huang-Huai-Hai Plain from 1995 to 2018

Chunshan Zhou [1], Rongrong Zhang [1], Xiaoju Ning [2],* and Zhicheng Zheng [3]

1. School of Geography and Planning, Sun Yat-sen University, Guangzhou 510275, China; zhoucs@mail.sysu.edu.cn (C.Z.); zhangrr5@mail2.sysu.edu.cn (R.Z.)
2. School of Resource and Environment, Henan University of Economics and Law, Zhengzhou 450000, China
3. School of Environment and Planning, Henan University, Kaifeng 475000, China; zzc3148@163.com
* Correspondence: nxj0655@163.com

Received: 30 October 2020; Accepted: 7 December 2020; Published: 9 December 2020

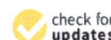

Abstract: The Huang-Huai-Hai Plain is the major crop-producing region in China. Based on the climate and socio-economic data from 1995 to 2018, we analyzed the spatial–temporal characteristics in grain production and its influencing factors by using exploratory spatial data analysis, a gravity center model, a spatial panel data model, and a geographically weighted regression model. The results indicated the following: (1) The grain production of eastern and southern areas was higher, while that of western and northern areas was lower; (2) The grain production center in the Huang-Huai-Hai Plain shifted from the southeast to northwest in Tai'an, and was distributed stably at the border between Jining and Tai'an; (3) The global spatial autocorrelation experienced a changing process of "decline–growth–decline", and the area of hot and cold spots was gradually reduced and stabilized, which indicated that the polarization of grain production in local areas gradually weakened and the spatial difference gradually decreased in the Huang-Huai-Hai Plain; (4) The impact of socio-economic factors has been continuously enhanced while the role of climate factors in grain production has been gradually weakened. The ratio of the effective irrigated area, the amount of fertilizer applied per unit sown area, and the average per capita annual income of rural residents were conducive to the increase in grain production in the Huang-Huai-Hai Plain; however, the effect of the annual precipitation on grain production has become weaker. More importantly, the association between the three factors and grain production was found to be spatially heterogeneous at the local geographic level.

Keywords: grain production; spatial–temporal characteristic; influencing factors; the Huang-Huai-Hai Plain

1. Introduction

China is an important food-producing country in the world, as well as a large food consumer. China's food self-sufficiency rate has reached more than 95% [1]. Although the current grain supply and demand in China maintains a balance of total quantity and a surplus in harvest, the small per capita arable land area, low mechanization level, and family-based business units determine that the current arable land has an extremely limited potential for increasing grain production [2,3]. From 1850–1900 to 2006–2015, the mean land surface air temperature increased by 1.53 °C [4]. Climate change has already affected food security due to warming, changing precipitation patterns, and the greater frequency of some extreme events [4]. Under the dual constraints of climate change and the process of urbanization, unpredictable meteorological disasters, limited arable land resources, huge population pressure, and the diversified consumer demand of residents directly generated strong demands for stable grain production [5,6]. Additionally, the outbreak of COVID-19 in 2019 led to labor shortages and supply chain disruptions, which affected the food security of some countries and regions [7]. Certain countries have even banned the export of food, leading to large fluctuations in global food prices and casting a shadow over the world's food crisis. Although China's major food crops, such as rice and wheat, are less dependent on the international market and national food security will not be affected by the agricultural trade restrictions brought about by the COVID-19, ensuring China's food security in the later period of the epidemic is of great strategic significance for domestic economic recovery and social stability.

The Huang-Huai-Hai Plain (HHH), located in the north of the country, is a high-yield agricultural region [8], accounting for 70% of wheat and 30% of maize production in China [9]. Because of its importance in grain production and China's self-sufficiency in food, it is known as the 'Breadbasket of China' [10,11]. Changes in grain production in the HHH can have direct impacts on both the national economy and food security of China [12]. Therefore, it is of great significance to understand its temporal and spatial characteristics and the influencing factors of grain production in the Huang-Huai-Hai plain in order to ensure national food security.

Previous studies have pointed out that while grain production in the Huang-Huai-Hai Plain is increasing, the difference in grain yields in various regions is gradually shrinking, but the spatial distribution pattern of grain production in the southern region of the Huang-Huai-Hai Plain is higher than that in the northern region, which remains unchanged [13–15]. Later studies attribute the distribution characteristics of grain production in the HHH to socio-economic factors [13,14,16]. The increase in grain production in the HHH is mainly due to the improvements of crop varieties, fertilizers and effective irrigation area. For example, the amount of fertilizer used has increased by about 400% and the effective irrigation area has increased by about 20% [10]. Liu, Tang [15] used the spatial lag model to reveal the factors affecting the differentiation in grain yield in the HHH from 1995 to 2010, and found that farmers' per capita net income, effective irrigation area ratio, and industrial structure had significant positive effects on grain yield. At the same time, studies have also found that although grain production and fertilizer input in the HHH are still significantly positively correlated, the current application of fertilizers in actual production is extremely unbalanced and unreasonable [17]. It is essentially important to improve fertilizer use efficiency in order to save resources as well as increase yield [10].

A number of studies have also emphasized the role of climate factors, especially precipitation, in grain production in the HHH [18–22]. Qu, Li [20] indicated that the increase in precipitation in the HHH can significantly increase the food production in the HHH, but the increase in thermal resources will increase the shortage of water resources and offset the impact of the increase in temperature. Xiao, Qi [23] reveled that climate change reduced the potential winter wheat yield of 80% of the stations by 2.3–58.8 kg·yr^{-1}, while at the same time it is pointed out that increasing the heat time of the wheat growth period is essential to alleviate the impact of the shortening of the growth period caused by warming climatic conditions. However, if the advancement of agricultural technology and other non-climatic factors are taken into account, for every 1 °C increase in the average temperature of the Huang-Huai-Hai Plain, the winter wheat yield in the north will increase by 2.1%, and the yield in the south will decrease by 4.0% [22].

Therefore, most of the previous research on grain production in the Huang-Huai-Hai Plain mainly focuses on the factors affecting grain production, that is, mainly from two aspects: socio-economic factors and climatic factors. Further, these studies are only carried out on one level, which separates the comprehensive impacts of climate and socio-economic factors on grain production. This will inevitably affect the final assessment results. To complete these data, this paper aims to explore the influencing factors of grain production in HHH by incorporating the climate factors and socio-economic factors into the models so as to provide a reference for ensuring food security and relevant departments to make decisions.

2. Study Area and Data Sources

2.1. Study Area

The Huang-Huai-Hai Plain (HHH), the second largest plain in China, is located at 32°–40° N and 114°–121° E, with a land area of about 4×10^5 km^2, spanning seven provinces and cities of Beijing, Tianjin, Hebei, Shandong, Henan, Anhui, and Jiangsu (Figure 1). The HHH belongs to the warm temperate semi-humid monsoon climate zone and is one of the most sensitive areas to climate change in China. The winter climate in this area is typically dry and cold, spring is dry, with less rain and much evaporation, and summer is characterized by high temperatures and heavy rainfall, including high intense rainfall that often leads to summer floods [24]. As an important agricultural region, this area has a long history of farming and is an important grain production base for food security in China, with its sown area of 20.4% of the nation's farmland and 23.6% of the whole nation's grain yield [25].

Here, wheat and maize occupy a larger proportion in the structure of grain production. The annual double-cropping system of winter wheat and summer maize is the most popular planting pattern. In addition, the yield of wheat and maize accounts for approximately 61% and 31% of the total national output, respectively [26]. Therefore, it is necessary to determine the pattern change rules and influencing factors of grain production in upgrading HHH grain production and ensuring national food security.

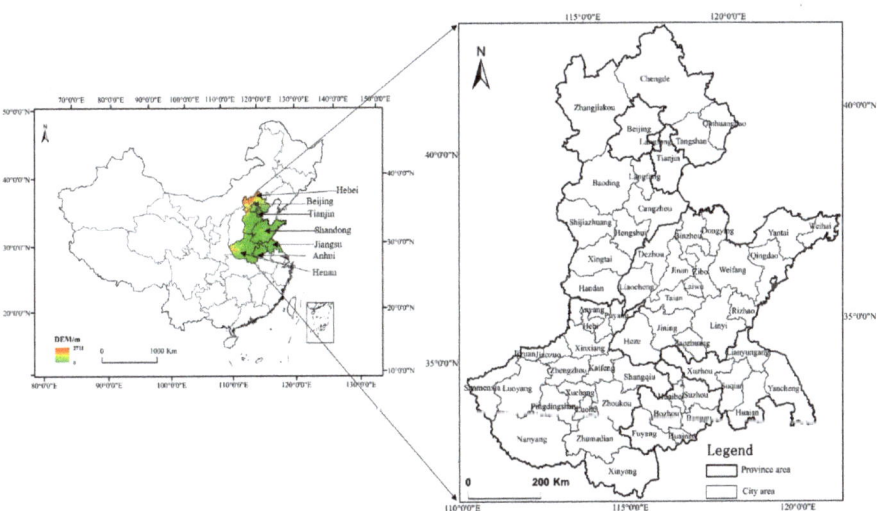

Figure 1. Location map of the Huang-Huai-Hai Plain (HHH).

2.2. Data Sources and Processing

The historical socio-economic data used in this paper were collected from the Statistical Yearbook published by the National Bureau of Statistics of China, which includes annual data on the grain yield per unit area, the sown area of grain crops, the amount of agriculture fertilizer application, the amount of effective irrigation area, the amount of pesticide application, the amount of mechanical power, and the per capita annual income of rural residents in the HHH from 1995 to 2018. According to China's statistics, grain production includes corn, rice, soybeans, wheat, potatoes, and sweet potatoes.

The historical climate data were collected from the Chinese meteorological data hub (https://data.cma.cn), including the annual precipitation, annual temperature, and annual sunshine duration of 123 meteorological stations in the HHH from 1995 to 2018. The meteorological data need to be processed by SQL-Server (Microsoft Corporation, Redmond, WA, USA) and ArcGIS10.2 software (Environmental

Systems Research Institute Inc, Redlands, CA, USA), which can analyze the average annual temperature, annual precipitation, and average annual sunshine hours of each city in different years.

Grain production is influenced by a variety of natural and socio-economic factors. In this paper, based on the previous literature [27–29], the grain yield per unit sown area (kg/km^2) was taken as the dependent variable, and climate and socio-economic factors were taken as the independent variables. Among them, the climate indexes included the annual average temperature (°C), the annual average precipitation (mm), and the annual average sunshine duration (h), and the social-economic factors included the proportion of effective irrigation area (%), amount of fertilizer application per unit sown area (t/km^2), amount of pesticide application per unit sown area (t/km^2), amount of mechanical power per sown area (kw/km^2), and per capita annual income of rural residents (RMB). Table 1 summarizes the data used in this study.

Table 1. Index selection and specific treatment methods.

Data Type	Data Name	Processing Method	
Climate Data	Annual average temperature (TEM)	Kriging interpolation	°C
	Annual average precipitation (PRE)	Kriging interpolation	mm
	Annual average sunshine duration (SSD)	Kriging interpolation	h
Socio-economic Data	Proportion of effective irrigation area (EIA)	Effective irrigation area/arable land area	%
	Amount of fertilizer application per unit sown area (AFA)	Total fertilizer application/crop sown area	t/km^2
	Amount of pesticide application per unit sown area (APA)	Total pesticide application/crop sown area	t/km^2
	Mechanical power per sown area (MPA)	Agricultural machinery power/crop sown area	kw/km^2
	Per capita annual income of rural residents (PCI)	/	RMB/per

3. Methods

3.1. Exploratory Spatial Data Analysis (ESDA)

Exploratory spatial data analysis is a collection of techniques for describing and visualizing spatial distributions, determining atypical locations or spatial outliers, discovering spatial associations, clusters, or hot spots, and to infer spatial characteristics or other forms of space heterogeneity [30]. In general, global and local spatial autocorrelation (or hot spots analysis) is often used to explore the spatial characteristics of observations [31].

3.1.1. Global Spatial Autocorrelation

Global spatial autocorrelation is used to test the spatial correlation of the observations of spatial units within the study area [32], and is mainly measured by the Global Moran's I, which was first proposed by Moran [33]. The Moran's I can be calculated using Equation (1):

$$I = \frac{n \sum_{i=1}^{n} \sum_{j=1}^{n} w_{ij}(x_i - \bar{x})(x_j - \bar{x})}{\sum_{i=1}^{n} \sum_{j=1}^{n} w_{ij} \sum_{i=1}^{n} (x_i - \bar{x})^2} \quad (1)$$

where I represents Moran's I, n is the number of spatial units (in this study, n = 59), x_i and x_j are the observations of spatial units I and j, respectively, $\bar{x}$ is the average value of observations of spatial units, and wij is the spatial weight matrix, where w_{ij} = 1 if spatial units I and j share a common border and w_{ij} = 0 otherwise. The values of Global Moran's I range from −1 to 1. If I < 0, it means there is a negative spatial correlation in the space, while if I > 0, it means there is a positive spatial correlation, an d if I = 0, it means there is no spatial correlation.

The significance of Moran's I is usually measured by Z statistics using Equation (2):

$$Z(I) = \frac{I - E(I)}{\sqrt{Var(I)}} \quad (2)$$

where $E(I)$ and $Var(I)$ are the expected value and variance of Moran's I, respectively.

3.1.2. Hot Spot (Getis-Ord G_i^*) Analysis

The Getis-Ord G_i^* is commonly used for hot spot analysis, which can identify clustering relationships at different spatial locations. Compared with the local spatial autocorrelation, the Getis-Ord G_i^* is more sensitive to the identification of cold and hot spots, and can fully reflect the high or low value distribution relationship between a certain geographic element and other surrounding elements [34]. The formula is [34–37]:

$$G_i^* = \frac{\sum_{j=1}^{n} w_{ij}(x_j - \bar{x})}{\sqrt{\frac{1}{n}\sum_{j=1}^{n} x_j^2 - \bar{x}^2} \cdot \sqrt{\frac{n}{n-1}\sum_{j=1}^{n} w_{ij}^2 - \frac{n}{n-1}\left(\sum_{j=1}^{n} w_{ij}\right)^2}} \quad (3)$$

where $\bar{x} = \frac{1}{n}\sum_{j=1}^{n} x_j$, n is the number of spatial units (in this study, $n = 59$), and w_{ij} is the spatial weight matrix, where $w_{ij} = 1$ if spatial units I and j share a common border and $w_{ij} = 0$ otherwise.

The significance of G_i^* is usually measured by Z statistics using Equation (4):

$$Z(G_i^*) = \frac{[G_i^* - E(G_i^*)]}{\sqrt{Var(G_i^*)}} \quad (4)$$

where $E(G_i^*)$ and $Var(G_i^*)$ are the expected value and variance of G_i^*, respectively. If $Z(G_i^*)$ is significantly positive, it indicates that the observations around the spatial unit i are relatively high (higher than the average), and are high-value clusters in the space, belonging to hot spots; on the contrary, if $Z(G_i^*)$ is significantly negative, it indicates that the observations around the spatial unit i are relatively low (lower than the mean), and are low-value clusters in the space, belonging to cold spots. The larger (or smaller) the $Z(G_i^*)$ is, the more intense the clustering of high (or low) values. A $Z(G_i^*)$ near zero indicates no apparent spatial clustering.

3.2. Gravity Center Model

The gravity center model is used to measure the overall distribution of a certain attribute in a region. It can provide a concise and accurate feature of the distribution of the attribute in the space, and can indicate the general trend and central location of its distribution. We assumed that a large region (such as an administrative region) consists of several subregions, and so the gravity center of grain production in the region could be calculated by the grain production and geographic coordinates of each sub-region. The formula is [38]:

$$X = \frac{\sum_{i=1}^{n} M_i X_i}{\sum_{i=1}^{n} M_i}; \quad Y = \frac{\sum_{i=1}^{n} M_i Y_i}{\sum_{i=1}^{n} M_i} \quad (5)$$

In Equation (2), X_i and Y_i represent the geographic coordinates of the ith subregion. M_i represents the grain yield per unit sown area of the subregion. X and Y represent the gravity center of grain production in a large region. Using formula (3), the moving distance of the gravity center in grain production can be obtained, which can reflect the evolution of the gravity center of a property in a region;

$$D_{ij} = R \times \sqrt{(X_i - X_j)^2 + (Y_i - Y_j)^2} \quad (6)$$

In Equation (3), D_{ij} is the gravity center movement distance (km) of grain production from j to i years. (X_i, Y_i) and (X_j, Y_j) are the gravity center coordinates of grain production in the i and j years. R is typically 111.111, which represents the coefficient of the spherical longitude and latitude coordinates converted to plane distance.

3.3. Spatial Panel Data Model

When the data have spatial autocorrelation effects, the residuals are no longer independent of each other; thus, it is not appropriate to use the ordinary least square regression (OLS) model. Instead, the spatial lag model (SLM) or the spatial error model (SEM) should be used for analysis. The formula is [39–41]:

$$\text{SLM}: \quad y = \rho w_{ij} y + x\beta + \mu \tag{7}$$

$$\text{SEM}: \quad \begin{cases} y = x\beta + \varepsilon \\ \varepsilon = \lambda w_{ij} + \mu \end{cases} \tag{8}$$

In Equations (4) and (5), y is the dependent variable, x is the explanatory variables, W_{ij} is the space weight matrix, ρ is the spatial hysteresis parameter, β is the parameter vector, μ is the random interference term, ε is the regression residual vector, and λ is the autoregression parameter.

3.4. Geographically Weighted Regression (GWR) Model

Geographically weighted regression models are superior to traditional regression models such as ordinary least squares (OLS). The geographical weighted regression (GWR) model can fully consider the spatial characteristics of each influencing factor, and more accurately show the spatial relationship between independent and dependent variables [42]. The form of a GWR model is as follows:

$$Y_i = \beta_0(u_i, v_i) + \sum_\lambda^n \beta_\lambda(u_i, v_i) X_{i\lambda} + \varepsilon \tag{9}$$

In Equation (6), Y_i represents the grain production in region i, $\beta_{0(u_i,v_i)}$ represents a constant, $\beta_{\lambda(u_i,v_i)}$ represents the regression coefficient, (u_i,v_i) represents the geographic location of the cities i, $X_{i\lambda}$ represents the parameter value of the λ independent variable of city i, and ε represents the random error. The optimal bandwidth distance can be obtained automatically in GWR4.0 corrected by finite correction of the Akaike Information Criterion (AICc). The smaller the AICc value, the higher the goodness of fit of the model will be [43].

4. Results

4.1. Temporal Changes of Grain Production in the HHH

From 1995 to 2018, the grain yield per unit of sown area in the HHH has shown a steady increase (Figure 2), which can be divided into three stages, as follows: the fluctuating growth stage (1995–2005), the steady growth stage (2005–2015), and the slow descent stage (2015–2018). Firstly, in the fluctuating growth stage (1995–2005), although the grain yield per unit sown area has increased in this stage, the fluctuation range is relatively large and the grain yield per unit of sown area gradually stabilized in 2005. Secondly, during the steady growth stage (2005–2015), the grain yield per unit of sown area showed a characteristic of small fluctuation growth. Finally, a slow decline began to appear in the grain yield per unit of sown area in the HHH during the slow descent stage (2015–2018).

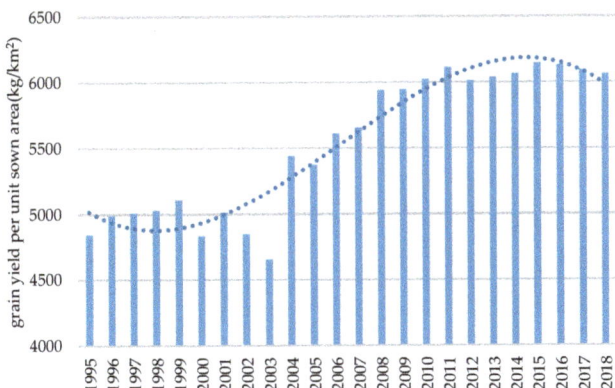

Figure 2. The temporal changes of grain production in the HHH from 1995 to 2018.

4.2. Spatial Characteristics of Grain Production in the HHH

We classified the grain yield data of each urban unit of sown area into four types according to 2000–3500, 3500–5000, 5000–6500, and 6500–8000 kg/km^2 using ArcGIS10.2 software. For the convenience of analysis, four time sections of 1995, 2005, 2015, and 2018 were selected for study, for which the spatial distribution characteristics of the grain production pattern were discussed (Figure 3).

It can be seen from Figure 3 that the spatial variation in grain yield per unit of sown area in each city is very significant, and the overall grain yield shows an increasing trend. Specifically, the number of cities in the HHH where the grain yield per unit of sown area remained within the range of 2000–3500 kg/km^2 continued to decrease, and was mainly distributed in Zhangjiakou, Cangzhou, Zhengzhou, Luoyang, Nanyang, Sanmenxia, and Bozhou in 1995, Zhangjiakou and Sanmenxia in 2005, and only in Zhangjiakou in 2015. In 2018, the number of cities of this type decreased to zero.

The number of cities within the range of grain yield per unit of sown area of 3500 to 5000 kg/km^2 also showed a downward trend, and the type area shrank from 30 cities in 1995 to 5 cities in 2018, and presented a layout trend of agglomeration to dispersion in spatial distribution.

The number of cities in the range of 5000–6500 kg/km^2 showed a rising–falling–rising trend. Among them, the number of cities in this type of area increased from 19 to 35 in 1995–2005, reduced from 35 to 28 in 2005–2015, and increased from 28 to 40 in 2015–2018. The spatial distribution of this type overall showed a tendency varying between scattered and clustered development, and appeared roughly from east to west, and from south to north.

The trend of unit of area sown to grain production maintained in the 6500–8000 kg/km^2 interval of urban change was different from the above three kinds. In 1995, the number of cities within this range was 3, which increased to 5 in 2005 and 24 in 2015, and reduced to 14 in 2018, which reflects a characteristic of a sharp increase followed by a slow decline. However, they were still mainly distributed in the central and southern parts of the HHH.

In terms of spatial distribution, the areas with high grain yield per unit of sown area in the Huang-Huia-Hai Plain were mainly distributed in the east and south, while the areas with low grain yield per unit of sown area were mainly distributed in the west and north of the HHH, which indicated that the grain production capacity of the eastern and southern regions of the HHH was higher, while that of the northern and western regions was lower.

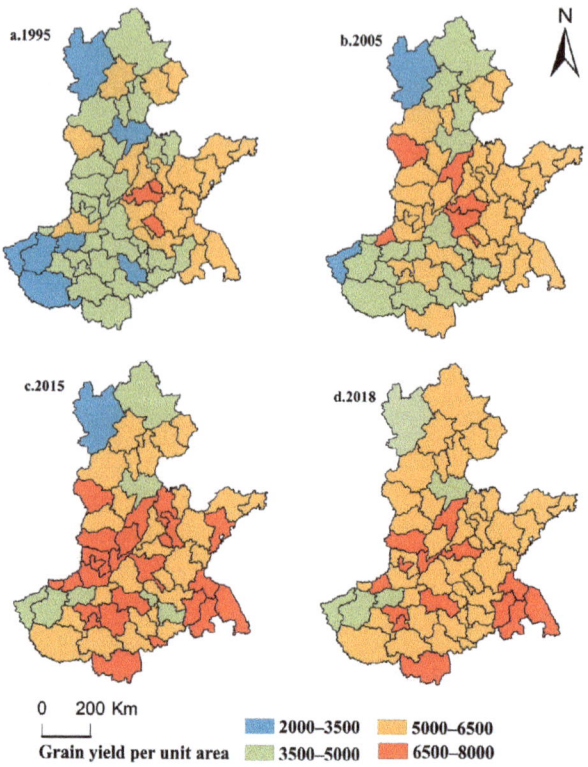

Figure 3. The spatial distribution of grain production in the HHH in (**a**) 1995, (**b**) 2005, (**c**) 2015, and (**d**) 2018.

4.3. Dynamic Change of Barycenter of Grain Production in the HHH

Figure 3 reflects the static distribution pattern of grain production in the HHH in 1995, 2005, 2015, and 2018, but does not reflect the dynamic change trend. Therefore, we used Equation (2) to calculate the barycenter of grain production in the HHH from 1995 to 2018 (Figure 4), and then used Equation (3) to calculate the barycenter movement distance (Table 2) to analyze the dynamic change characteristics of the grain production pattern.

According to Figure 4, the grain production center in the HHH generally shifted from southeast to northwest in Tai'an, and gradually stabilized in the central area of the HHH with the passage of time. Specifically, from 1995 to 1997, the grain production center of HHH was distributed in Jining city, which moved first to the northwest and then to the southwest. From 1998 to 2000, the movement direction of the barycenter in grain production remained highly stable; that is, it continued to move in the northwest direction. The barycenter of grain production began to enter Tai'an City. From 2000 to 2001, the movement direction of the barycenter in grain production was reversed and shifted to the southeast.

In 2001–2003, the barycenter of grain production shifted first to the southwest and then to the northeast, and in 2003–2005, it shifted first to the southwest and then to the southeast. From 2005 to 2011, the barycenter of grain production fluctuated in all directions. From 2011 to 2013, the grain production center assumed a similar change trend to that from 2001 to 2003. From 2013 to 2015, the grain production center first moved to the northeast and then to the northwest.

From 2015 to 2018, the grain production center of gravity showed characteristics of moving from southeast to northwest, but it was still stable in the territory of Tai'an City, that is, the southeast of the

HHH. The dynamic shift in the grain production center in the HHH indicates that the regional grain production capacity has the characteristics of non-stationarity in time and non-equilibrium in space at the same time, and the shift in the grain production center from southeast to northwest indicates that the grain production capacities in the western and northern parts of the HHH were continuously enhanced. In addition, the grain production center in the HHH tended to be stable over time, and it was concentrated in the border area between Jining and Tai'an.

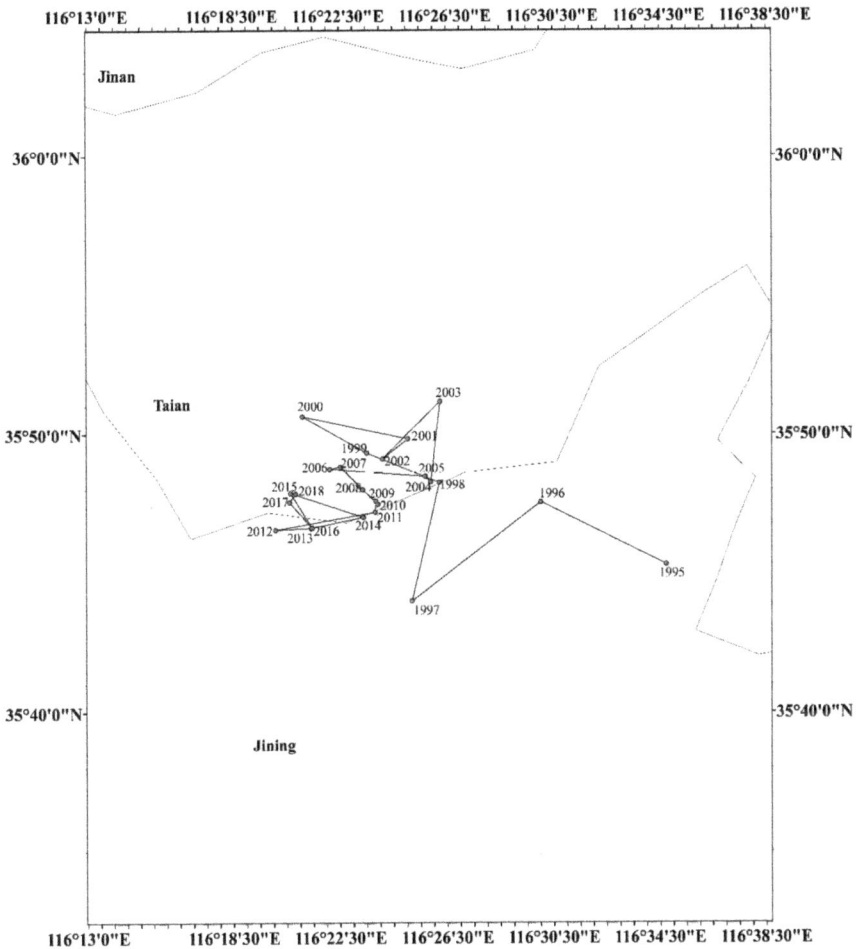

Figure 4. The track of the gravity center of grain production in the HHH from 1995 to 2018.

Table 2 shows that the barycenter of grain production in the HHH as a whole moved from the southeast to northwest from 1995 to 2005, with a distance of 17.7 km. From 2005 to 2018, the barycenter of grain production moved to the northwest with a distance of 9.4 km, which was significantly smaller than that from 1995 to 2005, which confirmed that the barycenter of grain production in the HHH showed good time-stability characteristics over time; however, this could not cover up the disequilibrium in the spatial characteristics of grain production. On the whole, from 1995 to 2018, the center of gravity of grain production moved 26.1 km to the northwest. The center was still stable in the territory of Tai'an city, that is, to the southeast of the HHH.

Table 2. The gravity center changes in grain production in 1995–2018.

Year	Gravity Center of Grain Production			Year	Gravity Center of Grain Production		
	Longitude	Latitude	Moving Distance/km		Longitude	Latitude	Moving Distance/km
1995	116.58 E	35.75 N	-	2007	116.38 E	35.81 N	0.774593
1996	116.50 E	35.79 N	9.663716	2008	116.39 E	35.80 N	2.163265
1997	116.42 E	35.73 N	11.05526	2009	116.40 E	35.79 N	1.415176
1998	116.44 E	35.80 N	8.099253	2010	116.40 E	35.79 N	0.261293
1999	116.39 E	35.82 N	5.382058	2011	116.40 E	35.79 N	0.747488
2000	116.35 E	35.84 N	5.081014	2012	116.33 E	35.78 N	7.035403
2001	116.42 E	35.83 N	7.488652	2013	116.36 E	35.78 N	2.505761
2002	116.41 E	35.82 N	2.213499	2014	116.39 E	35.78 N	3.691162
2003	116.44 E	35.85 N	5.510654	2015	116.34 E	35.80 N	5.316664
2004	116.43 E	35.80 N	5.391599	2016	116.36 E	35.78 N	2.751065
2005	116.43 E	35.80 N	0.532014	2017	116.34 E	35.79 N	2.319260
2006	116.37 E	35.81 N	6.620709	2018	116.35 E	35.80 N	0.697832

"-" means the item does not exist.

4.4. Spatial Correlation Characteristics of Grain Production Pattern in the HHH

4.4.1. Global Spatial Correlation Characteristics

Based on the grain yield data per unit sown area, the Moran's I value, Z statistic, and P-value were calculated using Geoda software, and the spatial correlation characteristics of grain production are shown in Table 3.

It can be seen from Table 3 that the Moran's I values from 1995 to 2018 were all greater than 0 and significant at the threshold level of 5%, indicating that the grain yield per unit sown area in the HHH was not randomly distributed but positively correlated. This indicates that the grain production layout showed strong spatial clustering characteristics. From 1995 to 1997, the Moran's I value decreased from 0.4114 to 0.1718. This indicates that the agglomeration and development trend in grain production in the HHH weakened during this period. From 1997 to 2002, the Moran's I value showed a fluctuating trend, ranging from 0.1718 to 0.3356. In this period, the grain production experienced a process of both agglomeration and dispersion development, but the change trend was small.

Table 3. Moran's I value of grain production in HHH.

Year	Moran's I	Z-Score	p	Year	Moran's I	Z-Score	p
1995	0.4114	5.0799	0.001 ***	2007	0.2371	3.0493	0.01 **
1996	0.3186	3.9572	0.001 ***	2008	0.2416	3.0646	0.01 **
1997	0.1718	2.2349	0.01 **	2009	0.2751	3.5401	0.001 ***
1998	0.3356	4.1347	0.001 ***	2010	0.2852	3.5766	0.001 ***
1999	0.3257	4.0797	0.001 ***	2011	0.2897	3.6144	0.001 ***
2000	0.3429	4.2799	0.001 ***	2012	0.2401	3.0216	0.01 **
2001	0.3286	4.1561	0.001 ***	2013	0.2529	3.1792	0.01 **
2002	0.2511	3.2294	0.001 ***	2014	0.3727	4.5792	0.001 ***
2003	0.5243	6.2996	0.001 ***	2015	0.3498	4.3184	0.001 ***
2004	0.2998	3.7368	0.001 ***	2016	0.2833	3.7924	0.001 ***
2005	0.3008	3.7651	0.001 ***	2017	0.2602	3.5101	0.001 ***
2006	0.2397	3.0403	0.01 **	2018	0.2315	3.1292	0.01 **

*** means significant at the 1% threshold level; ** means significant at the 5% threshold level.

From 2002 to 2006, the Moran's I value showed "up–down" fluctuation characteristics twice, and the change trend was more intense. This indicates that the grain production pattern of the HHH was greatly changed during this period. From 2007 to 2011, the increase in Moran's I value indicated that the grain production distribution in the HHH was in an increasingly concentrated state in this period. From 2011 to 2012, the Moran's I value changed from 0.2897 to 0.2401, a decrease by 0.0496 units, indicating that the clustering characteristics of grain production layout weakened during this period.

The Moran's I value showed a continuous rising trend, indicating that the clustering characteristics of grain production distribution were enhanced from 2012 to 2014. The value of Moran's *I* changed from 0.3727 to 0.2315 in 2014–2018, indicating that the agglomeration characteristics of grain production distribution during this period weakened. On the whole, the Moran's *I* value experienced a change process of "down–up–down" in this period; however, the agglomeration and distribution characteristics of grain production did not change.

4.4.2. Local Spatial Correlation Characteristics

The evaluation of the global spatial correlation feature has the defect of ignoring the instability of local spatial processes. Therefore, the local spatial correlation characteristics of grain production in the HHH can be analyzed by observing the G_i^* index in 1995, 2005, 2015, and 2018 (Figure 5).

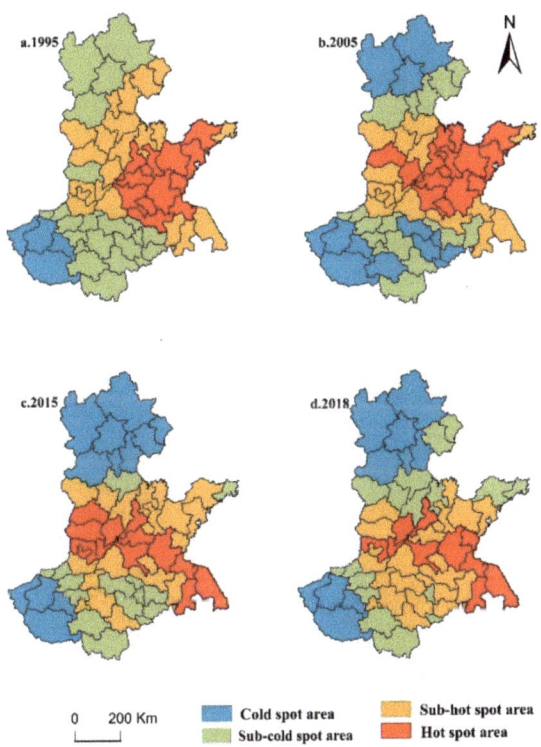

Figure 5. Spatial correlation characteristics of grain production in the HHH. (**a**) 1995, (**b**) 2005, (**c**) 2015, and (**d**) 2018.

According to Figure 5, the numbers of hot spots, sub-hot spots, sub-cold spots and cold spots were 13, 21, 21, and 4, respectively, in 1995, and the cold spots were mainly distributed in Sanmenxia, Luoyang, and Nanyang. The sub-cold spots were distributed in Beijing, Zhangjiakou, Chengde, Baoding, Jiaozuo, Xinxiang, Zhengzhou, Kaifeng, Zhoukou, Zhumadian, Xinyang, Fuyang, Bengbu, Huainan, and Bozhou. Sub-hot spots were concentrated in Tianjin, Qinhuangdao, Langfang, Cangzhou, Hengshui, Xingtai, Shijiazhuang, Dezhou, Binzhou, Dongying, Heze, Anyang, Hebi, and Puyang. Hot spots were distributed in the eastern part of the HHH. In particular, Yantai, Qingdao, Weifang, Jinan, Rizhao, Linyi, Zaozhuang, Jining, Lianyungang and Xuzhou were the most typical ones.

In 2005, the numbers of cities in the four categories were 16, 14, 16, and 13. Compared with 1995, the number of cities in hot spots and cold spots increased, indicating that the agglomeration of grain production increased from 1995 to 2005. The cold spots were concentrated in the north and southwest of the HHH. The sub-cold spots were distributed in Qinhuangdao, Tangshan, Tianjin, Langfang, Baoding, Xinyang, Fuyang, Zhoukou, Xuchang, Zhengzhou, and Jiaozuo. The sub-hot spots continued to shrink, and were mainly distributed in Shijiazhuang, Cangzhou, and Hengshui. The spatial distribution of hot spots is clear, and the main distribution was in the middle and eastern part of the HHH. In 2015, the numbers of hot spots, sub-hot spots, sub-cold spots, and cold spots were 13, 20, 14, and 12 cities, respectively.

Compared with 2005, the number of cities in hot spots and cold spots decreased by 3 and 1, respectively, indicating that the local spatial clustering characteristics of grain production in the HHH were weakened from 2005 to 2015. In 2018, the hot spots, sub-hot spots, sub-cold spots, and cold spots included 10, 17, 22, and 10 cities, respectively. Compared with 2015, the number of cities in hot spots and cold spots decreased by three and two, and the number of cities in sub-hot spots increased by eight. This indicates that the local spatial agglomeration characteristics of grain production in the Huang-Huai-Hai Plain gradually weakened from 2005. In general, hot spots spread from the east of the HHH to the southeast and the central region, and sub-hot spots were mainly distributed in the central region. The cold spots and sub-cold spots were mainly distributed in the north and south regions.

4.5. Influencing Factors for the Changes of Grain Production in the HHH

4.5.1. Analysis of the Spatial Spillover Effect of the Influencing Factors

First, SPSS software was used to eliminate the collinearity of variables, and finally four indexes were extracted, namely, the effective irrigation area (EIA), amount of fertilizer application per unit of sown area (AFA), per capita annual income of rural residents (PCI), and annual average precipitation (PRE). In addition, 3.3 proves that the grain production pattern in the HHH has dependent characteristics; therefore, the influence of the spatial spillover effect cannot be ignored. Secondly, the GeoDa software was used to obtain the parameter estimation results of the spatial lag model, spatial error model, and OLS model. Finally, the statistical values of LMLAG and R-LMLAG in the OLS results were significantly higher than those of LMERR and R-LMERR at the 10% level; as such, it was appropriate to use the spatial lag model to explore the key factors affecting grain production (Table 4).

According to Table 4, the coefficients of EIA were 0.505, 0.415, 0.532, and 0.588 in 1995, 2005, 2015, and 2018, respectively, and were effective at the 1% threshold level. This indicates that there was a positive correlation between the EIA and grain yield; that is, an increase in the EIA will bring about an increase in the grain yield. At the same time, the coefficient of EIA on the whole was on the rise, indicating that it has a stronger positive effect on grain yield. The continuous improvement of irrigation and water conservancy facilities in the HHH is the reason for this phenomenon.

The coefficients of fertilizer application per unit of sown area in 1995 and 2005 were 0.008 and 0.208, respectively, which were both significant at the 1% threshold level, and the coefficients in 2015 and 2018 were 0.124 and 0.023, respectively, and were significant at the 5% threshold level. This shows that the positive effect of chemical fertilizer application per unit of sown area on grain production experienced a changing process of decline after rising first, reflecting that the increase in chemical fertilizer application per sown area from 1995 to 2005 significantly increased the grain production in the HHH.

From 2005 to 2018, the boosting effect on grain production was alleviated. The reason for this phenomenon may be that the increase in the use of chemical fertilizers in the low-level agricultural development stage has a significant effect on increasing grain production. As the amount of fertilizer input remains at a high level, the effect of increasing the amount of fertilizer input in the future is limited as regards improving the grain yield. The coefficients of rural residents' per capita annual income in the four time sections were 0.405, 0.170, 0.124, and 0.050, which passed the significance tests at the critical value levels of 1%, 5%, 10%, and 10%, respectively.

The increase in per capita annual income continued to weaken the boost to grain production. The reason is that agriculture has been the main source of income for Chinese farmers to maintain their livelihoods for a long time. As farmers' income levels increase, they have more funds to purchase agricultural machinery, fertilizers, pesticides, seeds, and other production materials, thereby achieving the goal of increasing grain yield. With the rapid advancement of urbanization, farmers' income channels have become increasingly diversified, which has greatly reduced their dependence on agriculture, and the tendency of farmers to invest in non-agriculture has become more obvious. Therefore, to some extent, the increase in PCI has an inhibitory effect on grain output.

The coefficient of PRE was 0.508 in 1995 and passed the significance test of the 1% critical value level, indicating that the increase in PRE in that year played a promoting role in grain production. The coefficients of PRE were 0.016 and 0.148 in 2005 and 2015, both of which failed to pass the 10% significance test, indicating that the PRE increase did not have an obvious positive promotion effect on grain production. The underlying reason may be that with the continuous improvement of irrigation facilities, the impact of changes in PRE on grain production became weaker.

Table 4. Regression analysis results of the spatial lag model.

Model Variables	1995		2005		2015		2018	
	Coefficient	Standard Deviation	Coefficient	Standard Deviation	Coefficient	Standard Deviation	Coefficient	Standard Deviation
Constant	0.036	1.433	5.516	0.914	5.215 ***	1.155	8.665 ***	1.749
EIA	0.505 ***	0.072	0.415 ***	0.048	0.532 ***	0.081	0.588 ***	0.099
AFA	0.008 **	0.004	0.208 ***	0.053	0.124 **	0.053	0.023 **	0.029
PCI	0.405 ***	0.109	0.170 **	0.068	0.124 *	0.090	0.050 *	0.069
PRE	0.508 ***	0.170	0.016	0.794	0.148	0.099	0.022	0.061
R^2	0.729		0.779		0.656		0.529	
AIC	−34.039		−87.236		−85.007		−95.487	

*** means significant at the 1% threshold level; ** means significant at the 5% threshold level; * means significant at the 10% threshold level.

4.5.2. Analysis of Spatial Heterogeneity of Influencing Factors

Based on the above research findings, the EIA, AFA, and PCI had a significant impact on the grain production in the HHH. However, SLM cannot explain the specific degree and scope of the impact of these three factors in space, and so a GWR model was explored to investigate the spatial difference in the influence of these three factors. The three factors—EIA, AFA, and PCI—were put into the model according to the criteria of AICc minimization.

The spatial distribution of Local R-squared values derived from the GWR model is displayed in Figure 6. The GWR results show that three factors explain 81.1% of the variance in grain production. Geographic variations in these factors describe a difference in the combined statistical influence of the three variables on grain production across cities in the HHH, from a very weak relationship (near 0.30) to a strong relationship (>0.80). We found that 50.94% of cities maintained local R-squared values of more than 50%. The predictive power of the model shows characteristics of increasing from east to west. The local R-squared map suggests that the predictive power of the analysis was greatest in relation to the northern part (Chengde, Baoding, and Zhangjiakou) and the southwestern part (Jiaozuo, Jiyuan, and Sanmenxia). The lower R-squared values demonstrate a poorer regression fit in the eastern parts of the HHH, such as Weihai, Yantai, and Qingdao.

To explore the strength of the influence of each of the three factors on grain production, we created maps for each factor, which represent the geographic distribution of their regression coefficient values across HHH, according to the results of the GWR modeling. The mapped regression coefficients are divided into five classifications through Natural Breaks. In Figure 7, white is used to indicate cities without data, and gradient shading is used to show cities with a significant relationship between variables and grain production.

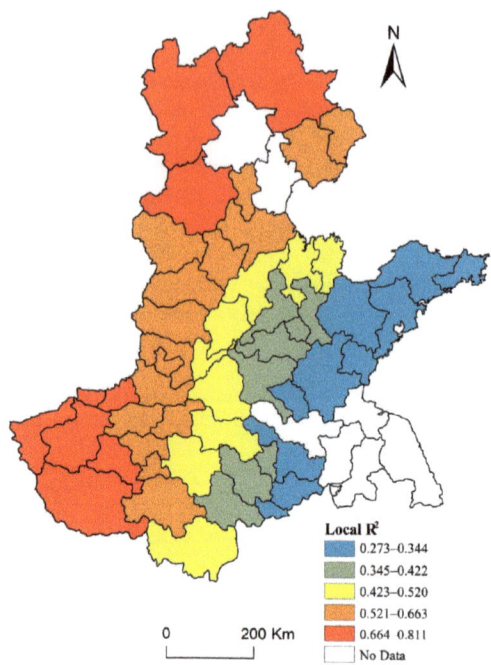

Figure 6. R-squared values derived from the geographical weighted regression (GWR) model.

The proportion of the effective irrigated area had a positive impact on grain production in the HHH, and its impact intensity presents a spatial distribution characteristic of "low west and high east". A total of 75.47% of the cities showed a significant positive relationship between the effective irrigate area and production, mainly in Hebei and Henan provinces. The reason may be that these two provinces are mostly inland, with relatively drier climate and less rainfall; therefore, irrigation is mainly used to supply the water requirement of crops.

AFA had a positive effect on 94.34% of the cities in the HHH, which can significantly increase the food production of 39.62% of the cities, mainly in the central, northern, and southern regions of the HHH, such as Zhangjiakou, Puyang, and Fuyang. AFA had a negative effect on 5.66% of the cities, mainly in the eastern part of the HHH, such as Qingdao and Weifang. The impact of AFA on grain production is limited. In particular, with the long-term investment of chemical fertilizers by Chinese farmers on cultivated land, the impact of various chemical fertilizers applied by farmers on soil fertility has become nearly saturated. The majority of the chemical fertilizers play a role in maintaining soil fertility after application, so even if the input of chemical fertilizers is increased, the positive effect on crop yield is not clear enough.

The per capita income of rural residents had a positive impact on 86.79% of the cities in the HHH, of which only 9.43% passed the significance test, mainly in the northeastern part of the HHH, such as Chengde, Qinhuangdao, Tangshan, Langfang, and Cangzhou. The per capita income of rural residents had a negative impact on 13.21% of cities, and was concentrated in the southwestern region of HHH, that is, the western and southern regions of Henan Province, such as Sanmenxia, Nanyang, and Xinyang. As rural residents flow into developed urban areas, the non-agricultural income they earn from moving into cities has gradually become an important source of livelihood, and their dependence and emphasis on agriculture has gradually decreased; abandonment can even occur, which causes a huge negative impact on grain production.

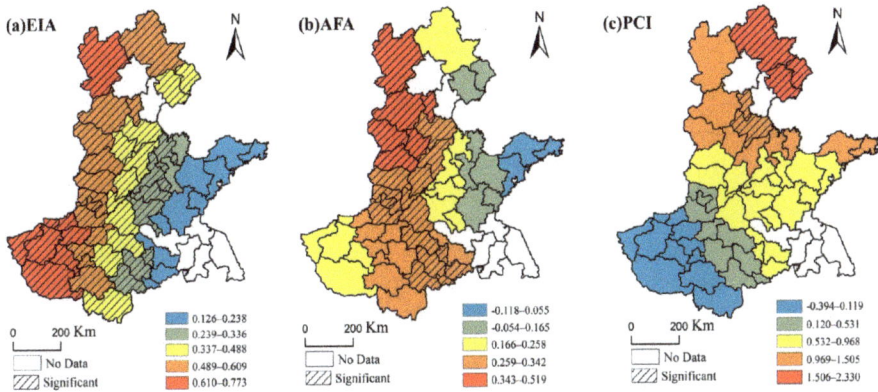

Figure 7. The spatial distribution of regression coefficients for the three factors based on a GWR model for 2018 in the HHH.

5. Discussions

Even our results suggested that the effect of precipitation on grain production became weaker, we should also be aware of the relationship between rainfall and groundwater; that is, rainfall becomes groundwater through infiltration, providing sufficient water for irrigating crops. With the improvement in irrigation facilities, irrigation has gradually become an indispensable and important means for stable grain production. This may also be the reason why the direct impact of PRE on grain production is gradually weakening and why the EIA is gradually increasing. Future research should focus on related research in this area. The reasons for the insignificant effect of temperature and sunshine duration may be attributed to two points: first, compared with precipitation, the heat resources of the HHH can well meet the growth needs of winter wheat and summer corn, and the yield is less affected by temperature and sunshine duration. At the same time, an increase in temperature and sunshine duration may increase evaporation, thereby offsetting the effect of precipitation. It is also possible to attribute this effect to precipitation rather than temperature and sunshine duration. Second, it may be that the crops in the research area are not subdivided. Different crops have inconsistent requirements for temperature and sunshine duration, which may weaken the effects of temperature and sunshine duration. This will also be the focus of future research. China's food self-sufficiency rate has reached more than 95%. The concept of "with grain in the hand, the heart is unharried" has been made reality. However, in the face of the impact of global warming and COVID-19, as well as the requirements of new urbanization, as a country with one of the largest populations in the world, ensuring the stability of China's food supply is not only related to national security, but is also related to the stability of the world.

Therefore, based on the results of this paper, the following policy suggestions are put forward to increase grain production in the HHH, an important grain production base for food security in China to maintain China's food security. The suggestions include the following: to increase the construction investment for basic farmland infrastructures, such as irrigation facilities; to cultivate and promote good varieties and treatments, and implement soil testing and formula fertilization; to standardize the rural land market; to promote the transfer of rural land in an orderly manner; and to realize the large-scale management of cultivated land.

However, the impact of relevant agricultural policies issued by the country also needs to be considered in the future. From 1995 to 2018, the overall increase in grain production in HHH and the gradual reduction in spatial differences well reflects the background and national policies of the country in different periods. Since 1995, with the advancement of agricultural technology, the agricultural development of the HHH has been weakened by natural conditions, and the grain production has increased significantly [13]. At the same time, due to the popularization of fertilizers, pesticides, and irrigation, the gap in grain production in various regions in HHH is also narrowing.

Due to rapid urbanization, the conversion of fertile irrigated land to non-agricultural land seems to pose a potential threat to the food security of the HHH, and even to the whole of China [10]. Moreover, farmers are gradually migrating to cities in search of higher incomes due to the urban–rural development gap [44], which has caused the arable land in the HHH to be abandoned, resulting in the expansion of spatial differences in grain production in different regions in the HHH, and also threatening national food security. In order to ensure national food security, the central government proposed the construction of "high-standard basic farmland projects" and "agricultural modernization" to promote the large-scale, intensive, and modernized management of arable land in the HHH, thereby increasing the grain production of the HHH, and promoting the development of sustainable agriculture.

At the same time, we should not ignore the resistance, created by resource endowments, to sustainable agriculture in the HHH. In particular, the precipitation cannot meet the water demand of the crops [8,45], and water shortage is one of the major factors threatening the high and stable production of wheat [20]. The water consumption greatly exceeds the precipitation, and groundwater must be extracted to make up for the deficiency so as to maintain high yields [21]. Some areas in the HHH even appear salinized due to unreasonable irrigation [10], which poses huge challenges for the minimization of environmental impacts and the development of sustainable agriculture [46,47]. Therefore, the government must not only build irrigation facilities, but more importantly, must promote water-saving irrigation technologies, improve water resource utilization efficiency, implement drip irrigation and sprinkler irrigation [46], etc., so as to achieve sustainable agricultural production in the HHH. At the same time, in the long run, in the face of the encroachment of arable land in the promotion of urbanization, the amount of arable land in the future will also face severe challenges [10]. Promoting intensive agricultural production and improving the level of intensive use of agricultural production are also of great significance to ensure future food production [48]. Moreover, these actions can also enhance the ability to respond to natural disasters in the future. However, a sustainable food and agriculture system is one which is environmentally sound, economically viable, socially responsible, nonexploitative, and which serves as the foundation for future generations [49–51]. With the long-term development of intensive agriculture production in the Huang-Huai-Hai Plain, agricultural practices ranging from the development of irrigation projects to the use of agrichemicals have often had negative environmental impacts, such as wildlife kills, pesticide residues in drinking water, soil erosion, groundwater depletion, and salinization [52]. Substituting environmentally sound inputs for those which are damaging is an important step in addressing these problems [49]. In view of this, the Ministry of agriculture of China started the construction of the Key Laboratory of Agricultural Environment in the Huang-Huai-Hai Plain, with the objectives of scientific research, environmental monitoring, detection analysis and technical services, in 2012, aiming to carry out research on regional agricultural pollution prevention by means of agricultural non-point source pollution prevention, the environmental protection of producing areas, and the development and application of environment-friendly inputs. However, for the farmers who are the main body of agricultural production, whether these agricultural technology inputs will increase agricultural production costs and reduce agricultural income will be an important factor affecting the promotion of agricultural technology and the development of sustainable agriculture. Therefore, whether the economic, social and environmental benefits generated by agricultural production in the Huang-Huai-Hai Plain under the influence of agriculture technology can achieve a balance will be the focus of our future research.

6. Conclusions

In this paper, exploratory spatial data analysis, the gravity center model, and the spatial lag model were used to explore the spatial–temporal variation and influencing factors of the grain production pattern in the HHH from 1995 to 2018. The main conclusions were drawn as follows:

The grain production pattern in the HHH has the characteristics of being non-equilibrated in space and non-stationary in time. The spatial non-equilibrium is reflected in the shift of the grain production center from the southeast to the northwest of Tai'an city. The high-level areas of grain production capacity were mainly distributed in the east and south, while the low-level areas were distributed in the west and north. The non-stationarity of time is reflected in the rising trend in the grain production capacity and the weakening of the non-stationarity of time in the grain production center over time;

The global and local spatial agglomeration characteristics of grain production in the HHH were significant. The global spatial correlation characteristics underwent a "decrease–growth–decrease" change process, and the local spatial correlation characteristics demonstrated a concentrated distribution. Specifically, the hot spots were mainly distributed in the central and eastern regions of the HHH, and the cold spots were distributed in the north and southwest. The global and local spatial autocorrelation characteristics showed that the polarization of grain production in local areas has gradually weakened and the spatial difference has gradually decreased in the HHH, which indicates that its agricultural production has gradually shifted in the direction of sustainable development;

The impact of social–economic factors on grain production was constantly strengthened and the influence of climate factors on grain production was gradually weakened. EIA, AFA, and PCI helped to increase the grain yield per unit of sown area in the HHH; however, the effect of the PRE on grain production became weaker as time went on. We adopted the GWR model to prove that the EIA, AFA, and PCI had clear spatial heterogeneity in the intensity and direction of the local scale. The results showed that the EIA had a larger impact on grain production in the HHH compared with other factors, with the percentage of significance at 75.47%.

Author Contributions: C.Z. and X.N. developed the main ideas of the study, gathered the data, performed the model construction and estimation, and wrote the manuscript. R.Z. helped to collect and process data. Z.Z. participated in revising the manuscript and proofreading the article. All authors have read and agreed to the published version of the manuscript.

Funding: This research was funded by National Natural Science Foundation of China [41771190].

Conflicts of Interest: The authors declare no conflict of interest.

References

1. Mingzhi, Y.; Yuansheng, P.; Xudong, L. Study on grain self-sufficiency rate in China: An analysis of grain, cereal grain and edible grain. *J. Nat. Resour.* **2019**, *34*, 881–889.
2. Gandhi, V.P.; Zhou, Z. Food demand and the food security challenge with rapid economic growth in the emerging economies of India and China. *Food Res. Int.* **2014**, *63*, 108–124. [CrossRef]
3. Maitra, C.; Rao, D.S.P. Poverty–Food Security Nexus: Evidence from a Survey of Urban Slum Dwellers in Kolkata. *World Dev.* **2015**, *72*, 308–325. [CrossRef]
4. Climate Change and Land: An IPCC Special Report on Climate Change, Desertification, Land Degradation, Sustainable Land Management, Food Security, and Greenhouse Gas Fluxes in Terrestrial Ecosystems. Available online: https://www.ipcc.ch/srccl/ (accessed on 8 December 2020).
5. Wang, J.; Zhang, Z.; Liu, Y. Spatial shifts in grain production increases in China and implications for food security. *Land Use Policy* **2018**, *74*, 204–213. [CrossRef]
6. Zhang, J.; Zhang, F.; Zhang, D.; He, D.; Zhang, L.; Wu, C.; Kong, X. The grain potential of cultivated lands in Mainland China in 2004. *Land Use Policy* **2009**, *26*, 68–76. [CrossRef]
7. Xie, Z.; Qin, Y.; Li, Y.; Shen, W.; Zheng, Z.; Liu, S. Spatial and temporal differentiation of COVID-19 epidemic spread in mainland China and its influencing factors. *Sci. Total Environ.* **2020**, *744*, 140929. [CrossRef] [PubMed]
8. Tuan, N.T.; Qiu, J.-J.; Verdoodt, A.; Li, H.; Van Ranst, E. Temperature and Precipitation Suitability Evaluation for the Winter Wheat and Summer Maize Cropping System in the Huang-Huai-Hai Plain of China. *Agric. Sci. China* **2011**, *10*, 275–288. [CrossRef]
9. Yang, J.-Y.; Mei, X.-R.; Huo, Z.-G.; Yan, C.; Ju, H.; Zhao, F.-H.; Liu, Q. Water consumption in summer maize and winter wheat cropping system based on SEBAL model in Huang-Huai-Hai Plain, China. *J. Integr. Agric.* **2015**, *14*, 2065–2076. [CrossRef]
10. Shi, W.; Tao, F.; Liu, J. Changes in quantity and quality of cropland and the implications for grain production in the Huang-Huai-Hai Plain of China. *Food Secur.* **2012**, *5*, 69–82. [CrossRef]

11. He, J.; Shi, Y.; Zhao, J.; Yu, Z. Strip rotary tillage with subsoiling increases winter wheat yield by alleviating leaf senescence and increasing grain filling. *Crop J.* **2020**, *8*, 327–340. [CrossRef]
12. Wang, P.; Wu, D.; Yang, J.; Ma, Y.; Feng, R.; Huo, Z. Summer maize growth under different precipitation years in the Huang-Huai-Hai Plain of China. *Agric. For. Meteorol.* **2020**, *285–286*, 107927. [CrossRef]
13. Liu, Y.; Gao, B.; Pan, Y.; Ren, X. Influencing factor decomposition of grain production at county level in Huang-Huai-Hai region based on LMDI. *Trans. Chin. Soc. Agric. Eng.* **2013**, *29*, 1–10.
14. Liu, Y.; Liu, J.; Zhang, J.; Chen, Y.; Xu, M.; Wang, C. A Study on the Driving Factors of Food Production in Huang-Huai-Hai Plain Based on Path Analysis. *Asain Agric. Res.* **2015**, *7*, 27–32.
15. Liu, Y.; Tang, X.; Pan, Y.; Tang, L. Analysis on spatial spillover effect and influence factors of grain yield per hectare at county level in Huang-Huai-Hai region. *Trans. Chin. Soc. Agric. Eng.* **2016**, *32*, 299–307.
16. Ge, D.; Long, A.H. Coupling Relationship Between Land Use Transitions and Grain Yield in the Huang-Huai-Hai Plain, China. *Comput. Sci.* **2017**, 1–6. [CrossRef]
17. Wu, L.; Chen, F.; Ou, Y.; Zhang, Q. The relationship between grain output and fertilizer input in wheat-corn cropping area of the Huang-Huai-Hai plain. *Plant Nutr. Fertilizer Sci.* **2003**, *9*, 257–263.
18. Tao, F.; Xiao, D.; Zhang, S.; Zhang, Z.; Rötter, R.P. Wheat yield benefited from increases in minimum temperature in the Huang-Huai-Hai Plain of China in the past three decades. *Agric. For. Meteorol.* **2017**, *239*, 1–14. [CrossRef]
19. Liu, Y.; Wang, E.; Yang, X.; Wang, J. Contributions of climatic and crop varietal changes to crop production in the North China Plain, since 1980s. *Glob. Chang. Biol.* **2009**, *16*, 2287–2299. [CrossRef]
20. Qu, C.-H.; Li, X.-X.; Ju, H.; Liu, Q. The impacts of climate change on wheat yield in the Huang-Huai-Hai Plain of China using DSSAT-CERES-Wheat model under different climate scenarios. *J. Integr. Agric.* **2019**, *18*, 1379–1391. [CrossRef]
21. Tang, X.; Song, N.; Chen, Z.; Wang, J.; He, J. ETc of winter wheat across HuangHuai-Hai Plain in the future with the modfied DSSAT model. *Sci. Rep.* **2018**, *8*, 15370. [CrossRef]
22. Chen, C.-Q.; Lu, W.-T.; Sun, X.-S.; Yu, H. Regional Differences of Winter Wheat Phenophase and Grain Yields Response to Global Warming in the Huang-Huai-Hai Plain in China Since 1980s. *Int. J. Plant Prod.* **2017**, *12*, 33–41. [CrossRef]
23. Xiao, D.; Qi, Y.; Li, Z.; Wang, R.; Moiwo, J.P.; Liu, F. Impact of thermal time shift on wheat phenology and yield under warming climate in the Huang-Huai-Hai Plain, China. *Front. Earth Sci.* **2017**, *11*, 148–155. [CrossRef]
24. Li, Y.; Xie, Z.; Qin, Y.; Zhou, S. Spatio-temporal variations in precipitation on the Huang-Huai-Hai Plain from 1963 to 2012. *J. Earth Syst. Sci.* **2018**, *127*, 101. [CrossRef]
25. Yin, J.; Yan, D.; Yang, Z.; Yuan, Z.; Yuan, Y.; Zhang, C. Projection of extreme precipitation in the context of climate change in Huang-Huai-Hai region, China. *J. Earth Syst. Sci.* **2016**, *125*, 417–429. [CrossRef]
26. Alam, M.; Siwar, C.; Jaafar, A.; Talib, B.A.; Salleh, K. Agricultural Vulnerability and Adaptation to Climatic Changes in Malaysia: Review on Paddy Sector. *Curr. World Environ.* **2013**, *8*, 1–12. [CrossRef]
27. Wei, X.; Erda, L.I.N.; Jinhe, J.; Yan, L.I.; Yinlong, X.U. An Integrated Analysis of Impact Factors in Determining China's Future Grain Production. *Acta Geogr. Sin.* **2010**, *65*, 397–406.
28. Ning, X.; Qin, Y.; Cui, Y.; Li, X.; Chen, Y. The spatio-temporal change of agricultural hydrothermal conditions in China from 1951 to 2010. *Acta Geogr. Sin.* **2015**, *70*, 364–379.
29. Zhang, R.; Ning, X.; Qin, Y.; Zhao, K.; Li, Y. Analysis of sensitivity of main grain crops yield to climate change since 1980 in Henan Province. *Resour. Sci.* **2018**, *40*, 137–149.
30. Haining, R. *Spatial Data Analysis in the Social and Environmental Sciences*; Cambridge University Press: Cambridge, UK, 1997.
31. Ye, W.F.; Ma, Z.Y.; Ha, X.Z. Spatial-temporal patterns of PM2.5 concentrations for 338 Chinese cities. *Sci. Total Environ.* **2018**, *631–632*, 524–533. [CrossRef]
32. Anselin, L. *Spatial Econometrics: Methods and Models*; Kluwer Academic Publishers: Boston, MA, USA, 1988.
33. Moran, P.A.P. The interpretation of statistical maps. *J. R. Stat. Soc. Ser. B Methodol.* **1948**, *10*, 243–251. [CrossRef]
34. Getis, J.K.O.A. Local spatial autocorrelation statistics: Distributional issues and an application. *Geogr. Anal.* **1995**, *27*, 286–306.
35. Li, C.Y.; Wang, X.H.; Xie, Z.X.; Qin, M.Z. Evolution of Patterns in the Ratio of Gender at Birth in Henan province, China. *Probl. Ekorozw.* **2018**, *13*, 59–67.

36. Wang, Y.Z.; Duan, X.J.; Wang, L. Spatial-Temporal Evolution of $PM_{2.5}$ Concentration and its Socioeconomic Influence Factors in Chinese Cities in 2014–2017. *Int. J. Environ. Res. Public Health* **2019**, *16*, 18. [CrossRef] [PubMed]
37. Rong, P.J.; Zhang, L.J.; Qin, Y.C.; Xie, Z.X.; Li, Y.N. Spatial differentiation of daily travel carbon emissions in small- and medium-sized cities: An empirical study in Kaifeng, China. *J. Clean. Prod.* **2018**, *197*, 1365–1373. [CrossRef]
38. Golpira, H.; Messina, A.R. A Center-of-Gravity-Based Approach to Estimate Slow Power and Frequency Variations. *IEEE Trans. Power Syst.* **2018**, *33*, 1026–1035. [CrossRef]
39. Elhorst, J.P. Applied Spatial Econometrics: Raising the Bar. *Spat. Econ. Anal.* **2010**, *5*, 9–28. [CrossRef]
40. Lu, J.F.; Zhang, L.J. Evaluation of Parameter Estimation Methods for Fitting Spatial Regression Models. *For. Sci.* **2010**, *56*, 505–514.
41. Baltagi, B.H.; Bresson, G.; Etienne, J.M. Hedonic Housing Prices In Paris: An Unbalanced Spatial Lag Pseudo-Panel Model With Nested Random Effects. *J. Appl. Econom.* **2015**, *30*, 509–528. [CrossRef]
42. Tobler, W.R. A Computer Movie Simulating Urban Growth in the Detroit Region. *Econ. Geogr.* **1970**, *46* (Suppl. S1), 234–240. [CrossRef]
43. Chen, J.; Zhou, C.; Wang, S.; Hu, J. Identifying the socioeconomic determinants of population exposure to particulate matter ($PM_{2.5}$) in China using geographically weighted regression modeling. *Environ. Pollut.* **2018**, *241*, 494–503. [CrossRef]
44. Liu, Y.; Zhang, R.; Li, M.; Zhou, C. What Factors Influence Rural-To-Urban Migrant Peasants to Rent out Their Household Farmland? Evidence from China's Pearl River Delta. *Land* **2020**, *9*, 418. [CrossRef]
45. Zhang, H.; Wang, X.; You, M.; Liu, C. Water-yield relations and water-use efficiency of winter wheat in the North China Plain. *Irrig. Sci.* **1999**, *19*, 37–45. [CrossRef]
46. Khan, S.; Hanjra, M.A.; Mu, J. Water management and crop production for food security in China: A review. *Agric. Water Manag.* **2009**, *96*, 349–360. [CrossRef]
47. Tilman, D.; Cassman, K.G.; Matson, P.A.; Naylor, R.; Polasky, S. Agricultural sustainability and intensive production practices. *Nature* **2002**, *418*, 671–677. [CrossRef] [PubMed]
48. Tan, R.; Beckmann, V.; Berg, L.V.D.; Qu, F. Governing farmland conversion: Comparing China with the Netherlands and Germany. *Land Use Policy* **2009**, *26*, 961–974. [CrossRef]
49. Allen, P.; Dusen, D.V.; Lundy, J.; Gliessman, S. Expanding the Definition of Sustainable Agriculture. *Sustain. Balance* **1991**, *3*, 1–8.
50. Velten, S.; Leventon, J.; Jager, N.W.; Newig, J. What is Sustainable Agriculture? A Systematic Review. *Sustainability* **2015**, *7*, 7833–7865. [CrossRef]
51. Pretty, J. Agricultural sustainability: Concepts, principles and evidence. *Philos. Trans. R Soc. Lond. B Biol. Sci.* **2008**, *363*, 447–465. [CrossRef]
52. Garnett, T.; Appleby, M.C.; Balmford, A.; Bateman, I.J.; Benton, T.G.; Bloomer, P.; Burlingame, B.; Dawkins, M.; Dolan, L.; Fraser, D.; et al. Sustainable Intensification in Agriculture: Premises and Policies. *Science* **2013**, *341*, 33–34. [CrossRef]

Publisher's Note: MDPI stays neutral with regard to jurisdictional claims in published maps and institutional affiliations.

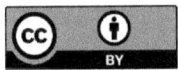

© 2020 by the authors. Licensee MDPI, Basel, Switzerland. This article is an open access article distributed under the terms and conditions of the Creative Commons Attribution (CC BY) license (http://creativecommons.org/licenses/by/4.0/).

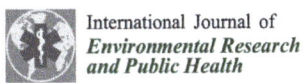

Article

Crepis vesicaria L. subsp. *taraxacifolia* Leaves: Nutritional Profile, Phenolic Composition and Biological Properties

Sónia Pedreiro [1,2], Sandrine da Ressurreição [3,4], Maria Lopes [1,2], Maria Teresa Cruz [1,5], Teresa Batista [1,6], Artur Figueirinha [1,2,*] and Fernando Ramos [1,2]

1. Faculty of Pharmacy, University of Coimbra, 3000-548 Coimbra, Portugal; soniaraquel_pedreiro@sapo.pt (S.P.); mlopes108@gmail.com (M.L.); trosete@ff.uc.pt (M.T.C.); mtpmb@ff.uc.pt (T.B.); framos@ff.uc.pt (F.R.)
2. LAQV, REQUIMTE, Faculty of Pharmacy, University of Coimbra, Azinhaga de Santa Comba, 3000-548 Coimbra, Portugal
3. Polytechnic of Coimbra, Coimbra Agriculture School, Bencanta, 3045-601 Coimbra, Portugal; sandrine@esac.pt
4. Research Centre for Natural Resources, Environment and Society (CERNAS), Escola Superior Agrária de Coimbra, Bencanta, 3045-601 Coimbra, Portugal
5. CNC-Center for Neuroscience and Cell Biology, University of Coimbra, 3000-548 Coimbra, Portugal
6. CIEPQPF, FFUC, Pólo das Ciências da Saúde, Azinhaga de Santa Comba, University of Coimbra, 3000-548 Coimbra, Portugal
* Correspondence: amfigueirinha@ff.uc.pt

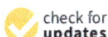

Abstract: *Crepis vesicaria* subsp. *taraxacifolia* (Cv) of Asteraceae family is used as food and in traditional medicine. However there are no studies on its nutritional value, phenolic composition and biological activities. In the present work, a nutritional analysis of Cv leaves was performed and its phenolic content and biological properties evaluated. The nutritional profile was achieved by gas chromatography (GC). A 70% ethanolic extract was prepared and characterized by HLPC-PDA-ESI/MS^n. The quantification of chicoric acid was determined by HPLC-PDA. Subsequently, it was evaluated its antioxidant activity by DPPH, ABTS and FRAP methods. The anti-inflammatory activity and cellular viability was assessed in Raw 264.7 macrophages. On wet weight basis, carbohydrates were the most abundant macronutrients (9.99%), followed by minerals (2.74%) (mainly K, Ca and Na), protein (1.04%) and lipids (0.69%), with a low energetic contribution (175.19 KJ/100 g). The Cv extract is constituted essentially by phenolic acids as caffeic, ferulic and quinic acid derivatives being the major phenolic constituent chicoric acid (130.5 mg/g extract). The extract exhibited antioxidant activity in DPPH, ABTS and FRAP assays and inhibited the nitric oxide (NO) production induced by LPS (IC$_{50}$ = 0.428 ± 0.007 mg/mL) without cytotoxicity at all concentrations tested. Conclusions: Given the nutritional and phenolic profile and antioxidant and anti-inflammatory properties, Cv could be a promising useful source of functional food ingredients.

Keywords: *Crepis vesicaria* L. subsp. *taraxacifolia*; nutritional value; phenolic profile; chicoric acid; antioxidant; anti-inflammatory

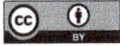

1. Introduction

The genus *Crepis* belongs to the Asteraceae family comprising about 200 species, and is widely distributed in the Northern Hemisphere, Africa and also in South East Asia [1]. The aerial parts and roots from the plants of the genus *Crepis* are widely used in foods like salads [2], infusions [3], decoctions [4], omelettes, pasta dough and pan-fried [2]. The plants of this genus are also used in traditional medicine to treat jaundice [5], hepatic disorders [6], cardiovascular diseases [7], cough [3,6], catarrh [3], cold [3], diabetes [4], kidney stones [8], eye diseases [6], abdominal colic [6], depurative, blood cleaning, laxative and as a diuretic [2]. It can be used externally in wound healing, bruises and inflammations [8].

Biological properties and phenolic composition have been evaluated for some species. Aerial part and root extracts of *Crepis foetida* L. subsp. *rhoeadifolia* showed antioxidant activity in DPPH and thiobarbituric acid reactive substances (TBARS) assays. In these extracts phenolic compounds to which antioxidant activity has been attributed were identified, namely chlorogenic acid and luteolin in the aerial parts and chlorogenic acid in the roots [7]. A methanolic extract from the flowers of this species showed that chlorogenic acid was the major phenolic compound. This extract presented high antiproliferative activity in HEPG-2, Caco-2, MCF-7 and MCF-10A cells, antioxidant (in DPPH, ABTS, nitric oxide and superoxide radical scavenging assays), anticholinesterase and antityrosinase activities [9]. Aqueous and ethanolic extracts of *Crepis japonica* L. showed antiproliferative activity against leukemia and sarcoma. Moreover, the ethanolic extract presented antiviral activity against respiratory syncytial vírus (anti-RSV). The phenolic content, including hydrolysable tannins may be responsible for this activity [10]. The 3,4-dicaffeoylquinic acid, 3,5-dicaffeoylquinic acid and luteolin-7-O-glucoside were isolated from the *Crepis japonica* ethanolic extract. The first two compounds exhibited significant anti-RSV activity. Moreover these three compounds together showed some antibacterial activity against *Vibrio cholerae* and *Vibrio parahaemolyticus* [11]. Besides these activities in this plant, anti-inflammatory, immunosuppressive, antiallergic, antioxidant, analgesic, central nervous system depressant and nematicidal activities were also reported [12].

It is known that reactive oxygen species (ROS), when unregulated, are related to several pathologies such as inflammation, through NF-kB signaling pathway activation [13]. The NF-kB transcription factor is present in the cytoplasm and is in its inactive state due to its association with the inhibitor complex of nuclear factor kappa B kinase (IKK). When this kinase is activated, NF-kB is released and enters the nucleus by activating the transcription of a variety of genes that participate in inflammatory and immune responses [14], such as interleukines IL-1β, IL-6 and IL-8, tumor necrosis factor-α (TNF-α) [15], prostaglandins [16], chemokine ligand 5 (CCL5), transcription of inducible nitric oxide synthase (iNOS), leading to the production of nitric oxide (NO) [17], and cyclooxygenase-2 (COX-2) [18], among others. Phenolic compounds such as phenolic acids, flavonoids and tannins have been identified as good radical scavengers [17]. The mechanisms by which they act in the radical scavenging are involved in signaling pathways of inflammation activation [13]. Phenolic acids presented anti-inflammatory activity acting mainly at the level of the proteasome, inhibiting this and, also, the activation of the NF-kB, since it maintains the phosphorylation levels of IkBα. These mechanisms were attributed to the action of chlorogenic acid, since this was identified as main phenolic acid together with *p*-coumaric acid derivatives [17]. These derivatives have been found to have the ability to inhibit iNOS-dependent NF-kB and COX-2 expression [19]. Phenolic acids from *Lippia* genus inhibited the carrageenan-induced pro-inflammatory cytokine production, namely IL-1β, IL-33 and TNF-α and consequently suppressed the NF-kB activation [16]. Polyphenols from *Ilex latifolia* Thunb. ethanolic extract showed high antioxidant and anti-inflammatory activities, through decreasing the production of NO, COX-2 and pro-inflammatory cytokines via inhibitions of MAPKs, namely ERK and JNK, and NF-kB activation [20]. In LPS-induced acute lung injury rats model, chlorogenic acid decreased the activity of iNOS and suppressing the activation of NF-kB [16]. Others phenolic compounds decreased TLR-4 upregulation, NOX activation and NF-kB activation in LPS-induced renal inflammation rat model [16]. The antioxidant and anti-inflammatory activities of rice bran (RB) phenolic compounds were evaluated in human umbilical vein endothelial cells (HUVECs) with induced oxidative stress. The RB extract regulated antioxidant genes, namely Nrf2, NQO1, HO1 and NOX4, as well anti-inflammatory genes (ICAM1, eNOS, CD39 and CD73). This activities were attributed to synergistic interactions between phenolic acids including *p*-coumaric acid, vanillic acid, caffeic acid, ferulic and syringic acid [21]. These studies support the correlation between oxidative stress and inflammation as well the biological effects of phenolic compounds on these.

There are no studies on phytochemical composition and biological activities of *Crepis vesicaria* L. subsp. *taraxacifolia* (Cv). Commonly known as beaked hawk's beard [2], this plant is used traditionally in foods and the treatment of diverse ailments. The cooking water of Cv young leaves are traditionally used as depurative, blood cleaning, diuretic and laxative [2]. Therefore it's important to study this phytoconstituents and to evaluate its health impact. In the present work, there was evaluated the phenolic and nutritional composition of Cv, as well assessed the antioxidant and anti-inflammatory activities.

2. Material and Methods

2.1. Plant Material and Extract Preparation

Crepis vesicaria L. subsp. *taraxacifolia* (Cv) plant was collected and identified by J. Paiva (Botany Department, University of Coimbra, Coimbra, Portugal). A voucher specimen (A. Figueirinha, 175) was deposited in the herbarium of the University of Coimbra, Faculty of Pharmacy. The leaves, dried in a circulating air drying oven, were milled in a knife mill (KSM 2, BRAUN, Frankfurt, Germany), avoiding the overheating of the sample, and sieved through a 60 mesh sieve. Subsequently, extracts were prepared from the powdered material with different solvents in a proportion of 1:100 (w/v). In order to improve the extraction of more active compounds, several extractions of Cv leaves (10 mg of dry plant/mL) were made with ethanol/water in various grades: 10%, 30%, 55%, 70% and 100% EtOH. The results of three independent assays showed that the reduction percentage of DPPH radical for the different extracts at 0.33 mg/mL was: 100% EtOH (28.22 ± 0.1575%) < 15% EtOH (66.92 ± 1.083%) < 30% EtOH (91.83 ± 0.602%) < 55% EtOH (90.96 ± 2.205%) < 70% EtOH extract (91.87 ± 2.066%). Thus, a leaves infusion of Cv (ICv) prepared according to its ethomedicinal uses, and 70% ethanol extracts were obtained. These extracts were filtered under vacuum, concentrated in a rotavapor at 40 °C, frozen, freeze-dried and kept at −20 °C in the dark until use. In the leaves 70% ethanol Cv extract (Cv 70% EtOH), a yield of 22.85% of dry plant was obtained. Relatively to ICv the yield of dry plant obtained was 30.1%. Both extracts were rich in soluble phenolics.

2.2. Chemical Characterization

2.2.1. Nutrient Composition Analysis

Proximate composition parameters were measured according to the international standards methods of Official Methods of Analysis of AOAC International [22], except neutral detergent fiber (NDF), acid detergent fiber (ADF) and acid detergent lignin (ADL) for calculation of cellulose, hemicellulose and lenhin, respectively [23]. Moisture evaluation was performed by oven drying sample at 105 °C until constant weight. Protein was determined by Kjeldahl method, using a protein conversion factor of 6.25. Lipids were gravimetrically quantified after a continuous extraction process in a Soxhlet apparatus by diethyl ether. Fatty acids were analysed by gas phase chromatography (GC-FID) of fatty acid methyl esters, and the quantification was performed by Supelco standards (Sigma-Aldrich, St Louis, MO, USA). The total dietary fiber, soluble and insoluble dietary fiber contents were determined using the Supelco enzyme kit TDF100A (Sigma-Aldrich). Crude fiber was gravimetrically quantified after chemical digestion and solubilisation of other materials. The fiber residue weight was then corrected for ash content. Ash was obtained by incineration of all organic matter of the sample in a muffle furnace at 550 °C. The Nitrogen-free extractives were estimated, considering the following equation: Nitrogen-free extractives = 100 − (moisture + ash + lipids + protein + crude fiber). The total carbohydrates were estimated, considering the following equation: Total carbohydrates = 100 − (moisture + ash + lipids + protein). Quantification and sugars were performed by High Performance Liquid Chromatography with refractive index detection (HPLC-RI). The separation column used was HC-75 Ca^{2+} 305 × 7.8 mm (Hamilton, Energy Way Reno, NV, USA) with ultrapure water with traces of sodium azide mobile phase, at a flow rate of 0.6 mL/min, at 80 °C. The quantification was performed by BioUltra standards (Sigma-Aldrich). The available carbohydrates were estimated, based on the following equation:

Available Carbohydrates = 100 − (moisture + ash + lipids + protein + dietary fiber). Quantification of sugars were performed by high performance liquid chromatography (HPLC), using BioUltra standards (Sigma-Aldrich). Energy values are expressed in Kcal and KJ/100 g and were calculated according to Regulation (EU) n° 1169/2011 of the European Parliament and of the Council of 25 October 2011. Minerals were determined by flame atomic absorption spectrometry (FAAS), with the exception of cadmium and lead traces, which were determined by graphite furnace atomic absorption spectrometry (GFAAS). Mercury traces was analysed by an AMA254 Mercury Analyzer (Leco, St Joseph, MI, USA) and phosphorus, by spectrophotometry.

2.2.2. Phenolic Profile HPLC-PDA-ESI/MS^n

The phenolic profile of Cv (ethanol 70% extract) was carried out on a liquid chromatograph (Finnigan Surveyor, THERMO, Waltham, MA, USA) with a Spherisorb ODS-2 column (150 × 2.1 mm i.d.; particle size, 3 μm; Waters Corp., Milford, MA, USA) and a Spherisorb ODS-2 guard cartridge (10 × 4.6 mm i.d.; particle size, 5 μm; Waters Corp. Milford, MA, USA). The separation occurred at 25 °C with a mobile phase constituted by 2% aqueous formic acid (v/v) (A) and methanol (B) in a discontinuous gradient of 5–15% B (0–10 min), 15–25% B (10–15 min), 25–50% B (15–40 min), 50–80% B (40–50 min), followed by an isocratic elution (50–60 min), a gradient 80–100% B (60–65 min) and other isocratic elution for 5 min, at a flow rate of 200 μL/min.

The first detection was done with a PDA detector ((Finnigan Surveyor, THERMO, Waltham, MA, USA)) at a wavelength range 200–400 nm, followed by a second detection using an Linear Ion Trap Mass Spectrometer (LIT-MS) (LTQ XL, Thermo Waltham, MA, USA). Mass spectra were obtained in the negative ion mode. The mass spectrometer acquired three consecutive spectra: full mass (m/z 125–1500), MS^2 of the most abundant ion in the full mass and MS^3 of the most abundant ion in the MS^2. Source voltage was 4.5 kV and the capillary temperature and voltage were 250 °C and −10 V, respectively. The sheath and auxiliary gas used was nitrogen at 20 Finnigan arbitrary units with helium as collision gas with a normalized energy of 45%. XCALIBUR software (Thermo, Waltham, MA, USA) was used for data treatment.

2.2.3. Quantification by HPLC-PDA

Quantification of L-chicoric acid in Cv 70% EtOH was performed in a chromatograph with a photodiode array (PDA) detector (Gilson Electronics SA, Villiers le Bel, France). The analysis were performed on a Spherisorb S5 ODS-2 column (250 × 4.6 mm i.d., 5 μm) (Waters Milford, MA, USA) with a C18 guard cartridge (30 × 4 mm i.d., 5 μm) (Nucleosil, Macherey-Nagel, Düren, Germany), at 24 °C. The mobile phase was constituted by methanol 100% (B) and formic acid 5% (A). The elution was made at a flow rate of 1 mL/min. The gradient used was: 5–15% B (0–10 min), 15–25% B (10–15 min), 25–50% B (15–40 min), 50–80% B (40–50 min) followed by an isocratic elution of 80% B (50–60 min), 80–100% B (60–70 min) and finally, an isocratic elution of 100% B (70–85 min). The volume of the sample injected was 100 μL. The UV-Visible spectra acquisition was performed between 200–600 nm and the chromatographic profiles were recorded at the wavelengths 280 and 320 nm. Data treatment was carried out with Unipoint®, version 2.10 software (Gilson, Middleton, WI, USA).

Quantification of the L-chicoric acid was performed using commercial standard dissolved in methanol (10 to 150 μg/mL) as external standard L-chicoric acid (Sigma Aldrich St. Louis, MO, USA). The chicoric acid present in the Cv 70% EtOH extract was quantified by the absorbance recorded in the chromatogram relative to this standard (330 nm). Three independent injections (100 μL) were performed in duplicate for each sample. The least-squares regression model was used to assess the correlation between peak area and concentration. The detection (LOD) and quantification (LOQ) limits were calculated from the calibration curve. The quantification of the chicoric acid in Cv 70% EtOH extract (identified first by HPLC-PDA-MS^n) was made using the standard calibration curve and the peak area of the compound.

2.3. Antioxidant Activity

2.3.1. 2,2-Diphenyl-1-Picrylhydrazyl Radical Assay (DPPH)

Free radical-scavenging activity of the infusion and ethanol/water Cv extracts was evaluated using the *DPPH* method previously described [24]. Briefly, aliquots of samples (100 µL) were assessed by their reactivity with methanolic solution of 500 µM *DPPH* (500 µL) in the presence of 100 mM acetate buffer, pH 6.0 (100 µL). The reaction mixtures (300 µL) were kept for 30 min at room temperature, in the dark. The decreases in the absorbance were measured at 517 nm, in a Thermo scientific multiskan FC plate reader. The % of reduction of *DPPH* of the Cv extracts were determined by:

$$\% \ reduction \ of \ DPPH = 100 - \frac{Abs \ sample - Abs \ control}{Abs \ control} \quad (1)$$

Posteriorly, the obtained values were plotted in a graph % of DPPH reduction vs. concentration in µg/mL. The IC_{50} was interpolated in the graph for the correspondent value of 50% reduction.

The results were expressed as Trolox equivalent (TE), defined as the concentration of the extract with antioxidant capacity equivalent to 1 mM of Trolox solution. This value was obtained interpolating the absorbance of 1 mM Trolox in the graph % of DPPH reduction vs. concentration. All the determinations were performed in triplicate.

2.3.2. Ferric Reducing Antioxidant Power Assay (FRAP)

Ferric reducing ability was evaluated with slight modifications [25]. The FRAP reagent was prepared by mixing 300 mM acetate buffer, 10 mL TPTZ (Sigma–Aldrich St. Louis, MO, USA) in 40 mM HCl and 20 mM $FeCl_3.6H_2O$ (Merck, Darmstadt, Germany) in the proportion of 10:1:1 ($v/v/v$). The extract (100 µL) was added to 3 mL of the FRAP reagent. An intense blue color complex was formed when ferric tripyridyl triazine (Fe^{3+} TPTZ) complex was reduced to ferrous (Fe^{2+}) form. The absorbance was measured at 593 nm, against a reagent blank, after incubation at room temperature for 6 min. The results were expressed as trolox equivalent (TE) values obtained using a calibration curve for Trolox (31.25–1000 mM). All the determinations were performed in triplicate.

2.3.3. 2,2'-Azinobis-(3-ethylbenzothiazoline-6-sulfonate) Assay (pH = 7) (ABTS)

The ABTS assay described by [26], consisted in generating the ABTS•+ radical by the oxidation of ABTS (7 mM) with potassium persulphate (2.45 mM) (Merck) in water. After 12–16 h in dark and at room temperature, this solution was diluted with phosphate buffered saline (PBS) at pH 7 to give an absorbance of 0.7 ± 0.02 at 734 nm. The extract (50 µL) was mixed with 2 mL of the ABTS + solution and vortexed for 10 s. After 4 min of reaction, the absorbance was measured at 734 nm. The IC_{50} value was interpolated in a graph % of ABTS reduction vs. concentration in µg/mL for the correspondent value of 50% reduction. The results were expressed as TE, obtained interpolating the absorbance of 1 mM trolox in the graph % of ABTS reduction vs. concentration. Three independent experiments in triplicate were performed for each of the assayed extracts.

2.4. Anti-Inflammatory Activity Evaluation

2.4.1. Nitrite Production by Griess Assay

Raw 264.7, a mouse leukemic monocyte macrophage cell line from American Type Culture Collection (Manassas, VA, USA), and kindly supplied by Dr. Otília Vieira (Center for Neurosciences and Cell Biology, University of Coimbra, Portugal), was cultured in Iscove's Modified Dulbecco's Eagle medium supplemented with 10% non-inactivated fetal bovine serum, 100 U/mL penicillin, and 100 µg/mL streptomycin at 37 °C in a humidified atmosphere of 95% air and 5% CO_2. The cells were monitored to detect any morphological change. For the experiments, the cells were plated (0.6×10^5 cells/well) with culture medium and allowed to stabilize for 12 h. Then the cells were incubated during 24 h at 37 °C in culture medium (control) or stimulated with 1 µg/mL of bacteria lipopolysaccharide (LPS) (Sigma) with or without different concentrations of extract (0.1–2.0 mg/mL).

The anti-inflammatory activity was determined by the nitric oxide production, measured indirectly by the accumulation of nitrite in the supernatant through a colorimetric assay with Griess reagent [0.1% (m/v) of N-(1-naphthyl)-ethylenediamine dihydrocloride and 1% (m/v) of sulfanilamide with 5% of phosphoric acid] [27]. To perform the assay, it was used 100 µL of the supernatant and 100 µL of Griess's reagent and then stored away from light during 30 min. The absorbance at 550 nm was measured in an automated plate reader (Synergy HT, BioTek Instruments SAS, Colmar, France). Culture medium was used as blank and nitrite concentration was determined from a regression analysis using serial dilutions of sodium nitrite as standard.

2.4.2. Assessment of Cell Viability by Resazurin Assay

In order to evaluate the cytotoxicity it was performed the resazurin assay [28]. After the incubation with the samples, the cells were incubated with 100 µL of a resazurin solution (10 µM in culture medium) during 2 h at 37 °C in a humid atmosphere with 5% CO_2/95% air. Quantification of resorufin was performed using a plate reader (Synergy HT, BioTek, Instruments SAS, Colmar, France) at 570 nm, with an optical filter for 620 nm.

2.5. Statistical Analysis

All samples were analysed, at least, in triplicates and the results were expressed as mean ± standard deviation (SD). To calculate the IC_{50} values for the anti-inflammatory activity, the linearization of the dose-response curve was performed as described by Chou [29].

The statistical analysis of the cellular viability and anti-inflammatory activity was performed in GraphPad Prism program (version 5.02, GraphPad Software, San Diego, CA, USA). For the comparison between treatment conditions and control it was used two-sided unpaired t-test. To evaluate the effect of different treatments to LPS-stimulated cells it was performed One-way ANOVA followed by Bonferroni's test. The limit of significance was set at *** $p < 0.001$.

3. Results and Discussion

3.1. Nutrient Composition of C. vesicaria

The knowledge of the nutritional properties of wild plants is crucial to assess their suitability for human consumption. In this study, the nutritional profile of Crepis vesicaria subsp. taraxacifolia leaves was analyzed.

3.1.1. Nutritional Analysis of Crepis vesicaria subsp. taraxacifolia Leaves

The nutritive content of Cv leaves was determined (Table 1). The proximate composition revealed high moisture content, even though all foods contain water; those with a higher content are more prone to the rapid occurrence of microbial spoilage phenomena, enzymatic degradation and other moisture-dependent chemical deterioration reactions. Therefore, precautions should be considered to prevent rapid deterioration during storage, such as drying or freezing.

Table 1. Nutritive content of *Crepis vesicaria* subsp. *taraxacifolia* leaves (mean ± SD; n = 3).

Composition		Raw Matter	Dry Matter
Energy (KJ/100 g)		175.190 ± 0.259	1211.80 ± 2.11
Energy (Kcal/100 g)		41.840 ± 0.062	289.43 ± 0.50
Moisture (g/100 g)		85.540 ± 0.006	-
Protein (g/100 g)		1.040 ± 0.003	7.18 ± 0.02
Dietary fiber (g/100 g)		4.240 ± 0.015	29.35 ± 0.11
Insoluble Dietary fiber (g/100 g)		3.490 ± 0.026	24.14 ± 0.18
Acid detergent fiber (ADF) (g/100 g)		3.120 ± 0.011	21.59 ± 0.08
Cellulose (g/100 g)		2.550 ± 0.002	17.61 ± 0.02
Crude fiber (g/100 g)		2.460 ± 0.009	17.00 ± 0.06
Hemicellulose (g/100 g)		0.620 ± 0.012	4.27 ± 0.09
Lignin (g/100 g)		0.440 ± 0.013	3.03 ± 0.09
Acid detergent lignin (ADL) (g/100 g)		0.430 ± 0.006	2.99 ± 0.04
Nitrogen-free extractives (g/100 g)		7.530 ± 0.010	52.11 ± 0.07
Carbohydrates	Maltose (g/100 g)	2.470 ± 0.015	17.11 ± 0.11
	Fructose (g/100 g)	0.940 ± 0.012	6.53 ± 0.08
	Glucose (g/100 g)	0.340 ± 0.012	2.37 ± 0.08

Total carbohydrates, calculated by difference, were the most abundant macronutrients (9.99 g/100 g wet weight (w/w)), followed by ash, protein and lipids. Carbohydrates play a major role in human diet. They are the main source of energy, and also help to maintain glycemic homeostasis and gastrointestinal integrity, among other functions. A healthy adult diet should include about 130 g of carbohydrates per day [30]. Cv leaves contain an important amount of carbohydrates, which is in line with what has been reported for other wild Asteraceae plants traditionally consumed in the Mediterranean region, such as *Taraxacum obovatum*, *Chondrilla juncea*, *Sonchus oleraceus*, *Cichorium intybus*, *Scolymus hispanicus* and *Silybum marianum* [31]. An important fraction of the total carbohydrates content in Cv leaves is fiber. In this study, different fiber measurement methods were used and the results showed that the chosen method has an impact on the values observed for different fiber parameters. Weende's crude fiber analysis determines cellulose, lignin and some hemicellulose, pectin, gums and mucilages. The acid detergent lignin (ADL) measures lignin, the acid detergent fiber (ADF) determines cellulose and lignin, and the neutral detergent fiber (NDF) consists mainly in the measurement of cellulose, hemicelluloses and lignin [32]. Regardless of the method, the results reveal that Cv leaves are an interesting dietary fiber source, with insoluble dietary fiber being the major fraction. It is well established that the daily consumption of about 25–30 g of fiber, for an adult, markedly reduces the risk of cardiovascular and digestive diseases [30]. Also, Cv leaves may contain insoluble-bound phenolics present in the cell wall plant components. These insoluble-bound form can contribute for to protection of cardiovascular health [33]. Thus, the use of this plant, either individually or added to other foods, may contribute to a desired increase in fiber intake with the associated health benefits.

With regard to the available carbohydrates, the estimated value was 5.75 g/100 g (w/w). The total sugars content found was 3.76 g/100 g (w/w), with maltose as the main sugar (2.47 g/100 g, w/w), followed by fructose and glucose. Protein makes up 1.04 g/100 g, w/w of Cv leaves. This value is considerably lower than that reported by Barnett and Crawford [34]. Variations in protein levels may be due to differences between species, environmental and climatic factors, or a mixture of both.

3.1.2. Lipid and Fatty Acids Composition of *Crepis vesicaria* subsp. *taraxacifolia* Leaves

According to Table 2, the lipid content was moderate, 0.69 g/100 g, w/w (4.78 g/100 g dry weight (dw)), higher than that reported for *C. Juncea*, the highest lipid content Asteraceae (0.79 g/100 g, w/w) analyzed in the study of García-Herrera [31]. The fatty acid profile of Cv leaves showed a predominance of polyunsaturated fatty acids (PUFA) (402.84 mg/100 g, w/w), mainly comprised by α-linolenic acid (343.24 mg/100 g). Total saturated fatty acids (SFA) concentration was 159.82 mg/100 g, w/w, with the main constituent being palmitic acid (108.75 mg/100 g, w/w). For a nutritional "good quality", including beneficial effects in terms of cardiovascular risk reduction, the PUFA/SFA ratio should be > 0.45, whilst n-3/n-6 fatty acids ratio should be > 4 [35]. In the present study, the PUFA/SFA ratio was 2.52 and the n-3/n-6 fatty acids ratio was 5.76. The presence of considerable amounts of oleic acid (60.49 mg/100 g, w/w) should also be highlighted, given the beneficial properties that have been attributed to it in the context of the immunomodulation, prevention and treatment of several pathologies such as cancer, cardiovascular and autoimmune diseases, and metabolic disturbances [36].

Table 2. Lipid and fatty acids composition of *Crepis vesicaria* subsp. *taraxacifolia* leaves (mean ± SD; $n = 3$).

Composition	Raw Matter	Dry Matter
Fatty acids, total polyunsaturated (mg/100 g)	402.840 ± 0.146	2786.53 ± 1.01
Fatty acids, total saturated (mg/100 g)	159.820 ± 0.207	1105.48 ± 1.44
Fatty acids, total monounsaturated (mg/100 g)	123.710 ± 0.063	855.75 ± 0.44
α-Linolenic acid (C18:3n-3) (mg/100 g)	343.240 ± 0.065	2374.30 ± 0.57
Linoleic acid (C18:2n-6) (mg/100 g)	59.600 ± 0.084	412.23 ± 0.45
Oleic acid (C18:1n-9) (mg/100 g)	60.490 ± 0.087	418.43 ± 0.58
Palmitic acid (C16:0) (mg/100 g)	108.750 ± 0.004	752.26 ± 0.56
Gondoic acid (C20:1) (mg/100 g)	63.220 ± 0.086	437.32 ± 0.59
Arachidic acid (C20:0) (mg/100 g)	17.490 ± 0.091	121.00 ± 0.63
Stearic acid (C18:0) (mg/100 g)	21.520 ± 0.047	148.84 ± 0.60
Margaric acid (C17:0) (mg/100 g)	12.050 ± 0.081	83.38 ± 0.33
Lipids (g/100 g)	0.690 ± 0.004	4.78 ± 0.03

3.1.3. Minerals and Heavy Metal Composition of Cv Leaves

Given the results in Table 3, *Crepis vesicaria* L. subsp. *taraxacifolia* leaves exhibited moderate levels of ash (2.74 g/100 g, w/w). This value is within the recommended range for human consumption and reveals considerable mineral richness, which is corroborated by studies on similar species, such as *C. commutata* and *C. vesicaria* [37]. The mineral fraction is an aspect of greater relevance in the use of edible plants in human nutrition. The inappropriate intake of minerals (macrominerals and trace minerals) is the cause of multiple degenerative and chronic diseases. Calcium (Ca), phosphorous (P), magnesium (Mg), sodium (Na), potassium (K) and iron (Fe) are essential elements and their intake is necessary at mg/kg level to keep the human body healthy. Zinc (Zn), copper (Cu), manganese (Mn), chromium (Cr), and nickel (Ni) are required at trace levels in the diet [38]. Concerning the macrominerals composition of Cv leaves, K, Ca and Na were the most abundant (591.29 mg/100 g, w/w; 309.93 mg/100 g, w/w; 76.78 mg/100 g, w/w, respectively). The macromineral profile found was identical to that reported for *C. vesicaria* (K > Ca > Na > P > Mg), but different from that observed in *C. commutata* (K > P > Na > Mg > Ca) [37]. When compared to other wild Asteraceae, such as *S. hispanicus*, K and Ca contents are lower, but Cv can still be considered a remarkable source of these minerals, better than many conventional vegetables [31]. Zn and Mn were found as major trace minerals (0.86 mg/100 g, w/w and 0.83 mg/100 g, w/w, respectively). The most abundant trace minerals in *C. vesicaria* and *C. commutate* were Fe and Mn. *Crepis* spp. seem to be a good source of Mn. The contaminants cadmium (Cd), lead (Pb) and mercury (Hg) were detected. These toxic metallic elements can induce damage to multiple organs and have carcinogenic effects [39]. Pb levels are below the maximum values legislated, 0.30 mg/kg, w/w. However, the concentration of Cd coincides with the maximum level of contamination that is considered safe, 0.2 mg/kg, w/w [40]. Overall, the results indicate that, when located in polluted areas, these plants can accumulate toxic metals in concentrations that may represent a risk to the consumer's health.

Table 3. Minerals and heavy metal composition of *Crepis vesicaria* subsp. *taraxacifolia* leaves (mean ± SD; n = 3).

Composition		Raw Matter	Dry Matter
Ash (g/100 g)		2.740 ± 0.007	18.94 ± 0.05
Minerals	Potassium (mg/100 g)	591.290 ± 0.058	4090.07 ± 0.31
	Calcium (mg/100 g)	309.930 ± 0.090	2143.84 ± 0.62
	Sodium (mg/100 g)	76.780 ± 0.084	531.12 ± 0.42
	Phosphorus (mg/100 g)	59.910 ± 0.074	412.33 ± 0.51
	Magnesium (mg/100 g)	45.460 ± 0.066	314.46 ± 0.34
	Zinc (mg/100 g)	0.860 ± 0.012	5.97 ± 0.09
	Manganese (mg/100 g)	0.830 ± 0.006	5.71 ± 0.04
	Iron (mg/100 g)	0.590 ± 0.003	4.05 ± 0.02
	Copper (mg/100 g)	0.420 ± 0.012	2.89 ± 0.09
	Nickel (mg/100 g)	0.110 ± 0.011	0.79 ± 0.08
	Chromium (mg/100 g)	0.020 ± 0.003	0.11 ± 0.02
Heavy metals	Cadmium (µg/100 g)	19.300 ± 0.076	133.52 ± 0.53
	Lead (µg/100 g)	2.300 ± 0.094	15.92 ± 0.65
	Mercury (µg/100 g)	0.050 ± 0.002	0.36 ± 0.01

3.2. Screening for Antioxidant/Scavenging Activity

The ability of ROS to activate the inflammation signaling pathway, through activation of pro-inflammatory cytokines is well known. The literature describes that colorimetric methods to assess antioxidant activity like DPPH and ABTS, are a good tool to select the extracts more promising [41]. Also, it was reported that phenolic extracts bearing higher radical scavenging towards DPPH and ABTS, present higher inhibition of NF-kB activation mediated by ROS [41]. Given the correlation between antiradical activity and inhibition of the NF-kB signaling pathway, the antioxidant activity of the extracts was screened using the DPPH and ABTS colorimetric methods. Based on the results obtained, it was chosen the extract that demonstrated the greatest activity in these tests.

The infusion (10 mg of dry plant/mL) was screened for antioxidant activity as it is the form of use in traditional medicine. However, the percentage of reduction observed was 20.27%. As the Cv 70% EtOH extract was the most active extract it was lyophilized (previously described in Material and Methods) and characterized relatively to its phenolic profile, and antioxidant and anti-inflammatory activities.

Regarding antioxidant activity, the infusion presented an IC_{50} of 103.22 ± 5.61 µg/mL and a TEAC of 441.980 ± 0.058 mg/mL. The IC_{50} of Cv 70% EtOH was 26.20 ± 1.86 µg/mL and TEAC of 111.980 ± 0.041 mg/mL meaning that this extract is more active than the infusion. Subsequently, the antioxidant activity of the 70% ethanol extract was assessed by FRAP and ABTS methods (Table 4). The ABTS and DPPH methods are based on electron and H atom transfer while the FRAP is based on electron transfer reaction [42]. Attending to the results, the Cv extract present reducing power besides their ability in scavenging free radicals. The results shown that the Cv 70% EtOH extract has a good radical-scavenging activity and antioxidant activity.

Table 4. Antioxidant activity of ethanolic extract (Cv 70% EtOH) from *Crepis vesicaria* L. subsp. *taraxacifolia*.

	IC_{50} (µg/mL)	TE *
DPPH•	26.20 ± 1.86	111.980 ± 0.041
ABTS• (pH = 7)	18.92 ± 2.24	21.670 ± 0.012
FRAP	-	0.678 ± 0.168

* TE (Trolox Equivalent): Amount of the samples (µg/mL) that has the same anti-radical activity of Trolox 1 mM. The results are expressed as mean ± SD of three independent experiments.

3.3. Phenolic Profile of 70% Ethanolic Extract from Crepis vesicaria subsp. taraxacifolia

Based on the given results relatively to the antioxidant activity, the 70% EtOH from Cv extract is the most active. Therefore, the phenolic profile by HPLC-PDA-MS^n of this extract was assessed (Figure 1).

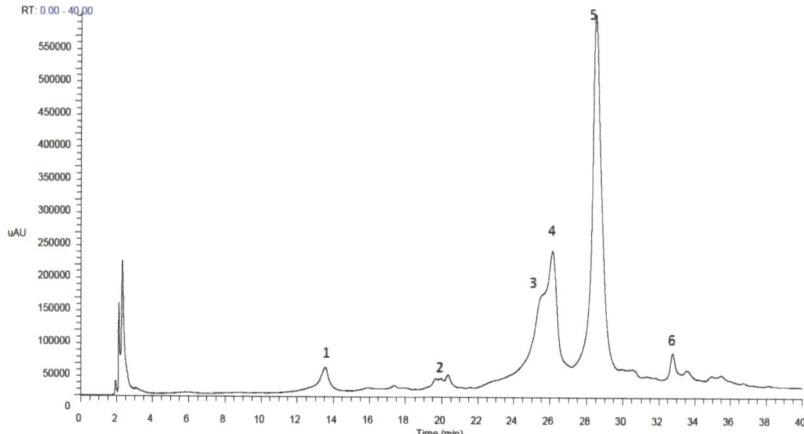

Figure 1. HPLC-PDA-ESI/MS^n profile of 70% ethanol extract from Cv recorded at 280 mn. It was used the gradient 2 described in Material and Methods section. (The chromatogram of the extract is not shown up to 40 min as no further compounds were eluted after this time period. Peaks 1–6 identification is showed in Table 5).

According to the absorption spectra, the 70% EtOH Cv extract is mainly composed of phenolic acids, generally presenting a shoulder at 295 nm and a maximum wavelength of 330 nm (Table 5), indicating to be caffeic or ferulic acids derivatives [43].

Table 5. Compounds identified in Cv 70% ethanol extract by HPLC-PDA-ESI/MS ^{n}.

Compound	Partial Identification	R_t (min.)	λ_{max} by HPLC/PDA (nm)	[M-H]$^-$	MS ^{2}	MS ^{3}
1	Caffeic acid [44]	13.54	238, 251, 291 sh, 299 sh, 328	179	[179]: 135 (100)	[179 135]: 151 (13), 135 (61), 125 (11), 107 (24), 91 (100)
2	Quinic acid [44]	20.33	238, 253, 291 sh, 300 sh, 326	191	[191]: 173 (82), 171 (24), 147 (12), 127 (100), 111 (45), 109 (27), 93 (46), 87 (14), 85 (66)	—
3	Chicoric acid isomer [45]	25.59	238, 251, 291 sh, 299 sh, 329	473	[473]: 311 (100), 293 (80)	[473 311]: 179 (62), 149 (100)
4	Chicoric acid isomer [45]	26.12	238, 251, 292 sh, 300 sh, 329	473	[473]: 311 (100), 293 (80)	[473 311]: 179 (58), 149 (100)
5	Chicoric acid isomer [45]	28.47	238, 251, 292 sh, 299 sh, 330	473	[473]: 311 (100), 293 (80)	[473 311]: 179 (61), 149 (100)
6	Feruloyl hexosylpentoside [46]	32.77	238, 253, 292 sh, 299 sh, 329	487	[487]: 325 (100), 307 (46), 293 (77)	[487 325]: 193 (100)

Identification based on the UV-Vis spectra, molecular weight and fragmentation patterns, which are according to authors referred.

In an attempt to identify the compounds of this extract, HPLC-PDA-ESI/MS^n was performed. The results (Table 5) showed that the extract consisted mainly of phenolic acids, namely caffeic and ferulic acid derivatives as well as chicoric acid isomers. The chicoric acid was identified as the main compound of the Cv 70% ethanol extract.

Compound 1. MS analysis showed a molecular ion [M-H]$^-$ at m/z 179 and a fragmentation pattern typical of caffeic acid. MS^2 data presented fragments at m/z 135 indicating a decarboxylated caffeic acid moiety [(M-H-CO$_2$)]$^-$. The compound 1 was tentatively identified as caffeic acid [44].

Compound 2. This compound presents a molecular ion [M-H]$^-$ at m/z 191. MS^2 most abundant fragments are m/z 173 indicating a dehydrated quinic acid moiety [M-H-H$_2$O]$^-$. This compound was tentatively identified as quinic acid [44].

Compounds 3, 4 and 5. The molecular ion [M-H]$^-$ occurs at m/z 473. The MS^2 presents a fragment at m/z 311, indicating the presence of deprotonated caftaric acid [M-H-C$_{13}$H$_{12}$O$_9$]$^-$ and m/z 293 corresponding to the neutral loss of caffeic acid [M-H-C$_9$H$_8$O$_4$]$^-$. MS^3 profiles have a fragment at m/z 149 corresponding to the tartaric acid and at m/z 179 corresponding to a deprotonated molecule of caffeic acid [M-H-C$_9$H$_8$O$_4$]$^-$. Based on this fragmentation pattern, these compounds were tentatively identified as chicoric acid isomers [47]. Accordingly with the literature, the most abundant chicoric acid isomer is L-chicoric acid [47]. The quantification by HPLC-PDA of this isomer was performed using a standard. The peak of the L-chicoric acid standard has approximately the same retention time of peak 5. Therefore, peak 5 was tentatively identified as L-chicoric acid.

Compound 6. This compound has a molecular ion [M-H]$^-$ at m/z 487. MS^2 showed fragments at m/z 325 (loss of 162 Da) indicating the loss of a hexose [M-H-C$_6$H$_{12}$O$_6$]$^-$ and at 307 that indicates the subsequent loss of water [M-H-C$_6$H$_{12}$O$_6$-H$_2$O]$^-$. The MS^3 fragment m/z 193 indicates the presence of ferulic acid [48], that can be probably associated to a hexosylpentosyl residue. All the data suggest that compound 6 was tentatively identified as feruloyl hexosylpentoside [46].

3.4. Quantification of Chicoric Acid

The major constituents in *Crepis vesicaria* subsp. *taraxacifolia* were chicoric acid derivatives and the evaluated activities were attributed to these compounds. Therefore, the L-chicoric acid was quantified by HPLC-PDA. The equation of calibration curve of L-chicoric acid was y = 4011236.2307 × −36474316.1324 (r^2 = 0.99). Based on this equation, the concentration of L-chicoric acid in the Cv 70% EtOH extract was 130.5 ± 4.2 mg/g extract of Cv 70% EtOH. The LOD and LOQ were 19.74 ± 3.33 mg/g extract and 44.58 ± 2.96 mg/g extract, respectively.

3.5. Assessment of Cell Viability of the Cv 70% EtOH Extract

The citotoxicity of the Cv 70% EtOH extract in macrophages was evaluated. The results (Figure 2) showed that none of the tested concentrations were cytotoxic.

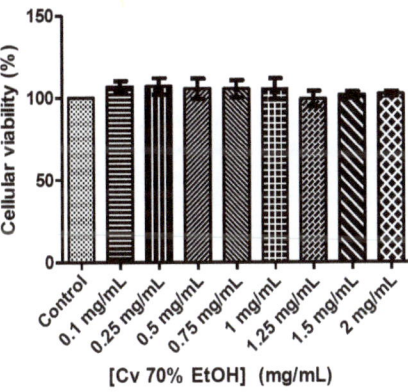

Figure 2. Effect of *Crepis vesicaria* subsp. *taraxacifolia* ethanolic extract on macrophages cell viability (RAW 264.7 cells). Each result represents the mean ± SD (minimum of three independent assays, performed in duplicate). The statistical tests were performed with $p < 0.05$ compared to control.

The cytotoxicity of chicoric acid in macrophages (Raw 264.7 cells) has also been was tested. The studies performed have shown that this compound is not cytotoxic [49]. There are few cell viability studies in normal cells with Cv extracts. However, some researchers studied the effects of a methanol extract of Cv flowers on tumor (HEPG-2, Caco-2 and MCF-7) and non-tumor (MCF-10A) cells. The Cv extract was not cytotoxic to the non-tumor cell line and cytotoxic to the tumor lines and therefore had some selectivity over tumor cells [9].

3.6. Antioxidant and Anti-Inflammatory Activity of the Cv 70% Ethanol Extract

The results showed that Cv 70% ethanol extract inhibited NO production in a dose-dependent manner (Figure 3) and the IC_{50} was 0.428 ± 0.00669 mg/mL. Cv extract is little active in inflammation compared to the results obtained in antioxidant activity.

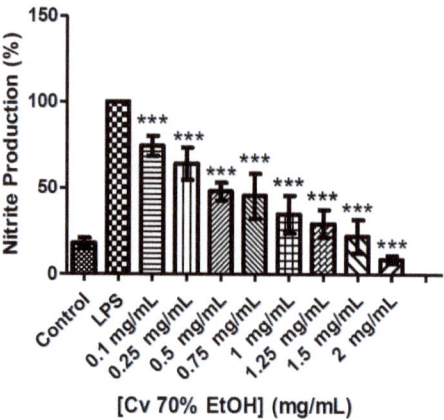

Figure 3. Effect of *Crepis vesicaria* subsp. *taraxacifolia* ethanolic extract on NO production in macrophages (RAW 264.7 cells). Each result represents the mean $\pm$ SD (minimum of three independent assays). *** $p < 0.001$ compared with the LPS group.

Reactive oxygen species are involved in various pathologies including inflammation. Cv extract was shown to have a high antioxidant activity. According to the characterization of the extract by HPLC-PDA-ESI/MS^n, the extract has phenolic acids namely caffeic and ferulic acid derivatives as well as chicoric acid isomers. The mechanisms involved in the antioxidant activity by which phenolic compounds act are based on: ability to chelate metals, such as copper and iron, that participate in the Fenton reaction generating hydroxyl radicals; interrupt signaling pathways triggered by free radicals; interfere with enzyme activity [50]. It is known that the antioxidant activity of phenolic compounds is directly related to the number of hydroxyl groups. Chicoric acid was identified as the major compound present in the extract. This compound has two caffeic acid moieties which are responsible for the high activity observed relatively to caffeic acid [51]. Some authors relate high molecular weight phenolic compounds, such as chicoric acid, with antioxidant activity [52]. Therefore, the observed antioxidant activity by H transfer and electron transfer reaction can be mostly attributed to chicoric acid.

Other plants of the genus *Crepis* are reported to have various biological activities including anti-inflammatory activity [6]. Chicoric acid has been reported to have that activity inhibiting activated immune cells, nitric oxide synthase and cyclooxygenase-2 through its inhibitory effects on nuclear factor NF-κB and TNF-α [53–55]. However, the results of Cv 70% EtOH extract weren't satisfactory in the anti-inflammatory activity. This fact can be due to the extract matrix [53] or antagonistic interactions between the matrix compound [56]. Moreover, this extract have chicoric acid isomers, and the observed activity can be due to this isomers. Further studies are needed to understand the inherent mechanisms of these compounds in anti-inflammatory activity.

4. Conclusions

The 70% ethanol *Crepis vesicaria* subsp. *taraxacifolia* leaves extract presents antioxidant and anti-inflammatory activities. Besides its biological activities, the Cv leaves extract demonstrated to have a high content of lipids and fatty acids. Given the observed antioxidant activity, Cv extract may be used as a functional food to prevent oxidative stress and its associated pathologies. In fact, Cv leaves displayed an interesting nutritional composition, with a low energetic contribution of 41.84 kcal/100 g, w/w. Some potential uses for this plant's leaves may be the development of new additives for human and/or animal consumption or food supplements that contribute to a balanced diet. In a context of food insecurity, their incorporation as an ingredient in recipes may also be of interest to increase their nutritional and functional value. From another perspective, to increase the consumption of this abundant and under-exploited plant, it is important to investigate its nutritional value and antioxidant and anti-inflammatory properties, but also to ensure that its consumption is safe, i.e., without neglecting the risk of contamination by toxic metals.

Author Contributions: S.P. contributed to the methodology, formal analysis and original draft preparation. A.F., T.B., M.T.C. and F.R. contributed to the project's administration, conceptualization and review and editing. S.d.R. and M.L. participated in the nutritional analysis and its interpretation. All authors have read and agreed to the published version of the manuscript.

Funding: This research was funded by PT national funds (FCT/MCTES, Fundação para a Ciência e Tecnologia and Ministério da Ciência, Tecnologia e Ensino Superior) through grant UIDB/50006/2020 and by Programa de Cooperación Interreg V-A España–Portugal (POCTEP) 2014–2020 (project 0377_IBERPHENOL_6_E).

Institutional Review Board Statement: Not applicable. This work didn't performed in vivo studies in animals or humans.

Informed Consent Statement: Not applicable. This work didn't performed human's assays.

Data Availability Statement: All data is available based on "MDPI Research Data Policies" at https://www.mdpi.com/ethics.

Acknowledgments: We are grateful to Laboratory of Mass Spectrometry (LEM) of UC Node integrated in the National Mass Spectrometry Network (RNEM) of Portugal, for MS analyses.

Conflicts of Interest: The authors state no conflict of interest

Abbreviations

GC-FID: gas chromatography-flame ionization detector; HPLC-PDA-ESI-MS^n: high performance liquid chromatography-photodiode array-electrospray ionization-mass spectrometry; HPLC-PDA: high performance liquid chromatography-photodiode array; DPPH: 2,2-diphenyl-1-picrylhydrazyl radical; ABTS: 2,2'-azinobis-(3-ethylbenzothiazoline-6-sulfonate); FRAP: ferric reduction antioxidant power.

References

1. Enke, N.; Gemeinholzer, B. Babcock revisited: New insights into generic delimitation and character evolution in *Crepis* L. (Compositae: Cichorieae) from ITS and matK sequence data. *Taxon* **2008**, *57*, 756–768. [CrossRef]
2. Sansanelli, S.; Tassoni, A. Wild food plants traditionally consumed in the area of Bologna (Emilia Romagna region, Italy). *J. Ethnobiol. Ethnomed.* **2014**, *10*, 1–12. [CrossRef] [PubMed]
3. Orhan, D.D.; Özçelik, B.; Hoşbaş, S.; Vural, M. Assessment of antioxidant, antibacterial, antimycobacterial, and antifungal activities of some plants used as folk remedies in Turkey against dermatophytes and yeast-like fungi. *Turk. J. Biol.* **2016**, *36*, 672–686.
4. Dalar, A. Plant taxa used in the treatment of diabetes in Van Province, Turkey. *Int. J. Second. Metab.* **2018**, *5*, 170–184. [CrossRef]
5. Singh, K.; Lal, B. Ethnomedicines used against four common ailments by the tribal communities of Lahaul-Spiti in western Himalaya. *J. Ethnopharmacol.* **2008**, *115*, 147–159. [CrossRef]
6. Ebada, S.S.; Al-Jawabri, N.A.; Youssef, F.S.; Albohy, A.; Aldalaien, S.M.; Disi, A.M.; Proksch, P. In vivo antiulcer activity, phytochemical exploration, and molecular modelling of the polyphenolic-rich fraction of *Crepis sancta* extract. *Inflammopharmacology* **2019**, *28*, 321–331. [CrossRef]

7. Bakar, F.; Acikara, Ö.B.; Ergene, B.; Nebioğlu, S.; Çitoğlu, G.S. Antioxidant activity and phytochemical screening of some Asteraceae plants. *Turk. J. Pharm. Sci.* **2015**, *12*, 36–45. [CrossRef]
8. Rahman, M. An ethnobotanical investigation on Asteraceae family at Rajshahi, Bangladesh. *Acad. J. Med. Plants* **2013**, *1*, 92–100.
9. Zengin, G. *Crepis foetida* L. subsp. *rhoeadifolia* (Bieb.) Celak. as a source of multifunctional agents: Cytotoxic and phytochemical evaluation. *J. Funct. Foods* **2015**, *17*, 698–708. [CrossRef]
10. Ooi, L.S.; Wang, H.; Luk, C.-W.; Ooi, V.E. Anticancer and antiviral activities of *Youngia japonica* (L.) DC (Asteraceae, Compositae). *J. Ethnopharmacol.* **2004**, *94*, 117–122. [CrossRef]
11. Ooi, L.S.; Wang, H.; He, Z.; Ooi, V.E. Antiviral activities of purified compounds from *Youngia japonica* (L.) DC (Asteraceae, Compositae). *J. Ethnopharmacol.* **2006**, *106*, 187–191. [CrossRef] [PubMed]
12. Munira, S.; Kabir, H.; Bulbul, I.J.; Nesa, L.; Muhit, A.; Haque, I. Pharmacological activities of *Youngia japonica* extracts. *Annu. Res. Rev. Biol.* **2018**, *25*, 1–14. [CrossRef]
13. Forrester, S.J.; Kikuchi, D.S.; Hernandes, M.S.; Xu, Q.; Griendling, K.K. Reactive oxygen species in metabolic and inflammatory signaling. *Circ. Res.* **2018**, *122*, 877–902. [CrossRef] [PubMed]
14. Xu, H.; Zheng, Y.-W.; Liu, Q.; Liu, L.-P.; Luo, F.-L.; Zhou, H.-C.; Isoda, H.; Ohkohchi, N.; Li, Y.-M. Reactive oxygen species in skin repair, regeneration, aging, and inflammation. In *Reactive Oxygen Species (ROS) in Living Cells*; Intech: London, UK, 2018.
15. Rapa, S.F.; Di Iorio, B.; Campiglia, P.; Heidland, A.; Marzocco, S. Inflammation and oxidative stress in chronic kidney disease—potential therapeutic role of minerals, vitamins and plant-derived metabolites. *Int. J. Mol. Sci.* **2019**, *21*, 263. [CrossRef] [PubMed]
16. Leyva-Jiménez, F.J.; Lozano-Sánchez, J.; Cádiz-Gurrea, M.D.L.L.; Arráez-Román, D.; Segura-Carretero, A. Functional ingredients based on nutritional phenolics. A Case Study against inflammation: Lippia Genus. *Nutrients* **2019**, *11*, 1646. [CrossRef] [PubMed]
17. Francisco, V.; Costa, G.; Figueirinha, A.; Marques, C.; Pereira, P.; Neves, B.M.; Lopes, M.C.; García-Rodríguez, C.; Cruz, M.T.; Batista, M.T. Anti-inflammatory activity of *Cymbopogon citratus* leaves infusion via proteasome and nuclear factor-κB pathway inhibition: Contribution of chlorogenic acid. *J. Ethnopharmacol.* **2013**, *148*, 126–134. [CrossRef] [PubMed]
18. Francisco, V.L.G.; Figueirinha, A.; Neves, B.M.; García-Rodríguez, C.; Lopes, M.C.; Cruz, M.T.; Batista, M.T. *Cymbopogon citratus* as source of new and safe anti-inflammatory drugs: Bio-guided assay using lipopolysaccharide-stimulated macrophages. *J. Ethnopharmacol.* **2011**, *133*, 818–827. [CrossRef]
19. Yen, G.-C.; Duh, P.-D.; Huang, D.-W.; Hsu, C.-L.; Fu, T.Y.-C. Protective effect of pine (*Pinus morrisonicola* Hay.) needle on LDL oxidation and its anti-inflammatory action by modulation of iNOS and COX-2 expression in LPS-stimulated RAW 264.7 macrophages. *Food Chem. Toxicol.* **2008**, *46*, 175–185. [CrossRef]
20. Zhang, T.-T.; Hu, T.; Jiang, J.-G.; Zhao, J.-W.; Zhu, W. Antioxidant and anti-inflammatory effects of polyphenols extracted from *Ilex latifolia* Thunb. *RSC Adv.* **2018**, *8*, 7134–7141. [CrossRef]
21. Saji, N.; Francis, N.; Blanchard, C.L.; Schwarz, L.J.; Santhakumar, A.B. Rice bran phenolic compounds regulate genes associated with antioxidant and anti-inflammatory activity in human umbilical vein endothelial cells with induced oxidative stress. *Int. J. Mol. Sci.* **2019**, *20*, 4715. [CrossRef] [PubMed]
22. Cunniff, P. *Official Methods of Analysis of AOAC International*; AOAC International: Gaithersburg, MD, USA, 1997.
23. Van Soest, P.J.; Robertson, J.B.; Lewis, B.A. Methods for dietary fiber, neutral detergent fiber, and nonstarch polysaccharides in relation to animal nutrition. *J. Dairy Sci.* **1991**, *74*, 3583–3597. [CrossRef]
24. Boly, R.; Boly, R.; Lamkami, T.; Lompo, M.; Dubois, J.; Guissou, I. DPPH free radical scavenging activity of two extracts from *Agelanthus dodoneifolius* (Loranthaceae) Leaves. *Int. J. Toxicol. Pharmacol. Res.* **2016**, *8*, 29–34. Available online: www.ijtpr.com (accessed on 27 January 2020).
25. Benzie, I.F.F.; Strain, J.J. The ferric reducing ability of plasma (FRAP) as a measure of 'antioxidant power': The FRAP assay. *Anal. Biochem.* **1996**, *239*, 70–76. [CrossRef] [PubMed]
26. Re, R.; Pellegrini, N.; Proteggente, A.; Pannala, A.; Yang, M.; Rice-Evans, C. Antioxidant activity applying an improved ABTS radical cation decolorization assay. *Free Radic. Biol. Med.* **1999**, *26*, 1231–1237. [CrossRef]
27. Green, L.; Wagner, D.A.; Glogowski, J.; Skipper, P.L.; Wishnok, J.S.; Tannenbaum, S.R. Analysis of nitrate, nitrite, and [15N]nitrate in biological fluids. *Anal. Biochem.* **1982**, *126*, 131–138. [CrossRef]
28. Rampersad, S.N. Multiple Applications of Alamar Blue as an indicator of metabolic function and cellular health in cell viability bioassays. *Sensors* **2012**, *12*, 12347–12360. [CrossRef]
29. Chou, T.-C. Theoretical basis, experimental design, and computerized simulation of synergism and antagonism in drug combination studies. *Pharmacol. Rev.* **2006**, *58*, 621–681. [CrossRef]
30. Trumbo, P.; Schlicker, S.; Yates, A.A.; Poos, M. Dietary reference intakes for energy, carbohydrate, fiber, fat, fatty acids, cholesterol, protein and amino acids. *J. Am. Diet. Assoc.* **2002**, *102*, 1621–1630. [CrossRef]
31. García-Herrera, P.; Sanchezmata, M.C.; Cámara, M.; Fernandezruiz, V.; Díez-Marqués, C.; Molina, M.G.A.; Tardio, J. Nutrient composition of six wild edible Mediterranean Asteraceae plants of dietary interest. *J. Food Compos. Anal.* **2014**, *34*, 163–170. [CrossRef]
32. Opitz, B.; Smith, P.M.; Kienzle, E.; Earle, K.E.; Maskell, I.E. The measurement of dietary fibre in pet food: A comparison of methods. *J. Anim. Physiol. Anim. Nutr.* **1998**, *79*, 146–152. [CrossRef]
33. Albishi, T.; Banoub, J.H.; De Camargo, A.C.; Shahidi, F. Wood extracts as unique sources of soluble and insoluble-bound phenolics: Reducing power, metal chelation and inhibition of oxidation of human LDL-cholesterol and DNA strand scission. *J. Food Bioact.* **2019**, *8*. [CrossRef]

34. Barnett, J.K.; Crawford, J.A. Pre-Laying Nutrition of Sage Grouse Hens in Oregon. *J. Range Manag.* **1994**, *47*, 114. [CrossRef]
35. Guil, J.L.; E Torija, M.; Giménez, J.J.; Rodríguez, I. Identification of fatty acids in edible wild plants by gas chromatography. *J. Chromatogr. A* **1996**, *719*, 229–235. [CrossRef]
36. Sales-Campos, H.; De Souza, P.R.; Peghini, B.C.; Da Silva, J.S.; Cardoso, C.R. An overview of the modulatory effects of oleic acid in health and disease. *Mini Rev. Med. Chem.* **2013**, *13*, 201–210. [PubMed]
37. Zeghichi, S.; Kallithraka, S.; Simopoulos, A.P.; Kypriotakis, Z. Nutritional composition of selected wild plants in the diet of Crete. *World Rev. Nutr. Diet.* **2003**, *91*, 22–40. [PubMed]
38. Mir-Marqués, A.; Cervera, M.; De La Guardia, M. Mineral analysis of human diets by spectrometry methods. *TrAC Trends Anal. Chem.* **2016**, *82*, 457–467. [CrossRef]
39. Tchounwou, P.B.; Yedjou, C.G.; Patlolla, A.K.; Sutton, D.J. Heavy Metal Toxicity and the Environment. *Mol. Ecol. Evol. Approaches Appl.* **2012**, *101*, 133–164. [CrossRef]
40. Commission of the European Communities. Commission Regulation (EC) No 1881/2006 of 19 December 2006 setting maximum levels for certain contaminants in foodstuffs. *Off. J. Eur. Union* **2006**, *364*. Available online: https://www.ecolex.org/details/legislation/commission-regulation-ec-no-18812006-setting-maximum-levels-for-certain-contaminants-in-foodstuffs-lex-faoc068134/ (accessed on 23 December 2020).
41. Falcão, H.G. Optimizing the potential bioactivity of isoflavones from soybeans via ultrasound pretreatment: Antioxidant potential and NF-κB activation. *J. Food Biochem.* **2019**, *43*, e13018. [CrossRef]
42. El Jemli, M.; Kamal, R.; Marmouzi, I.; Zerrouki, A.; Cherrah, Y.; Alaoui, K. Radical-Scavenging activity and ferric reducing ability of *Juniperus thurifera* (L.), *J. oxycedrus* (L.), *J. phoenicea* (L.) and *Tetraclinis articulata* (L.). *Adv. Pharmacol. Sci.* **2016**, *2016*. [CrossRef]
43. Costa, G.; Ferreira, J.P.; Vitorino, C.; Pina, M.E.T.; Sousa, J.; Figueiredo, I.; Batista, M.T. Polyphenols from *Cymbopogon citratus* leaves as topical anti-inflammatory agents. *J. Ethnopharmacol.* **2016**, *178*, 222–228. [CrossRef] [PubMed]
44. Li, Y.; Liu, Y.; Liu, R.; Liu, S.; Zhang, X.; Wang, Z.; Lu, J. HPLC-LTQ-Orbitrap MS^n profiling method to comprehensively characterize multiple chemical constituents in Xiao-er-qing-jie granules. *Anal. Methods* **2015**, *7*, 7511–7526. [CrossRef]
45. Vukovic, N.; Vukic, M.D.; Đelić, G.T.; Kačániová, M.; Cvijovic, M. The investigation of bioactive secondary metabolites of the methanol extract of eryngium amethystinum. *Kragujev. J. Sci.* **2018**, 113–129. [CrossRef]
46. Ferreres, F.; Bernardo, J.; Andrade, P.B.; E Sousa, C.A.; Gilizquierdo, A.; Valentão, P. Pennyroyal and gastrointestinal cells: Multi-target protection of phenolic compounds against t-BHP-induced toxicity. *RSC Adv.* **2015**, *5*, 41576–41584. [CrossRef]
47. Lee, J.M.; Scagel, C. Chicoric acid: Chemistry, distribution, and production. *Front. Chem.* **2013**, *1*. [CrossRef] [PubMed]
48. Wang, S.-P.; Liu, L.; Wang, L.; Hu, Y.; Zhang, W.-D.; Liu, R. Structural characterization and identification of major constituents in Jitai tablets by High-Performance Liquid Chromatography/Diode-Array Detection Coupled with Electrospray Ionization Tandem Mass Spectrometry. *Molecules* **2012**, *17*, 10470–10493. [CrossRef]
49. Zhu, X.; Huang, F.; Xiang, X.; Fan, M.; Chen, T. Evaluation of the potential of chicoric acid as a natural food antioxidant. *Exp. Ther. Med.* **2018**, *16*, 3651–3657. [CrossRef]
50. Biskup, I.; Golonka, I.; Gamian, A.; Sroka, Z. Antioxidant activity of selected phenols estimated by ABTS and FRAP methods. *Adv. Hyg. Exp. Postępy Hig. Med. Doświadczalnej* **2013**, *67*, 958–963. [CrossRef]
51. Jabłońska-Trypuć, A.; Krętowski, R.; Kalinowska, M.; Świderski, G.; Cechowska-Pasko, M.; Lewandowski, W. Possible mechanisms of the prevention of doxorubicin toxicity by cichoric acid—antioxidant nutrient. *Nutrients* **2018**, *10*, 44. [CrossRef]
52. Petropoulos, S.A.; Fernandes, Â.; Barros, L.; Ferreira, I.C. A comparison of the phenolic profile and antioxidant activity of different *Cichorium spinosum* L. ecotypes. *J. Sci. Food Agric.* **2017**, *98*, 183–189. [CrossRef]
53. Peng, Y.; Sun, Q.; Park, Y. The bioactive effects of chicoric acid as a functional food ingredient. *J. Med. Food* **2019**, *22*, 645–652. [CrossRef] [PubMed]
54. Liu, Q.; Chen, Y.; Shen, C.; Xiao, Y.; Wang, Y.; Liu, Z.; Liu, X. Chicoric acid supplementation prevents systemic inflammation-induced memory impairment and amyloidogenesis via inhibition of NF-κB. *FASEB J.* **2017**, *31*, 1494–1507. [CrossRef] [PubMed]
55. Ding, H.; Ci, X.; Cheng, H.; Yu, Q.; Li, D. Chicoric acid alleviates lipopolysaccharide-induced acute lung injury in mice through anti-inflammatory and anti-oxidant activities. *Int. Immunopharmacol.* **2019**, *66*, 169–176. [CrossRef] [PubMed]
56. Yan, H.; Zhang, B.; Li, S.; Zhao, Q. A formal model for analyzing drug combination effects and its application in TNF-α-induced NFκB pathway. *BMC Syst. Biol.* **2010**, *4*, 50. [CrossRef] [PubMed]

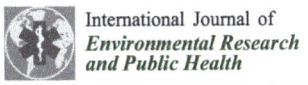

Article

Food Insecurity among Low-Income Food Handlers: A Nationwide Study in Brazilian Community Restaurants

Ingrid C. Fideles [1], Rita de Cassia Coelho de Almeida Akutsu [2,*], Rosemary da Rocha Fonseca Barroso [1], Jamacy Costa-Souza [1], Renata Puppin Zandonadi [2], António Raposo [3,*] and Raquel Braz Assunção Botelho [2]

1. Department of Food Science, School of Nutrition, Federal University of Bahia, Salvador 40110-150, Brazil; ingridfideles@gmail.com (I.C.F.); rosemary.fonseca2017@gmail.com (R.d.R.F.B.); jamacy@ufba.br (J.C.-S.)
2. Department of Nutrition, Faculty of Health Sciences, University of Brasilia, Brasilia 70910-900, Brazil; renatapz@yahoo.com.br (R.P.Z.); raquelbabotelho@gmail.com (R.B.A.B.)
3. CBIOS (Research Center for Biosciences and Health Technologies), Universidade Lusófona de Humanidades e Tecnologias, Campo Grande 376, 1749-024 Lisboa, Portugal
* Correspondence: rita.akutsu@gmail.com (R.d.C.C.d.A.A.); antonio.raposo@ulusofona.pt (A.R.); Tel.: +55-61-3107-1781 (R.d.C.C.d.A.A.)

Abstract: This study aims to evaluate food insecurity (FI) among Brazilian Community restaurant food handlers and its associated factors. This cross-sectional study was performed with a representative sample of 471 food handlers working in community restaurants (CR) from all Brazilian regions. Participants are mostly female (62.2%), ≤40 years old (67.7%), with a partner (52.0%), and with up to eight years of education (54.1%). Predictors of participants' socioeconomic status and CR geographic location are associated with the household food insecurity categories ($p < 0.05$). The predictors of socioeconomic conditions are associated with mild and moderate/severe FI category. Workers with less education are twice as likely to belong to the category with the highest FI severity. Lower per capita household income increased the chances of belonging to the mild insecurity category by 86%. It more than doubled the chance to be in the category of moderate/severe insecurity. Predictors of health status, lifestyle, and work are not associated with any multinomial outcome categories. However, working in the South, Southeast, or Midwest regions of Brazilian decreased the chances of belonging to one of the FI categories, with significance only for the mild category. Variables that show an association for this population are per capita household income for the different levels of FI and the CR region for mild FI. A high prevalence of FI in this population points to the need for more studies with low-income workers to prevent FI and its health consequences.

Keywords: Brazil; community restaurants; food handlers; food insecurity; low-income

1. Introduction

Food insecurity is a global public health problem, affecting more than 2 billion people worldwide [1]. Food security is a basic need covering access to safe, sufficient, and proper nutritional food [2,3]. Among adults, food insecurity is related to the high prevalence of chronic health problems that compromise this population's quality of life and longevity. It is strongly linked to economic vulnerability [1,4]. In Brazil, the estimation is that more than 14 million households have some food insecurity level [5]; additionally, people eat more outside their homes because they have less time to prepare meals. In Brazil, to the low-income population, eating out tends to represent an intake of cheaper and fast snacks, usually representing inadequate nutrient intake that influences their health outcomes increasing the risk of chronic diseases and nutrient deficits [2,6–8].

In Brazil, people with no or limited access to adequate, safe, and nutritional food are characterized in food insecurity situations (FIS) [5]. FIS can generate fear of the inability to obtain food (influencing quantity or quality of food choice) or generate hunger in the most severe cases due to the scarcity of food at home [5]. The FIS determinants can present social, economic, and political nature, affecting populations' health. The living and working conditions of individuals and population groups are related to their health situation [9]. Among the factors associated with FIS, mainly in the moderate and severe categories of FI, income, and weight excess have been highlighted [10]. Women in developed countries have higher chances of being overweight and obese when in FIS [11].

Based on this information, the Brazilian Government developed the community restaurant (CR) program as a strategy to face the FIS. CRs were created to offer safe, cheap, and healthy meals to the low-income population [12,13]. The CR Program is one of the programs integrated into the "Fome Zero" network of actions, a social inclusion policy established in 2003 [13]. From the beginning, the Government planned to increase the number of CR distributed throughout the Brazilian territory located in regions with more significant numbers of low-income people, reaching 135 CRs in 2020 [13,14]. The production and distribution of CR involve professionals with different education and income levels [15], highlighting the food handlers that directly produce meals [13]. Among food handlers, it is common to have weight excess [15–18], low education levels, and low-income [15,19], making them more susceptible to FIS [10] even though they work in places that produce a great amount of food. Godoy et al. [20] studied food insecurity among CR customers. Despite a high percentage of FI (40.6% for males and 43.8% for females), there were no significant associations between FI and Body Mass Index or body fat percentage. There were significant associations between FI and household income and educational levels. There was also an association with Brazilian's regions among females, FI being worse in the North and Northeast regions.

Few studies evaluated FIS among workers in Brazil [21–23] and in the world [24–27]. However, only three of these studies were performed with professionals working in food service. A study showed a high prevalence of FIS perception among these professionals in Canada compared to other professionals [24]. The two studies conducted in Brazil only evaluated food handlers in a specific region without a nationwide Brazilian representative sample of food handlers [21,22]. Studies with the population of food handlers demonstrate their susceptibility to food insecurity [21,22], to excess weight [22,28], to management in foodservice with a greater focus on the costs involved with the production of meals than with the health of workers [29]. Even though the studies found in Brazil were both developed in the format of case studies [30–32], geographically delimited to institutional spaces, such as universities, Brazilian states or municipalities [21–23,28,31–33], food insecurity is multifactorial and, in CR, we hypothesize that socioeconomic and demographic factors of food handlers are associated with food insecurity. Since the program tends to increase the number of CR in Brazilian territory, more CRs open over the country, possibly resulting in more opportunities to decrease FI among customers and more work opportunities for food handlers. However, these food handlers need to be closely investigated because of their well-being, quality of life, and food security to guarantee motivation to work and meals safely produced. Therefore, the objective was to evaluate nationwide the food insecurity among Brazilian CR food handlers and its associated factors. As it has an exploratory character, the study sought to answer the following question: What are the factors associated with food insecurity among food handlers in Brazilian CR? We expect to provide data allowing to promote interventions to reduce food insecurity among this vulnerable group that works inside foodservices but does not overcome FI inside their families.

2. Materials and Methods

2.1. Design, Settings, and Participants

This cross-sectional study was performed in Brazilian CR (focused on the low-income Brazilian population offering meals from Monday to Friday). It was conducted according to the Declaration of Helsinki guidelines and approved by the University of Brasília Research Ethics Committee (#037210). Written informed consent was obtained from all participants.

The basis of the sample calculation was the official list of all existing CR throughout the Brazilian territory at the moment of data collection [13]. With CR nationwide selection, food handlers in different Brazilian regions and similar work conditions were evaluated. Researchers were allowed to enter all of the CR with nationwide permission. The restaurant inclusion criteria were to be part of the Brazilian CR program, sign the Institutional Acknowledgement Agreement by the CR responsible, and offer daily more than 500 meals. With more than 500 meals, CR allowed researchers to evaluate many workers, helping to achieve a representative sample. Restaurants that provide less than 500 daily meals are considered small and present fewer food handlers than medium or large restaurants that offer more than 500 daily meals [34]. There were 65 existing CR in Brazil, and all of them met the inclusion criteria.

From the 65 CR, a sampling plan was calculated considering a level of significance (α) of 5% [35] using the "survey select" of the SAS 9.1.3 program (SAS Institute Inc., Cary, NC, USA). Therefore, a minimum of 31 CR existing in each of the five Brazilian regions (North, Northeast, Midwest, South, and Southeast) was randomly selected to be part of the study. The final sample of 36 restaurants was used, respecting the stratification criteria by the Brazilian region. The distribution of randomly drawn CRs was proportional to the number of CR in each region. The researchers visited 36 CR and included them in the sample (4 in North, 10 in Northeast, 1 in Midwest, 15 in Southeast, and 6 in South). All of the working food handlers in the 36 drawn CR were invited to participate in this study ($n = 1062$). Data collection was carried out over four consecutive days to cover the various work schedules to guarantee access to the largest possible number of handlers in each CR. Therefore, from the total of 1062 handlers working on the selected CRs, 970 met the inclusion criteria (e.g., not being pregnant, and workers on vacation or not working due to medical issues). From them, 471 (48.6%) agreed to participate and completed the study.

Some handlers refused to participate in the research because they did not want to stop working or worried about employability. Even though researchers explained that participation would not influence their work, some decided not to participate in the study. A total of 383 individuals was necessary to be a representative sample stratified in the five Brazilian regions according to the number of food handlers in each region. Participants were not compensated for the participation. They were just informed about the importance of the study for their category. The study used a 95% confidence interval and an error of 4%, respecting the minimum handlers' sample per Brazilian region [35]. Therefore, it was necessary to achieve a minimum of 11% of the handlers from the North, 28% from the Northeast, 3% from the Midwest, 41% from the Southeast, and 17% from the South.

2.2. Data Collection

Trained researchers performed data collection using standardized instruments to identify socio-demographic characteristics and the Brazilian Food Insecurity Scale (EBIA/BFIS) [36]. The socio-demographic variables were gender, age, educational level, per capita household income, marital status, smoking status, participation in a governmental program, and how many years or months the individual has worked in the CR. The presence of diagnosed non-communicable diseases (NCDs) (by a physician) was self-reported. The information was recorded in a specific form showing the presence or absence of one or more than one of the following NCDs: Systemic arterial hypertension (SAH), type 2 diabetes mellitus (DM), and others (cancer, dyslipidemia, cardiovascular diseases, respiratory diseases, depression). The self-reported NCD data was used because population studies widely use this method for its convenience and economy [37,38].

The individuals who agreed to participate signed the consent form after receiving information about the research. Before participants' lunch in a reserved room, weight and height were measured with a Plenna® (São Paulo, Brazil) weighing scale (150 kg) and a stadiometer (220 cm). Participants had to take off their shoes and coats. After that, the body mass index (BMI) was calculated [39]. The anthropometric status based on body mass index classification [39] was dichotomized on weight excess (0. No; 1. Yes). The cut-off point used to indicate excess weight was a BMI value ≥ 25 kg/m^2, which covers both the category of overweight and obesity.

2.3. Dependent Variable

The study's outcome, household food security situation (HFSS), was obtained through EBIA/BFIS adapted and validated for the Brazilian population [40,41]. The EBIA/BFIS seeks to assess the perception and experience of household residents' hunger in the three months before the instrument application. The positive answers to the 14 questions of the instrument categorize the level of food security/insecurity (considering the age of the residents) in food security (0 points); mild food insecurity (1–5 points in the presence of residents <18 years old, or 1–3 points in the absence of residents <18 years old); moderate food insecurity (6–9 points in the presence of residents <18 years old, or 4–5 in the absence of residents <18 years old) and, severe food insecurity (10–14 points in the presence of residents <18 years old, or 6–8 points in the absence of residents <18 years). Based on the methodology adopted by Panigassi et al. [42], for this study, the HFSS categories were grouped into food security, mild food insecurity, and moderate/severe food insecurity.

2.4. Statistical Analysis

The data were analyzed with the STATA 15.0® (StataCorp LP, College Station, TX, USA), using frequencies to describe the categorical variables and Pearson's chi-square test (χ^2) to identify associations (p-value < 0.05).

The outcome with three categories of HFSS, multinomial (polytomous) logistic regression models were used. They are applicable for outcomes with three or more levels [43]. For this study, the category "food security" was chosen as a reference. In this type of analysis, the logistic model will have two logit functions: the ratio between Y = 1 and Y = 0 and the ratio between Y = 2 and Y = 0, with Y = 0 as the referent. The numbers 0, 1, and 2 represent the food security status classification for statistical analysis—(0) Food Security—the household has regular and permanent access to food in sufficient quantity and quality without compromising access to other needs; (1) Mild food insecurity—at this level there is uncertainty regarding access to food in the future, with a change in the quality of food, but without compromising the amount of food; (2) includes the levels of moderate food insecurity and severe, in which there is already a quantitative reduction in access to food, causing changes in the dietary pattern of residents at home. These categories were grouped to enable comparison with population data given that national food insecurity assessment studies [44] and international [45] present their analyses considering the grouped on these two levels.

Bivariate multinomial regression models, with HFSS as the dependent variable, were applied to all predictor variables. This stage helped to understand the initial associations of the determinant factors for the HFSS of this population and the magnitude of each predictor's effect by calculating the gross Odds Ratio (OR) and their respective 95% Confidence Intervals (CI). The predictor variables were included in the multivariate model based on two assumptions. The first assumption was the theoretical basis underlying the HFSS. The second one was the statistical decision based on the bivariate multinomial model result with a value of $p < 0.20$ [16]. Thus, the multivariate multinomial model was composed of the predictors that met the assumptions and were adjusted together, without considering hierarchical order or determination level.

The backward stepwise procedure was used for the selection in the final model. The Likelihood Ratio Test (LRT) was used to test hypotheses about the significance of the predictor variables, that is, to evaluate the effect at all levels of the outcome simultaneously, which affects the number of parameters tested and the degrees of freedom associated with the test [46]. Thus, the comparison of the observed and the expected values using the likelihood function was based on the expression:

$$D = -2lnL_{reduced} - \left(-2lnL_{full}\right) \sim \chi^2$$

The full model corresponds to the complete multivariate model and the reduced model to the model without a corresponding predictor, following a chi-square distribution with degrees of freedom equal to the number of set parameters (defined as zero under the null hypothesis—H0). Statistically significant results ($p < 0.05$) reject H0 and indicate that the predictor is significant for the model, being maintained in the final model.

3. Results

The socioeconomic and demographic characteristics, health status, HFSS, and aspects related to food handlers' work in CR are in Table 1. The sample was composed mainly of women (62.2%), aged ≤40 years old (67.7%), with a partner (52.0%), and with up to eight years of education (54.1%). In most households, there were up to two people employed (78.8%), less than six rooms (64.4%), per capita household income below half a minimum wage (40%), and 19.3% of the workers in government programs. Among the health risk behaviors or conditions, overweight and alcohol use was more prevalent (60.8% and 46%, respectively) when compared to the smoking habit (17.2%) and the presence of NCDs (19.1%). More than half of these professionals were working in the CR for ≥12 months (57.3%) (Table 1). For most of the factors in Table 1, the median value was used to split the sample and perform the analysis.

Predictors of socioeconomic status (education, per capita household income, and participation in governmental programs) and geographic location of the CR were associated with the HFSS categories by the chi-square test ($p < 0.05$) (Table 1).

There was no significant association between mild FI and the demographic variables in the bivariate multinomial analysis. In contrast, the predictors of socioeconomic conditions were associated with both the mild and the moderate/severe FI category. Workers with less education were twice as likely to belong to the category with the highest severity of food insecurity (OR: 2.17; 95% CI: 1.25–3.77). Having lower per capita household income increased the chances of belonging to the category of mild insecurity by 86% (OR: 1.86; 95% CI: 1.20–2.88) and more than doubled the chance to be in the category of moderate/severe Insecurity (OR: 3.8; 95% CI: 2.18–6.60) in addition to participating in governmental programs (OR: 3.17; 95% CI: 1.75–5.74). Living in households with fewer rooms was also associated with the most severe food insecurity category (OR: 1.87; 95% CI: 1.05–3.34) (Table 2).

Predictors of health status, lifestyle, and work were not associated with any of the multinomial outcomes' categories at a 5% significance level. However, working in the South, Southeast, or Midwest regions of Brazilian decreased the chances of belonging to one of the Food Insecurity categories between 21% to 42%, with significance only for the mild category (OR: 0.58; 95% CI: 0.38–0.88) (Table 2).

The bivariate multinomial regression models confirmed the associations of education, per capita income, participation in a governmental program, and the Brazilian region with the categories of HFSS, with an increase in the number of rooms among the predictors. Besides, variables that showed association with any of the categories of HFSS (p-value < 0.20) were also included in the multivariate multinomial model (gender, number of people working at home, and the presence of NCDs) (Table 2).

Table 1. Descriptive analysis of the study population, considering the distribution in Household Food Security Situation of demographic, socioeconomic characteristics, health status and lifestyle, and work-related aspects.

Variables	% (n)	Food Security % (n)	Food Insecurity Mild % (n)	Food Insecurity Moderate/Severe % (n)	p-Value *
		Gender (n = 471)			
Female	62.2 (293)	53.9 (158)	29.01 (85)	17.06 (50)	0.44
Male	37.8 (178)	58.4 (104)	28.65 (51)	12.92 (23)	
		Age group (n = 471)			
≤40 years old	67.7 (319)	54.23 (173)	30.41 (97)	15.36 (49)	0.56
>40 years old	32.3 (152)	58.55 (89)	25.66 (39)	15.79 (24)	
		Education level (n = 471)			
≤08 years of study	54.1 (255)	51.37 (131)	29.02 (74)	19.61 (50)	0.02
>08 years of study	45.9 (216)	60.65 (131)	28.70 (62)	10.65 (23)	
		Marital status (n = 471)			
With partner	52.0 (245)	55.1 (135)	31.02 (76)	13.88 (34)	0.43
Without a partner	48.0 (226)	56.2 (127)	26.55 (60)	17.26 (39)	
		Number of workers in the family (n = 471)			
1 or 2 work	78.8 (364)	53.8 (196)	28.85 (105)	17.31 (63)	0.15
Above 2 workers	21.2 (98)	63.3 (62)	26.53 (26)	10.2 (10)	
		Income (per capita minimum wage) [1] (n = 451)			
>1/2 MW	60.1 (271)	64.6 (175)	25.8 (70)	9.6 (26)	0.00
≤1/2 MW	39.9 (180)	43.3 (78)	32.22 (58)	24.44 (44)	
		Governmental program participation (n = 471)			
No	80.7 (380)	59.2 (225)	28.16 (107)	12.63 (48)	0.00
Yes	19.3 (91)	40.7 (37)	31.87 (29)	27.47 (25)	
		Number of rooms at home (n = 463)			
<6 rooms	35.6 (165)	61.8 (102)	26.67 (44)	11.52 (19)	0.07
≥6 rooms	64.4 (298)	52.0 (155)	29.87 (89)	18.12 (54)	
		Health status and lifestyle			
		NCD (n = 471)			
Yes	19.1 (90)	62.2 (56)	20.0 (18)	17.78 (16)	0.19
No	80.9 (381)	54.1 (206)	30.97 (118)	14.96 (57)	
		Weight excess (n = 469)			
Yes	60.8 (285)	53.7 (153)	29.82 (85)	16.49 (47)	0.52
No	39.2 (184)	58.7 (108)	27.72 (51)	13.59 (25)	

Table 1. Cont.

Variables	% (n)	Food Security % (n)	Food Insecurity Mild % (n)	Food Insecurity Moderate/Severe % (n)	p-Value *
		The habit of drinking alcohol (n = 470)			0.99
No	54.0 (254)	55.5 (141)	29.13 (74)	15.35 (39)	
Yes	46.0 (216)	55.6 (120)	28.70 (62)	15.74 (34)	
		Smoking habit (n = 470)			0.25
No	82.8 (389)	55.0 (214)	30.33 (118)	14.65 (57)	
Yes	17.2 (81)	58.0 (47)	22.22 (18)	19.75 (16)	
		Work-related aspects			
		Time working at the CR (n = 471)			0.58
<12 months	42.7 (201)	58.2 (117)	27.86 (56)	13.93 (28)	
≥12 months	57.3 (270)	53.7 (145)	29.63 (80)	16.67 (45)	
		Management model (n = 471)			0.79
Direct management	38.0 (179)	53.6 (96)	30.17 (54)	16.2 (29)	
Outsourced	62.0 (292)	56.8 (166)	28.1 (82)	15.07 (44)	
		Brazilian region of CR (n = 471)			0.03
North/Northeast	45.7 (215)	49.8 (107)	34.42 (74)	15.81 (34)	
Midwest/South/Southeast	54.4 (256)	60.6 (155)	24.22 (62)	15.23 (39)	

* Pearson's chi-square p-value. [1] Minimum wage (MW): 175.90 USD per month.

Table 2. Bivariate multinomial logit model with odds ratio (OR) estimation between household food security situation (reference group: food security) and demographic, socioeconomic, health, lifestyle predictors, and those related to work in a Community Restaurant in all the Brazilian regions.

Predictor Variables	Mild Insecurity				Moderate/Severe Insecurity			
	OR	SE	p-Value	IC95%	OR	SE	p-Value	IC95%
Gender (n = 471)								
Female	1.1	0.24	0.67	0.72–1.68	1.43	0.4	0.20	0.82–2.49
Marital status (n = 471)								
Without partner	0.84	0.18	0.41	0.55–1.27	1.22	0.32	0.45	0.73–2.05
Age group (n = 471)								
>40 years old	0.78	0.18	0.28	0.50–1.23	0.95	0.27	0.86	0.55–1.65
Education level (n = 471)								
Elementary Education (complete/incomplete)	1.19	0.25	0.40	0.79–1.81	2.17	0.61	0.00	1.25–3.77
Income (per capita minimum wage) (n = 451)								
≤1/2 MW	1.86	0.42	0.00	1.20–2.88	3.8	1.07	0.00	2.18–6.60
Number of rooms								
<6 rooms	1.33	0.30	0.20	0.86–2.07	1.87	0.55	0.03	1.05–3.34
Number of workers in the family								
1 or 2 work	1.28	0.34	0.35	0.76–2.14	1.99	0.74	0.06	0.96–4.12
Governmental program participation (n = 471)								
Yes	1.65	0.45	0.07	0.96–2.82	3.17	0.96	0.00	1.75–5.74
Health status and lifestyle								
Weight excess (n = 469)								
Yes	1.18	0.26	0.45	0.77–1.80	1.33	0.37	0.31	0.77–2.29
NCD (n = 471)								
No	1.78	0.52	0.05	1.00–3.17	0.97	0.31	0.92	0.52–1.82
Smoking habit (n = 470)								
Yes	0.69	0.21	0.22	0.39–1.25	1.28	0.42	0.45	0.68–2.42
The habit of drinking alcohol (n = 470)								
Yes	0.98	0.21	0.94	0.65–1.49	1.02	0.27	0.93	0.61–1.72
Work aspects								
Time working at CR (n = 471)								
≥12 months	1.15	0.25	0.51	0.76–1.75	1.3	0.35	0.34	0.76–2.21
Management model (n = 471)								
Outsourced	0.88	0.19	0.55	0.57–1.34	0.88	0.24	0.63	0.52–1.49
Brazilian region (n = 471)								
Midwest/South/Southeast	0.58	0.12	0.01	0.38–0.88	0.79	0.21	0.381	0.47–1.33

OR: Odds ratio; SE: standard error. * Chi-Square test statistic p-value. ¹ Minimum wage (MW): 175.90 USD per month.

Table 3 shows the results of the multivariate model containing eight predictors selected in the previous steps. They were associated with at least one of the categories of HFSS with a value of $p < 0.20$. In the complete crude model, per capita income (Mild Insecurity—OR: 1.64; 95% CI: 1.01–2.66/Moderate/Severe Insecurity—OR: 2.7; 95% CI: 1.48–4.94); participation in a governmental program (Moderate/Severe Insecurity—OR: 2.02; 95% CI: 1.04–3.92) and CR region (Mild insecurity—OR: 0.5; 95% CI: 0.31–0.80) maintained an association with HFSS, increasing the chances of a CR worker belonging to one of the risk categories for food insecurity when in unfavorable socioeconomic situations, and compared to those with better socioeconomic conditions.

A stepwise backward method was applied to the multinomial model to adjust the final HFSS model. Calculating the odds ratios and standard errors and the model's goodness adjustment indexes guided the model's choice that best-suited data. Reduced models with smaller Akaike information criterion (AIC) than the previous model indicated the removal of the tested variable, as well as the p-value (>0.05) of the LRT (Table 4). The variables per capita household income, number of rooms, and number of people working (at the same home), in addition to the CR Brazilian region, remained in the model (Table 5).

Despite being maintained in the final model, considering the LRT results, the number of rooms and the number of people working did not maintain the association with food insecurity in the adjusted model. When tested, they were not confirmed (range of estimates < 10%). The multivariate model results confirmed the statistical significance of per capita household income as a predictor of HFSS. Food handlers with per capita household income equal to or less than half the minimum wage were 1.77 times more likely to be in a situation of mild food insecurity (OR: 1.77; CI95: 1.12–2.80) and around three times more likely to be in a situation of moderate/severe food insecurity (OR: 3.52; CI95: 2.00–6.19) when compared to individuals belonging to the food security category. In the adjusted model, the association with the CR Brazilian region was maintained in mild food insecurity. Therefore, the food handlers working in CR located in the Midwest/Southeast/South regions were 47% less likely to experience mild food insecurity (OR: 0.53; CI95: 0.34–0.83) compared to individuals in food security (Table 5).

Table 3. Multivariate multinomial logit model for predictors of Household Food Security Situation (reference group: food security) in food handlers of community restaurants.

Variables	Mild Insecurity				Moderate/Severe Insecurity			
	OR	SE	p-Value	IC95%	OR	SE	p-Value	IC95%
Incomplete/complete elementary education	1.27	0.3	0.32	0.79–2.02	1.76	0.54	0.07	0.96–3.22
Gender: Female	1.27	0.31	0.32	0.79–2.05	1.23	0.38	0.50	0.67–2.26
Income: ≤1/2 MW	1.64	0.4	0.04	1.01–2.66	2.7	0.83	0.001	1.48–4.94
Number of rooms ≥ 6	0.83	0.20	0,45	0.52–1.34	0.65	0.21	0,18	0.35–1.22
1 or 2 work in the family	1.02	0.29	0.93	0.59–1.79	1.22	0.48	0.61	0.56–2.64
Government program participation: Yes	1.29	0.39	0.41	0.71–2.34	2.02	0.68	0.04	1.04–3.92
NCD: No	1.62	0.51	0.12	0.88–2.98	1.07	0.38	0.85	0.53–2.15
Brazilian region: Midwest/South/Southeast	0.5	0.12	0.004	0.31–0.80	0.68	0.2	0.20	0.38–1.22

OR: Odds ratio; SE: standard error.

Table 4. Comparison of the complete and incomplete model performed using the Likelihood Ratio Test (LRT)—stepwise backward method.

LRT (Complete and Incomplete Model)	Obs.	ll(Nulo)	ll (Model)	gl	AIC	BIC	X² (LR X² (2))	p > X²
Complete Model backward	439	−427.5	−402.8	18	841.70	915.20	49.31	0.00
Model without education	439	−427.49	−404.65	16	841.296	906.649	3.63	0.16
Model without education and gender	439	−427.49	−405.11	14	838.211	895.394	4.54	0.34
Model without education, gender, and income	458	−447.10	−431.27	12	886.54	936.066	56.88	0.00
Model without education, gender, and number of workers	443	−431.19	−409.68	12	843.359	892.48	13.69	0.03
Model without education, gender, and government program	439	−427.49	−407.51	12	839.028	888.042	9.36	0.15
Model without education, Gender, government program, and number of rooms	443	−430.49	−412.33	10	844.652	885.588	18.98	0.01
Model without education, Gender, government program, and Region	439	−427.49	−411.20	10	842.407	883.252	16.74	0.03
Model without education, Gender, government program, and NCD	439	−427.49	−408.64	10	837.273	878.118	11.61	0.17

LRT: Likelihood Ratio Test; ll = Log likelihood; gl = degrees of freedom; AIC = Akaike information criterion; BIC = Bayesian information criterion.

Table 5. An adjusted multivariate model of the Household Food Security Situation (HFSS) (reference group: food security) determinants among food handlers in Brazilian community restaurants.

HFSS Model Adjusted	Mild Insecurity				Moderate/Severe Insecurity			
	OR	SE	p-Value	IC95%	OR	SE	p-Value	IC95%
Income ≤ 1/2 MW	1.77	0.41	0.02 *	1.12–2.80	3.52	1.02	0.00 *	2.00–6.19
Number of rooms < 6	0.77	0.18	0.27	0.48–1.23	0.58	0.18	0.08	0.31–1.07
Number of workers: 1 or 2	1.08	0.30	0.79	0.62–1.87	1.37	0.53	0.42	0.64–2.92
Brazilian region: Midwest/South/Southeast	0.53	0.12	0.01 *	0.34–0.83	0.76	0.21	0.32	0.43–1.32

Model adjusted for income, number of rooms, and workers in the household and region of the CR. 95% CI: 95% confidence interval; OR: Odds Ratio; SE: standard error. * significance level $p < 0.05$.

4. Discussion

Food insecurity is a public health problem, affecting individuals in all parts of the world. The latest survey conducted in 2018 by the Food and Agriculture Organization of the United Nations (FAO) showed that about two billion people suffered from moderate or severe food insecurity, representing 26.4% of the world population [1]. In Latin America, including Brazil, 188 million people had the perception of moderate to severe food insecurity, representing 30.9% of the population [1]. In Brazil, the last populational study that assessed food insecurity in households was the National Household Sample Survey (PNAD/NHSS), carried out in 2013 and showed a prevalence of 22.6% of food insecurity in the population [36].

In Brazil, the foodservice market employs about 250 thousand food handlers [47], who work in several foodservice segments, such as this study's locus (the CR). The findings can be extended to others in the foodservice segment, such as the food handlers working in hospitals, industrial or commercial food services. The activities of workers in the Brazilian foodservice sector revolve around a common goal, the production of meals for groups, whether healthy or sick [47], and, in the case of CR handlers, they provide meals for groups in social vulnerability [13]. The results of this study can be extended to the population of food handlers, given the peculiarities of this sector that include: (a) the composition of teams with professionals from different levels of educational background and with different and complementary activities [31]; (b) by workers from the different foodservice segments with a high prevalence of excess weight [30,32,48–50]; (c) by workers without professional training to carry out the activities, the in-service learning process takes place, which also leads to high turnover in the sector [31]; (d) inadequate work conditions, characterized by the requirement of long hours, rhythm and intense efforts with work overload, tasks such as repetitive movements, leading to absenteeism and high turnover of workers and the prevalence of work-related diseases [31]. This scenario reinforces the importance of the study and its scope.

Our results showed a total prevalence of 44.4% of food insecurity, much higher than the general population [51]. Moderate/severe food insecurity was almost twice the prevalence of the Brazilian population. In this study, socio-demographic characteristics showed that most food handlers were females in the age group ≤40 years old, similar to previous studies carried out with food handlers [15,16,18,22].

Two studies on food handlers from CR, the first in the city of Rio de Janeiro (n = 273 individuals from 7 CR) [21] and the second in the city of Belo Horizonte (n = 180 individuals from 4 CR) [22] showed a prevalence of total food insecurity of 53.7% and 24%, respectively. This prevalence, as in our study, is higher than food insecurity for the Brazilian population. It is worth mentioning that in these studies [21,22], most food handlers perceived themselves in mild food insecurity, according to the EBIA/BFIS classification [36]. There is a concern with access to food in the future, and it may impact the quality of the diet, choosing to buy cheaper foods [52].

In our study, an association was found between income and food insecurity, maintained in the regression model. Of the study participants, 39.9% had a per capita income at home equal to or less than half the minimum wage, classified as low-income families, according to the Brazilian Government [53]. Moreover, income showed a more significant impact on households with moderate to severe insecurity. Low-income families were about three times more likely to have food insecurity than workers with income above half the minimum wage. Other variables related to household income were associated with food insecurity as the number of rooms in the house and the number of individuals working, also maintained in the final regression model. Another variable related to household income that showed an association with food insecurity was the participation in a governmental program. Almost 40% of participants presented the requirements to receive governmental benefits [53], but only 19.3% of the participants received any benefit. Godoy et al. [20] also showed differences in food insecurity prevalence and income and education for CR customers. Among males, food insecurity prevalence was 64.2% when per capita income was below $\frac{1}{4}$ minimum wage and 54.8% from $\frac{1}{4}$ to half of the minimum wage. Females showed similar results, with 61.5% in food insecurity when per capita income was lower than $\frac{1}{4}$ minimum wage, and 54.8% when income was between $\frac{1}{4}$ to half of the minimum wage. CR customers with less than eight years of education also presented higher food insecurity for males and females (51% and 56.3%, respectively) [20].

In a previous study with the Brazilian population, 54.8% of households with moderate to severe food insecurity received per capita income up to half a minimum wage [51]. In the study carried out with food handlers in the CR in Rio de Janeiro, 59.4% of workers reported having another job to increase their income [21]. Per capita household income showed an inverse association with food insecurity in a study developed with food handlers in CR in Belo Horizonte/Brazil [22].

In a study that assessed food insecurity among workers in Canada, multivariate regression revealed that increased income independently decreases the chances of food insecurity in Canadian families, as well as having more workers in the family or at home. Income was considered a significant factor for the chances of food insecurity at home [24]. Some studies show an association between FI lower per capita income at home [53–55].

Schooling was associated with food insecurity at home in the bivariate analysis (p = 0.02), not remaining in the final regression model. In our study, 54.1% of the participants had an education level equal to or less than eight years, in agreement with other studies conducted with this professional category, identifying the highest percentage of individuals with educational level up to eight years of formal study (equivalent to elementary school) [19,21,34]. In general, education is associated with food insecurity among the general Brazilian population [51], in which a higher level of education relates to the lower prevalence of moderate or severe insecurity. Since food handlers in Brazil receive low salaries and present fewer years of formal education, they are more related to food insecurity even though working with food production.

In the study by Falcão et al. [21], an association was found between education and food insecurity in food handlers' homes. In the studied sample, the risk of those who had up to nine years of formal study was almost three times more likely to find themselves in a food insecurity situation than those with higher education.

Another variable that showed association with food insecurity was the region of the CR. Food handlers from the Midwest-South regions perceived themselves in household food security. The National Household Sample Survey (PNAD/NHSS) [47] identified a higher prevalence of food insecurity in the North and Northeast regions (30%) than the Midwest/Southeast/South regions (less than 20%). Bezerra et al. [54] also demonstrated higher FI in the North (40.3%) and the Northeast (46.1%) with positive and moderate correlation between FI and the percentage of the extremely poor population. Gubert et al. [55] demonstrated a reduction in FI prevalence in all Brazilian states from 2004 and 2013, higher in the Northeast region. Santos et al. [56] evaluated the tendency and associated factors of food insecurity in Brazil, analyzing the NHSS from 2004, 2009, and 2013. These researchers verified that even though there was a reduction in food insecurity levels with time, there was an increase in the association force between food insecurity and regions North and Northeast of Brazil. Residents from these regions had three to four more chances of having moderate to severe food insecurity. With CR customers, only for females, there was an association between region and food insecurity, with higher prevalence in the north and northeast regions [20].

This study did not show an association between food security and excess weight, contrary to other studies [57–60] that showed an association between food insecurity and excess weight. Shamah-Levy et al. [60] associated food insecurity with undernutrition and obesity, discussing that both situations come from poor eating habits. In children, Kac et al. [58] discussed a less consistent association with overweight, but Franklin et al. [57] studying women presented a higher prevalence of excess weight with food insecurity. Godoy et al. [61] did not find a significant association between food insecurity and BMI or body fat percentage for CR's male or female customers. Even though obesity is included in the NCDs, excess weight was not included as NCD for this study's associations. There was an association between food insecurity and NCDs; however, it was not maintained in the model.

One of this study's contributions is the confirmation of the dichotomy between FI and the performance in the food field. In the case of this study, places designed to promote access to food (CR) to prevent the occurrence of food insecurity also constitute a workspace for people in FI. Besides, the geographic location of the CRs act as protectors, confirming that regional inequalities in Brazil affect the same population group differently and confirming their claim that income is associated with FI. It is important to emphasize that the mean income from the North and Northeast regions is almost half of the income from workers from the South and Southeast regions in Brazil. This inequality is also observed in this food handler group and needs to be discussed inside a governmental program.

5. Conclusions

In Brazil, few studies assess workers' food insecurity. Food handlers play an essential role in promoting food security as responsible for producing and supplying meals in hygienic and nutritional conditions suitable for the population using this state equipment. These workers have characteristics, confirmed in the study, as low education and low income, which places them both as actors and target population of public policies aimed at food insecurity. This study is the first to assess food handlers nationwide, and a high prevalence of food insecurity was observed, higher than that of the general population. For moderate/severe food insecurity, it was almost twice the Brazilian population. Based on the study design, it is not possible to establish a causal link between the variables, but the study shows paths for further studies. The variables that showed an association for this population were the household income per capita for the different levels of food insecurity and the CR region for mild food insecurity. The high prevalence of food insecurity in this population and the return of the increase in the prevalence of food insecurity in the Brazilian and worldwide population point to the need for further studies on the theme with categories of workers, mainly low-income, which allow identifying factors related to the work environment and developing policies and interventions aimed at preventing food insecurity and its consequences for health.

Author Contributions: Conceptualization, I.C.F.; R.d.C.C.d.A.A.; R.d.R.F.B.; J.C.-S.; methodology, I.C.F.; R.d.C.C.d.A.A.; R.d.R.F.B.; J.C.-S.; R.P.Z.; R.B.A.B.; validation, I.C.F.; R.d.C.C.d.A.A.; R.d.R.F.B.; J.C.-S.; formal analysis, I.C.F.; R.d.C.C.d.A.A.; R.d.R.F.B.; J.C.-S.; R P.Z.; R.B.A.B.; investigation, I.C.F.; R.d.C.C.d.A.A.; R.P.Z.; R.B.A.B.; data curation, I.C.F.; R.d.C.C.d.A.A.; writing—original draft preparation, I.C.F.; R.d.C.C.d.A.A.; R.P.Z.; R.B.A.B.; writing—review and editing, I.C.F.; R.d.C.C.d.A.A.; R.P.Z.; A.R.; R.B.A.B.; visualization, A.R.; supervision, R.d.C.C.d.A.A.; project administration, R.d.C.C.d.A.A.; R.B.A.B.; funding acquisition, A.R. All authors have read and agreed to the published version of the manuscript.

Funding: This research received no external funding.

Institutional Review Board Statement: The study was conducted according to the guidelines of the Declaration of Helsinki, and approved by the Ethics Committee of University of Brasília (protocol code #037210).

Informed Consent Statement: Written informed consent was obtained from all participants.

Data Availability Statement: Data sharing is not applicable to this article.

Acknowledgments: The authors acknowledge the support of "Ministério do Desenvolvimento Social".

Conflicts of Interest: The authors declare no conflict of interest.

References

1. FAO; IFAD; UNICEF; WFP; WHO. *El Estado de la Seguridad Alimentaria y la Nutrición en el Mundo 2019*; FAO: Roma, Italy, 2019. Available online: http://www.fao.org/publications/es (accessed on 25 January 2020).
2. Araújo, F.R.; Santos, D.F.; Araújo, M.A.D. O direito humano à alimentação adequada promovido por políticas de acesso a alimentos: O caso da unidade Natal-RN do Projeto Café do Trabalhador. *Rev. Políticas Públicas* **2011**, *15*, 267–276. Available online: http://www.periodicoseletronicos.ufma.br/index.php/rppublica/article/view/842 (accessed on 15 April 2019).
3. General Assembly of the United Nations. *Universal Declaration of Human Rights*; United Nations Organization: New York, NY, USA, 1948. Available online: http://www.un.org/en/universal-declaration-human-rights/ (accessed on 9 July 2018).
4. Brown, E.M.; Tarasuk, V. Money speaks: Reductions in severe food insecurity follow the Canada Child Benefit. *Prev. Med.* **2019**, *129*, 105876. [CrossRef] [PubMed]
5. IBGE. *Segurança Alimentar*; Instituto Brasileiro de Geografia e Estatística: Rio de Janeiro, Brazil, 2013. Available online: https://biblioteca.ibge.gov.br/visualizacao/livros/liv91984.pdf (accessed on 25 June 2020).
6. Godoy, K.C.; Sávio, K.E.O.; Akutsu, R.d.C.; Gubert, M.B.; Botelho, R.B.A. Perfil e situação de insegurança alimentar dos usuários dos Restaurantes Populares no Brasil. *Cad. Saude. Publica* **2014**, *30*, 1239–1249. [CrossRef] [PubMed]
7. Bezerra, I.N.; Sichieri, R. Características e gastos com alimentação fora do domicílio no Brasil. *Rev. Saude. Publica* **2010**, *44*, 221–229. [CrossRef]
8. Lachat, C.; Nago, E.; Verstraeten, R.; Roberfroid, D.; Van Camp, J.; Kolsteren, P. Eating out of home and its association with dietary intake: A systematic review of the evidence. *Obes. Rev.* **2012**, *13*, 329–346. [CrossRef]
9. Buss, P.M.; Pellegrini Filho, A. A saúde e seus determinantes sociais. *Physis Rev. Saúde Coletiva* **2007**, *17*, 77–93. [CrossRef]
10. Food and Agriculture Organization of the United Nations. *The State of Food Security and Nutrition in the World 2019. Safeguarding against Economic Slowdowns and Downturns*; FAO: Rome, Italy, 2019.
11. Laraia, B.A. Food Insecurity and Chronic Disease. *Adv. Nutr.* **2013**, *4*, 203–212. [CrossRef]
12. Carrijo, A.P.; Botelho, R.B.A.; Akutsu, R.C.C.A.; Zandonadi, R.P. What Low-Income Brazilians Are Eating in Popular Restaurants Contributing to Promote Their Health? *Nutrients* **2018**, *10*, 414. [CrossRef]
13. Brasil. *Manual-Programa Restaurante Popular*; Ministério do Desenvolvimento Social e Combate à Fome: Brasília, Brazil, 2004. Available online: http://bvsms.saude.gov.br/bvs/publicacoes/projeto_logico_restaurante_popular.pdf (accessed on 22 October 2018).
14. Brazil. Mais de 130 Restaurantes Populares Garantem Alimentação Saudável Para População Vulnerável. 2020; pp. 1–5. Available online: https://www.gov.br/cidadania/pt-br/noticias-e-conteudos/desenvolvimento-social/noticias-desenvolvimento-social/mais-de-130-restaurantes-populares-garantem-alimentacao-saudavel-para-populacao-vulneravel (accessed on 27 December 2020).
15. Fideles, I.C.; Akutsu, R.d.C.C.d.A.; Costa, P.R.F.; Costa-Souza, J.; Botelho, R.B.A.; Zandonadi, R.P. Brazilian community restaurants' low-income food handlers: Association between the nutritional status and the presence of non-communicable chronic diseases. *Sustainability* **2020**, *12*, 3467. [CrossRef]
16. Boclin, K.d.L.S.; Blank, N. Prevalência de sobrepeso e obesidade em trabalhadores de cozinhas dos hospitais públicos estaduais da Grande Florianópolis, Santa Catarina. *Rev. Bras. Saúde. Ocup.* **2010**, *35*, 124–130. [CrossRef]
17. Scarparo, A.L.S.; Amaro, F.S.; Oliveira, A.B. Caracterização e Avaliação Antropométrica dos Trabalhadores dos Restaurantes Universitários da Universidade Federal do Rio Grande do Sul | Scarparo | Clinical & Biomedical Research. 2010, p. 30. Available online: https://seer.ufrgs.br/hcpa/article/view/15382 (accessed on 10 December 2019).
18. Simon, M.I.S.d.S.; Garcia, C.A.; Lino, N.D.; Forte, G.C.; Fontoura, I.d.D.; Oliveira, A.B.A.d. Avaliação nutricional dos profissionais do serviço de nutrição e dietética de um hospital terciário de Porto Alegre. *Cad. Saúde Coletiva* **2014**, *22*, 69–74. [CrossRef]
19. Cavalli, S.B.; Salay, E. Gestão de pessoas em unidades produtoras de refeições comerciais e a segurança alimentar. *Rev. Nutr.* **2007**, *20*, 657–667. [CrossRef]
20. Godoy, K.; Sávio, K.E.d.O.; Akutsu, R.d.C.; Gubert, M.B.; Botelho, R.B.A. Insegurança alimentar e estado nutricional entre indivíduos em situação de vulnerabilidade social no Brasil. *Cienc. Saude Coletiva* **2017**, *22*, 607–616. [CrossRef]
21. Falcão, A.C.M.L.; de Aguiar, O.B.; da Fonseca, M.d.J.M. Association of socioeconomic, labor and health variables related to food insecurity in workers of the popular restaurants in the city of Rio de Janeiro. *Rev. Nutr.* **2015**, *28*, 77–87. [CrossRef]
22. Costa, B.V.d.L.; Horta, P.M.; Ramos, S.A. Food insecurity and overweight among government-backed economy restaurant workers. *Rev. Nutr.* **2019**, *32*. [CrossRef]
23. Sobrinho, F.M.; Silva, Y.C.; Abreu, M.N.S.; Pereira, S.C.L.; Júnior, C.S.D. Fatores determinantes da insegurança alimentar e nutricional: Estudo realizado em Restaurantes Populares de Belo Horizonte, Minas Gerais, Brasil. *Cienc. Saude Coletiva* **2014**, *19*, 1601–1611. [CrossRef]
24. McIntyre, L.; Bartoo, A.C.; Emery, J.C.H. When working is not enough: Food insecurity in the Canadian labour force. *Public Health Nutr.* **2014**, *17*, 49–57. [CrossRef]
25. Sharkey, J.R.; Johnson, C.M.; Dean, W.R. Less-healthy eating behaviors have a greater association with a high level of sugar-sweetened beverage consumption among rural adults than among urban adults. *Food Nutr. Res.* **2011**, *55*. [CrossRef]
26. Oyefara, J.L. Food insecurity, HIV/AIDS pandemic and sexual behaviour of female commercial sex workers in Lagos metropolis, Nigeria. *SAHARA J.* **2007**, *4*, 626–635. [CrossRef]
27. Hill, B.G.; Moloney, A.G.; Mize, T.; Himelick, T.; Guest, J.L. Prevalence and predictors of food insecurity in migrant farmworkers in Georgia. *Am. J. Public Health* **2011**, *101*, 831–833. [CrossRef]

28. Colares, L.G.T.; De Freitas, C.M. Work process and workers' health in a food and nutrition unit: Prescribed versus actual work. *Cad. Saude Publica* **2007**, *23*, 3011–3020. [CrossRef] [PubMed]
29. Matos, C.H.d.; Proença, R.P.d.C. Condições de trabalho e estado nutricional de operadores do setor de alimentação coletiva: Um estudo de caso. *Rev. Nutr.* **2003**, *16*, 493–502. [CrossRef]
30. Isosaki, M.; Cardoso, E.; Glina, D.M.R.; Pustiglione, M.; Rocha, L.E. Intervention in a hospital foodservice and its effects on musculoskeletal symptoms. *Rev. Nutr.* **2011**, *24*, 449–462. [CrossRef]
31. Dos Santos, J.; Ferreira, A.A.; Meira, K.C.; Pierin, A.M.G. Excess weight in employees of food and nutrition units at a university in São Paulo State. *Einstein* **2013**, *11*, 486–491. [CrossRef]
32. De Aguiar, O.B.; Valente, J.G.; da Fonseca, M.d.J.M. Descrição sócio-demogŕfica, laboral e de saúde dos trabalhadores do setor de serviços de alimentaçõ dos restaurantes populares do estado do Rio de Janeiro. *Rev. Nutr.* **2010**, *23*, 969–982. [CrossRef]
33. Boclin, K.d.L.S.; Blank, N. Excesso de peso: Característica dos trabalhadores de cozinhas coletivas? *Rev. Bras. Saúde. Ocup.* **2006**, *31*, 41–47. [CrossRef]
34. Antunes, M.T.; Dal Bosco, S.M. Gestão em Unidades de Alimentação e Nutrição da Teoria à Prática. Editora Appris. 2020. Available online: https://books.google.com.br/books?id=gbfRDwAAQBAJ&pg=PT195&lpg=PT195&dq=uan+500+refeições&source=bl&ots=b59PT4BwP3&sig=ACfU3U3Lo0T7ytQ1uAKAwZbIDrzvFx3Sfg&hl=pt-BR&sa=X&ved=2ahUKEwjCx8bE78boAhUMGLkGHTzlDuIQ6AEwBXoECAwQLA#v=onepage&q=uan500refeições&f=fal (accessed on 1 April 2020).
35. Cochran, W.G. *Sampling Techniques*; John Wiley & Sons: Hoboken, NZ, USA, 2007.
36. Brasil; de Insegurança, E.B. Alimentar-EBIA: Análise Psicométrica de Uma Dimensão da Segurança Alimentar e Nutricional Ministériododesenvolvimentosociale Combate à Fomesecretariadeavaliaçãoe, G.E.S.T.Â.O.D.A.I.N.F.O.R.M.A.Ç.Ã.O. Brasília. 2014. Available online: www.mds.gov.br/sagi (accessed on 25 June 2020).
37. Ministério da Saúde. Vigitel: O Que é, Como Funciona, Quando Utilizar e Resultados. *Vigitel* **2019**, *1*. Available online: http://portalms.saude.gov.br/saude-de-a-z/vigitel (accessed on 18 March 2019).
38. Malta, D.C.; Bernal, R.T.I.; Andrade, S.S.C.d.A.; da Silva, M.M.A.; Velasquez-Melendez, G. Prevalence of and factors associated with self-reported high blood pressure in Brazilian adults. *Rev. Saude Publica* **2017**, *51*. [CrossRef]
39. WHO. *Mean Body Mass Index (BMI)*; WHO: Geneva, Switzerland, 2017.
40. Segall-Corrêa, A.M.; Marin-Leon, L. A segurança alimentar no Brasil: Proposição e usos da escala brasileira de medida da insegurança alimentar (EBIA) de 2003 a 2009. *Segurança Aliment Nutr.* **2015**, *16*, 1–19. [CrossRef]
41. Pérez-Escamilla, R.; Segall-Corrêa, A.M. Food Insecurity Measurement and Indicators. *Rev. Nutr.* **2008**, *21*, 15s–26s. Available online: https://www.scielo.br/scielo.php?pid=S1415-52732008000700003&script=sci_arttext&tlng=en (accessed on 25 June 2020). [CrossRef]
42. Panigassi, G.; Segall-Corrêa, A.M.; Marin-León, L.; Pérez-Escamilla, R.; Sampaio, M.D.F.A.; Maranha, L.K. Insegurança alimentar como indicador de iniquidade: Análise de inquérito populacional. *Cad. Saude Publica* **2008**, *24*, 2376–2384. [CrossRef] [PubMed]
43. Kleinbaum, D.G.; Klein, M. *Introduction to Logistic Regression*; Springer: Berlin, Heidelberg, Germany, 2010; Chapter 12. [CrossRef]
44. IBGE. *Pesquisa de Orçamentos Familiares 2017–2018: Análise do Consumo Alimentar no Brasil*; Instituto Brasileiro de Geografia e Estatística: Rio de Janeiro, Brazil, 2020.
45. FAO. *Food Security and Nutrition in the World*; FAO: Rome, Italy, 2020.
46. Hosmer, D.; Lemeshow, S. *Applied Logistic Regression*, 2nd Ed. ed; John Wiley: New York, NY, USA, 2000. Available online: http://resource.heartonline.cn/20150528/1_3kOQSTg.pdf (accessed on 26 September 2019).
47. IBGE. *Pesquisa Nacional por Amostra de Domicílio Contínua (PNAD Contínua)*; IBGE: Rio de Janeiro, Brazil, 2020.
48. ABERC. Mercado Real. Assoc. Bras. das Empres. Refeições Coletivas. 2020. Available online: https://www.aberc.com.br/mercadoreal.asp?IDMenu=21 (accessed on 27 December 2020).
49. Brazil. Art. 4 do Decreto 6135/07. Casa civil. 2007. Available online: https://www.jusbrasil.com.br/topicos/10827947/artigo-4-do-decreto-n-6135-de-26-de-junho-de-2007 (accessed on 25 June 2020).
50. Lopes, T.S.; Sichieri, R.; Salles-Costa, R.; Veiga, G.V.; Pereira, R.A. Family food insecurity and nutritional risk in adolescents from a low-income area of RIO de Janeiro, Brazil. *J. Biosoc. Sci.* **2013**, *45*, 661–674. [CrossRef] [PubMed]
51. Souza, N.N.D.; Dias, M.D.M.; Sperandio, N.; Franceschini, S.D.C.C.; Priore, S.E. Perfil socioeconômico e insegurança alimentar e nutricional de famílias beneficiárias do Programa Bolsa Família no município de Viçosa, Estado de Minas Gerais, Brasil, em 2011: Um estudo epidemiológico transversal. *Epidemiol. Serviços. Saúde* **2012**, *21*, 655–662. [CrossRef]
52. Lawrence, M.A.; Friel, S.; Wingrove, K.; James, S.W.; Candy, S. Formulating policy activities to promote healthy and sustainable diets. *Public Health Nutr.* **2015**, *18*, 2333–2340. [CrossRef]
53. IBGE-Instituto Brasileiro de Geografia e estatística. *Características Gerais dos Domicílios e dos Moradores: 2018*; IBGE: Rio de Janeiro, Brazil, 2019.
54. Bezerra, M.S.; Jacob, M.C.M.; Ferreira, M.A.F.; Vale, D.; Mirabal, I.R.B.; Lyra, C.D.O. Food and nutritional insecurity in Brazil and its correlation with vulnerability markers. *Cienc. Saude. Coletiva* **2020**, *25*, 3833–3846. [CrossRef]
55. Gubert, M.B.; dos Santos, S.M.C.; Santos, L.M.P.; Perez-Escamilla, R. A Municipal-level analysis of secular trends in severe food insecurity in Brazil between 2004 and 2013. *Glob. Food Sec.* **2017**, *14*, 61–67. [CrossRef]
56. Santos, T.G.; Cardoso Da Silveira, J.A.; Longo-Silva, G.; Ramires, E.K.N.M.; Menezes, R.C.E.D. Tendência e fatores associados à insegurança alimentar no Brasil: Pesquisa Nacional por. *Cad. Saúde Pública* **2018**, *34*, 66917. [CrossRef]

57. Franklin, B.; Jones, A.; Love, D.; Puckett, S.; Macklin, J.; White-Means, S. Exploring mediators of food insecurity and obesity: A review of recent literature. *J. Community Health* **2012**, *37*, 253–264. [CrossRef]
58. Kac, G.; Schlüssel, M.M.; Pérez-Escamilla, R.; Velásquez-Melendez, G.; da Silva, A.A.M. Household Food Insecurity Is Not Associated with BMI for Age or Weight for Height among Brazilian Children Aged 0–60 Months. *PLoS ONE* **2012**, *7*, e45747. [CrossRef]
59. Kac, G.; Velasquez-Melendez, G.; Schlüssel, M.M.; Segall-Côrrea, A.M.; Silva, A.A.; Pérez-Escamilla, R. Severe food insecurity is associated with obesity among Brazilian adolescent females. *Public Health Nutr.* **2012**, *15*, 1854–1860. [CrossRef]
60. Shamah-Levy, T.; Mundo-Rosas, V.; Rivera-Dommarco, J.A. La magnitud de la inseguridad alimentaria en México: Su relación con el estado de nutrición y con factores socioeconómicos. *Salud. Pública Méx* **2014**, s79–s85. Available online: http://www.scielosp.org/scielo.php?script=sci_arttext&pid=S0036-36342014000700012 (accessed on 2 July 2020). [CrossRef]
61. Godoy, K.C.; Sávio, K.E.; Gubert, M.B.; Botelho, R.B. Socio-demographic and food insecurity characteristics of soup-kitchen users in Brazil. *Cad. Saude Publica* **2014**, *30*, 1239–1249. [CrossRef] [PubMed]

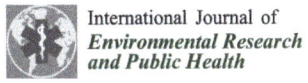

Article

Food Acquisition and Daily Life for U.S. Families with 4- to 8-Year-Old Children during COVID-19: Findings from a Nationally Representative Survey

Mackenzie J. Ferrante [1], Juliana Goldsmith [1], Sara Tauriello [1], Leonard H. Epstein [1,2], Lucia A. Leone [2,3] and Stephanie Anzman-Frasca [1,2,*]

1. Jacobs School of Medicine and Biomedical Sciences, University at Buffalo, Buffalo, NY 14214, USA; ferrant2@buffalo.edu (M.J.F.); jmgoldsm@buffalo.edu (J.G.); sarataur@buffalo.edu (S.T.); lhenet@buffalo.edu (L.H.E.)
2. Center for Ingestive Behavior Research, University at Buffalo, Buffalo, NY 14214, USA
3. School of Public Health and Health Professions, University at Buffalo, Buffalo, NY 14214, USA; lucialeo@buffalo.edu
* Correspondence: safrasca@buffalo.edu; Tel.: +1-716-829-6692

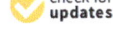

Citation: Ferrante, M.J.; Goldsmith, J.; Tauriello, S.; Epstein, L.H.; Leone, L.A.; Anzman-Frasca, S. Food Acquisition and Daily Life for U.S. Families with 4- to 8-Year-Old Children during COVID-19: Findings from a Nationally Representative Survey. *Int. J. Environ. Res. Public Health* **2021**, *18*, 1734. https://doi.org/10.3390/ijerph18041734

Academic Editor: António Raposo

Received: 23 December 2020
Accepted: 3 February 2021
Published: 10 February 2021

Publisher's Note: MDPI stays neutral with regard to jurisdictional claims in published maps and institutional affiliations.

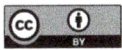

Copyright: © 2021 by the authors. Licensee MDPI, Basel, Switzerland. This article is an open access article distributed under the terms and conditions of the Creative Commons Attribution (CC BY) license (https://creativecommons.org/licenses/by/4.0/).

Abstract: Evidence of short-term impacts of the coronavirus disease 2019 (COVID-19) pandemic on family life is emerging. Continued research can shed light on potential longer-term impacts. An online survey of U.S. parents with 4- to 8-year-old children (n = 1000) was administered in October 2020. The survey examined parent-reported impacts of COVID-19 on lifestyle (e.g., work, child-care, grocery shopping), as well as current family food acquisition and eating behaviors (e.g., cooking, restaurant use). Descriptive statistics were calculated, incorporating sampling weights based on sociodemographics. In terms of COVID-19 impacts, parents reported increases in working from home, decreased work hours, and increased child care and instruction, with most children attending school or receiving care at home. Parents reported increased home cooking and online grocery shopping; only 33% reported increased take-out or delivery from restaurants. About half of parents reported that their child dined at restaurants, 62% reported getting take-out, and 57% reported delivery from restaurants at least 2–3 times per month. About half viewed dining at restaurants as safe, while take-out and delivery were seen as safe by around three-quarters. Approximately two-thirds reported recent food insecurity. These nationally-representative results illustrate possible longer-lasting shifts in family life, with the potential to impact health and well-being. Sociodemographic differences and research and policy implications are discussed.

Keywords: COVID-19; families; children; food acquisition; restaurants

1. Background

The coronavirus disease 2019 (COVID-19) pandemic caused sudden and drastic lifestyle changes across the globe. In the United States (U.S.), protection measures were implemented beginning in March 2020 to halt the spread of the virus, closing restaurants, businesses, schools, and child-care facilities around the country and sending more than 50 million children back to their homes to finish the school year [1–3]. Families' day-to-day lives were upended, as many suddenly needed to provide child care and schooling at home, often in combination with remote work or job loss as unemployment rates increased [4,5]. Evidence of short-term impacts of these drastic changes on energy-balance-related health behaviors, such as physical activity and screen time, in the early months of the pandemic is beginning to emerge. More than six months later, the COVID-19 pandemic continues, but in many regions, restaurants, businesses, and schools are now open under new restrictions [6]. Information on families' behaviors under this "new normal" is limited. Examining families' daily lives as the COVID-19 pandemic progresses is important, as potential new family routines and behaviors may have lasting positive, or negative, impacts on the health of families, as well as implications for research and policy.

Recently published survey data suggest that the early months of the pandemic brought changes in many energy-balance-related behaviors. In the initial months of the pandemic, there were reported increases in sedentary behavior and less time spent on physical activity for both adults and children [7–9]. This was coupled with increased screen time and sleep for children [7] and increased levels of stress and anxiety for adults, particularly parents [4,8,10]. In addition, almost 35% of households in the U.S. with children under the age of 18 indicated some form of food insecurity early in the pandemic, a substantial change from 11% in 2018/2019 [11–13]. Increased food insecurity early in the pandemic may be connected to increases in unemployment, which in the U.S. reached over 14% in April of 2020 with almost 19 million unemployment claims filed [5,14]. Food insecurity has been linked with unhealthy dietary and weight outcomes for children, highlighting that these impacts of COVID-19 have the potential to affect children's eating and health in the long term [15,16].

Prior to the start of the pandemic, U.S. children had a notably poor diet quality, consumed few nutrient-dense foods such as whole grains, fruits, and vegetables, and frequently ate restaurant foods [17,18]. U.S. families spent a significant amount of their food dollars on restaurant foods and fewer food dollars on groceries and home cooked meals, a trend documented since the 1970s [19,20]. This trend in food spending translated to families eating out frequently and preparing less food at home [21,22], a trend that has also been observed across the world [23,24]. However, there is evidence that the pandemic may be reversing this trend. Surveys administered during stay-at-home orders indicated significant increases in meals prepared at home, and data from the Economic Research Service indicated an increase in food purchasing from retail stores [8,25]. Families also shifted where and how they shopped for food (e.g., altering the typical location of grocery trips and making more use of freezers and pantry staples) [10]. It is estimated that almost three-quarters of American households avoided restaurant food in the initial months of the pandemic, and household expenditures for restaurant foods were about 30% lower than they had been in March 2019 [13,25]. However, the initial months of the pandemic also brought increases in snacking and intake of foods such as sugar-sweetened beverages, potato chips, and red meat [7,9]. While results from the initial COVID-19 pandemic studies illustrate shifts in food acquisition and eating behavior, the extent to which these trends translate into longer-lasting changes for families is unknown. Research on family food acquisition and eating behavior during COVID-19 has primarily focused on the initial months of the pandemic and involved convenience samples. In addition, food acquisition from restaurants via take-out and delivery is understudied, both during COVID-19 and in general. Therefore, nationally representative studies examining families' current behaviors related to food acquisition and restaurant use are warranted.

Taken together, emerging evidence suggests that the drastic lifestyle changes of the pandemic's early months brought changes in energy-balance-related behaviors for children and families. However, little is known about whether these changes have persisted more than six months into the pandemic. A description of current behaviors can elucidate the extent to which COVID-19 may have longer-lasting impacts on families' energy-balance-related behaviors and health. Therefore, in Fall 2020, we examined the following among a nationally representative sample of U.S. parents with at least one 4- to 8-year-old child: (1) parent-reported impacts of COVID-19 on various aspects of daily life, including food acquisition, physical activity, child care, and employment; and (2) families' current food acquisition and eating behaviors, including preparation of meals at home, children's consumption of restaurant foods in-person and via take-out and delivery, and factors affecting restaurant meal choices.

2. Methods

2.1. Participants

Invitations to participate in this study were sent to a stratified random sample identified as U.S. residents 18 years of age or older with at least one 4- to 8-year-old child in the household ($n = 1000$). Participants were recruited using the Harris Poll Online opt-in panel (https://theharrispoll.com/), which includes millions of respondents who have agreed to participate in survey research. To be eligible, individuals needed to be English-speaking, at least 18 years of age, a parent/caregiver (referred to herein as parents) with at least one 4- to 8-year-old child, and have internet access. Possible participants were sent a password-protected email invitation to participate in the survey.

2.2. Procedures

A 61-item survey was developed by researchers at the University at Buffalo in order to understand how parents with at least one 4- to 8-year-old child describe daily life and energy-balance-related behaviors during the COVID-19 pandemic. Harris Interactive was commissioned to disseminate the survey and incorporate sampling weights based on parent age, sex, race and ethnicity, education, income, region, marital status, household size, and number of children under 18 years, so results would be representative of the U.S. population of parents with 4- to 8-year-old children. Participating parents completed the survey at one time during October 2020. Participants with multiple 4- to 8-year-old children were asked to complete child-focused survey questions about their child with the most recent birthday. Study procedures were approved by the University at Buffalo Institutional Review Board.

2.3. Measures

The survey was created using previously-developed measures from the existing literature as well as newly-developed items. Validated scales were used to measure perceived stress and food insecurity as described below. No changes were made to the former, while the latter's time frame was modified to fit with the present study's focus on the COVID-19 pandemic (i.e., specifying that responses should reflect experiences in the past two months, rather than the past year). Other survey items were adapted or created for this study as described herein. Overall, the main modification to existing items was to specify that responses should reflect experiences during the past two months where appropriate. Other minor modifications to existing items are described below.

2.3.1. Participant Demographics and Context

Parents reported their age, gender, height, weight, marital status, highest level of education, household income, employment status, race/ethnicity, and whether the household received any government benefits (e.g., the Supplemental Nutrition Assistance Program (SNAP), which provides nutritional assistance to supplement food budgets, or Medicaid, which assists low-income individuals with health costs). Parents also reported characteristics of their 4-to-8-year-old child, including age, gender, race/ethnicity, and eligibility for free or reduced-price school meals. Additionally, they indicated who in the household was the most familiar with the child's daily activities (responses included: I am, another parent/guardian, another parent/guardian and I are equally familiar). A brief validated 2-item screen was administered to identify households at risk for food insecurity [26], specifying that respondents should answer based on the past two months. Items assessed how often in the prior two months the household has 'worried whether food would run out before we got money to buy more' and 'the food that we bought just didn't last and we didn't have money to get more.' Responses included: often, sometimes, or never. Food insecurity is indicated when participants respond often or sometimes to at least one of the two items. Cronbach's alpha for this 2-item screen in the present sample was 0.84.

Parents were also asked a series of questions developed by the research team about the extent of current COVID-19 related protection measures in their town/city, including if mask wearing was mandated and whether there were restaurant-related restrictions. Children's schooling and care in the last week (in-person elementary school, virtual elementary school, home school, and/or in- or out-of-home non-parental child care) was also assessed. Parental stress during the previous month was measured using the short version of the validated Perceived Stress Scale (PSS-4) [27]. Participants completed four questions, administered verbatim from the original scale, assessing the degree to which they perceived situations in their life to be stressful (e.g., 'how often have you felt that you were unable to control the important things in your life?'). Items were rated on a five-point scale from never (0) to very often (4). Cronbach's alpha for the PSS-4 in this sample was 0.56. The correlation between food insecurity and perceived stress scores was also examined as an indicator of convergent validity and was 0.31 ($p < 0.0001$).

2.3.2. Daily Life Changes during the Coronavirus Disease 2019 (COVID-19) Pandemic

Parent-reported changes in daily life and energy-balance-related behaviors were assessed using questions adapted from The Epidemic–Pandemic Impacts Inventory (EPII), establishing who in the household was affected by changes related to care of, instruction of, and quality time with children, and care for other family members [28]. Parents were also asked whether or not (yes or no) their work had been affected in a variety of ways, including job loss and increased or decreased work hours, using a question and response options from the National Institute of Health's Environmental influences on Child Health Outcomes (ECHO) questionnaire [29]. The extent to which the COVID-19 pandemic resulted in changes in various lifestyle behaviors was also assessed using questions adapted from the ECHO questionnaire [29]. Participants indicated how often they engaged in the following behaviors: getting physical exercise, spending time outdoors in nature, spending time on screens or devices (e.g., phone, video games, TV), eating home-cooked meals, eating takeout/delivered food, going to the grocery store, going to farmer's markets, using farm shares or community-supported agriculture, and using online grocery shopping/grocery delivery, relative to their behaviors pre-pandemic. For these questions, we modified the original response scale, so that participants indicated whether they engaged in each behavior: more often, less often, no change, or N/A. We began with behaviors from the ECHO questionnaire and then added some additional behaviors of interest, specific to food acquisition (e.g., use of online grocery shopping, farmer's markets).

2.3.3. Current Food Acquisition and Eating Behaviors

Parents were asked how frequently meals were prepared at home during the past two months with response options including 0–1 times per week, 2–3 times, 4–5 times, and more than 5 times per week [8]. Restaurant use was assessed by asking parents how often their child ate food from restaurants during the past two months in three different contexts: dine-in, take-out, or delivery. Response options included: never, once a month or less, 2–3 times a month, once a week, 2–3 times a week, and 4 or more times a week. Parents were also asked to indicate how safe they felt it was to obtain food from a restaurant as dine-in, take-out, or delivery (response options included: very unsafe, somewhat unsafe, somewhat safe, very safe). For each mode of restaurant use, parents also reported typical behaviors over the past 2 months, including who typically selected the child's restaurant meal (the child, the responding parent, the responding parent and child together, another adult, or another adult and the child together) and the most important (1) to least important (7) reasons for the child's typical restaurant meal selection (taste, habit, cost, nutrition, appeal, treat, something new). These items were generally administered verbatim from previous restaurant research [30], with exceptions being the aforementioned change to the time frame of interest (i.e., the past two months), as well as asking participants to rank order the reasons for the child's meal choice rather than having them select all reasons that applied. In addition, the perceived restaurant safety item was newly developed for the present study.

Three additional restaurant-related items were developed for the present study. Parents reported what was typically ordered for the child when ordering restaurant food for take-out or delivery: their own kid's meal, their own adult meal, shared food with other family members, or other. Parents also ranked their top five reasons for deciding to order restaurant food for take-out or delivery and the top five reasons affecting their choice of restaurant from a list of options (e.g., no time, no groceries, cost, promotion, treat for child, treat for self, appeal, taste, nutrition, something new, habit, convenience, technology, support for restaurants).

2.4. Data Analysis

Frequencies (for categorical variables) and means and standard errors (for continuous variables) were calculated for demographic/contextual variables. Items from the PSS-4 were reverse-scored as appropriate and then summed, resulting in a composite score ranging from 0–16, with higher scores indicating higher stress. Frequencies (for categorical variables) and means and standard errors (for continuous variables) were calculated to describe: (1) parent-reported impacts of COVID-19 on various aspects of daily life and energy-balance-related behaviors, including employment, child care and instruction, physical activity, screen time, grocery shopping, cooking, and ordering take-out or delivery; as well as (2) families' current food acquisition and eating behaviors. These included: frequency of preparation of meals at home, children's consumption of restaurant foods (frequency of dining in, take-out, and delivery), perceived safety of restaurant foods, who chose children's restaurant meals and types of meals chosen, and factors affecting children's meal choices and restaurant choices. Analysis of factors affecting children's meal choices were restricted to parents who reported playing a role in deciding the child's meal order (determining it themselves or with the child), as those not playing any role in the decision would not be expected to know which factors contributed to the decision.

Given the potential for differential impacts of COVID-19, we also explored whether current food acquisition behaviors differed by sociodemographics. We tested models that considered parent age, sex, race/ethnicity, education, and family income as predictors of: the frequency of home cooking, dining out, take-out, and delivery, as well as the perceived safety of each mode of restaurant use. Linear regression models were used unless distributions of residuals violated normality assumptions, in which case outcomes were dichotomized, with logistic regression used to predict meaningful outcomes (e.g., rating restaurant dining as safe vs. unsafe). Backwards deletion was used to arrive at final models, retaining independent variables that predicted outcomes at $p < 0.05$. All analyses incorporated sampling weights, so that results were representative of U.S. parents with 4- to 8-year-old children. Sampling weights were based on parent age, sex, race and ethnicity, education, income, region, marital status, household size, and number of children under 18 years. Data were analyzed using SAS 9.4 (Cary, NC, USA).

3. Results

3.1. Participant Demographics, Characteristics, and Context

A majority of responding parents were married or living with their partner (83%), with a median of 2 children in the household. Most parents (95%) reported being a primary caregiver of the target child, indicated by reporting that they were the parent or guardian in the household who is the most familiar with the child's daily activities, or that they and another parent or guardian were equally familiar. Despite variability in family income, reported food insecurity was very common among families over the past two months. More than two-thirds (69%) of parents met the criteria for food insecurity by reporting that they had often or sometimes felt that they might run out of food and not have money to purchase more (66%); or that it was often or sometimes true that the food they had purchased hadn't lasted and they didn't have money to purchase more (56%).

In terms of current COVID-related protection measures, a majority of parents reported that masks were mandated in the city or town where they resided (90%), and that in most cases, at least some closures had been reversed, with very few (38%) or some (44%) businesses closed at the time of survey administration. About half of parents reported that restaurants were open for both indoor and outdoor dining at a reduced capacity, while approximately one-third (29%) reported restaurants in their town or city could only offer take-out or delivery. In many cases, changes to children's schooling persisted: parents reported that 47% of children were attending school virtually, and 31% were being homeschooled, while 21% attended in-person elementary school, and 19% received care outside the home (including preschools, after-school programs, and child-care centers). Parents reported an average stress level of 7.2 (standard error of the mean (SEM) = 0.14) on the PSS-4's 0–16 scale. Additional demographic and contextual variables are reported in Table 1.

Table 1. Participant characteristics for study sample (n = 1000) (weighted frequencies and means).

Sociodemographic Variables	%	Mean (SEM)	Sociodemographic Variables Cont.	%	Mean (SEM)
Gender			**Race/ethnicity**		
Female	55		White	69	
Male	45		Black or African American	12	
Transgender	1		Asian	11	
Other	0		Other	8	
Marital status			Hispanic	22	
Now Married/Living with Partner	83		**Highest level of education completed**		
Single/Never Married	9		≤High School/GED [a]	20	
Divorced/Separated/Widowed	8		Some college/Tech/Associates	37	
Age (years)		38.8 (9.5)	Bachelor's Degree	17	
18–24	2		≥Graduate Degree	26	
25–34	31		**Government benefits received at any point in 2020**		
35–44	45		SNAP [b]	42	
45–54	14		WIC [c]	30	
55+	8		Medicaid	46	
Body mass index			Disability	21	
25.0–29.9 (overweight)	33		TANF [d]	25	
≥30.0 (obese)	17		**Number of children in the household**		2.4 (1.2)
Current employment status			1	18	
Employed Full Time	63		2	45	
Employed Part Time	6		3	24	
Self-employed	6		4+	12	
Not employed	7		**4–8-year-old child with most recent birthday**		
Homemaker/Stay-at-home	14		Age (years)		6.2 (1.4)
Household income (per year)			Gender—% Male	55	
<$24,999	10		Gender—% Female	45	
$25,000–$34,999	7		**Child eligible for free or reduced-price school meals (n = 593 due to age range)**		
$35,000–$49,999	11				
$50,000–$74,999	16		Yes	59	
$75,000–$99,999	15		No	31	
>$100,000	41		Don't know	9	
Coronavirus disease 2019 (COVID-19)-related restrictions in place in parent's town or city					
General restrictions			**Restaurant restrictions**		
Most businesses are closed	18		Can offer take-out or delivery	29	
Some businesses are closed	44		Can dine in: Outdoors only	15	
Very few businesses are closed	38		Both outdoors and indoors: reduced capacity	50	
Masks mandated (public places, indoors)			Both outdoors and indoors: full capacity	6	
Yes	90				

[a] GED – General Educational Development Test. [b] SNAP—Supplemental Nutrition Assistance Program. [c] WIC—Special Supplemental Nutrition Program for Women, Infants, and Children (31). [d] TANF—Temporary Assistance for Needy Families.

3.2. Daily Life Changes during the COVID-19 Pandemic

Parents reported changes to employment as a result of the COVID-19 pandemic, including that one-third (38%) moved to working remotely (from home) while 14% lost their job permanently. One-third (30%) of parents also indicated that their job put them at an increased risk for getting COVID-19. Parent-reported impacts on employment appear in Table 2. The pandemic impacted daily home life such that a majority of parents reported either themselves, another person in the home, or a combination of the two had to take over teaching or instruction of the child, and a substantial proportion of parents (48%) reported spending more quality time with children than they had prior to COVID-19. Table 3 illustrates further parent-reported impacts of COVID-19 on child care and schooling and care for others in the household.

Table 2. Parent-reported impacts of the COVID-19 pandemic on employment (n = 1000).

Employment Changes	Yes (%)	No (%)
Moved to working remotely/from home	38	62
Permanent job loss	14	86
Temporary job loss	20	80
Got a new job	14	86
Reduced work hours	38	62
Increased work hours	25	75
Laid off employees	16	84
Work was affected in some other way	39	61
Put at increased risk for getting COVID-19	30	70
Did not have a paying job before COVID-19	10	90

Table 3. Parent-reported impacts of the COVID-19 pandemic on child-care, schooling, and care of other family members (n = 1000).

Family Care Changes	Yes (Me) (%)	Yes (Person in Household) (%)	Yes (Me & Person in Household) (%)	No (%)	N/A (%)
Took over teaching/instruction of child	47	16	20	12	4
Child care or babysitting unavailable	25	14	13	30	18
More quality time with child(ren)	48	14	29	7	1
More time spent caring for other family members	38	15	17	23	7

Parent-reported impacts of COVID-19 on energy-balance-related behaviors—physical activity, screen time, grocery shopping, cooking, and ordering take-out and delivery—appear in Table 4. Two-thirds of parents (66%) reported spending more time on screens or devices while only a small percentage (13%) reported less time spent on screens or devices. Parent-reported impacts on time spent exercising and in nature were more varied, with substantial percentages of respondents each reporting increases and decreases in these behaviors (Table 4). A majority of parents reported eating home-cooked meals more often than before the pandemic (64%). Almost half of parents (44%) reported eating take-out and delivery less often, while 22% reported no change from before the pandemic. Half of parents (48%) reported going to the grocery store less often than they did pre-pandemic, with about one-quarter (26%) indicating increased frequency. About half of parents (49%) reported increases in use of online grocery shopping.

Table 4. Parent-reported impacts of COVID-19 on physical activity, outdoor time, screen time, food acquisition, and cooking (n = 1000).

Lifestyle Behavior Changes	More Often (%)	Less Often (%)	No Change (%)	N/A (%)
Physical Exercise	40	29	27	4
Time spent: outdoors/in nature	36	40	22	2
Time spent: on screens/devices	66	13	19	2
Eat home-cooked meals	64	12	23	1
Eat take-out/delivery	33	44	22	1
Go to the grocery store	26	48	25	2
Go to farmer's markets	20	34	21	25
Use of farm shares or community supported agriculture	19	23	22	36
Used online grocery shopping	49	11	19	20

3.3. Food Acquisition and Eating Behaviors

Recent food acquisition and eating behaviors are reported in Table 5. Almost three-quarters of parents (71%) reported preparing meals at home at least four days per week during the last two months. Parent-reported frequency of dining-in at restaurants by children during that same period revealed that around one-quarter (27%) were dining-in at least once per week, and around one-third had restaurant food via take-out (37%) and delivery (34%) at least once per week. Just under half of parents (47%) reported that they felt dining-in at a restaurant was either very safe or somewhat safe while take-out and delivery were reported to be either somewhat safe or very safe by approximately three-quarters of parents. Over half of parents were involved in deciding what their child ordered to eat from restaurants, either making the decision on their own or together with their child. Parents reported that when ordering take-out or delivery, over three-quarters of children (77%) had their own children's meal, while one-quarter of children had their own adult meal (26%), and one-third (31%) shared food with other family members (selecting all options that applied). When it came to ranking reasons for choosing the child's meal, on average, parents who had a hand in the decision (46.7%) reported that taste was the most important reason, followed closely by nutrition (Table 6). When asked about reasons for deciding to order take-out or delivery, the most popular selections were convenience and taste. Table 7 displays all reasons for take-out and delivery choices.

Table 5. Parent-reported restaurant use and ordering for their 4- to 8-year-old-child and perceived restaurant safety ($n = 1000$ *).

Frequency	How Often Child Ate at/from Restaurants (Past 2 Months)		
	In-person (%)	Take-out (%)	Delivery (%)
Never	28	14	23
<1×/month	24	24	20
2–3×/month	21	25	23
1×/week	13	19	15
2–3×/week	11	14	15
>4/week	3	4	4
	Who Typically Decided What to Order for Child (Past 2 Months)?		
	In-person (%)	Take-out (%)	Delivery (%)
Mother (Reporting Parent)	12	16	18
Father (Reporting Parent)	17	16	18
The child	33	28	23
Parent and child together	28	34	34
Another adult	5	4	4
Child and another adult	4	2	3
	How Safe Do You Currently Feel That It Is to:		
	Dine indoors at a restaurant (%)	Eat take-out food (%)	Eat delivered food (%)
Very unsafe	21	9	6
Somewhat unsafe	32	16	16
Somewhat safe	29	45	46
Very safe	18	29	31

* All 1000 parents responded to restaurant frequency questions (for dining in-person, take-out, and delivery). Parents who responded "never" to these were not asked to respond to the subsequent questions about that mode of restaurant use.

In terms of individual differences in current food acquisition behaviors, parent gender was the only significant predictor of cooking at home in the tested multivariable models, with female parents cooking at home more than other respondents (t = 2.6, $p < 0.01$). Being a female parent also predicted a lower frequency of the child consuming food at restaurants (t = −3.1, $p < 0.01$), as did lower income (t = 4.5, $p < 0.0001$; R^2 for final multivariable model = 0.08). Parent education was the only significant predictor of children's frequency of take-out consumption in the tested multivariable models, such that parents with lower education levels reported less take-out (t = 5.9, $p < 0.0001$; R^2 = 0.05). Lower parent education was also linked with less restaurant delivery (t = 2.52, $p < 0.05$), as were lower income (t = 2.60, $p < 0.01$) and non-Hispanic Asian race (t = 2.01, $p < 0.05$; R^2 = 0.09). Race and ethnicity was the main predictor of variability in the reported safety of restaurant use: using dummy-coded indicators of race/ethnicity, Hispanic (t = −4.3, $p < 0.0001$), non-Hispanic Black (t = −5.4, $p < 0.0001$), and non-Hispanic Asian (t = −3.0, $p < 0.01$) respondents were all less likely to view in-person dining as safe, as were respondents with lower education (t = 2.3, $p < 0.05$). Hispanic respondents were less likely than respondents in other race/ethnicity categories to report that restaurant delivery was safe as well (t = −2.4, $p < 0.05$). Other demographic factors were unrelated to perceived restaurant safety.

Table 6. Parent ranking of the importance of different factors when choosing a restaurant meal for their child over the past 2 months (n = 467) [a,b].

Reasons for Meal Choice	Dining in-Person	Ordering Take-Out	Ordering Delivery
	Mean (SEM)	Mean (SEM)	Mean (SEM)
Taste—child likes the foods in the meal	3.2 (0.1)	3.2 (0.1)	3.3 (0.1)
Habit—what the child typically orders	3.7 (0.1)	3.6 (0.1)	4.1 (0.1)
Cost—price of the meal	4.6 (0.1)	4.5 (0.1)	4.5 (0.1)
Nutrition—health of the meal	3.5 (0.1)	3.6 (0.1)	3.8 (0.1)
Appeal—the meal looks good	4.2 (0.1)	4.2 (0.1)	4.0 (0.1)
Treat—my child doesn't get it often	4.3 (0.1)	4.1 (0.1)	4.0 (0.1)
New—trying a new flavor	4.5 (0.1)	4.7 (0.1)	4.5 (0.1)

Parents ranked factors shown above on a 7-point scale, where 1 was the most important reason, and 7 was least important. The means depict the average rank for each reason, with lower means indicating that the reason was more important on average. [a] All 1000 parents responded to restaurant frequency questions (for dining in-person, take-out, and delivery). Parents who responded "never" to these were not asked to respond to the subsequent questions about that mode of restaurant use. [b] In addition, only parents who reported playing a role in deciding the child's meal order (determining it themselves or with the child) were included in this analysis, as those not playing any role in the decision would not be expected to know which factors contributed to the decision.

Table 7. Reasons behind parents' take-out and delivery orders over the past 2 months.

Reasons for Take-Out/Delivery	Participants Selecting This Reason (%) [a]	Mean (SEM)
Convenience: it was fast/easy	50.1	2.7 (0.1)
Taste: the meal would taste good	43.1	3.1 (0.1)
Treat self: to treat myself	41.6	3.0 (0.1)
Treat child: to treat my child(ren)	41.8	3.1 (0.1)
No time: I wanted to save time/didn't have time to cook	40.5	2.5 (0.1)
Promotion: because of a special such as a discount	29.3	3.3 (0.1)
Support: trying to support restaurants that my family likes	28.7	3.0 (0.1)
Cost: because of its price	27.1	3.1 (0.1)
Appeal: the meal looked good in the picture on the menu/website	26.2	3.3 (0.1)
Something new: trying new foods/flavors	26.0	3.3 (0.1)
Habit: it is what I usually do	25.5	3.2 (0.1)
Nutrition: the meal would be healthy	24.7	2.9 (0.1)
Technology: Able to order using an online delivery service	23.6	3.0 (0.1)
No groceries: did not have groceries or ingredients to cook	22.2	2.8 (0.1)
Reasons for restaurant choice		
Taste: my family likes the food from that restaurant	59.4	2.8 (0.1)
Convenience: it is fast/easy	53.7	2.8 (0.1)
Cost: because of its price	47.0	3.0 (0.1)
Treat: it is a treat that my family does not get often	44.6	3.1 (0.1)
Habit: it is a restaurant we usually order from	41.1	3.1 (0.1)
Promotion: because of a special such as a discount	37.7	3.1 (0.1)
Support: trying to support restaurants that my family likes	36.2	3.1 (0.1)
Appeal: the food at that restaurant looked good in the picture	35.5	3.3 (0.1)
Nutrition: because it offers healthy food	34.3	3.0 (0.1)
Technology: able to order using an online delivery service	33.4	3.1 (0.1)
Something new: trying a new flavor	27.2	3.1 (0.1)

[a] Here, parents ranked their top 5 reasons in each category. The (weighted) percent of parents endorsing each option is shown, as well as the average rank order for each option among parents endorsing it.

4. Discussion

The COVID-19 pandemic is changing the way families in the U.S. eat, work, and live. Such periods of drastic flux can potentially lead to the establishment of new behaviors and habits, for better or worse. Evidence of short-term impacts of COVID-19 on families' energy-balance-related behaviors has emerged, but to date, little is known about potential longer-term impacts. The present nationally representative survey of U.S. parents was administered in Fall 2020, a time during which many initial protection measures and restrictions had been lifted, thus offering a glimpse into families' potential "new normal". Results suggest there may be some longer-lasting impacts of COVID-19, including on children's schooling and time spent at home, as well as the reported prevalence of food insecurity, which remains high. Families reported increased home food preparation while still using restaurants a few times each month. Take-out and delivery were perceived as safer than dining in and were used at higher rates, with some sociodemographic differences in restaurant use and perceived safety. Understanding families' behaviors during this phase of the pandemic can provide insight into potential lasting impacts on families' lifestyles and health and can inform future research and policy.

Surveys of families in many nations have contributed evidence of short-term impacts of COVID-19 on energy-balance-related behaviors. For example, changes in the home food environment and increases in food insecurity were reported in a survey study of 584 U.S. parents of children ages 5 to 18 [31], and in a survey study of 254 families with young children in Ontario, Canada, substantial percentages of parent respondents reported eating more snack foods, eating less fast food or take-out food, spending more time cooking, and eating more meals with their children [32]. Both of these surveys were fielded in April and May 2020, and these apparent short-term impacts may be tied to broader contextual changes, including COVID-19-related changes to work and family life.

In the present study, parents' self-reported impacts of COVID-19 revealed that they were working from home more and taking greater part in the care and instruction of their children, with many reporting reduced work hours. Notably, more than six months into the pandemic, the majority of respondents' children were either attending school virtually or being homeschooled. In 2019, only 3% of children were homeschooled while the remaining 97% of the 50 million children enrolled in primary or secondary education in the U.S. attended school in person, highlighting an ongoing, drastic change to family routines [33]. It is not surprising that levels of reported stress were higher than previously-established norms [34,35], consistent with findings from other nations that reflect high levels of stress during COVID-19 [32,36]. High stress may impact decision-making, including decisions about energy-balance related behaviors, as research supports the idea that stress can catalyze a change from analytical to intuitive decision-making [37]. Under ongoing high levels of stress, food-related decisions may be governed by heuristics (i.e., short-cuts, such as: what is the habitual, automatic, or convenient choice?) or emotions (what will make me feel better?). In addition to potential links with stress, persisting changes in childcare and schooling may be linked to energy-balance-related variables reported herein, as children spending more time at home could impact food security, acquisition, and/or preparation.

The present results suggest that high levels of food insecurity persist among families more than six months into the pandemic. Over two-thirds of parents indicated they had experienced some form of food insecurity in the previous two months. While the current 2-item food insecurity screening tool may be limited compared to longer measures, the general point that very high proportions of families are suffering from food insecurity during COVID-19 is consistent with other research, including prior findings that more than half of surveyed families reported some form of food insecurity during COVID-19, a significant increase from prior to the pandemic [31]. Persistent food insecurity has implications for child health, as food insecurity has been linked with poor dietary intake and unhealthy weight outcomes [15]. During the initial months of the pandemic, increases in snacking behavior and low nutrient quality foods were seen [7,15]. It has also been well documented that many children in the U.S. already ate few nutrient dense foods, like fruits and vegetables, prior to the pandemic and ate at restaurants frequently [17,18]. Mitigation of food insecurity is an important research and policy target.

While families juggle ongoing contextual challenges, parents reported acquiring food from various sources. Similar to earlier studies, the majority of parents in the present nationally-representative sample reported more home cooking, with a substantial percentage also reporting less restaurant take-out and delivery as a result of the pandemic. Early reports stated that restaurant purchasing was down 30% in March 2020 compared to the previous year, and another study reported that in the early months of the pandemic, people were avoiding restaurants completely [13,25]. Yet the present results do suggest that restaurant dining may be moving toward pre-pandemic levels for many families. Overall reported frequencies of restaurant use showed that around half of children were eating restaurant food at least a few times each month via in-person, take-out, and delivery, in the context of two-third of families reporting that in-person dining was currently available in their area. Studies examining children's frequency of eating at restaurants in-person or via take-out from years prior to the COVID-19 pandemic show similar patterns (e.g., 56% of children ate at restaurants at least 2–3 times per month) [30]. In particular it appears higher-income, higher-education families are more likely to be returning to pre-COVID-19 restaurant habits.

However, there is a subset of parents who do not view restaurant dining as safe, with the present results indicating that perceived safety is lower among parents with lower education and among Hispanic, non-Hispanic Black, and non-Hispanic Asian parents. These differing perspectives could reflect different sources of information (e.g., engagement with varying types of media) and/or varying lived experiences as different demographic groups may occupy different spaces (e.g., with variable mitigation measures in place, variable levels of exposure among essential workers). Generally, a larger percentage of parents in the present study viewed take-out and delivery as safe, compared to dining-in, highlighting a need for more research on individual differences, as well as on these understudied modes of restaurant dining in the future.

Convenience and taste were the primary reported reasons for take-out and delivery choices, and taste and nutrition were highly ranked reasons for child meal choices from restaurants overall. Surprisingly, cost was not one of the higher-ranked choices for children's meal choices. Research prior to COVID-19 has shown that for many low-income families, cost is a dominant factor in meal selection, even after the decision to eat out is reached [38], while in higher socioeconomic status families, taste and cost are both important [39]. The current findings are consistent with prior research showing that liking and taste are important factors for children's meal selection [30]. Perhaps in the context of the COVID-19 pandemic, families may be particularly motivated to seek convenient options and provide their child with a tasty meal when they do decide to dine out.

Limitations of the present study include the use of a self-report measure, which can be subject to social desirability bias. Minor modifications to some existing survey items were made to fit with the aims of the present study (e.g., changing the time frame to the past two months). Furthermore, the short versions of some survey instruments were used (i.e., food insecurity, perceived stress). While demonstrations of the validity of these short forms are present in the literature, the long-form versions of these measures generally have superior psychometrics. In the present study, the PSS-4 had a relatively low Cronbach's alpha, as observed in some prior research [40], suggesting that longer versions of the Perceived Stress Scale may be preferable when feasible. A strength of the study is the use of sampling weights to achieve a nationally representative sample of families with 4- to 8-year-old children in the U.S. The study was conducted in October of 2020, more than six months after the pandemic was recognized. Evidence of shorter-term impacts of the pandemic on energy-balance-related behaviors and daily life may reflect the novel nature of the pandemic and stringent initial lockdowns. As the pandemic continues, and restrictions have relaxed in many areas, it is possible that families may show some returns to pre-pandemic lifestyles, while other changes may be longer-lasting. Results from the present study illustrate ongoing impacts on children's schooling and food insecurity, with a possible return to pre-pandemic behaviors in other areas, such as restaurant use, among many families. These findings have implications for future energy balance-related intervention research, as such work must take place in the context of families' realities. For example, current healthy eating interventions in restaurants would need to be feasible and acceptable in the context of families' varied use of and perceived safety of restaurant dining.

Continued surveillance can elucidate lasting shifts in behavior as a result of the pandemic and guide interventions to be safe, feasible, and relevant in the future. Nationally representative studies allow for generalizable conclusions, and examination of individual differences can facilitate targeted research and policy efforts to promote health and provide support to those most impacted. Research and policy efforts to address food insecurity are also of paramount importance.

5. Conclusions

Key goals of the present study were to describe parent-reported impacts of COVID-19 and current family food acquisition and eating behaviors more than six months into the pandemic. Results suggest continuing impacts of COVID-19 in many areas (e.g., schooling at home, food insecurity) and a potential move toward normalcy in other areas (e.g., restaurant dining) among some families, with some evidence of sociodemographic differences. Most parents reported that their child was consuming food from restaurants at least 2–3 times per month, with lower use of restaurants and lower reported perceived safety among some sociodemographic groups. These observations have implications for future research as the pandemic progresses, as well as intervention and policy efforts as scientists and policymakers consider the best ways to improve health and well-being among families in the COVID-19 era.

Author Contributions: S.A.-F., J.G., S.T., L.H.E., and L.A.L. designed the study; M.J.F. and S.A.-F. analyzed and interpreted the data; M.J.F. drafted the manuscript; all authors provided critical feedback; S.A.-F. had responsibility for final content. All authors have read and agreed to the published version of the manuscript.

Funding: This research was funded by NIH R01HD096748 (PI: S.A.-F.). In addition, S.T. is supported by an Ingestive Behavior Research Scholarship from the Center for Ingestive Behavior Research at the University at Buffalo.

Institutional Review Board Statement: The study was conducted according to the guidelines of the Declaration of Helsinki and approved by the University at Buffalo Institutional Review Board (STUDY00004723, 8 September 2020).

Informed Consent Statement: Informed consent was obtained from all subjects involved in the study.

Data Availability Statement: Access to study data can be provided by the corresponding author upon reasonable request after the study team has completed planned data analyses.

Acknowledgments: The authors would like to thank Lily McGovern for help with survey testing.

Conflicts of Interest: The authors declare no conflict of interest.

Abbreviations

U.S.	United States
PSS-4	Perceived Stress Scale: 4-item version
EPII	The Epidemic—Pandemic Impacts Inventory
ECHO	Environment Influences on Child Health Outcomes

References

1. Decker, S.; Peele, H.; Riser-Kositsky, M.; Kim, H.; Patti Harris, E. The coronavirus spring: The historic closing of US schools. Education Week. Available online: https://www.edweek.org/ew/section/multimedia/thecoronavirus-spring-the-historic-closing-of.html (accessed on 31 January 2021).
2. Dutta, M. COVID-19 and impact of school closures on the children of the United States; a point of view with an empirical analysis. *Soc. Sci. Humanit. Open* **2020**. [CrossRef]
3. Leone, L.A.; Fleischhacker, S.; Anderson-Steeves, B.; Harper, K.; Winkler, M.; Racine, E.; Baquero, B.; Gittelsohn, J. Healthy Food Retail during the COVID-19 Pandemic: Challenges and Future Directions. *Int. J. Environ. Res. Public Health* **2020**, *17*, 7397. [CrossRef]
4. Cameron, E.; Joyce, K.; Delaquis, C.; Reynolds, K.; Protudjer, J.; Roos, L. Maternal psychological distress & mental health service use during the COVID-19 pandemic. *J. Affect. Disord* **2020**. [CrossRef]
5. United States Bureau of Labor Statistics. The Employment Situation-October 2020. Bureau Labor Statistics. 2020; Contract No. USDL-20-2033. Available online: https://www.bls.gov/news.release/pdf/empsit.pdf (accessed on 31 January 2021).
6. The New York Times. See Coronavirus Restrictions and Mask Mandates for All 50 States. *The New York Times*. 2020. Available online: https://www.nytimes.com/interactive/2020/us/states-reopen-map-coronavirus.html (accessed on 31 January 2021).
7. Pietrobelli, A.; Pecoraro, L.; Ferruzzi, A.; Heo, M.; Faith, M.; Zoller, T.; Antoniazzi, F.; Piacentini, G.; Fearnbach, S.N.; Heymsfield, S.B. Effects of COVID-19 lockdown on lifestyle behaviors in children with obesity living in Verona, Italy: A longitudinal study. *Obesity* **2020**, *28*, 1382–1385. [CrossRef] [PubMed]
8. Flanagan, E.W.; Beyl, R.A.; Fearnbach, S.N.; Altazan, A.D.; Martin, C.K.; Redman, L.M. The impact of COVID-19 stay-at-home orders on health behaviors in adults. *Obesity* **2020**. [CrossRef]
9. Robinson, E.; Boyland, E.; Chisholm, A.; Harrold, J.; Maloney, N.G.; Marty, L.; Mead, B.R.; Noonan, R.; Hardman, C.A. Obesity, eating behavior and physical activity during COVID-19 lockdown: A study of UK adults. *Appetite* **2020**. [CrossRef] [PubMed]
10. Benker, B. Stockpiling as resilience: Defending and contextualising extra food procurement during lockdown. *Appetite* **2020**. [CrossRef]
11. Coleman-Jensen, A.; Gregory, C.; Singh, A. Household food security in the United States in 2013-Economic Research Report. The United States Department of Agriculture, Economic Research Service. 2014 (173). Available online: https://www.ers.usda.gov/webdocs/publications/45265/48787_err173.pdf (accessed on 31 January 2021).
12. Bauer, L. The COVID-19 Crisis Has Already Left Too Many Children Hungry in America. Brookings. 6 May 2020. Available online: https://www.brookings.edu/blog/up-front/2020/05/06/the-covid-19-crisis-has-already-left-too-many-children-hungry-in-america/ (accessed on 31 January 2021).
13. Wozniak, A.; Benz, J.; Hart, N. Social, Economic, Health Impacts Persist as Americans Grapple with Convergence of Pandemic and Civil Unrest. Chicago, IL: National Opinion Research Center. 2020. Available online: https://www.covid-impact.org/blog/social-economic-health-impacts-persist-as-americans-grapple-with-convergence-of-pandemic-and-civil-unrest (accessed on 31 January 2021).
14. Cheng, W.; Carlin, P.; Carroll, J.; Gupta, S.; Rojas, F.L.; Montenovo, L.; Nguyen, T.D.; Schmutte, I.; Scrivner, O.; Simon, K.I.; et al. Back to business and (re)employing workers? Labor market activity during state COVID-19 reopenings Report No. 0898-2937. *Natl. Bur. Econ. Res.* **2020**. [CrossRef]
15. Metallinos-Katsaras, E.; Must, A.; Gorman, K. A Longitudinal Study of Food Insecurity on Obesity in Preschool Children. *J. Acad. Nutr. Diet.* **2012**, *112*, 1949–1958. [CrossRef]
16. Rundle, A.G.; Park, Y.; Herbstman, J.B.; Kinsey, E.W.; Wang, Y.C. COVID-19–Related School Closings and Risk of Weight Gain Among Children. *Obesity* **2020**, *28*, 1008–1009. [CrossRef] [PubMed]
17. Ford, C.N.; Slining, M.M.; Popkin, B.M. Trends in dietary intake among US 2-to 6-year-old children, 1989–2008. *J. Acad. Nutr. Diet.* **2013**, *113*, 35–42.e6. [CrossRef] [PubMed]
18. Banfield, E.C.; Liu, Y.; Davis, J.S.; Chang, S.; Frazier-Wood, A.C. Poor Adherence to US Dietary Guidelines for Children and Adolescents in the National Health and Nutrition Examination Survey Population. *J. Acad. Nutr. Diet.* **2016**, *116*, 21–27. [CrossRef] [PubMed]
19. United States Department of Agriculture, Economic Research Service. Food Ex-Penditures, Table 3–Food Away from Home: Total Expenditures. 2016. Available online: https://www.ers.usda.gov/data-products/food-expenditures.aspx (accessed on 31 January 2021).
20. Saksena, M.J.; Okrent, A.M.; Anekwe, T.D.; Cho, C.; Dicken, C.; Effland, A.; Elitzak, H.; Guthrie, J.; Hamrick, K.S.; Hyman, J.; et al. *America's Eating Habits: Food Away From Home*; United States Department of Agriculture, Economic Research Service: Washington, DC, USA, 2018.
21. Wootan, M.G. Children's meals in restaurants: Families need more help to make healthy choices. *Child. Obes.* **2012**, *8*, 31–33. [CrossRef] [PubMed]
22. Zick, C.D.; Stevens, R.B. Trends in Americans' food-related time use: 1975–2006. *Public Health Nutr.* **2010**, *13*, 1064–1072. [CrossRef] [PubMed]
23. Ma, H.; Huang, J.; Fuller, F.; Rozelle, S. Getting Rich and Eating Out: Consumption of Food Away from Home in Urban China. *Can. J. Agric. Econ.* **2006**, *54*, 101–119. [CrossRef]

24. Adams, J.; Goffe, L.; Brown, T.; Lake, A.A.; Summerbell, C.; White, M.; Wrieden, W.; Adamson, A.J. Frequency and sociodemographic correlates of eating meals out and take-away meals at home: Cross-sectional analysis of the UK national diet and nutrition survey, waves 1–4 (2008–12). *Int. J. Behav. Nutr.* **2015**, *12*, 51. [CrossRef] [PubMed]
25. United States Department of Agriculture, Economic Research Service. Eating-out expenditures in March 2020 were 28 percent below March 2019 expenditures. 2020. Available online: https://wwwersusdagov/data-products/chart-gallery/gallery/chart-detail/?chartId=98556 (accessed on 31 January 2021).
26. Hager, E.R.; Quigg, A.M.; Black, M.M.; Coleman, S.M.; Heeren, T.; Rose-Jacobs, R.; Cook, J.T.; de Cuba, S.A.E.; Casey, P.H.; Chilton, M.; et al. Development and validity of a 2-item screen to identify families at risk for food insecurity. *Pediatrics* **2010**, *126*, e26–e32. [CrossRef]
27. Cohen, S.; Kamarck, T.; Mermelstein, R. A global measure of perceived stress. *J. Health Soc. Behav.* **1983**, *24*, 385–396. [CrossRef] [PubMed]
28. Grasso, D.J.; Briggs-Gowan, M.J.; Carter, A.S.; Goldstein, B.; Ford, J.D. A Person-Centered Approach to Profiling COVID-Related Experiences in the United States: Preliminary Findings from the Epidemic-Pandemic Impacts Inventory (EPII). *PsyArXiv Prepr.* **2020**. [CrossRef]
29. The National Institutes of Health (Kim et al.) Environmental Influences on Child Health Outcomes (ECHO) COVID-19 Task Force. Environmental Influences on Child Health Outcomes (ECHO) COVID-19 questionnaire-Adult Primary Version. 2020. Available online: https://www.nlm.nih.gov/dr2/C19-aPV_COVID-19_Questionnaire-Adult_Primary_Version_20200409_v01.30.pdf (accessed on 31 January 2021).
30. Anzman-Frasca, S.; Dawes, F.; Sliwa, S.; Dolan, P.R.; Nelson, M.E.; Washburn, K.; Economos, C.D. Healthier side dishes at restaurants: An analysis of children's perspectives, menu content, and energy impacts. *Int. J. Behav. Nutr. Phys. Act.* **2014**, *11*, 81.
31. Adams, E.L.; Caccavale, L.J.; Smith, D.; Bean, M.K. Food Insecurity, the Home Food Environment, and Parent Feeding Practices in the Era of COVID-19. *Obesity* **2020**, *28*, 2056–2063. [CrossRef]
32. Carroll, N.; Sadowski, A.; Laila, A.; Hruska, V.; Nixon, M.; Ma, D.W.L.; Haines, J.; On Behalf Of The Guelph Family Health Study. The Impact of COVID-19 on Health Behavior, Stress, Financial and Food Security among Middle to High Income Canadian Families with Young Children. *Nutrients* **2020**, *12*, 2352. [CrossRef]
33. Riser-Kositsky, M. Education Statistics: Facts about American Schools. 2020. Available online: https://www.edweek.org/ew/issues/education-statistics/index.html. (accessed on 31 January 2021).
34. Warttig, S.L.; Forshaw, M.J.; South, J.; White, A.K. New, normative, English-sample data fort he Short Form Perceived Stress Scale (PSS-4). *J. Health Psychol.* **2013**, *18*, 1617–1628. [CrossRef] [PubMed]
35. Vallejo, M.A.; Vallejo-Slocker, L.; Fernández-Abascal, E.G.; Mañanes, G. Determining Factors for Stress Perception Assessed with the Perceived Stress Scale (PSS-4) in Spanish and Other European Samples. *Front. Psychol.* **2018**, *9*, 37. [CrossRef]
36. Jia, R.; Ayling, K.; Chalder, T.; Massey, A.; Broadbent, E.; Coupland, C.; Vedhara, K. Mental health in the UK during the COVID-19 pandemic: Cross-sectional analyses from a community cohort study. *BMJ Open* **2020**, *10*, e040620. [CrossRef] [PubMed]
37. Yu, R. Stress potentiates decision biases: A stress induced deliberation-to-intuition (SIDI) model. *Neurobiol. Stress* **2016**, *3*, 83–95. [CrossRef] [PubMed]
38. Cohen, J.F.; Rimm, E.B.; Davison, K.K.; Cash, S.B.; McInnis, K.; Economos, C.D. The Role of Parents and Children in Meal Selection and Consumption in Quick Service Restaurants. *Nutrients* **2020**, *12*, 735. [CrossRef]
39. Anzman-Frasca, S.; Folta, S.C.; Glenn, M.E.; Jones-Mueller, A.; Lynskey, V.M.; Patel, A.A.; Tse, L.L.; Lopez, N.V. Healthier children's meals in restaurants: An exploratory study to inform approaches that are acceptable across stakeholders. *J. Nutr. Educ. Behav.* **2017**, *49*, 285–295. [CrossRef]
40. Lee, E.-H. Review of the Psychometric Evidence of the Perceived Stress Scale. *Asian Nurs. Res.* **2012**, *6*, 121–127. [CrossRef]

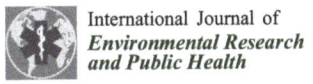

International Journal of *Environmental Research and Public Health*

Article

Impact of Ginger Root Powder Dietary Supplement on Productive Performance, Egg Quality, Antioxidant Status and Blood Parameters in Laying Japanese Quails

Zabihollah Nemati [1,*], Zahra Moradi [1], Kazem Alirezalu [2], Maghsoud Besharati [1] and António Raposo [3,*]

1. Department of Animal Science, Ahar Faculty of Agriculture and Natural Resources, University of Tabriz, Tabriz 5166616471, Iran; zahra.moradi81@yahoo.com (Z.M.); m_besharati@hotmail.com (M.B.)
2. Department of Food Science and Technology, Ahar Faculty of Agriculture and Natural Resources, University of Tabriz, Tabriz 5166616471, Iran; kazem.alirezalu@tabrizu.ac.ir
3. CBIOS (Research Center for Biosciences and Health Technologies), Universidade Lusófona de Humanidades e Tecnologias, Campo Grande 376, 1749-024 Lisboa, Portugal
* Correspondence: znnemati@yahoo.com or znemati@tabrizu.ac.ir (Z.N.); antonio.raposo@ulusofona.pt (A.R.)

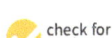

Citation: Nemati, Z.; Moradi, Z.; Alirezalu, K.; Besharati, M.; Raposo, A. Impact of Ginger Root Powder Dietary Supplement on Productive Performance, Egg Quality, Antioxidant Status and Blood Parameters in Laying Japanese Quails. *Int. J. Environ. Res. Public Health* **2021**, *18*, 2995. https://doi.org/10.3390/ijerph18062995

Academic Editors: María José Benito and Paul B. Tchounwou

Received: 9 January 2021
Accepted: 11 March 2021
Published: 15 March 2021

Publisher's Note: MDPI stays neutral with regard to jurisdictional claims in published maps and institutional affiliations.

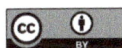

Copyright: © 2021 by the authors. Licensee MDPI, Basel, Switzerland. This article is an open access article distributed under the terms and conditions of the Creative Commons Attribution (CC BY) license (https://creativecommons.org/licenses/by/4.0/).

Abstract: Medicinal plants with antibacterial effects have been used by humans for centuries. In the recent decade, due to the development of antibiotic resistant strains, many studies have focused on the use of natural compounds as feed additives in livestock. Ginger, among all, have repetitively shown numerous biological activities, antibacterial, and antibiotic properties. This study was conducted to evaluate the effects of ginger root powder (GP) on the performance, egg quality, and blood parameters of Japanese quail. A total of 240 10-weeks old female quails were used in a completely randomized design with 4 treatments, 4 replicates, and 15 birds per replicate. Dietary treatment were basal diet (control) and basal diet containing 0.5, 1, and 1.5 g/kg of ginger root powder. Growth performance and exterior and interior quality of egg were measured biweekly over eight-week period. At the end of experiment blood parameters were evaluated. The results showed that diet supplementation with different levels of GP had no significant effect on egg production, egg mass weight, and egg weight ($p > 0.05$). However, feed intake and feed conversion ratio were significantly lower in the treatment group than the control in the whole period ($p < 0.05$). Egg Quality traits (shape index, albumen index, the percentage of albumen, yolk and shell, yolk pH, and shell thickness and strength) were not affected by the supplements in the whole trial period. Addition of GP significantly increased the albumen height, Haugh unit, and albumen pH in comparison with the control treatment ($p < 0.05$). GP reduced blood triglyceride level yet was ineffective on blood total antioxidant capacity and malondialdehyde. In conclusion, dietary supplementation with GP, could improve productive performance and the egg quality of Japanese quails. Nonetheless a comprehensive study needs to be performed in order to evaluate the impact of quail dietary ginger supplementation on productive performance and egg quality and their stability during storage time for commercial use.

Keywords: antioxidant; egg quality traits; ginger; immunity; Japanese quail performance

1. Introduction

Today, many phytochemical rich medicinal herbs are considered as potential alternatives to antibiotics and growth promoters due to the ban of antibiotics use in livestock in the European union [1]. Aromatic plants have been successfully used to improve antioxidant capacity in poultry industry [2,3]. Ginger *(zingiber officinale roscoe)* belongs to the Zingiberaceae family, including 47 genera and 1400 species [4]. Ginger is a native tropical plant in Southeast Asia and its commercial cultivation is not limited to Asia as is grown worldwide [4]. The global production of ginger was 3.3 million tons in 2016 [5]. The ginger can be consumed as fresh produce, dehydrated, and or processed product. Fresh rhizome is widely used as a spice and food condiment whether in the form of powder, extract, supplement, and or medicine [6]. Not only that the ginger rhizome is nutrient rich (amino acids, fatty acids, vitamins, and minerals) but the produce also contains compounds such as gingerol, gingerdiol, gingerdione, and shagaol that are potent intestinal mucous membrane and digestion stimulators [7]. The gingerols and shagaols are responsible for the pungency of fresh ginger and dried ginger, respectively [8].Ginger containing different phenolic component and they exhibited many bioactivities such as antioxidant [9], anti-anxiety [10], anti- Nausea [11], anti-inflammation [12], glucose-lowering [13], and health benefiting effects by reducing free radicals damage and improving cardiovascular status [14,15]. Furthermore, ginger is used for its various medicinal properties and alleviation and treatment of different symptoms such as animal mycotoxicosis [16], vomiting, pain, indigestion, and upper respiratory tract infection [17].

Throughout the production of ginger drink, powder, flakes and or ginger extract, significant amount of process discards, and byproducts are produced every year that could potentially be used as inexpensive feed additive in animal industry [18,19]. In a recent study, ginger supplement in broiler chicken diets stimulated the immune and digestive systems of the birds considerably [20]. In another study, Yusuf et al. [21] showed that, ginger in combination with probiotic and organic acid (citric acid) in laying Japanese quail diets improved the laying performances, feed conversion ratio (FCR), egg quality, bone characteristics, and reproductive indexes. Accordingly, diet supplementation with ginger powder increased total superoxide dismutase and glutathione peroxidase (Gpx) activities while it reduced malondialdehyde (MDA) and cholesterol concentrations in serum of broiler chickens at 21 and 42 days of age [22]. Ginger has also been reported to increase gastrointestinal secretion, digestive enzymes, improve circulation and intestinal movements [23]. It has been reported that using 4 and 8 g/kg of ginger powder of diet reduced feed intake but improved weight gain compared with control group [24]. In a study, ginger powder at 0.05 g/kg of diet, increased the egg production, hatching, reproductive performance, and economic efficiency of Japanese quail [25]. Other studies have reported that the addition of ginger essential oils at 300 µL/kg of diet, increased egg shell weight and shell thickness in laying hens [26]. Supplementation of broiler chickens diet with ginger reduced MDA and cholesterol concentration in serum of chickens at 21 and 42 days of age [22]. The effects of ginger supplementation in diets of broiler chicks at 64 weeks of age at 0.2, 0.4, and 0.6% showed a significant improvement in the feed conversion ratio in the treatment group containing 0.4% ginger powder [25]. Ibtisham et al. [27] have shown improvement of the production rate and feed intake of ginger powder and Chinese herbal medicine fed laying hens. They also concluded that ginger powder could be a suitable alternative to the antibiotic in poultry feed. In another study, Habibi et al. [28] reported that ginger powder and essential oils may be a vital replacement for synthetic antioxidants in broiler diets. Additionally, these researchers stated that ginger powder might be better than extracted essential oil for improving antioxidant status in broiler. The effect of diet supplementation with extract from thyme and ginger on the egg quality of laying hen was investigated by Damaziak et al. [29], who demonstrated that hen diet supplementation was improved Haugh unit of albumen and yolk color of fresh and hard boiled eggs. Recent studies suggest that Haugh unit and yolk color are important in the commercial production of table eggs which affected by dietary composition (e.g., protein sources and pigments) [30]. Color is an important qualitative feature of food acceptability as it affects consumers' perceptions of quality and flavor helping those making decisions about the purchase. Most consumers find yolk color related to the age and health of the animal and the quality of egg and its derivatives. Generally, edible additives and feeding methods are the main factors in the egg yolk color. For instance, natural pigments of plants such as carotenoids play an important role in the development of egg yolk color [25]. However, to the best of our knowledge, information regarding the potential benefits of these feed additive in the Japanese quail's diet is limited, so the present study was conducted to evaluate the effects of using different levels of ginger powder on the productive performance, eggs quality, and blood parameters in laying Japanese quails.

2. Materials and Methods

Animal welfare statement: All the methods and protocols used in this study were approved by the Research Bioethics Committee of Tabriz University (RBCT) for Use of Laboratory Animals of University of Tabriz (Approved number: IR.TABRIZU.REC.1399.032).

2.1. Experimental Birds and Management

A total of 240 laying Japanese quails (10 weeks old), after a two-week adaptation period, were randomly divided into 4 experimental groups (4 replicates each, 15 birds per pen). Dietary groups included the basal diet (control) and the basal diet supplemented with 0.5, 1, and 1.5 g ginger root powder per kg of diet. The birds were kept in a multi-story wired cages in a well-ventilated room with the temperature of 23–29 °C and 16L:8D light regime during experiment. Each cage had 3600 cm^2 floor space with size 45 × 45 cm^2 and was equipped with two nipple drinker and one feeder. The basal diet was formulated to meet the National Research Council (NRC) recommendations [31] as showed in Table 1. Quails received water and feed ad libitum throughout the experimental period.

Table 1. Ingredient and composition of the basal diet.

Item	Value (%)	Diet Composition	Value
Corn	45.38	ME (kcal/kg)	2900
Soybean meal	32.50	Crude protein (%)	20
Wheat bran	10.51	Ca (%)	2.5
Soybean oil	3.2	Available P (%)	0.39
Di calcium phosphate	1.8	Na	0.15
Calcium carbonate	5.3	Methionine (%)	0.7
Methionine	0.39	Lysine (%)	1.12
Sodium chloride	0.32	Sys (%)	0.34
Bicarbonate	0.1		
Vitamin [1]	0.3		
Trace mineral [2]	0.3		

[1] Supplied per kg of feed: vitamin B1, 2.16 mg; vitamin B2, 7.92 mg; pantothenic acid, 12 mg; nicotinic acid;36, vitamin B6, 3.6 mg; folic acid, 1.2 mg; biotin, 0.12 mg; vitamin K3, 2.4 mg; vitamin E, 21.6 IU; cholin chloride, 300; antioxidant, 120 mg; vitamin A, 10,800 IU; vitamin D3, 2400 IU and vitamin B12, 0.018 mg. [2] Supplied per kg feed: FeSO$_4$, 0.15 g; MnSO$_4$, 0.12 g; CuSO$_4$, 0.03 g; I, 1.2 mg and Se, 0.24 mg.

2.2. Preparation of Ginger Powder Samples

Fresh ginger root was purchased from the local market and then cut into slices. Ginger slices were air-dried (sunshade for 1 day) at room temperature and further oven-dried (at 40 °C for 40 h) (Memmert UNB400). Dehydrated slices were then processed by grinder device (IKA, MF 10 basic) to fine powder, and subsequently stored in moisture-controlled ziplock bags at 4 °C. Ethanolic ginger extract was prepared by mixing 2 g of ginger powder in the 100 mL of absolute ethanol. The mixture was processed for 30 min at 85 °C. The prepared extract was filtered by Whatman No. 1 filter paper. Dry extract (5 g) was dissolved in 10 mL of methanol solvent and sonicated for 30 min at 15 °C. Constituents of the extract were quantified by HPLC (Smartline, Knauer, Germany) method [32]. The contents of bioactive components were determined in the extract and the concentration of 6-gingerol, 8-gingerol, 10-gingerol, and 6-shogaol was 6163.1, 802.8, 783.9, and 839.9 mg/kg ginger (on dry weight basis), respectively. Nutrient compositions and total phenolic content of ginger root powder were analyzed according to standard method, Association of Official Analytical Chemists (AOAC) [33] and Nemati et al. [34], respectively and the results are given in Table 2.

Table 2. Nutrient composition of ginger powder (% DM) used in the experiment.

Item	Level (%)
Dry matter, DM	88.5
Phenol, component (g/100 gr)	0.703
Crude protein	5.5
Ash	11.75
Organic matter, OM	88.25
Ether extract, EE	1.35
Neutral detergent fiber, NDF	7.5
Acid detergent fiber, ADF	4.5
Natural detergent soluble fiber, NDS	92.5
Acid Detergent soluble fiber, ADS	95.5

2.3. Measurement of Productive Performance and Egg Quality

In this study, egg production was recorded daily; however, feed consumption and egg weight [25] were recorded weekly. Moreover, feed efficiency was calculated by dividing the total feed intake by total egg mass during each period. The feed conversion ratio (FCR) [35] was expressed as kilograms of feed consumed per kilogram of egg produced. Six eggs (per replicate) were randomly selected to determine the traits related to the characteristics of quail eggs at 0, 2, 4, 6, and 8 weeks. Egg length and width were measured with a 0.01 mm digital caliper (Mitutoyo). For Haugh unit measurements six eggs were weighed and then cracked separately. Albumen heights of three near yolk areas were measured with a 0.01 mm digital caliper. The Haugh unit [35] was calculated using egg weight and albumen height data of each 6 egg. Furthermore, the yolk height and width were measured by 0.01 mm digital caliper. For calculation of yolk to albumen ratio as well as yolk and albumen percentages, yolk and albumen were carefully separated from each other and subsequently weighed by 0.001 g digital scale (A&D N92) [36]. For color measurements using Roche color fan, eggs were individually broken onto a flat surface and then color was recorded [35]. Egg shell thickness was measured using a 0.01 mm micrometer at three different points. Average of three points was considered as final thickness of each eggshell. The eggshell percentages were calculated using washed and dried eggshell weights [35]. For pH analysis, yolk and albumen were completely mixed with a glass rod prior to measurement separately (pH meter; Hanna 211, Woonsocket, RI, USA) [34].

2.4. Blood Biochemical Parameters Analysis

At the end of the experiment, two birds from each replicate were randomly picked up for slaughter (6 birds per treatment). Blood samples were collected from the neck vein of the birds using sterilized needles and then centrifuged for 15 min at 3000 rpm to separate the serum. The collected serum was stored at $-20\ °C$ for the analysis of glucose (Catalog No: 117500), albumin (Catalog No: 5017) and total protein (Catalog No: 128500), cholesterol (Catalog No: 110500), and triglycerides (Catalog No: 132500). Blood biochemical parameters were measured by a spectrophotometric analysis, using commercially available kits (Pars Azmun Diagnostic, Tehran, Iran).

2.5. Antioxidant Status

Ferric reducing antioxidant power assay was used to assess the total antioxidant capacity (TAC) of blood samples [37]. TAC was quantified by the reaction of phenanthroline and Fe^{2+} using a spectrophotometer at 520 nm. TAC is defined as the amount of antioxidants required to increase the absorbance by 0.01, in 1 mL of blood sample at 37 °C. Concentration of MDA in the serum, as an index of lipid peroxidation and oxidative stress, was determined using the thiobarbituric acid reactive substances (TBARS) method [37]. The principle is that TBARS reacts with MDA to form a stable pink color that could be measured spectrophotometrically at 532 nm. The values of MDA were expressed as (nmol/mL).

2.6. Statistical Analysis

Data of production performance and egg quality were subjected to one-way analysis of variance (ANOVA) using MIXED procedure (Repeated Measurement), SAS (version 9) as a completely randomized design [38]. Tukey multiple comparison test was used to compare the averages at a 5% confidence level. The Shapiro–Wilk and Levene tests were used for model assumptions of homogeneity of variance and normality, respectively. The percentage data including egg mass, egg production rate, yolk index, egg yolk, eggshell and albumen relative weight, and egg shape were transformed by arcsine of the square root before analysis to achieve homogeneity of variance. No statistical difference was observed between the two sets of data thus results of statistical analysis on the original data are presented in this article.

The statistical design model is as follows:

$$Y_{ijkm} = \mu + T_i + W_j + TW_{ij} + \emptyset k_{(ji)} + E_{ijkm}.$$

In which Y_{ijkm} is observed parameters, μ is the mean of population, T_i is the treatment effect, W_j is the time effect, TW_{ij} is the treatment and time interactions, $\emptyset k_{(ji)}$ is the random factor (bird), and E_{ijkm} are residual effects.

Data of blood biochemical parameters and immune response were subjected to one-way ANOVA (general linear model (GLM) procedure), SAS following the statistical model. Comparison of means was performed using Duncan test at the confidence level of 5%. A level of $p < 0.05$ was used as the criterion for statistical significance.

$$Y_{ij} = \mu + T_i + E_{ij}.$$

In which Y_{ijk} is observed parameters (dependent variable), μ is the mean of population, T_i is the treatment effect and E_{ij} are residual effects.

3. Results

3.1. Productive Performance

The effect of dietary supplementation with natural additives of ginger powder on the productive performance is presented in Table 3. The results showed that the experimental treatments had no significant effect on egg production rate among the treatments during the experimental period ($p > 0.05$). Egg mass and egg weight were not significantly affected by the level of ginger powder used ($p > 0.05$). As shown in Table 3, addition of different levels of ginger significantly reduced feed intake during the whole experimental period ($p < 0.05$) compared with the control treatment. Ginger powder had dose-dependent effect since highest concentration of 1.5 g/kg of diet was most the potent treatment. The effect of treatment and time interaction was insignificant on the feed intake, egg weight and egg mass ($p > 0.05$). Nonetheless, the treatment x time interaction was significant on the FCR ($p < 0.05$). According to our results, Table 3, GP supplemented diet reduced FCR compared with the control group during experiment period ($p < 0.05$). High levels of ginger powder at 1.5 g/kg level decreased FCR compared with other groups. The experimental treatments significantly reduced FCR during breeding weeks. Moreover, the effect of time on the FCR was also significant.

Table 3. Effects of ginger powder supplementation on productive performance in Japanese quails.

Item		Feed Intake (g/day)	Feed Conversion Ratio (g:g)	Egg Production Rate (%)	Egg Weight (g)	Egg Mass (%)
Treat						
Control		33.87 [a]	3.03	92.99	12.01	11.16
GP0.5		32.93 [b]	2.88	94.10	12.13	11.41
GP1.0		32.19 [c]	2.77	94.42	12.31	11.62
GP1.5		31.33 [d]	2.72	94.77	12.15	11.51
SEM		0.17	0.02	1.19	0.13	0.13
Week 0		34.02	2.99	93.87	12.12	11.37
Time, w						
Week 2		34.21 [a]	2.95	94.51	12.25 [a]	11.58 [a]
Week 4		32.13 [b]	2.78	94.91	12.17 [a]	11.54 [a]
Week 6		32.06 [b]	2.85	93.84	11.99 [b]	11.25 [b]
Week 8		31.93 [b]	2.82	93.03	12.18 [a]	11.33 [b]
SEM		0.21	0.01	0.82	0.08	0.08
treat × Time						
Control	Week 2	34.71	3.02 [a,b]	93.92	12.22	11.48
Control	Week 4	34.45	3.01 [a,b,c]	94.10	12.13	11.41
Control	Week 6	33.66	3.1 [a]	92.32	11.77	10.85
Control	Week 8	32.68	2.99 [a,b,c,d]	91.61	11.91	10.91
GP0.5	Week 2	34.82	3.05 [a,b]	93.21	12.26	11.42
GP0.5	Week 4	32.11	2.81 [d,e,f]	94.46	12.08	11.39
GP0.5	Week 6	31.94	2.85 [b,c,d,e,f]	93.03	12.02	11.18
GP0.5	Week 8	32.84	2.82 [c,d,e,f]	95.71	12.15	11.63
GP1.0	Week 2	34.05	2.89 [b,c,d,e]	95.17	12.36	11.77
GP1.0	Week 4	31.19	2.69 [f,g]	94.28	12.26	11.56
GP1.0	Week 6	32.03	2.77 [e,f,g]	94.50	12.23	11.56
GP1.0	Week 8	31.50	2.71 [e,f,g]	93.75	12.37	11.59
GP1.5	Week 2	33.25	2.85 [b,c,d,e,f]	95.71	12.15	11.65
GP1.5	Week 4	30.80	2.61 [g]	96.78	12.19	11.80
GP1.5	Week 6	30.58	2.68 [f,g]	95.53	11.94	11.42
GP1.5	Week 8	30.69	2.74 [e,f,g]	91.07	12.31	11.19
SEM		0.42	0.03	1.64	0.16	0.17
Probability						
Treat		>0.0001	>0.0001	0.74	0.48	0.16
Time		>0.0001	>0.0001	0.32	0.001	0.007
Treat × Time		0.07	0.01	0.23	0.41	0.06

Different letters ([a, b, c, d, e, f] or [g]) after the means within a column indicate significant differences among treatments ($p < 0.05$).

3.2. Quality Traits of Eggs

The effects of diet supplementation with different levels of ginger powder on qualitative traits of eggs are given in Table 4. The results showed that the effects of ginger powder on egg weight, shape index, albumen weight, shell weight, albumen, yolk and shell percentage, yolk pH, and shell thickness and strength were insignificant ($p > 0.05$). Ginger supplementation improved yolk index; however, it did not increase yolk weight compared with the control treatment ($p > 0.05$). Nonetheless, effect of time on yolk index was significant ($p < 0.05$). The highest yolk color was related to the highest level of ginger in the diet. The effect of treatment × time interaction, as shown in Table 5, were significant on yolk color, albumen height and albumen index during experimental period ($p < 0.05$). The albumen and yolk pH were significantly reduced by ginger powder experimental diet compared with the control treatment ($p < 0.05$). Ginger diet improved Haugh unit relative to control group ($p < 0.05$), but egg specific gravity (ESG) did not differ (Table 4).

Table 4. Effect of different level of ginger root powder on egg quality of Japanese quails.

Traits	Experimental Diets				SEM	p Value		
	Ginger Powder (g/kg of Diet)					Treatment	Time	Treatment × Time
	0	0.5	1	1.5				
Shape index %	128.97	130.25	253.90	122.66	62.09	0.43	0.45	0.43
Albumen index %	10.36	10.74	10.89	10.79	0.23	0.46	0.01	0.009
Yolk index %	44.77 [c]	47.02 [a]	46.16 [a,b]	45.17 [b,c]	0.54	0.005	>0.001	0.13
Albumen height (mm)	3.81 [b]	3.99 [a]	4.11 [a]	4.04 [a]	0.04	0.004	0.21	0.02
Haugh unit	84.88 [b]	86.06 [a]	86.62 [a]	86.27 [a]	0.24	0.003	0.13	0.07
Albumen weight	7.45	7.49	7.52	7.53	0.09	0.93	0.49	0.15
Yolk colour	4.25 [b]	4.45 [b]	4.70 [a]	4.75 [a]	0.08	0.004	>0.001	>0.001
Shell weight (g)	0.965	0.966	0.987	0.989	0.01	0.56	0.59	0.98
Albumen percentage %	59.92	60.80	60.14	60.41	0.36	0.39	0.11	0.29
Yolk percentage %	32.31	31.35	31.95	31.64	0.30	0.20	0.03	0.44
Shell percentage %	7.76	7.84	7.90	7.93	0.11	0.73	0.59	0.29
Albumen to yolk	0.539	0.515	0.531	0.524	0.008	0.26	0.03	0.33
Yolk weight (g)	4.02	3.86	3.99	3.94	0.05	0.21	0.08	0.70
Yolk pH	5.87 [a]	5.84 [b]	5.81 [b]	5.85 [b]	0.01	0.02	>0.001	0.02
Albumen pH	8.91 [a]	8.78 [b]	8.77 [b]	8.83 [b]	0.02	0.01	>0.001	0.009
Egg specific gravity (g/cm^3)	1.0740	1.0745	1.0748	1.0750	0.0006	0.72	0.60	0.97
Shell thickness (mm × 10)^2	20.61	20.67	20.29	20.76	0.35	0.80	0.005	0.51
Shell strength (hg/cm^2)	19.51	19.71	19.86	19.94	0.28	0.73	0.59	0.97

Different letters ([a, b] or [c]) after the means within a row indicate significant differences among treatments ($p < 0.05$).

Table 5. Effect of treatment and time Interaction on egg albumen and yolk traits in Japanese quails fed different level of ginger root powder.

Treat	Time (Week)	Albumen Index	Albumen Height (mm)	Yolk Colour	Yolk pH	Albumen pH
Control	2	10.38 [a,b]	3.71 [b]	3.87 [d]	5.91 [a,b]	8.99 [a,b]
Control	4	9.75 [b]	3.68 [b]	4.56 [b,c]	5.85 [a,b,c,d]	9.10 [a]
Control	6	10.36 [a,b]	3.90 [a,b]	4.35 [b,c,d]	5.84 [a,b,c,d]	8.81 [c,d,e,f]
Control	8	10.95 [a,b]	3.94 [a,b]	4.20 [b,c,d]	5.89 [a,b,c]	8.75 [c,d,e,f]
GP0.5	2	9.98 [a,b]	4.01 [a,b]	4.20 [b,c,d]	5.81 [b,c,d]	8.73 [e,f,g]
GP0.5	4	11.09 [a,b]	4.001 [a,b]	4.12 [c,d]	5.82 [a,b,c,d]	8.91 [a,b,c,d]
GP0.5	6	10.86 [a,b]	3.91 [a,b]	4.56 [b,c,d]	5.85 [a,b,c,d]	8.74 [e,f,g]
GP0.5	8	11.02 [a,b]	4.04 [a,b]	4.91 [a,b]	5.88 [a,b,c]	8.72 [e,f,g]
GP1.0	2	10.99 [a,b]	4.26 [a]	4.29 [b,c,d]	5.76 [d]	8.76 [c,d,e,f]
GP1.0	4	10.33 [a,b]	3.98 [a,b]	4.41 [b,c,d]	5.81 [a,b,c,d]	8.90 [a,b,c,e]
GP1.0	6	11.50 [a]	4.25 [a]	4.54 [b,c,d]	5.81 [a,b,c,d]	8.72 [d,f,g]
GP1.0	8	10.71 [a,b]	3.94 [a,b]	5.56 [a]	5.86 [a,b,c,d]	8.70 [f]
GP1.5	2	10.24 [a,b]	4.05 [a,b]	4.35 [b,c,d]	5.85 [a,b,c,d]	8.81 [b,c,d,e,f]
GP1.5	4	10.45 [a,b]	4.04 [a,b]	4.50 [b,c,d]	5.79 [c,d]	8.89 [a,b,c,d,e,f]
GP1.5	6	11.26 [a,b]	4.06 [a,b]	4.58 [b,c,d]	5.84 [a,b,c,d]	8.76 [c,d,e,f]
GP1.5	8	10.87 [a,b]	4.02 [a,b]	5.56 [a]	5.92 [a]	8.86 [b,c,d,e,f]
SEM		0.34	0.08	0.13	0.02	0.04
p value		0.009	0.02	0.001	0.02	0.009

Different letters ([a, b, c, d, e, f] or [g]) after the means within a column indicate significant differences among treatments ($p < 0.05$).

3.3. Blood Parameters and Egg Yolk Phenolic Compounds

The effect of experimental diets on blood parameters of animals are presented in Table 6 and Figure 1. The results revealed that supplementation of ginger powder in the diet had significant effect on the level of triacylglycerol ($p < 0.05$). Nevertheless, serum albumin, cholesterol, glucose, MDA, and TAC were not affected by the diet ($p > 0.05$). Level of serum TAC only numerically elevated, while MDA level was reduced in birds fed medium level of ginger powder compared with the control group. The effect of experimental treatments on phenolic compounds of the yolk, as shown in Figure 1, was significant ($p < 0.05$). Highest concentration of ginger powder (1.5 g/kg diet) was the most effective treatment in stimulating the production of phenolic.

Table 6. Biochemical parameters in blood serum of Japanese quail fed diets with ginger powder supplementation.

Treatments	Protein (g dL^{-1})	Albumin (g dL^{-1})	Triacylglycerol (mg dL^{-1})	Cholesterol (mg dL^{-1})	Glucose (mg dL^{-1})
Control	5.80	1.60	453.1 [a]	243	195
Ginger (0.5 g/kg of diet)	5.70	1.43	351.8 [b]	247	242
Ginger (1 g/kg of diet)	5.73	1.56	336.8 [b]	210	173
Ginger (1.5 g/kg of diet)	6.15	1.70	342.6 [b]	219	221
SEM	0.28	0.1	23.03	22.18	21.80
p-value	0.64	0.39	0.01	0.58	0.17

Different letters ([a] or [b]) after the means within a column indicate significant differences among treatments ($p < 0.05$).

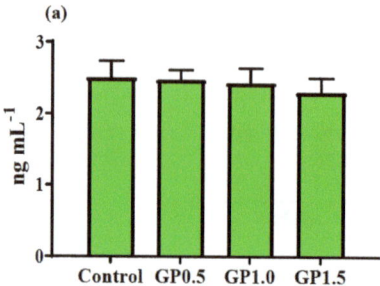 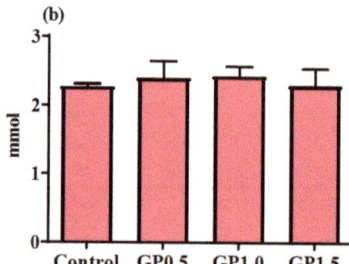

Figure 1. Concentrations of malondialdehyde (MDA) (**a**) and total antioxidant capacity (TAC) (**b**) in Japanese quails fed different levels of GP. Values (means ± SEM) within the same week with uncommon letters are significantly ($p < 0.05$) different.

4. Discussion

In general, inclusion of ginger powder in the diet of birds was effective on various productive parameters. In this experiment, production rate and egg mass were not influenced by the treatments, while feed intake and FCR decreased when birds received increasing levels of ginger powder. In agreement to our results, previous findings confirmed that dietary supplementation with ginger root improved FCR in broiler chickens [39] and decreased feed intake in guinea fowl [40]. Furthermore, ginger supplements had no adverse effect on the palatability of broiler feeds [39] and improved the digestibility of dry matter in guinea fowl [40]. Contrarily, Damaziak et al. [29] did not observe any positive effect of the ginger root on egg production rate in laying hens. However, findings of our study were not in agreement with the handful studies showing the insignificant effect of ginger powder [41] or ginger extract dietary supplementation [42] on the FCR. Akbarian et al. reported that using different levels of ginger (0.25, 0.5 and 0.75 g/100 g of diet) in laying hens during 30 weeks had insignificant effect on FI and FCR [43]. The disparity of this study with previous research results could be due to differences in ginger source, processing methods as well as poultry species [42,44]. Ginger contains many active compounds (e.g., brunel, camphon, limonene, humolin, gingerol, gingeron, gingerdiol, shogaols, some phenolic ketone derivatives, volatile oils, alkaloids, saponins, and flavonoids) [45] that could stimulate feed digestion and the digestive enzymes, thus increasing FI and FCR [38]. In the same way Platel and Srinivasan [46] stated that ginger enhanced the activity of pancreatic lipase, amylase, trypsin chymotrypsin, and bile acid secretion in albino rats. In fact, these enzymes, bile and biliary bile acids significantly affect the digestion and absorption of nutrients. In accord, Habibi et al. [28] indicated the stimulating effect of ginger root powder (7.5 g/kg of diet) on body weight and weight gain in broiler chicks at 22 days of the experiment. In another study, ginger powder increased production, hatchability, reproductive performance, and economic efficiency at a level of 0.05 g/kg diet while increasing egg weight and feed intake in Japanese quail [25]. In present study, ginger powder supplemented diet had no effect on egg production, egg weight, and total egg mass among the treatments during the experiment period. Our findings were in line with the results of Wen at al. [42] and Herve et al. [47] reporting the insignificant effect of ginger supplemented diet in laying hen and quail. Moreover, Wen et al. concluded that egg weight was improved in ginger powder fed laying hen [47]. The results of studies on the effect of ginger at increasing levels of 0, 5, 10, 15, and 20 g/kg of diet on the performance of laying hens at the age of 27 weeks showed that all laying hens were in good health and no mortality was recorded in the whole period of the experiment. Average egg weight and laying rate were similar in treatments containing ginger powder. Egg mass was positively affected by the treatments compared with the control group, which can be related to the positive effect of ginger powder on laying rate as well as egg weight [48]. In contrast to the current quail study, egg production rate was increased in ginger extract/powder fed laying hen [48,49] alone or in combination with medicinal herbs [27]. This means that the beneficial effect of ginger on performance depends on the bird species, dosage of ginger, and its derivatives and interaction with other dietary components. However, information about mechanism of action of ginger intake are scarce [50].

In this study ginger powder was beneficial on the reducing the blood triacylglyceride levels yet its effects were not significant on serum cholesterol and glucose levels. Other serum parameters including albumin, and protein were not significantly affected by ginger powder ($p > 0.05$). Consistent with these results, studies have shown that diet supplementation with ginger extract at 0.4 and 0.6 mg/g of diet, significantly decreased glucose, triglyceride, and cholesterol levels [51]. Akhany et al. [52] concluded that ginger extract significantly reduced blood glucose levels and increased insulin levels. Some of the essential minerals (calcium, zinc, potassium, manganese, and chromium) are related to the mechanism of insulin release [53]. In another study, ginger at concentrations up to 2% of the diet reduced cholesterol, triglyceride, and glucose levels in comparison with the control group, while the serum protein was not affected by the experimental treatments [38]. Ginger has previously shown strong anti-lipidemic effect on serum cholesterol and triglyceride levels [54]; hence, its mode of action may be related to the inhibition of cholesterol synthesis (e.g., β-hydroxy-β-methylglutaryl coenzyme A (HMG—CoA) [51]. Correspondingly, ginger is a potent HMGR-inhibiting drug, known to cause liver-specific inhibition of cholesterol synthesis [55]. In addition, other reports showed that diabetic therapy with insulin helps in reducing the plasma triglycerides by affecting lipoprotein lipase levels [56] Ginger has insulin-stimulating effect which could reduce plasma triglycerides [56]. Previous studies stated that phenols and flavonoids act as potent antioxidants [57]. Khalifa and Noseer [58] revealed that eggs produced by quail supplemented with combined ginger powder and probiotics had the lowest total cholesterol content in serum and yolk compared with the control, along with an increase in high-density lipoprotein (HDL) and decrease of low-density lipoprotein (LDL). Herve et al. [59] showed that total cholesterol and triglycerides, transaminases, and MDA decreased in quails supplemented with ginger essential oil at 50, 100, and 150 µL/kg body weight.

Haugh unit, albumen height, and yolk index are characterized as main reference associated with egg quality, which influenced by feed additive (e.g., green tea powder) [60]. In this study yolk index, albumen height, and Haugh unit of eggs were increased in diet supplemented with ginger powder. Several studies indicated that ginger supplementation in poultry diets significantly increased antioxidant enzymes as well as TAC and decreased MDA [22,28,43]. Improvement of egg yolk index and Haugh unit in the current study may be due to the effect of the phenolic compounds of ginger (gingerols and shagaol) which have antioxidant properties [61]. As discussed earlier, color of the yolk an acceptability and freshness feature of the egg, could be improved by natural products such as carotenoids. In this study, egg yolk color was positively affected by ginger powder consumption (1.5 mg/kg). However, others have reported the ineffectiveness of fermented ginger powder (10 and 50 mg/kg of diet concentrations) [23] and ginger extract [42] on the yolk color and yolk and albumen percentage. The intensity of egg yolk color depends on the presence and utilization of pigments in the diet, because laying hens have no ability to produce pigments through their biochemical processes [62]. The darker yolk color of eggs from quails received ginger is probably due to the natural pigments found in ginger, including 6-dehydrogingerdione, which causes a deep yellow color [63]. No difference in other quality traits of quail eggs indicates that ginger does not affect the egg shell quality or egg composition (percentage of albumen, yolk, and shell). The results of present experiment consistent with the result of Wen et al. 2019 [42] showing that the use of ginger root as an additive in Japanese quail diet had significant effect on Haugh unit and albumen height yet being ineffective on shell thickness, shell strength, and egg composition percentage. We, in this study, observed concentration dependent potency of ginger powder on many important parameters of fresh egg quality (e.g., Haugh unit, yolk index, and yolk color) in laying quails; however, other variables associated with egg shelf life should be tested for a final statement.

5. Conclusions

The results of this study suggest that the inclusion of ginger root powder in Japanese quail diet can partially improve the productive performance, antioxidant status, and blood parameters. Moreover, ginger could improve yolk color and albumen quality expressed in Haugh units. The effects on the quail production performance seemed to be dose dependent and ginger at the highest tested level (1.5 g/kg of ginger powder) was most effective treatment. However, further studies are needed to conclude on the effect of ginger on quality of the poultry products as well as its mechanism of action.

Author Contributions: Conceptualization, Z.N.; methodology, Z.N., Z.M., and K.A.; software, Z.N. and Z.M.; validation Z.N. and Z.M.; formal analysis, Z.N. and K.A; investigation and resources, Z.M. and Z.N.; data curation, Z.N.; writing—original draft preparation, Z.M and Z.N; writing—review and editing, A.R. and M.B.; project administration, Z.N.; funding acquisition, Z.N. and A.R. All authors have read and agreed to the published version of the manuscript.

Funding: This research was funded by The University of Tabriz (grant number: 11.934).

Institutional Review Board Statement: The study was conducted according to the guidelines of the National norms and standard for conducting medicinal research in Iran, and approved by the Research Bioethics Committee of Tabriz University (Approved number: IR.TABRIZU.REC.1399.032).

Informed Consent Statement: Not applicable.

Data Availability Statement: Qualified researchers can obtain the data from the corresponding author. The data are not publicly available due to privacy concerns imposed by the RBCT ethical principles.

Conflicts of Interest: The authors declare no conflict of interest.

References

1. Castanon, J. History of the Use of Antibiotic as Growth Promoters in European Poultry Feeds. *Poult. Sci.* **2007**, *86*, 2466–2471. [CrossRef]
2. Nemati, Z.; Mohammadi, R. The effects of different levels of dietary garlic powder on productive performance, egg quality traits and blood parameters of laying hens. *J. Anim. Prod.* **2017**, *19*, 657–670.
3. Zeng, Z.; Zhang, S.; Wang, H.; Piao, X. Essential oil and aromatic plants as feed additives in non-ruminant nutrition: A review. *J. Anim. Sci. Biotechnol.* **2015**, *6*, 7–17. [CrossRef]
4. Ravindran, P.; Nirmal, B. Ginger: The genus Zingiber. In *Medicinal and Aromatic Plant–Industrial Profile*; CRC Press: Boca Raton, FL, USA, 2005.
5. Food and Agriculture Organization of the United Nations, Statistics Division. Ginger production in 2016, Crops/ Regions/ World/ Production/ Quantity (from pick lists). 2017. Available online: http://www.fao.org/faostat/en/#data/QC/visualize (accessed on 2 March 2021).
6. Policegoudra, R.; Aradhya, S. Biochemical changes and antioxidant activity of mango ginger (Curcuma amada Roxb.) rhizomes during postharvest storage at different temperatures. *Postharvest Biol. Technol.* **2007**, *46*, 189–194. [CrossRef]

7. Dieumou, F.; Teguia, A.; Kuiate, J.; Tamokou, J.; Fonge, N.; Dongmo, M. Effects of ginger (Zingiber officinale) and garlic (Allium sativum) essential oils on growth performance and gut microbial population of broiler chickens. *Livest. Res. Rural Dev.* **2009**, *21*, 23–32.
8. Arablou, T.; Aryaeian, N.; Valizadeh, M.; Sharifi, F.; Hosseini, A.; Djalali, M. The effect of ginger consumption on glycemic status, lipid profile and some inflammatory markers in patients with type 2 diabetes mellitus. *Int. J. Food Sci. Nutr.* **2013**, *65*, 515–520. [CrossRef] [PubMed]
9. Chakraborty, D.; Mukherjee, A.; Sikdar, S.; Paul, A.; Ghosh, S.; Khuda-Bukhsh, A.R. [6]-Gingerol isolated from ginger attenuates sodium arsenite induced oxidative stress and plays a corrective role in improving insulin signaling in mice. *Toxicol. Lett.* **2012**, *210*, 34–43. [CrossRef] [PubMed]
10. Vishwakarma, S.L.; Pal, S.C.; Kasture, V.S.; Kasture, S.B. Anxiolytic and antiemetic activity of Zingiber officinale. *Phytother. Res.* **2002**, *16*, 621–626. [CrossRef] [PubMed]
11. Ernst, E.; Pittler, M.H. Efficacy of ginger for nausea and vomiting: A systematic review of randomized clinical trials. *Br. J. Anaesth.* **2000**, *84*, 367–371. [CrossRef]
12. Grzanna, R.; Lindmark, L.; Frondoza, C.G. Ginger—An Herbal Medicinal Product with Broad Anti-Inflammatory Actions. *J. Med. Food* **2005**, *8*, 125–132. [CrossRef] [PubMed]
13. Al-Amin, Z.M.; Thomson, M.; Al-Qattan, K.K.; Peltonen-Shalaby, R.; Ali, M. Anti-diabetic and hypolipidaemic properties of ginger (Zingiber officinale) in streptozotocin-induced diabetic rats. *Br. J. Nutr.* **2006**, *96*, 660–666. [CrossRef] [PubMed]
14. Verma, S.K.; Singh, M.; Jain, P.; Bordia, A. Protective effect of ginger, Zingiber officinale Rosc on experimental atherosclerosis in rabbits. *Indian J. Exp. Biol.* **2004**, *42*, 736–738.
15. Bosisio, E. Effect of the flavanolignans of Silybum marianum L. On lipid peroxidation in rat liver microsomes and freshly isolated hepatocytes. *Pharmacol. Res.* **1992**, *25*, 147–165. [CrossRef]
16. Vipin, A.V.; Raksha Rao, K.; Kurrey, N.K.; Anu Appaiah, K.A.; Venkateswaran, G. Protective effects of phenolics rich extract of ginger against Aflatoxin B1-induced oxidative stress and hepatotoxicity. *Biomed. Pharmacother.* **2017**, *91*, 415–424.
17. Wang, W.; Wang, Z. Studies of commonly used traditional medicine-ginger. *Zhongguo Zhong Yao Za Zhi China J. Chin. Mater. Med.* **2005**, *30*, 1569–1573.
18. Gao, Y.; Ozel, M.Z.; Dugmore, T.; Sulaeman, A.; Matharu, A.S. A biorefinery strategy for spent industrial ginger waste. *J. Hazard. Mater.* **2021**, *401*, 123400. [CrossRef]
19. Wiastuti, T.; Khasanah, L.U.; Kawiji, W.A.; Manuhara, G.J.; Utami, R. Characterization of active paper packaging incorporated with ginger pulp oleoresin. In *Proceedings of the IOP Conference Series: Materials Science and Engineering*; IOP Publishing: Bristol, UK, 2016; Volume 107, p. 012057.
20. Al-Shuwaili, M.A.; Ibrahim, E.; Naqi Al-Bayati, M. Effect of dietary herbal plants supplement in turkey diet on performance and some blood biochemical parameters. *Glob. J. Biosci. Biotechnol.* **2015**, *4*, 153–157.
21. Yusuf, M.; Hasan, M.; Elnabtiti, A.; Cui, H. Single dose of ginger powder, supported with organic acid or probiotic, maximizes the laying, egg quality hatchability and immune performances of laying Japanese quails. *Int. J. Recent Sci. Res.* **2015**, *6*, 6707–6711.
22. Zhang, G.F.; Yang, Z.B.; Wang, Y.; Yang, W.R.; Jiang, S.Z.; Gai, G.S. Effects of ginger root (Zingiber officinale) processed to different particle sizes on growth performance, antioxidant status, and serum metabolites of broiler chickens. *Poult. Sci.* **2009**, *88*, 2159–2166. [CrossRef]
23. Incharoen, T.; Yamauchi, K. Production Performance, Egg Quality and Intestinal Histology in Laying Hens Fed Dietary Dried Fermented Ginger. *Int. J. Poult. Sci.* **2009**, *8*, 1078–1085. [CrossRef]
24. Najafi, S.; Taherpour, K. Effects of dietary ginger (Zingiber Ofjicinale), cinnamon (Cinnamomum), synbiotic and antibiotic supplementation on performance of broilers. *J. Anim. Sci. Adv.* **2014**, *4*, 658–667.
25. Abd El-Galil, K.; Mahmoud, H.A. Effect of ginger roots meal as feed additives in laying Japanese quail diets. *J. Am. Sci.* **2015**, *2*, 233–234.
26. Nasiroleslami, M.; Torki, M. Including essential oils of fennel (Foeniculum vulgare) and ginger (Zingiber officinale) to diet and evaluating performance of laying hens, white blood cell count and egg quality characteristics. *Adv. Environ. Biol.* **2010**, *4*, 341–346.
27. Ibtisham, F.; Nawab, A.; Niu, Y.; Wang, Z.; Wu, J.; Xiao, M.; An, L. The effect of ginger powder and Chinese herbal medicine on production performance, serum metabolites and antioxidant status of laying hens under heat-stress condition. *J. Therm. Biol.* **2019**, *81*, 20–24. [CrossRef]
28. Habibi, R.; Sadeghi, G.; Karimi, A. Effect of different concentrations of ginger root powder and its essential oil on growth performance, serum metabolites and antioxidant status in broiler chicks under heat stress. *Br. Poult. Sci.* **2014**, *55*, 228–237. [CrossRef]
29. Damaziak, K.; Gozdowski, D.; Niemiec, J.; Riedel, J.; Róg, D.; Siennicka, A. Effects of ginger or ginger and thyme extract in laying hens feeding on productive results and eggs quality. *Ann. Wars. Univ. Life Sci. SGGW Anim. Sci.* **2018**, *57*, 5–18. [CrossRef]
30. Wang, X.; Wu, S.; Zhang, H.; Yue, H.; Qi, G.; Li, J. Effect of dietary protein sources and storage temperatures on egg internal quality of stored shell eggs. *Anim. Nutr.* **2015**, *1*, 299–304. [CrossRef]
31. NRC. *Nutrient Requirements of Poultry*; National Academy Press: Washington, DC, USA, 1994.
32. Nourbakhsh Amiri, Z.; Najafpour, G.; Mohammadi, M.; Moghadamnia, A. Subcritical water extraction of bioactive compounds from ginger (Zingiber officinale Roscoe). *Int. J. Eng.* **2018**, *31*, 1991–2000.
33. AOAC. *Official Methods of Analysis*; Association of Official Analytical Chemists: Washington, DC, USA, 1990.

34. Nemati, Z.; Alirezalu, K.; Besharati, M.; Holman, B.; Hajipour, M.; Bohrer, B. The Effect of Dietary Supplementation with Inorganic or Organic Selenium on the Nutritional Quality and Shelf Life of Goose Meat and Liver. *Animals* **2021**, *11*, 261. [CrossRef] [PubMed]
35. Nemati, Z.; Ahmadian, H.; Besharati, M.; Lesson, S.; Alirezalu, K.; Domínguez, R.; Lorenzo, J.M. Assessment of Dietary Selenium and Vitamin E on Laying Performance and Quality Parameters of Fresh and Stored Eggs in Japanese Quails. *Foods* **2020**, *9*, 1324. [CrossRef]
36. Ahmadian, H.; Nemati, Z.; Karimi, A.; Safari, R. Effect of different dietary selenium sources and storage temperature on enhancing the shelf life of quail eggs. *Anim. Prod. Res.* **2019**, *8*, 23–33. (In Persian)
37. Nemati, Z.; Alirezalu, K.; Besharati, M.; Amirdahri, S.; Franco, D.; Lorenzo, J.M. Improving the Quality Characteristics and Shelf Life of Meat and Growth Performance in Goose Fed Diets Supplemented with Vitamin E. *Foods* **2020**, *9*, 798. [CrossRef]
38. Mohamed, A.B.; Al-Rubaee, M.A.; Jalil, A.Q. Effect of Ginger (Zingiber officinale) on Performance and Blood Serum Parameters of Broiler. *Int. J. Poult. Sci.* **2012**, *11*, 143–146. [CrossRef]
39. Karangiya, V.K.; Savsani, H.H.; Patil, S.S.; Garg, D.D.; Murthy, K.S.; Ribadiya, N.K.; Vekariya, S.J. Effect of dietary supplementation of garlic, ginger and their combination on feed intake, growth performance and economics in commercial broilers. *Vet. World* **2016**, *9*, 245–250. [CrossRef] [PubMed]
40. Oso, A.O.; Awe, A.W.; Awosoga, F.G.; Bello, F.A.; Akinfenwa, T.A.; Ogunremi, E.B. Effect of ginger (Zingiber officinale Roscoe) on growth performance, nutrient digestibility, serum metabolites, gut morphology, and microflora of growing guinea fowl. *Trop. Anim. Health Prod.* **2013**, *45*, 1763–1769. [CrossRef] [PubMed]
41. Thayalini, K.; Shanmugavelu, S.; Saminathan, P.; SitiMasidayu, M.; Noridayusni, Y.; Zainmuddin, H.; Nurul Akmai, C.; Wong, H. Effects of Cymbopogon citratus leaf and Zingiber officinale rhizome supplementation on growth performance, ileal morphology and lactic acid concentration in broilers. *Malays. J. Anim. Sci.* **2011**, *14*, 43–49.
42. Wen, C.; Gu, Y.; Tao, Z.; Cheng, Z.; Wang, T.; Zhou, Y. Effects of Ginger Extract on Laying Performance, Egg Quality, and Antioxidant Status of Laying Hens. *Animals* **2019**, *9*, 857. [CrossRef] [PubMed]
43. Akbarian, A.; Golian, A.; Ahmadi, A.S.; Moravej, H. Effects of ginger root (Zingiber officinale) on egg yolk cholesterol, antioxidant status and performance of laying hens. *J. Appl. Anim. Res.* **2011**, *39*, 19–21. [CrossRef]
44. PR, S.A.; Prakash, J. Chemical composition and antioxidant properties of ginger root (Zingiber officinale). *J. Med. Plants Res.* **2010**, *4*, 2674–2679.
45. Hashimoto, K.; Satoh, K.; Murata, P.; Makino, B.; Sakakibara, I.; Kase, Y.; Ishige, A.; Higuchi, M.; Sasaki, H. Component of Zingiber officinale that Improves the Enhancement of Small Intestinal Transport. *Planta Med.* **2002**, *68*, 936–939. [CrossRef]
46. Platel, K.; Srinivasan, K. Influence of dietary spices and their active principles on pancreatic digestive enzymes in albino rats. *Food Nahrung* **2000**, *44*, 42–46. [CrossRef]
47. Herve, T.; Raphaël, K.J.; Ferdinand, N.; Victor Herman, N.; Willy Marvel, N.M.; Cyril D'Alex, T.; Laurine Vitrice, F.T. Effects of ginger (Zingiber officinale, Roscoe) essential oil on growth and laying performances, serum metabolites, and egg yolk antioxidant and cholesterol status in laying Japanese quail. *J. Vet. Med.* **2019**, *2019*. [CrossRef]
48. Zhao, X.; Yang, Z.B.; Yang, W.R.; Wang, Y.; Jiang, S.Z.; Zhang, G.G. Effects of ginger root (Zingiber officinale) on laying performance and antioxidant status of laying hens and on dietary oxidation stability. *Poult. Sci.* **2011**, *90*, 1720–1727. [CrossRef]
49. An, S.; Liu, G.; Guo, X.; An, Y.; Wang, R. Ginger extract enhances antioxidant ability and immunity of layers. *Anim. Nutr.* **2019**, *5*, 407–409. [CrossRef]
50. Kiyama, R. Nutritional implications of ginger: Chemistry, biological activities and signaling pathways. *J. Nutr. Biochem.* **2020**, *86*, 108486. [CrossRef]
51. Saeid, J.M.; Mohamed, A.B.; Al-Baddy, M.A. Effect of Aqueous Extract of Ginger (Zingiber officinale) on Blood Biochemistry Parameters of Broiler. *Int. J. Poult. Sci.* **2010**, *9*, 944–947. [CrossRef]
52. Akhani, S.P.; Vishwakarma, S.L.; Goyal, R.K. Anti-diabetic activity of Zingiber officinale in streptozotocin-induced type I diabetic rats. *J. Pharm. Pharmacol.* **2004**, *56*, 101–105. [CrossRef] [PubMed]
53. Kar, A.; Choudhary, B.K.; Bandyopadhyay, N.G. Preliminary studies on the inorganic constituents of some indigenous hypoglycaemic herbs on oral glucose tolerance test. *J. Ethnopharmacol.* **1999**, *64*, 179–184. [CrossRef]
54. Jang, I.; Ko, Y.; Kang, S.; Lee, C. Effect of a commercial essential oil on growth performance, digestive enzyme activity and intestinal microflora population in broiler chickens. *Anim. Feed Sci. Technol.* **2007**, *134*, 304–315. [CrossRef]
55. Manju, V.; Viswanathan, P.; Nalini, N. Hypolipidemic Effect of Ginger in 1,2-Dimethyl Hydrazine-Induced Experimental Colon Carcinogenesis. *Toxicol. Mech. Methods* **2006**, *16*, 461–472. [CrossRef] [PubMed]
56. Austin, G.E.; Maznicki, E.; Sgoutas, D. Comparison of phosphotungstate and dextran sulfate-Mg2+ precipitation procedures for determination of high density lipoprotein cholesterol. *Clin. Biochem.* **1984**, *17*, 166–169. [CrossRef]
57. Pietta, P.-G. Flavonoids as Antioxidants. *J. Nat. Prod.* **2000**, *63*, 1035–1042. [CrossRef]
58. Khalifa, M.I.; Noseer, E.A. Cholesterol quality of edible eggs produced by quail fed diets containing probiotic and/or ginger (Zingiber officinale). *Livest. Res. Rural Dev.* **2019**, *31*, 165–175.
59. Herve, T.; Raphaël, K.J.; Ferdinand, N.; Vitrice, F.T.L.; Gaye, A.; Outman, M.M.; Marvel, N.M.W. Growth Performance, Serum Biochemical Profile, Oxidative Status, and Fertility Traits in Male Japanese Quail Fed on Ginger (Zingiber officinale, Roscoe) Essential Oil. *Vet. Med. Int.* **2018**, *2018*, 1–8. [CrossRef] [PubMed]

60. Zhang, J.; Zhang, M.; Liang, W.; Geng, Z.; Chen, X. Green tea powder supplementation increased viscosity and decreased lysozyme activity of egg white during storage of eggs from Huainan partridge chicken. *Ital. J. Anim. Sci.* **2020**, *19*, 586–592. [CrossRef]
61. Hasan, H.A.; Raauf, A.M.R.; Razik, B.M.A.; Hassan, B.A.R. Chemical Composition and Antimicrobial Activity of the Crude Extracts Isolated from Zingiber Officinale by Different Solvents. *Pharm. Anal. Acta* **2012**, *3*, 1–5. [CrossRef]
62. Spasevski, N.; Puvača, N.; Pezo, L.; Tasić, T.; Vukmirović, Đ.; Banjac, V.; Čolović, R.; Rakita, S.; Kokić, B.; Džinić, N. Optimisation of egg yolk colour using natural colourants. *Eur. Poult. Sci.* **2018**, *82*, 2018–2035.
63. Ajileye, B.A.; Iteire, A.K.; Arigi, Q.B. Zingiber officinale (ginger) extract as a histological dye for muscle fibers and cytoplasm. *Int. J. Med. Sci.* **2015**, *4*, 1445–1448. [CrossRef]

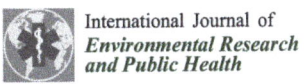

Article

Halal Food Performance and Its Influence on Patron Retention Process at Tourism Destination

Heesup Han [1], Linda Heejung Lho [1], António Raposo [2,*], Aleksandar Radic [3] and Abdul Hafaz Ngah [4]

[1] College of Hospitality and Tourism Management, Sejong University, 98 Gunja-Dong, Gwangjin-Gu, Seoul 143-747, Korea; heesup.han@gmail.com (H.H.); heeelho@gmail.com (L.H.L.)
[2] CBIOS (Research Center for Biosciences and Health Technologies), Universidade Lusófona de Humanidades e Tecnologias, Campo Grande 376, 1749-024 Lisboa, Portugal
[3] Independent Researcher, Gornji Kono 8, 20000 Dubrovnik, Croatia; aleradic@gmail.com
[4] Faculty of Business, Economy and Social Development, Universiti Malaysia Terengganu, Kuala Nerus 21030, Terengganu, Malaysia; hafaz.ngah@umt.edu.my
* Correspondence: antonio.raposo@ulusofona.pt

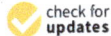

Citation: Han, H.; Lho, L.H.; Raposo, A.; Radic, A.; Ngah, A.H. Halal Food Performance and Its Influence on Patron Retention Process at Tourism Destination. *Int. J. Environ. Res. Public Health* **2021**, *18*, 3034. https://doi.org/10.3390/ijerph18063034

Academic Editors: Massimo Lucarini and Paul B. Tchounwou

Received: 4 January 2021
Accepted: 9 March 2021
Published: 16 March 2021

Publisher's Note: MDPI stays neutral with regard to jurisdictional claims in published maps and institutional affiliations.

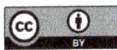

Copyright: © 2021 by the authors. Licensee MDPI, Basel, Switzerland. This article is an open access article distributed under the terms and conditions of the Creative Commons Attribution (CC BY) license (https://creativecommons.org/licenses/by/4.0/).

Abstract: Muslim tourism is one of the most rapidly developing sectors in the international tourism industry. Nevertheless, halal food performance and its relationship with international Muslim traveler decision-making and behaviors have not been sufficiently examined. The present research explored the influence of halal food performance, which encompasses availability, health/nutrition, accreditation, and cleanness/safety/hygiene factors, on the Muslim traveler retention process at a non-Islamic destination. A survey methodology with a quantitative data analytic approach was employed to achieve research goals. Our findings indicated that halal food performance increased destination trust and destination attachment, which in turn influenced Muslim traveler retention. Additionally, the efficacy of the higher-order framework of halal food performance was defined. Both destination trust and attachment mediated the effect of halal food performance on retention. A halal-friendly destination image included a moderating influence on the retention process. The effectiveness of the proposed theoretical framework for explicating Muslim traveler behaviors was uncovered. This research better introduces the importance of halal food performance and its attributes for the elicitation of Muslim traveler approach responses and behaviors at a non-Islamic destination to researchers and practitioners.

Keywords: halal food performance; availability; healthy/nutritional factor; accreditation; clean/safe/hygiene factor; trust; attachment; halal-friendly image; retention; muslim travelers

1. Introduction

Muslim travelers are undoubtedly an emerging tourist group in the global tourism industry [1–5]. As the competition in the international tourism marketplace is intensifying, many destinations are eager to develop halal-friendly products and make a Muslim-friendly tourism environment to attract a greater number of Muslim visitors [1,4]. Developing new halal-friendly marketing and retention strategies is irrefutably important in expanding the business volume related to Muslim tourism at tourist destinations [1,5,6]. Halal food is frequently regarded as one of the most significant halal-friendly products at many places [7–10]. Increasing the halal food availability and improving its attribute quality is indisputably becoming essential to fulfill Muslim travelers' halal-friendly tourism needs and provide them with pleasant tourism experiences, especially in non-Islamic countries and tourism destinations [10,11].

Despite the rapid growth of Muslim tourism for the past few decades in the global tourism sector, the competitiveness with many non-Islamic destinations in the marketplace is still not strong enough [4,5,10]. According to [12], such weak competitiveness is mostly relevant to Muslim travelers' experiences with restaurants and foods that are not sufficiently halal-friendly. Nevertheless, the empirical endeavor investigating the possible influence of halal food performance on Muslim traveler post-purchase behavior at non-Islamic destinations has hardly been made. In addition, the existing studies indicated the criticality of trust and attachment in explicating the traveler retention process [13–16]. Scant research has unearthed the possible linkages between halal food performance and these essential concepts. Moreover, destination image is irrefutably a crucial variable, affecting the entire traveler post-purchase decision-making procedure [17–19]. A halal-friendly destination image is vital in Muslim traveler behaviors [20]. Yet, how a halal-friendly destination image determines the magnitude of the relation strength between halal food performance and its outcome constructs has hardly been examined. That is, the particular role of a halal-friendly destination image as a moderator in the Muslim visitor retention process has not been thoroughly explored.

Taking this into account, the current research was devised to build a theoretical framework that explicates Muslim traveler retention formation in a clear manner. Many previous studies focused on defining what halal food is and what halal tourism is. Thus, the current research tried to take a step further from the latent literature and develop both the theoretical and the practical contribution of halal food to halal tourism. In particular, we aimed (1) to assess the possible impact of halal food performance, which comprises availability, health/nutrition, accreditation, and cleanness/safety/hygiene factors as its constituents, on the Muslim visitor retention process at a non-Islamic destination; (2) to uncover the appropriateness of a higher-order structure of halal food performance and its competence; (3) to investigate the convoluted relations among halal food performance, destination trust, and destination attachment, and the possible influence on retention; (4) to assess the mediating role of destination trust and attachment; and (5) to unearth the moderating role of a halal-friendly destination image within the proposed conceptual framework. The remaining parts of this research are the literature review, methodology, data analysis and results, and discussion and implications. Investigating these five aims, this research will be able to not only build a theoretical framework of Muslim traveler retention but also discover practical contributions for ways to retain Muslim travelers.

2. Literature Review
2.1. Halal Food and Its Performance

Halal is an Arabic term indicating, "which is allowed by Islamic teaching" [9,11]. Halal dietary laws were developed within Asia for Islamic followers to practice a nutritious and healthy lifestyle [21]. The foods permitted under these halal dietary laws are called halal food [21]. Muslim travelers' demand for overseas traveling is rapidly increasing, and their primary distress is the accessibility and quality of halal food in an international destination [1,9,11]. Indeed, [22] recently reported that halal food consumption is a key aspect of Muslim tourism. Little availability (or unavailability) and low performance of halal food at a destination lowers the quality of Muslims' overall tourism experiences and generates their avoidance behaviors for that place [2,10]. Due to the recent growth of the Muslim tourism market [7,23], halal food is becoming a fundamental topic in the international tourism industry [8,11,20].

According to [24], the term "performance" indicates that individuals' evaluation of the excellence of a product and its attributes as compared to other products available in the marketplace offered by rival firms. Consistently, halal food performance in this research refers to travelers' appraisal of the excellence of halal food and its essential attributes as compared to the halal foods offered by competing destinations. Halal food performance is constructed as an amalgamation of multiple dimensions that explicate an intricate aspect of food and beverage consumption in a halal-friendly way [11,12]. Halal food availability factors, halal food health/nutrition factors, halal food accreditation factors (e.g., accreditation with a halal certificate, halal logos), and halal food cleanness/safety/hygiene factors are all crucial constituents of assessing halal food performance at international destinations [9,20,25]. Indeed, [12] and [11] asserted that availability, health/nutrition, accreditation, and cleanness/safety/hygiene are the main things for Muslims to consider related to halal food consumption when planning and practicing halal-friendly tourism activities at non-Islamic destinations.

Research on halal food and understanding its influence on Muslim traveler behaviors is still in its infancy in many non-Islamic destinations [1,6]. In these destinations, halal food and beverage are relatively a new type of tourism product [11,26]. Muslim travelers can be somewhat skeptical about whether the foods provided in non-Islamic destinations are pure halal [11]. Although the authenticity and decency of halal food in such destinations is not entirely certain [27], the quality performance of halal food often inspires Muslim travelers' high level of trust for the food and the places [1,12], elicits their affection and attachment to the places [8,20], and affects approach behaviors for the destinations [2,28]. Simply put, halal food and its performance are strongly relevant to responses and behaviors among overseas Muslim travelers [8,28].

2.2. Destination Trust

Because of the intangible form of hospitality and tourism products, trust and reliability of the products/services often become an important subject in the hospitality and tourism marketplace [14,15]. Many hospitality/tourism products entail a certain level of uncertainty/risk, particularly in the international tourism context [14,29,30]. While the definition of trust varies in the existing literature, one of the most broadly accepted definitions in tourism is that trust is the degree to which travelers rely on a product, place, brand, or exchanging partner [15]. Similarly, [31] conceptualized destination trust as the travelers' level of confidence and reliability toward a tourist destination and its performance. It is broadly known that trust is a critical influence factor on travelers' emotional attachment and approach behaviors [13,15,29,31]. Thus, destination trust will positively affect destination attachment.

For instance, in consumer behavior, [32] found that trust is an essential driver of repurchase intention. In addition, [15] uncovered that trust in a place helps visitors attach to the place and plays a vital role in building their positive intentions for the place in the international tourism context. In recent decades, the importance of trust has been especially emphasized in the Muslim tourism/consumer behavior sector [10,13,14]. Such trust is likely formed based on a Muslim-friendly tourism environment at the destination [10]. In the Muslim tourism context, trust also generates travelers' emotional responses and reactions that are favorable for tourism destinations [28,33]. In other words, destination trust will positively affect Muslim traveler retention.

2.3. Destination Attachment

A comprehension of attachment has a meaningful implication for understanding traveler behavior [16,34–36]. Due to its hefty contribution to a surge of positive decision/behavior of visitors, attachment to a destination/place has broadly been a crucial concept in hospitality and tourism [36]. Generating such attachment can be described as the process of building an emotional connection between an individual and a destination [16]. Coherently, destination attachment in the present research indicates Muslim travelers' emotional ties to a specific tourism destination. Attachment plays a crucial role when individuals choose tourism/leisure products [34,36,37]. Findings in the extant literature demonstrated that the high tourist attachment to a tourism product/service/destination affects his/her post-purchase decision formation, inducing positive behaviors for the product/service/destination [35,38].

In the hospitality context, [39] explored the influence of patrons' attachment/involvement. In [38], the findings revealed that the patrons' purchase decision formation for a hospitality product is significantly impacted by their level of product attachment. In the cruise tourism sector, [35] investigated the intricate process of passenger loyalty generation. Their empirical finding showed that passenger loyalty formation is significantly triggered by passenger attachment to the cruise line. In the festival tourism sector, [36] discovered that visitors' attachment to a festival destination is significantly associated with their loyalty for the place. More recently, [37] uncovered that travelers' level of attachment to the tourism product/place increases their approach behaviors, such as retention and word-of-mouth activities. Travelers' strong attachment to a destination boosts their willingness to revisit the place, whereas travelers' weak attachment increases their avoidance decisions [16,36]. Therefore, destination attachment will positively affect Muslim traveler retention.

2.4. Halal-Friendly Destination Image

Image has long been believed a crucial dimension when explaining patrons' decision-making procedures and attitudes of consumption [17,18,39,40]. Image refers to patrons' overall perception of a firm and its product(s) based on the relations held in their memory [41]. Kotler et al. [42] provided a more precise conceptualization of it where image is the overall set of consumers' perceptions, opinions, and beliefs about a firm and its product(s). Coherently, in this research, destination image indicates the summation of perceptions, opinions, and beliefs that Muslim travelers have about a place and its halal-friendly attributes. Individuals' impressions/thoughts/beliefs of a particular object are formed ultimately based on attained and processed information [43]. Baloglu, McCleary [44] and Lee et al. [45] thus indicated that building an image of a place/product in the consumer behavior context is a subjective and cognitive process of assessing such information about a place/product.

Image and its potential influence have been well documented in consumer behavior and tourism literature [19,39,45]. It is widely believed that increasing an image of a firm/place eventually results in increased repeat business and loyalty for the firm/place [40,44,46]. According to [47], one's image of a place significantly impacts the formation of his/her revisit intention in the hospitality sector. More recently, [19] uncovered that destination image among travelers' social network members has a considerable effect on their choice behaviors. It is likely that the entire customer retention process becomes strong when a customer image of a place/product is favorable, whereas said process becomes weak when he/she has an unfavorable image of the place/product [18,40,45]. Likewise, while a positive image of a place/product often reinforces the formation of patrons' post-purchase decisions, a negative image often weakens their decision formation [18,39,47]. It is also evident that travelers' image, which is positive for a particular destination/tourism product, considerably influences the process of generating their favorable behavioral intentions toward the destination/tourism product [45]. Consequently, it can be concluded that a halal-friendly destination image includes a significant effect on the relation between halal food performance and destination trust and the relation between halal food performance and destination attachment.

2.5. Proposed Model and Hypothesis

The proposed model shown in Figure 1 encompassed (a) halal food performance whose first-order factors are availability, health/nutrition, accreditation, and cleanness/safety/hygiene; (b) destination trust; (c) destination attachment; (d) halal-friendly destination image; and (e) Muslim traveler retention. The model contained a total of seven research hypotheses. Hypotheses 1–6 concern the causal relationships among research constructs. In addition, Hypotheses 7a–7b pertain to the moderating impact of a halal-friendly destination image.

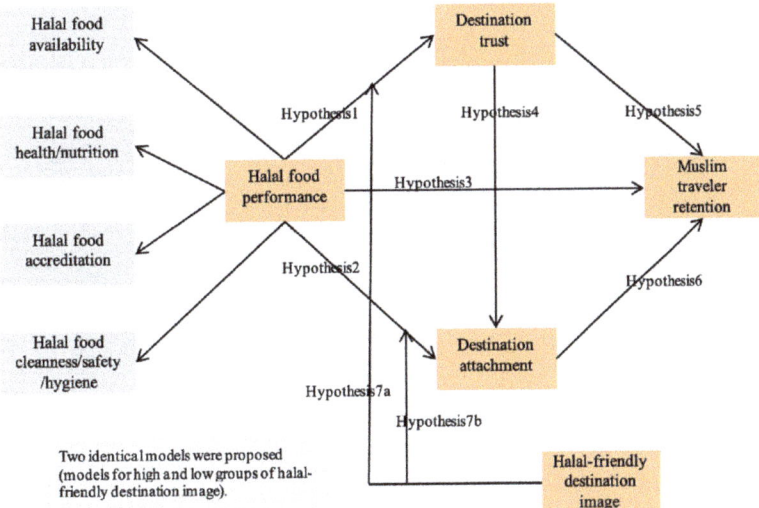

Figure 1. The proposed conceptual framework. H1: Halal food performance includes a positive effect on destination trust. H2: Halal food performance includes a positive effect on destination attachment. H3: Halal food performance includes a positive effect on Muslim traveler retention. H4: Destination trust includes a positive effect on destination attachment. H5: Destination trust includes a positive effect on Muslim traveler retention. H6: Destination attachment includes a positive effect on Muslim traveler retention. H7a: Halal-friendly destination image includes a significant effect on the relation between halal food performance and destination trust. H7b: Halal-friendly destination image includes a significant effect on the relation between halal food performance and destination attachment.

3. Method

Measures

The measurement items for the research factors used in this research were adopted from the existing studies [11,12,16,17,29,48,49] and adjusted to be appropriate to the current study context. All items were measured by a seven-point Likert scale. Additionally, multiple items were used to assess each construct. A total of six items were adopted to evaluate halal food performance. Specifically, two items for halal food availability (e.g., "Availability of halal food attracted me to visit tourist places"), two items for halal food health/nutrition (e.g., "Halal foods served in restaurants are healthy and nutritious"), two items for halal food accreditation (e.g., "Halal food providers in tourist sites are accredited with halal certification"), and two items for halal food cleanness/safety/hygiene (e.g., "Halal food and beverage offered in tourist sites/places were clean, safe, and hygienic") were utilized.

To measure destination trust, three items were used (e.g., "I have confidence in Korea as a halal-friendly destination"). Destination attachment was assessed with two items (e.g., "I feel emotionally attached to Korea as a tourist destination"). Additionally, we utilized three items to assess a halal-friendly destination image (e.g., "Overall, I have a good image of Korea as a Halal-friendly destination"). For assessing Muslim traveler retention, two items were utilized (e.g., "Korea as a Halal family-friendly place will be my first choice when it comes to choosing a destination"). The survey questionnaire comprising these measures was pre-tested with tourism researchers. A minor modification was adopted based on their feedback. The survey was then further modified by halal tourism specialists' reviews. All measures used in this research are exhibited in Appendix A.

4. Results

4.1. Data Collection and Sample Profiles

A field survey was conducted. The survey was carried out in many tourist places of Korea, which include restaurants, hotels, shopping malls, cultural districts, and tourist sites. Many international travelers prefer these places. The surveyors contacted Muslim tourists and asked if they were willing to fill out the survey. All survey participation was voluntary. Detailed information about the survey and its objectives were explained to all participants. The participants were asked to read the mandatory survey instructions thoroughly and answer the questions. All responses were returned onsite. Throughout this process, the researchers attained a total of 326 usable responses, which were used to analyze the data. Of 326 participants, 54.3% were female tourists, whereas 45.7% were male tourists. The participants' age range was 20–69 years old. The average age was 29.17 years old. When visit frequency was questioned, roughly 65.6% showed that they had visited Korea only once. About 89.3% indicated that they had visited Korea three times or less. A majority of the respondents classified themselves as pleasure travelers (55.2%), then education travelers (36.2%), and lastly business travelers/others (8.6%). About 77.9% indicated that their annual income is less than USD 39,999 (77.9%), followed by between USD 40,000 and USD 99,999 (20.3%), and then USD 100,000 or higher (1.8%). The sample respondents were, in general, highly educated. About 55.2% indicated they are college graduates, then graduate degree holders (28.8%), and then high school graduates or less (16.0%). Asking the following question, "For you, how important are halal-friendly food products when choosing a destination," most survey participants reported that halal foods are important or very important when selecting a tourism destination (87.1%).

4.2. Confirmatory Factor Analysis and Measurement Model Evaluation

A confirmatory factor analysis was performed (shown in Table 1). The measurement model contained a satisfactory level of goodness-of-fit statistics (χ^2 = 318.108, df = 107, $p < 0.001$, χ^2/df = 2.973, RMSEA = 0.078, CFI = 0.958, IFI = 0.958, TLI = 0.939). Each loading value was found significant at $p < 0.01$. A composite reliability test was conducted. All reliability values (halal food availability = 0.785, halal food health/nutrition = 0.903, halal food accreditation = 0.833, halal food cleanness/safety/hygiene = 0.737, destination trust = 0.945, destination attachment = 0.829, halal-friendly destination image = 0.949, and Muslim traveler retention = 0.732) were above the suggested threshold of 0.70 [50]. Therefore, the internal consistency of the construct measures was apparent. Additionally, the calculated average extracted values (halal food availability = 0.647, halal food health/nutrition = 0.824, halal food accreditation = 0.713, halal food cleanness/safety/hygiene = 0.584, destination trust = 0.852, destination attachment = 0.707, halal-friendly destination image = 0.861, and Muslim traveler retention = 0.579) were all higher than the recommended level of 0.50 [50]. Moreover, these values were higher than the correlations (squared) between factors (refer to Table 2). Hence, construct validity (convergent and discriminant) was evident in this research.

Table 1. A confirmatory factor analysis of measurement items ($n = 326$).

Measurement Items (Factor Loadings)	CR	AVE
HA1: Availability of halal food attracted me to visit tourist places. (0.739)	0.785	0.647
HA2: Halal food and beverage are served in restaurants and outlets in tourist sites/places. (0.865)		
HN1: Halal foods served in restaurants are healthy and nutritious. (0.921)	0.903	0.715
HN2: Halal foods that are available in tourist sites/places are healthy and nutritious. (0.894)		
HAC1: Halal food providers in tourist sites are accredited with halal certification. (0.843)	0.833	0.713
HAC2: Halal food outlets/restaurants in tourist sites clearly display a halal logo. (0.846)		
HC1: Halal food and beverage offered in tourist sites/places were clean, safe, and hygienic. (0.797)	0.737	0.584
HC2: Halal foods served in restaurants are clean, safe, and hygienic. (0.0.73)		
DT1: I think Korea as a halal-friendly destination is reliable. (0.901)	0.945	0.852
DT2: I have confidence in Korea as a halal-friendly destination. (0.963)		
DT3: I think that Korea as a halal-friendly destination has high integrity. (0.904)		
DA1: I like Korea more than other tourist destinations. (0.844)	0.829	0.707
DA2: I feel emotionally attached to Korea as a tourist destination. (0.838)		
HD1: My overall image of Korea as a Halal friendly destination is positive. (0.914)	0.949	0.861
HD2: My overall image of Korea as a halal friendly destination is positive. (0.951)		
HD3: Overall, I have a good image of Korea as a Halal-friendly destination. (0.918)		
MT1: I am willing to revisit Korea in the near future. (0.686)	0.732	0.579
MT2: Korea as a Halal family-friendly place will be my first choice when it comes to choosing a destination. (0.829)		

Note. HA: Halal food availability, HN: Halal food nutrition, HAC: Halal food accreditation, HC: Halal food cleanness, DT: Destination trust, DA: Destination attachment, HD: Halal friendly destination trust, MT: Muslim traveler retention.

Table 2. Measurement model and data quality assessment results ($n = 326$).

Constructs	(1)	(2)	(3)	(4)	(5)	(6)	(7)	(8)
(1) Halal food availability	1.000	–	–	–	–	–	–	–
(2) Halal food health/nutrition	0.715 [a] (0.511) [b]	1.000	–	–	–	–	–	–
(3) Halal food accreditation	0.659 (0.434)	0.715 (0.511)	1.000	–	–	–	–	–
(4) Halal food cleanness/safety/hygiene	0.653 (0.426)	0.628 (0.394)	0.751 (0.564)	1.000	–	–	–	–
(5) Destination trust	0.418 (0.175)	0.380 (0.144)	0.315 (0.099)	0.454 (0.206)	1.000	–	–	–
(6) Destination attachment	0.306 (0.094)	0.273 (0.075)	0.262 (0.069)	0.320 (0.102)	0.531 (0.282)	1.000	–	–
(7) Halal-friendly destination image	0.506 (0.256)	0.486 (0.235)	0.424 (0.180)	0.556 (0.309)	0.699 (0.487)	0.544 (0.296)	1.000	–
(8) Muslim traveler retention	0.465 (0.216)	0.406 (0.165)	0.370 (0.137)	0.470 (0.221)	0.654 (0.428)	0.585 (0.342)	0.759 (0.576)	1.000
Mean	4.824	4.399	4.747	4.848	4.405	4.704	4.432	4.432
Standard deviation	1.582	1.594	1.552	1.381	1.349	1.206	1.206	1.387

Note. Goodness-of fit statistics: $\chi^2 = 318.108$, $df = 107$, $p < 0.001$, $\chi^2/df = 2.973$, RMSEA = 0.078, CFI = 0.958, IFI = 0.958, TLI = 0.939.
[a] Between-construct correlations are below the diagonal. [b] Between-construct correlations (squared) are within parentheses.

4.3. Structural Model Analysis and Hypotheses Testing

A structural equation modeling was performed. The proposed model was found to have an acceptable level of goodness-of-fit statistics ($\chi^2 = 283.934$, df = 80, $p < 0.001$, $\chi^2/df = 3.549$, RMSEA = 0.089, CFI = 0.943, IFI = 0.944, TLI = 0.926). The details are exhibited in Table 3 and Figure 2. As exhibited in Figure 2, the higher-order model for halal food performance result indicated that the first-order dimensions (availability, health/nutrition, accreditation, and cleanness/safety/hygiene) and the higher-order latent construct are related in a significant manner ($p < 0.01$). Coefficient values (standardized) for such relationships were 0.918 (availability), 0.870 (health/nutrition), 0.938 (accreditation), and 0.964 (cleanness/safety/hygiene), correspondingly. The relations were all significant ($p < 0.01$). The first-order dimensions of availability ($R^2 = 0.843$), health/nutrition ($R^2 = 0.758$), accreditation ($R^2 = 0.880$), and cleanness/safety/hygiene ($R^2 = 0.929$) were sufficiently alleged to its global latent factor. The framework encompassing halal food performance dimensions as direct drivers of its outcome variables (the first-order formative research model) was run to compare it to the proposed higher-order model. However, the result indicated that most halal food performance factors within the first-order formative research model were not significantly associated with destination trust, destination attachment, and retention. Therefore, it was clear that the first-order variables related to one global factor of halal food performance.

Table 3. Structural equation modeling results and hypotheses testing ($n = 326$).

	Hypothesized Paths			Standardized Estimates	t-Values
H1	Halal food performance	→	Destination trust	0.461 **	7.799
H2	Halal food performance	→	Destination attachment	0.131 *	2.091
H3	Halal food performance	→	Muslim traveler retention	0.244 **	4.359
H4	Destination trust	→	Destination attachment	0.539 **	8.461
H5	Destination trust	→	Muslim traveler retention	0.439 **	6.547
H6	Destination attachment	→	Muslim traveler retention	0.379 **	4.884
	Halal food performance		Halal food availability	0.918 **	-
	Halal food performance		Halal food health/nutrition	0.870 **	14.754
	Halal food performance		Halal food accreditation	0.938 **	13.774
	Halal food performance		Halal food cleanness/safety/hygiene	0.964 **	12.606
Total variance explained:		Indirect impact on retention:		Total impact on RI:	

R^2 for Muslim traveler retention = 0.765
R^2 for destination attachment = 0.372
R^2 for destination trust = 0.213
R^2 for halal food availability = 0.843
R^2 for halal food health/nutrition = 0.758
R^2 for halal food accreditation = 0.880
R^2 for halal food cleanness/safety/hygiene = 0.929

$\beta_{trust-attachment-retention} = 0.204$ **

$\beta_{halal\ food\ performance-trust\ \&\ attachment-retention} = 0.346$ **

$\beta_{halal\ food\ performance-trust-attachment} = 0.248$ **

$\beta_{destination\ attachment} = 0.379$ **

$\beta_{destination\ trust} = 0.643$ **

$\beta_{halal\ food\ performance} = 0.590$ **

Note1. Goodness-of-fit statistics for the structural model (higher-order framework): $\chi^2 = 283.934$, $df = 80$, $p < 0.001$, $\chi^2/df = 3.549$, RMSEA = 0.089, CFI = 0.943, IFI = 0.944, TLI = 0.926, * $p < 0.05$, ** $p < 0.01$.

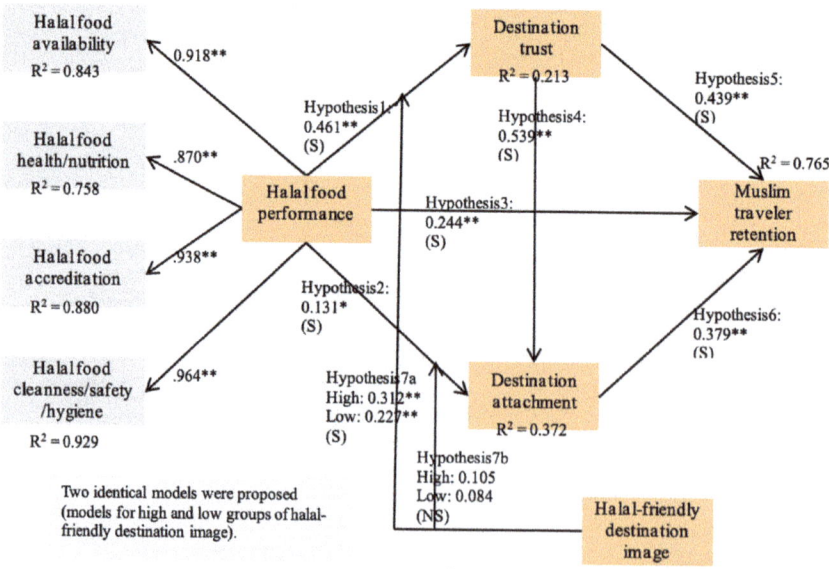

High = high group of halal-friendly destination image
Low = low group of halal-friendly destination image

Note1. Goodness-of-fit statistics for the structural model (higher-order model): $\chi^2 = 283.934$, $df = 80$, $p < 0.001$, $\chi^2/df = 3.549$, RMSEA = 0.089, CFI = 0.943, IFI = 0.944, TLI = 0.926
Note2. Goodness-of-fit statistics for the baseline model: $\chi^2 = 376.699$, $df = 168$, $p < 0.001$, $\chi^2/df = 2.242$, RMSEA = 0.062, CFI = 0.926, IFI = 0.927, TLI = 0.907
* $p < 0.05$, ** $p < 0.01$

Figure 2. The structural model results.

The proposed associations were tested. As expected, halal food performance exercised a significant influence on destination trust ($\beta = 0.461$, $p < 0.01$), destination attachment

($\beta = 0.131$, $p < 0.05$), and Muslim traveler retention ($\beta = 0.244$, $p < 0.01$). This outcome supported Hypotheses 1, 2, and 3. The hypothesized influence of destination trust was evaluated. Our finding showed the significant linkages between destination trust and destination attachment ($\beta = 0.539$, $p < 0.01$) and between destination trust and Muslim traveler retention ($\beta = 0.439$, $p < 0.01$). Hence, Hypotheses 4 and 5 were found true. In addition, as anticipated, destination attachment was a significant predictor of Muslim traveler retention. Hence, Hypothesis 6 was supported ($\beta = 0.379$, $p < 0.01$). Muslim traveler retention was satisfactorily accounted for by its antecedents ($R^2 = 0.765$). Moreover, about 37.2% and 21.3% of the total variance in destination attachment and destination trust were described by their predictors, respectively.

The indirect influence of research constructs was observed. As shown in Table 2, our result showed that trust significantly affected retention indirectly through destination attachment ($\beta = 0.204$, $p < 0.01$). In addition, halal food performance encompassed a significant indirect impact on destination attachment ($\beta = 0.248$, $p < 0.01$) and Muslim traveler retention ($\beta = 0.346$, $p < 0.01$). This finding indicated that both destination trust and attachment played a critical mediating role within the proposed model. Our further investigation showed that destination trust had the strongest total impact on Muslim traveler retention ($\beta = 0.643$, $p < 0.01$), halal food performance ($\beta = 0.590$, $p < 0.01$), and then destination attachment ($\beta = 0.379$, $p < 0.01$).

4.4. Baseline and Structural Invariance Model Results

A metric invariance test was carried out to uncover the proposed effect of a halal-friendly destination image. The obtained responses were split into high and low image groups. The high group contained 151 cases, whereas the low group included 175 cases. This group was completed on the basis of the K-means cluster analysis result. A baseline model comprising these two groups was created. The baseline model assessment results are shown in Table 4. The model contains a satisfactory level of goodness-of-fit statistics ($\chi^2 = 376.699$, $df = 168$, $p < 0.001$, $\chi^2/df = 2.242$, RMSEA = 0.062, CFI = 0.926, IFI = 0.927, TLI = 0.907). Within the model, all loadings were constrained to be equivalent across groups. We conducted a Chi-square test subsequently.

Table 4. Baseline and invariance model assessment results.

Paths	High Group of Halal-Friendly Destination Image ($n = 151$)		Low Group of Halal-Friendly Destination Image ($n = 175$)		Baseline Model (Freely Estimated)	Nested Model (Constrained to Be Equal)
	Coefficients	t-Values	Coefficients	t-Values		
Halal food performance → Trust	0.312 **	3.418	0.227 **	2.747	χ^2 (168) = 376.699	χ^2 (169) = 380.863 [a]
Halal food performance → Attachment	0.105	1.191	0.084	0.886	χ^2 (168) = 376.699	χ^2 (169) = 376.985 [b]
Chi-square difference test:						
[a] $\Delta\chi^2$ (1) = 4.164, $p < 0.05$ (H7a—supported)						
[b] $\Delta\chi^2$ (1) = 0.286, $p > 0.05$ (H7b—not supported)						

Note. Goodness-of-fit statistics for the baseline model: $\chi^2 = 376.699$, $df = 168$, $p < 0.001$, $\chi^2/df = 2.242$, RMSEA = 0.062, CFI = 0.926, IFI = 0.927, TLI = 0.907, ** $p < 0.01$.

The result of the comparison between the baseline model and the constrained model indicated that the path from halal food performance to trust was meaningfully different between the high and low groups of halal-friendly destination image ($\Delta\chi^2$ [1] = 4.164, $p < 0.05$). This result supported Hypothesis 7a. However, the linkages from halal food performance to attachment ($\Delta\chi^2$ [1] = 0.286, $p > 0.05$) were not meaningfully different between the high and low groups. Thus, Hypothesis 7b was rejected. Figure 2 and Table 3 include the specifics about the metric invariance test results.

5. Discussion

5.1. Higher-Order Framework of Halal Food Performance and Implications

One of the meaningful points in the present research is the higher-order framework of halal food performance. The four first-order variables, such as (1) availability, (2) health/nutrition, (3) accreditation, and (4) cleanness/safety/hygiene, belong to one inclusive latent factor of halal food performance. This means that the commonality underlying the four first-order variables was wholly extracted by its second-order construct. This empirical result and finding enrich the halal food literature by providing a hierarchical approach, which clearly apprehends the halal food performance. The parsimonious higher-order structure framework enlightens academics and practitioners about the competence of theorizing intricate halal food performance factors in a more succinct manner in the Muslim tourism sector.

Food cleanness/safety/hygiene and accreditation were two main factors of halal food performance. Therefore, for practitioners, assuring that halal foods served in restaurants and available in tourist sites are clean, safe, and hygienic is critical. Displaying a halal logo clearly and providing halal certified/accredited food/service is also essential. Such efforts would fulfill many crucial facets of overseas Muslim travelers' needs. In addition, food availability and health/nutrition were the other crucial dimensions of halal food performance. Boosting the availability of halal food and enhancing the healthy and nutritious facets of existing halal food are hence imperative for a non-Islamic destination product to appeal to Muslim visitors.

More than 20.0% of the food industry in the world is related to halal foods, and its volume is increasing with the constant growth of the international Muslim traveler population [20]. Many non-Muslim countries can also use halal foods as a tactic of their Muslim tourism development. As demonstrated in this research, halal food performance ultimately results in Muslim traveler retention. Improving the performance of halal food by centering on its cleanness/safety/hygiene, accreditation, availability, and health/nutrition can elicit approach behaviors for destinations, eventually increasing business opportunities, creating more jobs, and bringing monetary investment/benefit to the destinations. Theoretically, this research successfully explored halal food performance and its potential influence, which was weakly known. Accordingly, diverse aspects of halal food performance should be actively utilized when developing/building a theoretical framework for explicating international Muslim traveler responses and behaviors at non-Muslim destinations.

5.2. Implications Related to the Role of Destination Trust and Attachment

Prior research in the literature asserted that the influence of cognitive variable(s) on traveler post-purchase behaviors is likely to be strengthened by the mediating effect of trust or attachment [12,29,30,37]. In line with these studies, the present research finding demonstrated that destination trust and destination attachment significantly mediated the impact of halal food performance on Muslim traveler retention. This means that both destination trust and destination attachment acted as intensifiers of Muslim traveler retention within our proposed theoretical framework. Our results offer tourism academics and destination practitioners crucial information about the importance of escalating destination trust and enhancing destination attachment in order to induce the maximum impact of halal food performance on Muslim visitor retention. Given the elaborate theoretical mediating mechanism unearthed in the present research, it is imperative to deal with such mediator variables for the effectual increase in Muslim visitor approach behaviors for a non-Islamic tourism destination.

5.3. Moderating Effect of Halal-Friendly Destination Image and its Implications

Findings of our metric invariance test indicated that the relationship between halal food performance and destination trust is moderated by a halal-friendly destination image. In particular, the association strength was greater in the high group of destination image than in the low group (high group: $\beta = 0.312, p < 0.01$ vs. low group: $\beta = 0.227, p < 0.01$). This result implies that at a similar level of halal food performance, Muslim visitors who have a strong halal-friendly image of a non-Islamic location more heavily rely on the destination and its tourism environment than those who have an unfriendly image. Theoretically, this finding has a strong value as the present study is the first empirical research that provides evidence regarding the significance of a halal-friendly destination image in determining the magnitude of the influence of halal food performance on destination trust. Our evaluation and finding of the convoluted associations among food performance, destination image, and destination trust, which are especially crucial in the international Muslim tourism context, contribute to escalating academics' understanding of Muslim visitors' post-purchase formation regarding non-Islamic destination products. Our finding is also practically meaningful. As a halal-friendly image about a destination is decisive in Muslim visitors' retention process, practitioners should be more aware of its criticality. Offering superior services and developing/providing new products, which are entirely friendly for Muslim visitors, could generate a positive halal-friendly destination image.

6. Conclusions and Limitations

6.1. Conclusions

The rapid growth of Muslim tourism is evident in many Islamic and non-Islamic destinations [4,5,10]. Yet, our understanding of halal food performance and its influence on Muslim traveler approach behaviors for a destination was lacking. The present research has filled this gap. The hypothesized conceptual framework was wholly supported. Halal food performance was revealed to be a determinant of destination trust, destination attachment, and Muslim traveler retention. Destination trust and attachment contributed to making the best use of halal food performance in the retention process. A Halal-friendly destination image strengthened the influence of halal food performance on destination trust. Our findings help practitioners at non-Islamic destinations invent useful strategies to retain international Muslim visitors by utilizing halal food, trust, attachment, and image as important tools. Indubitably, a theoretical base pertinent to Muslim traveler behaviors at non-Islamic places is in the infant stage. From this perspective, our research that helps academics and practitioners increase their understanding of such behaviors contains high originality and value.

6.2. Limitations and Future Research Arena

Although these research findings have presented both theoretical and conceptual frameworks, this research had some limitations that provide some directions for potential studies. First, the present study centered on Muslim traveler behaviors at a non-Islamic destination. Their behaviors can possibly differ at an Islamic destination. Future research should conduct an empirical comparison of the Muslim traveler retention process and behavior across Islamic and non-Islamic destinations, which would be a meaningful extension of this study. Second, it would be true that a normative process such as social norms and moral/ethical obligation is also crucial when explicating Muslim traveler approach or avoidance behaviors. Indeed, some research denoted the criticality of normative factors in traveler behaviors [51]. Thus, future research should broaden the proposed conceptual model by integrating normative influence in order to improve the comprehensiveness and explanatory power of the model. Lastly, future research should consider the changes in travel options. For example, the accommodation option of Airbnb and/or other rental properties will allow travelers to cook their own meals during their travel so that they do not have to consider the halal-friendly options.

Author Contributions: Conceptualization, H.H. and L.H.L.; methodology, A.R. (Aleksandar Radic); writing—original draft preparation, H.H.; writing—review and editing, L.H.L. and (António Raposo); visualization, A.H.N. and A.R. (António Raposo); supervision, H.H., L.H.L. and A.R. (Aleksandar Radic); project administration, H.H., A.R. (Aleksandar Radic) and A.H.N. All authors have read and agreed to the published version of the manuscript.

Funding: This research received no external funding.

Data Availability Statement: The dataset used in this research are available upon request from the corresponding author. The data are not publicly available due to restrictions i.e., privacy or ethical.

Acknowledgments: The authors would like to thank Lorna Darelius for the meticulous review of the manuscript.

Conflicts of Interest: The authors declare no conflict of interest.

Ethics Statement: Because of the observational nature of the study, and in the absence of any involvement of therapeutic medication, no formal approval of the Institutional Review Board of the local Ethics Committee was required. Nonetheless, all subjects were informed about the study and participation was fully on a voluntary basis. Participants were ensured of the confidentiality and anonymity of the information associated with the surveys. The study was conducted in accordance with the Helsinki Declaration.

Appendix A

Halal Food Performance [2,11,12,17]
Halal Food Availability Factor
Availability of halal food attracted me to visit tourist places.
Halal food and beverage are served in restaurants and outlets in tourist sites/places.
Halal Food Health/Nutrition Factor
Halal foods served in restaurants are healthy and nutritious.
Halal foods that are available in tourist sites/places are healthy and nutritious
Halal Food Accreditation Factor
Halal food providers in tourist sites are accredited with halal certification.
Halal food outlets/restaurants in tourist sites clearly display a halal logo.
Halal Food Cleanness/Safety/Hygiene Factor
Halal food and beverage offered in tourist sites/places were clean, safe, and hygienic.
Halal foods served in restaurants are clean, safe, and hygienic.
Destination Trust [12,29]
I think Korea as a halal-friendly destination is reliable.
I have confidence in Korea as a halal-friendly destination.
I think that Korea as a halal-friendly destination has high integrity.
Destination Attachment [16,37]
I like Korea more than other tourist destinations.
I feel emotionally attached to Korea as a tourist destination.
Halal-friendly Destination Image [45]
My overall image of Korea as a Halal-friendly destination is positive.
The overall image I have of Korea as a Halal-friendly destination is favorable.
Overall, I have a good image of Korea as a Halal-friendly destination.
Muslim Traveler Retention [49]
I am willing to revisit Korea in the near future.
Korea as a Halal family-friendly place will be my first choice when it comes to choosing a destination.

References

1. Akhtar, N.; Sun, J.; Ahmad, W.; Akhtar, M.N. The effect of non-verbal message on Muslim tourists' interaction adaptation: A case study of Halal restaurants in China. *J. Dest. Mark. Manag.* **2019**, *11*, 10–22. [CrossRef]
2. Al-Ansi, A.; Han, H.; Kim, S.; King, B. Inconvenient experiences among Muslim travelers: An analysis of the multiple causes. *J. Travel Res.* **2020**. [CrossRef]
3. Han, H.; Al-Ansi, A.; Jung, H.; Jeong, E.; Jeong, D. Motivating Muslim travelers to visit Korea. *Int. J. Tour. Hosp. Res.* **2018**, *32*, 19–27. [CrossRef]
4. Jafari, J.; Scott, N. Muslim world and its tourisms. *Ann. Tour. Res.* **2014**, *44*, 1–19. [CrossRef]
5. Kim, S.; Im, H.H.; King, B.E.M. Muslim travelers in Asia: The destination preferences and brand perceptions of Malaysian tourists. *J. Vacat. Mark.* **2015**, *21*, 3–21. [CrossRef]
6. Ryan, C. Halal tourism. *Tour. Manag. Perspect.* **2016**, *19*, 121–123. [CrossRef]
7. Aziz, Y.; Chok, N. The role of halal awareness, halal certification, and marketing components in determining halal purchase intention among non-muslims in Malaysia: A structural equation modeling approach. *J. Int. Food Agribus. Mark.* **2013**, *25*, 1–23. [CrossRef]
8. Mannaa, M.T. Halal food in the tourist destination and its importance for Muslim travelers. *Curr. Issues Tour.* **2020**, *23*, 2195–2206. [CrossRef]

9. Mostafa, M.M. A knowledge domain visualization review of thirty years of halal food research: Themes, trends and knowledge structure. *Trends Food Sci. Technol.* **2020**, *99*, 660–677. [CrossRef]
10. Olya, H.G.; Al-ansi, A. Risk assessment of halal products and services: Implication for tourism industry. *Tour. Manag.* **2018**, *65*, 279–291. [CrossRef]
11. Jia, X.; Chaozhi, Z. Turning impediment into attraction: A supplier perspective in Halal food in non-Islamic destinations. *J. Dest. Mark. Manag.* **2021**, *19*, 1–11.
12. Al-Ansi, A.; Olya, H.G.T.; Han, H. Effect of general risk on trust, satisfaction, and recommendation intention for halal food. *Int. J. Hosp. Manag.* **2019**, *83*, 210–219. [CrossRef]
13. Artigas, E.M.; Yrigoyen, C.C.; Moraga, E.T.; Villalon, C.B. Determinants of trust towards tourist destinations. *J. Dest. Mark. Manag.* **2017**, *6*, 327–334.
14. Liu, J.; Wang, C.; Fang, S.; Zhang, T. Scale development for tourist trust toward a tourism destination. *Tour. Manag. Perspect.* **2019**, *31*, 383–397. [CrossRef]
15. Kim, S.H.; Song, M.K.; Shim, C. Storytelling by medical tourism agents and its effect on trust and behavioral intention. *J. Travel Tour. Mark.* **2020**, *37*, 679–694. [CrossRef]
16. Yuksel, A.; Yuksel, F.; Bilim, Y. Destination attachment: Effects on customer satisfaction and cognitive, affective and conative loyalty. *Tour. Manag.* **2010**, *31*, 274–284. [CrossRef]
17. Lee, S.; Park, H.; Ahn, Y. The influence of tourists' experience of quality of street foods on destination's image, life satisfaction, and word of mouth: The moderating impact of food neophobia. *Int. J. Environ. Res. Public Health* **2020**, *17*, 163. [CrossRef]
18. Lojo, A.; Li, M.; Xu, H. Online tourism destination image: Components, information sources, and incongruence. *J. Travel Tour. Mark.* **2020**, *37*, 495–509. [CrossRef]
19. Pan, X.; Rasouli, S.; Timmermans, H. Investigating tourist destination choice: Effect of destination image from social network members. *Tour. Manag.* **2021**, *83*, 1–11. [CrossRef]
20. Han, H.; Al-Ansi, A.; Olya, H.G.T.; Kim, W. Exploring halal-friendly destination attributes in South Korea: Perceptions and behaviors of Muslim travelers toward a non-Muslim destination. *Tour. Manag.* **2019**, *71*, 151–164. [CrossRef]
21. Aslan, I.; Aslan, H. Halal food awareness and future challenges. *Brit. J. Econ. Manag. Trade* **2016**, *12*, 1–20. [CrossRef]
22. Xiong, J.; Zhang, C.Z. "Halal tourism": Is it the same trend in non-Islamic destinations with Islamic destinations? *Asia Pacific J. Tour. Res.* **2020**, *25*, 189–204.
23. Ali, M.; Tan, K.; Ismail, M. A supply chain integrity framework for halal food. *Br. Food J.* **2017**, *119*, 20–38. [CrossRef]
24. Taylor, S.A.; Baker, T.L. An assessment of the relationship between service quality and customer satisfaction in the formation of consumers' purchase intentions. *J. Retail.* **1994**, *70*, 163–178. [CrossRef]
25. Ambali, A.R.; Bakar, A.N. People's awareness on Halal foods and products: Potential issues for policy-makers. *Procedia Soc. Behav. Sci.* **2014**, *121*, 3–25. [CrossRef]
26. Moira, P.; Sarchosis, D.; Mylonopoulos, D. The religious beliefs as parameter of food choices at tourist destination: The case of Mykonos. In Proceedings of the International Religious Tourism and Pilgrimage Conferences, Armeno, Orta Lake, Italy, 30 June 2017.
27. Shaikh, F.; Sharma, D. Islam and consumption: Religion interpretations and changing consumerism. In *Islamic Perspectives on Marketing and Consumer Behavior: Planning, Implementation and Control*; IGI Global: Hershey, PA, USA, 2015.
28. Jeaheng, Y.; Al-Ansi, A.; Han, H. Halal-friendly hotels: Impact of halal-friendly attributes on guest purchase behaviors in the Thailand hotel industry. *J. Travel Tour. Mark.* **2019**, *36*, 729–746. [CrossRef]
29. Abubakar, A.M.; Ilkan, M.; Al-Tal, R.M.; Eluwole, K.K. eWOM, revisit intention, destination trust and gender. *J. Hosp. Tour. Manag.* **2017**, *31*, 220–227. [CrossRef]
30. Tang, L.; Jang, S. Tourism information trust as a bridge between information value and satisfaction: An exploratory study. *Tour. Anal.* **2008**, *13*, 565–578. [CrossRef]
31. Sirdeshmukh, D.; Singh, J.; Sabol, B. Consumer trust, value, and loyalty in relational exchanges. *J. Mark.* **2002**, *66*, 15–37. [CrossRef]
32. Chiu, C.M.; Hsu, M.H.; Lai, H.; Chang, C.M. Reexamining the influence of trust on online repeat purchase intention: The moderating role of habit and its antecedents. *Decis. Support Syst.* **2012**, *53*, 835–845. [CrossRef]
33. Bonne, K.; Verbeke, W. Muslim consumer trust in halal meat status and control in Belgium. *Meat Sci.* **2008**, *79*, 113–123. [CrossRef]
34. Chen, C.; Luo, W.; Kang, N.; Li, H.; Yang, X.; Xia, Y. Serial mediation of environmental preference and place attachment in the relationship between perceived street walkability and mood of the elderly. *Int. J. Environ. Res. Public Health* **2020**, *17*, 4620. [CrossRef] [PubMed]
35. Han, H.; Hyun, S. Role of motivations for luxury cruise traveling, satisfaction, and involvement in building traveler loyalty. *Int. J. Hosp. Manag.* **2018**, *70*, 75–84. [CrossRef]
36. Kim, S.; Choe, J.Y.; Petrick, J.F. The effect of celebrity on brand awareness, perceived quality, brand image, brand loyalty, and destination attachment to a literary festival. *J. Dest. Mark. Manag.* **2018**, *9*, 320–329. [CrossRef]
37. Han, H.; Lee, K.-S.; Chua, B.; Lee, S.; Kim, W. Role of airline food quality, price reasonableness, image, satisfaction, and attachment in building re-flying intention. *Int. J. Hosp. Manag.* **2019**, *80*, 91–100. [CrossRef]
38. Kim, S.; Prideaux, B.; Chon, K. A comparison of results of three statistical methods to understand the determinants of festival participants' expenditures. *Int. J. Hosp. Manag.* **2010**, *29*, 297–307. [CrossRef]

39. Park, S.H.; Hsieh, C.-M.; Lee, C.-K. Examining Chinese college students' intention to travel to Japan using the extended Theory of Planned Behavior: Testing destination image and the mediating role of travel constraints. *J. Travel Tour. Mark.* **2017**, *34*, 113–131. [CrossRef]
40. Zhang, H.; Fu, X.; Cai, L.A.; Lu, L. Destination image and tourist loyalty: A meta-analysis. *Tour. Manag.* **2014**, *40*, 213–223. [CrossRef]
41. Keller, K.L. Conceptualizing, measuring, and managing customer-based brand equity. *J. Mark.* **1993**, *57*, 1–22. [CrossRef]
42. Kotler, P.; Haider, D.H.; Rein, I. *Marketing Places: Attracting Investment, Industry, and Tourism to Cities, States, and Nations*; The Free Press: New York, NY, USA, 1993.
43. Assael, H. *Consumer Behavior and Marketing Action*; Kent: Boston, MA, USA, 1984.
44. Baloglu, S.; McCleary, K.W. A model of destination image formation. *Ann. Tour. Res.* **1999**, *26*, 868–897. [CrossRef]
45. Lee, J.; Hsu, L.; Han, H.; Kim, Y. Understanding how consumers view green hotels: How a hotel's green image can influence behavioral intentions. *J. Sust. Tour.* **2010**, *18*, 901–914. [CrossRef]
46. Ostrowski, P.; O'Brien, T.; Gordon, G. Service quality and customer loyalty in the commercial airline industry. *J. Travel Res.* **1993**, *32*, 16–24. [CrossRef]
47. Han, H.; Hyun, S. Impact of hotel-restaurant image and quality of physical-environment, service, and food on satisfaction and intention. *Int. J. Hosp. Manag.* **2017**, *63*, 82–92. [CrossRef]
48. Hennig-Thurau, T. Customer orientation of service employees: Its impact on customer satisfaction, commitment, and retention. *Int. J. Serv. Indust. Manag.* **2004**, *15*, 460–478. [CrossRef]
49. Oliver, R.L. *Satisfaction: A Behavioral Perspective on the Consumer*, 2nd ed.; Routledge: New York, NY, USA, 2010.
50. Hair, J.F.; Black, W.C.; Babin, B.J.; Anderson, R.E. *Multivariate Data Analysis*; Prentice-Hall: Upper Saddle River, NJ, USA, 2010.
51. Sun, S.; Law, R.; Schuckert, M. Mediating effects of attitude, subjective norms and perceived behavioral control for mobile payment-based hotel reservations. *Int. J. Hosp. Manag.* **2020**, *84*, 102331. [CrossRef]

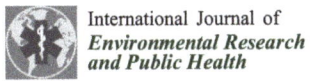

International Journal of *Environmental Research and Public Health*

Article

The Removal of Meat Exudate and *Escherichia coli* from Stainless Steel and Titanium Surfaces with Irregular and Regular Linear Topographies

Adele Evans [1], Anthony J. Slate [2], I. Devine Akhidime [1,3], Joanna Verran [1], Peter J. Kelly [1] and Kathryn A. Whitehead [1,3,*]

1. Faculty of Science and Engineering, Manchester Metropolitan University, Manchester M1 5GD, UK; Adele.Evans@mmu.ac.uk (A.E.); D.Akhidime@mmu.ac.uk (I.D.A.); j.verran@mmu.ac.uk (J.V.); peter.kelly@mmu.ac.uk (P.J.K.)
2. Department of Biology and Biochemistry, University of Bath, Claverton Down, Bath BA2 7AY, UK; ajs319@bath.ac.uk
3. Microbiology at Interfaces, Department of Life Sciences, Manchester Metropolitan University, Manchester M1 5GD, UK
* Correspondence: k.a.whitehead@mmu.ac.uk

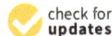

Citation: Evans, A.; Slate, A.J.; Akhidime, I.D.; Verran, J.; Kelly, P.J.; Whitehead, K.A. The Removal of Meat Exudate and *Escherichia coli* from Stainless Steel and Titanium Surfaces with Irregular and Regular Linear Topographies. *Int. J. Environ. Res. Public Health* **2021**, *18*, 3198. https://doi.org/10.3390/ijerph18063198

Academic Editor: Ki Hwan Park

Received: 18 February 2021
Accepted: 15 March 2021
Published: 19 March 2021

Publisher's Note: MDPI stays neutral with regard to jurisdictional claims in published maps and institutional affiliations.

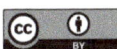

Copyright: © 2021 by the authors. Licensee MDPI, Basel, Switzerland. This article is an open access article distributed under the terms and conditions of the Creative Commons Attribution (CC BY) license (https://creativecommons.org/licenses/by/4.0/).

Abstract: Bacterial retention and organic fouling on meat preparation surfaces can be influenced by several factors. Surfaces with linear topographies and defined chemistries were used to determine how the orientation of the surface features affected cleaning efficacy. Fine polished (irregular linear) stainless steel (FPSS), titanium coated fine polished (irregular linear) stainless steel (TiFP), and topographically regular, linear titanium coated surfaces (RG) were fouled with *Escherichia coli* mixed with a meat exudate (which was utilised as a conditioning film). Surfaces were cleaned along or perpendicular to the linear features for one, five, or ten wipes. The bacteria were most easily removed from the titanium coated and regular featured surfaces. The direction of cleaning (along or perpendicular to the surface features) did not influence the amount of bacteria retained, but meat extract was more easily removed from the surfaces when cleaned in the direction along the linear surface features. Following ten cleans, there was no significant difference in the amount of cells or meat exudate retained on the surfaces cleaned in either direction. This study demonstrated that for the *E. coli* cells, the TiFP and RG surfaces were easiest to clean. However, the direction of the clean was important for the removal of the meat exudate from the surfaces.

Keywords: *Escherichia coli*; bacterial retention; surface topographies; meat exudate; wipe cleaning; conditioning film

1. Introduction

Modern food processing and production facilities provide an environment that promotes bacterial retention due to a myriad of factors, which include the surface properties of the equipment and the matrix of the food being processed [1,2]. The removal of bacteria and/or organic material from food production surfaces is important since its build up can result in microbial contamination of food products, which can have a significant effect on consumers, food companies, and food suppliers, for example, cross-contamination of food with pathogenic bacteria can result in food-borne illnesses [3–6]. The Food Standard Agency estimates that foodborne illness in the UK alone result in a financial loss of £1.5 billion per annum [7]. As such, biofouling in the food industry is a significant problem [8]. For certain bacteria, some of which are important human pathogens, there can be contamination of raw meat due to biofouling [9]. Contamination of beef with *Escherichia coli* O157:H7 has been linked to outbreaks of foodborne illnesses and concerns about *E. coli* O157:H7 contamination have resulted in a zero tolerance towards this microorganism in the food industry [10,11].

Once a surface is introduced into an environment, it will adsorb a variety of organic and inorganic matter, resulting in the formation of a conditioning film [12–14]. Surface conditioning is a process which starts within seconds of the substratum becoming immersed into liquids [15]. The structure and composition of a conditioning film is ultimately dependent upon the surrounding products and the properties of the surface and can result in physicochemical, chemical, and topographical alterations, affecting both the rate and extent of bacterial retention and therefore surface contamination [16–18]. With regards to the meat industry, the exudate of frozen raw meat has been identified as an important source of bacterial contamination on food processing surfaces [19]. It has also been shown that sterilized chicken juice is an ideal environment for survival of *Campylobacter jejuni* [20] and its presence may also increase biofilm formation [21].

The method and type of physical cleaning methods used will be dependent on the food industry and the surfaces involved [22]. Product contact surfaces may typically be cleaned several times per day, while environmental surfaces such as walls and hoods may be cleaned less frequently [23]. In the meat industry, chilled beef carcasses are cut into smaller pieces, which are deboned and made into cuts; such work takes place on flat surfaces that are regularly cleaned [24]. However, it has been suggested that bacterial recontamination during this meat fabrication process results in higher numbers of *E. coli* on the cuts and trimmings [25,26]. Hence, a better understanding is required of the mechanisms involved in the attachment and detachment of bacteria to meat processing surfaces and their removal following cleaning. To simulate more realistic conditions, cleaning assays need to be carried out in the presence of a meat exudate (or relevant conditioning film) to increase the understanding of surface hygiene and decrease transmission and hence potential public health risks [27].

The ideal conditions for a hygienic surface have been defined as easy to clean, able to resist wear and maintain their hygienic qualities over time [28]. The hygienic quality and cleanability of a surface has been linked to the surface properties including the topography [28–30], chemical composition [31] and physicochemical properties [32,33]. Thermodynamics are thought to play a central role in initial bacterial: substrata interactions where it has been suggested that bacterial cells will attach preferentially to hydrophobic materials (i.e., materials with a low surface energy), when the surface energy of the bacteria is greater than the surface energy of the surrounding liquid [34]. Due to the complexity of bacterial-substratum interactions, further research is required to fully elucidate the underpinning mechanisms of bacterial attachment, adhesion, and retention [35].

An approach to reduce microbial contamination, which is a prerequisite for biofilm formation, is the modification of surface topography. Microscale surface topographic features have been shown to both inhibit or promote bacterial retention depending on the size, shape, and density of the topographical features [36]. It has also been shown that surfaces with features on the same scale as bacterial cells (e.g., cocci-shaped *Staphylococcus aureus*; ~1 µm diameter) promote the strongest retention due to maximum binding at the cell-substrate contact areas [37,38]. In an industrial setting, the wear of the surfaces may introduce random features (i.e., scratches) of different dimensions and it has been suggested that an increase in the surface roughness may cause the entrapment of microorganisms within the surface features, which in turn will affect the cleanability and hence the hygienic status of the surface [39]. Bacteria and organic material that become entrapped in the topographical features of a surface are difficult to remove using standard cleaning procedures [40], and it has been proposed that the development of the micro-pattern materials may help in the reduction of viable bacteria on food contact surfaces [41]. However, most studies have not determined the effect of the presence of the conditioning film on surface cleaning, especially with regards to the influence of surface topographical features [20], or with regards to the direction of cleaning compared to the linear surface features.

Stainless steels are used widely throughout the food and beverage industry due to their resistance to corrosion, thermal conductivity, and their ability to be produced with a smooth surface finish [33]. Stainless steel grade 304 is most commonly used in the food industry [42]. Due to the production process of stainless steel, 'microniches' of heterogenous chemical composition may result in varying bacterial retention patterns [43]. Titanium has been incorporated into stainless steel alloys in the food industry to improve corrosion resistance because it forms stable carbides [44,45]. Titanium surfaces may also have a more homogenous chemical composition than stainless steel since it is comprised mainly of TiO_2 [46]. This work aimed to determine how surface attributes (chemistry and topography) and the direction of cleaning affected bacteria and meat exudate removal from surfaces.

2. Materials and Methods

2.1. Equipment and Material Suppliers

The following reagents and materials were used; stainless steel sheets (Outokumpu Stainless Ltd., Helsinki, Finland), sodium hydroxide, di-potassium hydrogen phosphate, potassium di-hydrogen phosphate, tri-sodium citrate ammonium sulphate, magnesium sulphate (Merck, Darmstradt, Germany), tryptone soya agar and tryptone soya broth (Oxoid, Basingstoke, UK) rolled beef brisket (Co-op, Manchester, UK), *Escherichia coli* CCL410 (Agence Francaise de Securite Sanitaire des Aliments, Paris, France), cleaning clothes (WYPALL® ×80 Kimberley-Clark, West Malling, UK), Rhodamine B, DAPI and glycerol (Merck, Darmstradt, Germany). The following equipment was purchased: Atomic force microscope (Quesant Instruments, Santa Cruz, CA, USA), Crockmeter (A.A.T.C.C Crockmeter, Model CM1, NC, USA), Epifluorescence microscope (Nikon, Tokyo, Japan), F-View II camera (Soft Imaging System Ltd., Olympus, Tokyo, Japan), and Cell F Image Analysis package (Olympus, Tokyo, Japan).

2.2. Production of Surfaces

Three different surfaces were used in this study, including stainless steel 304 with a fine polished finish (FPSS), 304 fine polished finished stainless steel coated with titanium (TiFP) and a linear, regular finished (RG) titanium surface. Fine polished, grade 304, stainless steel sheets were prepared as 10 mm × 10 mm sample squares using a guillotine. To ensure that the samples were examined in a pristine "as-manufactured" state, the manufacturer's protective plastic coating was only removed directly before experimentation.

The titanium surfaces with a regular topography were unwritten digital video discs stripped of their protective coats. The samples were cut into 10 mm × 10 mm squares using metal cutting shears and soaked overnight in 30% sodium hydroxide solution, followed by rinsing thoroughly with sterile distilled water and drying in a class 2 microbiological cabinet prior to coating with titanium.

Samples of the fine polished stainless steel surfaces and the stripped digital video discs were coated using titanium. The substrata were coated with titanium via magnetron sputtering in a modified Edwards E306A coating system rig using a single 150 mm diameter × 10 mm thick, 99.5% pure titanium target attached to an unbalanced magnetron (argon gas at a working pressure of 0.15 Pa; magnetron power of 0.5 kW; base pressure 10^{-4} Pa; time 15 min; substrate biased at −50 V) [47].

2.3. Atomic Force Microscopy (AFM)

The shape and depth of the surface features was determined using atomic force microscopy. The analysis was carried out in in contact mode using triangular shaped silicon nitride tips, with a spring constant of 0.12 N m^{-2}. The height and shape of the features were determined from five areas taken from different replicate surfaces.

2.4. Sample Organisms

This study was conducted with *Escherichia coli* strain CCL410. This strain was recovered by the laboratory of Dr C. Vernozy-Rozand (Unité de Microbiologie alimentaire et prévisionnelle, Ecole vétérinaire de Lyon, France) from heifers fecal samples. This strain was selected due to it being a non-pathogenic variant of *E. coli* O157:H7 (wild type strain). The pathogenicity of the bacteria was reduced due to the loss of *stx1* and *stx2* [48].

2.5. Bacterial Stock and Working Cultures

Stock cultures of E. coli were stored at −80 °C in a freezer mix, which was composed of a sterilised salt solution containing a mixture of autoclaved 12.6 g L^{-1} di-potassium hydrogen phosphate, 3.6 g L^{-1}, potassium di-hydrogen phosphate, 0.9 g L^{-1}, tri-sodium citrate 1.8 g L^{-1} ammonium sulphate and 300 g L^{-1} glycerol combined with a litre sterilised solution of 1.8 g L^{-1} magnesium sulphate [49]. In preparation for the cleaning assays, cultures of E. coli were prepared by inoculating E. coli onto Tryptone soya agar (TSA), at 37 °C overnight. A single colony of E. coli was inoculated into 10 mL of Tryptone soya broth (TSB) and incubated at 37 °C overnight. One hundred microlitres of overnight culture was inoculated into 100 mL TSB and incubated at 37 °C for 18 h with shaking (200 rpm). Following incubation, the bacterial cells were harvested by centrifuging at 1721× g for 10 min, washed once, and re-suspended in sterile distilled water using a vortex mixer for 30 s. The suspension was centrifuged at 1721× g for 10 min and the cells were resuspended to an optical density (OD) of 1.0 (±0.1) at 540 nm in sterile distilled water. This corresponded to ca. 1.88 ± 0.22 × 10^8 CFU mL^{-1}.

2.6. Meat Exudates

The production of meat exudates was adapted [50]. Commercially available, fresh rolled beef brisket was cut into 10 mm × 10 mm pieces, placed in a stainless steel tray and covered in aluminium foil. The meat was covered by another stainless steel tray and weighed down with 8.4 kg of stainless steel sheets and frozen at −20 °C for 24 h. The diced meat pieces were defrosted at room temperature, and the meat exudate produced was collected and stored at −20 °C until use.

2.7. Cleaning Assays

The substrata were inoculated with a bacterial/meat exudate mixture and dried in a microbiological class 2 cabinet. For the bacterial/meat exudate mixture, 100 µL of bacteria and 100 µL of meat exudate was placed into an Eppendorf tube, vortexed for 5 s and 10 µL of the preparation was pipetted onto the substratum, spread across the surface with a sterile plastic spreader, and dried in a class 2 flow hood at room temperature. A crockmeter was used for the wipe clean method to ensure that each wipe across the stainless steel surface was standardised. The substrata were placed on the steel specimen stage and a 45 mm × 45 mm piece of blue wipe cloth was folded and attached to the 16 mm diameter test finger. Sterile distilled water (1 mL) was pipetted onto the cloth and the hand crank was turned to simulate one wipe. The wipe cycles compromised one, five, or ten repeats. Following each cleaning cycle, the substrata were dried for 2 h in a class 2 microbiological cabinet. Three replicates were taken at each cleaning cycle point for each surface, and for each direction of clean (along or perpendicular to the linear features).

Following the cleaning assays, the percentage coverage of the bacteria and meat extract retained on the surfaces per field of view was analysed following differential staining and epifluorescence microscopy.

2.8. Preparation of Stains

[9-(2-carboxyphenyl)-6-diethylamino-3-xanthenylidene]-diethylammonium chloride (Rhodamine B) was prepared as a stock solution of 0.1 g mL^{-1} in ethanol (absolute) and used at a working concentration of 0.1 mg mL^{-1}. 4′, 6-diamidino-2-phenylindole (DAPI) was prepared as a stock solution of 0.3 g mL^{-1} in sterile distilled water and used at a working concentration of 0.1 mg mL^{-1}. Prior to use, the stains were refrigerated (4 °C) and stored in a dark environment.

2.9. Differential Staining of Meat Exudate and E. coli

A dual staining procedure was conducted as described previously [51]. Ten microlitres of DAPI was added to the samples and spread across the surface using a sterile plastic spreader to detect the bacteria and then 10 µL of Rhodamine B was applied to the substrate in the same manner to detect the retained meat extract [51]. Following staining, the samples were dried in the dark at room temperature in a microbiological class 2 flow hood.

The samples were viewed, and images obtained using an epifluorescence microscope with black and white digital camera and a Cell F Image Analysis package to measure the percentage coverage of the area of the stained material and to determine the percentage surface coverage of the bacteria and organic material. A filter wavelength of 330–380 nm was used to detect the DAPI stained cells, and a 590–650 nm filter was used to detect the Rhodamine B stained organic material. The retained material on the surfaces was measured using percentage coverage of the field size for randomly selected areas across the test substratum. Each of the three samples had 15 areas independently selected and analysed for the percentage coverage of bacteria and meat extract ($n = 45$).

2.10. Statistical Analysis

Statistical analysis was conducted by performing two-way ANOVA coupled with Tukey's multiple comparison tests for post hoc analysis using GraphPad Prism (version 8.4.2; GraphPad Software, San Diego, CA, USA) to determine significant differences at a confidence level of 95% ($p < 0.05$). Error bars represent the standard error of the mean. Asterisks denote significance, * $p \leq 0.05$, ** $p \leq 0.01$, *** $p \leq 0.001$, and **** $p \leq 0.0001$.

3. Results

Three surfaces were prepared to determine the effect of a linear surface topography (irregular and regular), and defined surface chemistry (stainless steel and titanium) on the removal of bacterial and meat exudate using a wipe clean assay. Atomic force microscopy (AFM) of the fine polished stainless steel (FPSS), titanium coated fine polished stainless steel (TiFP), and the regular linear featured titanium coated surface (RG) revealed that the surface features of the FPSS and TIFP surfaces demonstrated irregular, linear topographies. The Z height of the TiFP surface (Figure 1b) was higher than the FPSS surface (0.338 ± 0.017 µm and 0.284 ± 0.014 µm, respectively) (Figure 1a). Regular linear features were evident on the titanium coated surface (RG) and the z height of the titanium coated regular surface was 0.420 ± 0.021 µm. The FPSS demonstrated valley widths of ~1 µm to 5 µm, whilst the TiFP demonstrated valley demonstrated valley widths of ~0.5 µm to 5 µm. The RG surface demonstrated valley widths of 1.02 µm. The contact angles of the three surfaces were $82 \pm 3°$, $84 \pm 4.5°$, and $91 \pm 3.7°$ for the FPSS, TiFP and RG surfaces, respectively, and this indicated that the FPSS and TiFP were marginally more wettable than the RG surface.

The percentage coverage of the bacteria on the surfaces following initial fouling of the substrata before cleaning demonstrated that cells were retained in significantly higher amounts of bacteria on the FPSS (15.86%) or TiFP (18.52%) compared to the linear finished RG surface (0.81%) ($p < 0.0001$) (Figure 2).

Following one clean, fouling of the surfaces with different features and chemistries (FPSS, TiFP, RG), the amount of bacteria when cleaned along the linear features was significantly reduced (FPSS 6.98%; TiFP 1.91%; RG 0.17%) ($p < 0.0001$) (Figure 2a), whereas following one clean in the direction perpendicular to the linear features, there was only a significant difference in the amount of cells removed from the FPSS and RG surfaces (FPSS 5.49%; TiFP 1.51%; RG 0.21%) ($p > 0.05$) (Figure 2b). After five or 10 cleans, there was no significant difference in the amount of bacteria retained when the surfaces was cleaned along or perpendicular to the surface features (FPSS 6.98%, 5.49%; TiFP 1.91%, 1.51%; RG 0.17%, 0.21%) ($p > 0.05$). Overall removal of the cells from the surfaces in the direction of the linear features or perpendicular to the linear features demonstrated the same trend whereby the FPSS surface retained more bacteria than the TiFP surface, and the lowest amounts of bacteria was retained on the RG surface (Figure 2a,b).

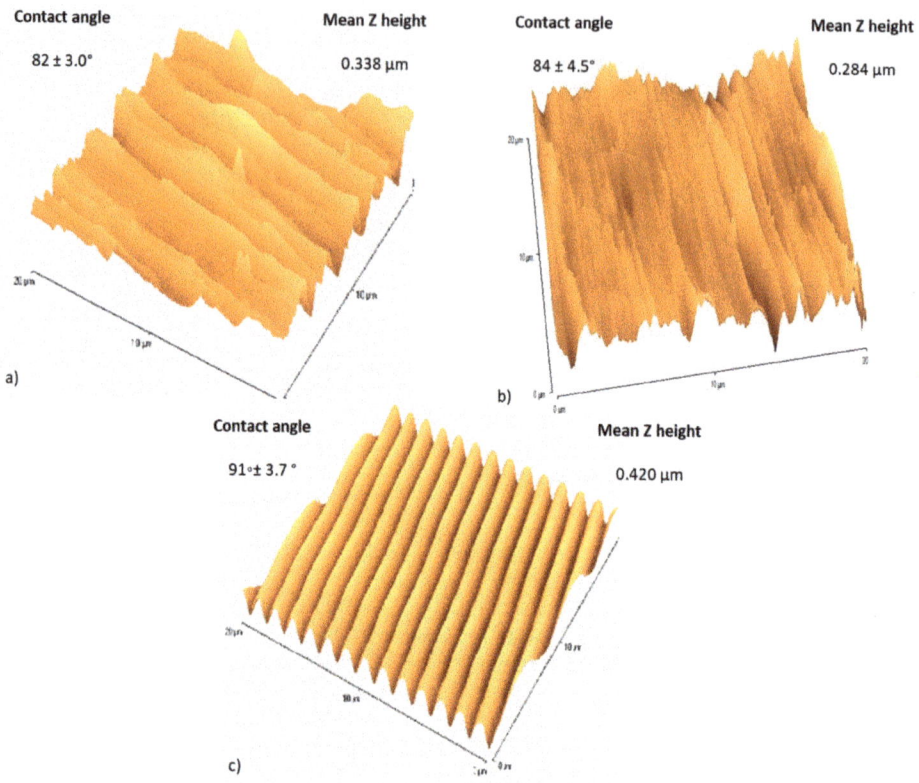

Figure 1. Atomic force microscopy (AFM) demonstrating the (**a**) fine polished stainless steel (FPSS), (**b**) titanium-coated fine polished stainless steel (TiFP), and (**c**) titanium coated regular linear featured surface (RG) (n = 15).

Detection of the meat exudate on the surfaces following the initial application demonstrated no significant differences in the amount of conditioning film retained on the different surfaces (FPSS, 76.2%; TiFP, 76.67% and RG, 83.20%) ($p > 0.05$) (Figure 3). The meat exudate was increasingly removed from the surfaces with increased number of cleans and this was evident for all surface types (Figure 3a,b). Following one and five cleans, there was a significant difference in the amount of meat exudate removed from the surfaces when cleaned along the linear features ($p < 0.0001$) and perpendicular to the linear features ($p > 0.05$). There was no significant difference in the amount of meat exudate retained on the different surfaces after ten cleans along (FPSS 1.4%, TiFP 0.7%, RG 0.9%), or perpendicular to (FPSS 3.6%, TiFP 1.5%, RG, 1.6%) the linear features ($p > 0.05$). However, when cleaned along the linear surface features, the overall trend was that most of the meat exudate was retained on the FPSS > TiFP > RG surface demonstrating the same trend as the removal of cells. When cleaned in the direction perpendicular to the linear features, the amount of meat exudate retained on the surfaces did not follow the same trend (one clean, FPSS > TiFP > RG; five cleans, TiFP > FPSS > RG; ten cleans, FPSS > RG > TiFP).

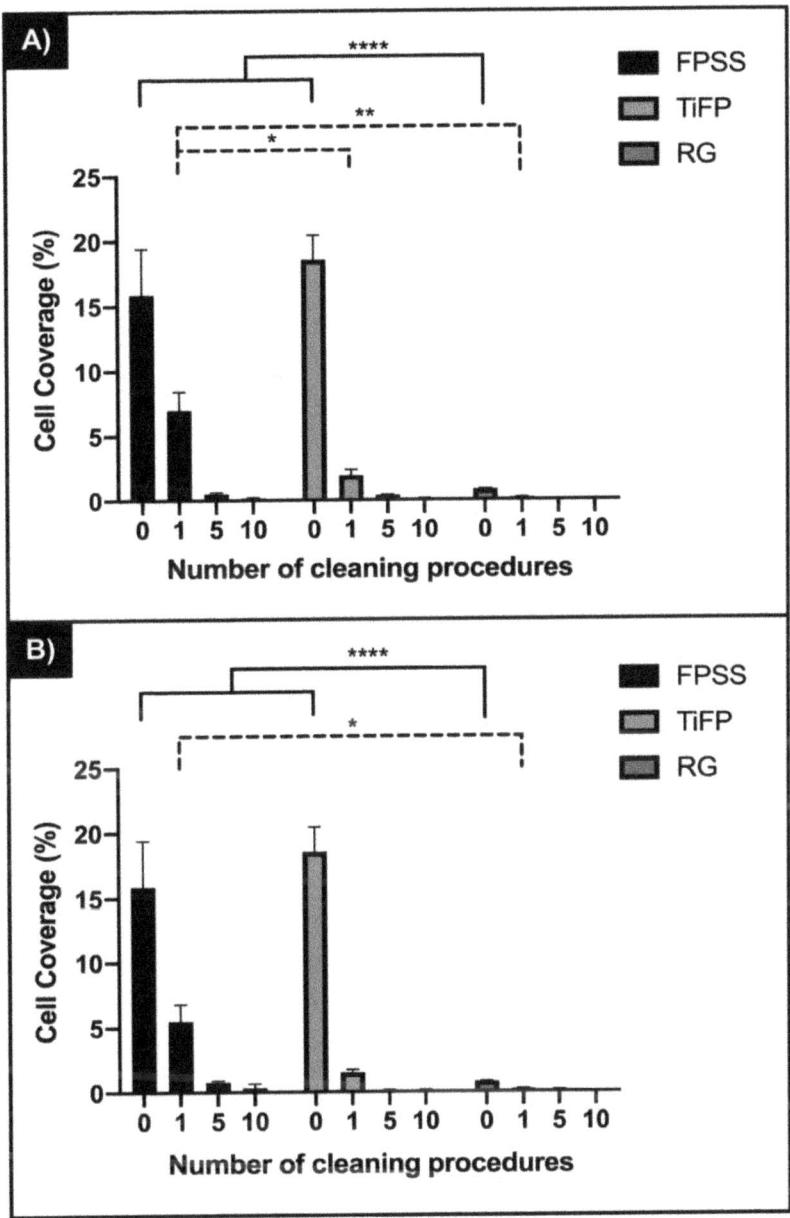

Figure 2. Percentage coverage bacteria retained on fine polished stainless steel (FPSS), titanium polished stainless steel (TiFP) and the regular linear featured titanium coated surface (RG) surface following 0, 1, 5 and 10 cleans (**A**) along the direction and (**B**) perpendicular to the surface features ($n = 45$). Asterisks denote significance, * $p \leq 0.05$, ** $p \leq 0.01$ and **** $p \leq 0.0001$.

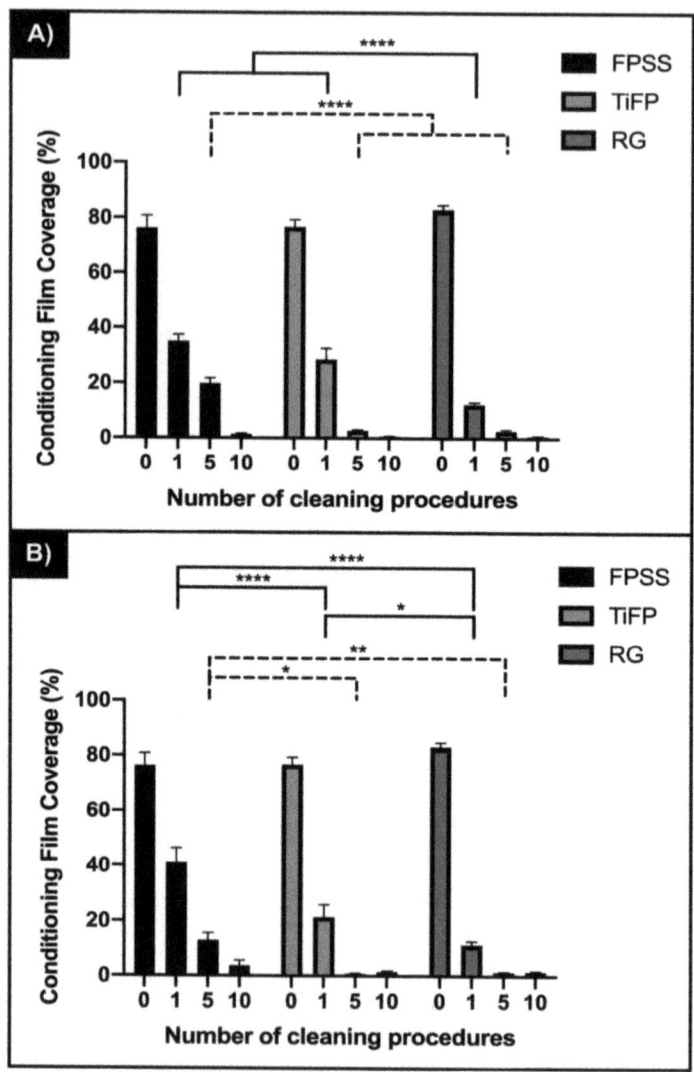

Figure 3. Percentage coverage of meat exudate retained on fine polished stainless steel (FPSS), titanium polished stainless steel (TiFP) and the regular linear featured titanium coated surface (RG) surface following 0, 1, 5 and 10 cleans (**A**) along the direction and (**B**) perpendicular to the surface features (n = 45). Asterisks denote significance, * $p \leq 0.05$, ** $p \leq 0.01$ and **** $p \leq 0.0001$.

The amount of bacteria and meat exudate removed from the surfaces following cleaning along linear features compared to cleaning in a perpendicular direction to the linear features, demonstrated that there was no significant difference ($p > 0.05$) in the removal of cells (with the exception five cleans on the FPTi). However, the meat exudate demonstrated a different trend whereby by ten cleans, the meat exudate was significantly more removed when the surfaces were cleaned in the direction along the surface features ($p < 0.05$). This result may have occurred due to the size of the bacterial cells and organic components of the meat exudate with respect to the size of the surface features (Figure 4).

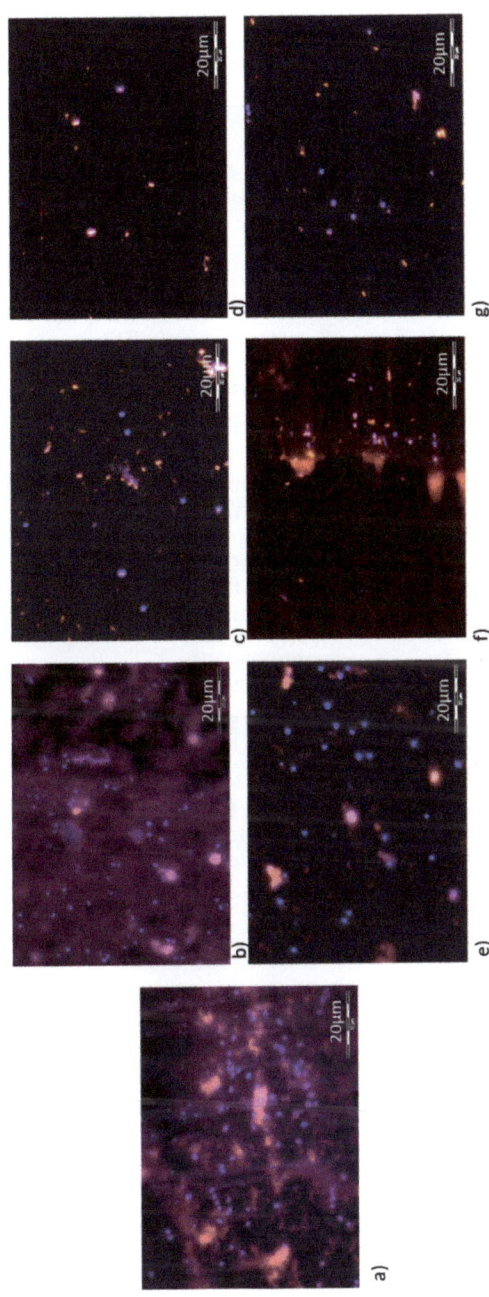

Figure 4. Meat exudate (red) and *E. coli* cells (blue) remaining on titanium coated fine polished stainless steel surface (TiFP) following (**a**) pre-cleaning procedure, (**b**) one wipe clean along, (**c**) five wipe cleans along, (**d**) ten wipe cleans along and (**e**) one wipe clean across, (**f**) five wipe cleans across and (**g**) ten wipe cleans across. Scale bar: 20 µm. Differential staining was conducted to visualise bacterial cells and the meat exudate on the surfaces and an example of the images on the TiFP surfaces is demonstrated (Figure 5). Prior to the cleaning procedure, the meat exudate (red) and bacterial cells (blue) can be observed in abundance (Figure 5a). The concentration of organic material and *E. coli* declined as the number of wipe cleans increased, both in the direction of, and perpendicular to the linear surface features (Figure 5).

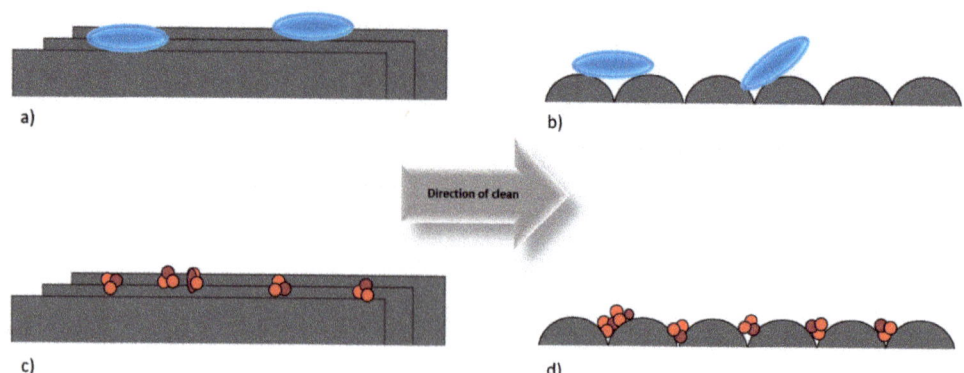

Figure 5. Schematic demonstrating how (a,b) the size of the bacteria (cylindrical) and (c,d) meat exudate (circles) influenced the efficacy of cleaning in the (a,c) direction of cleaning along the linear surface features or (b,d) in a direction perpendicular to the surface features.

A schematic representation of the bacteria retained, and the effect of the surface topography was produced. The bacteria were initially retained in higher amounts on the irregularly polished surfaces (FPSS and TiSS) being entrapped in the irregular surface features (Figure 6a). However, on the surfaces with regular surface features, the bacteria sat on the top, rather than inside the surface features (Figure 6b). This resulted in a lower binding of the bacteria on the surfaces and less bacterial retention.

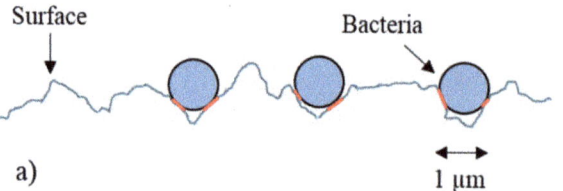

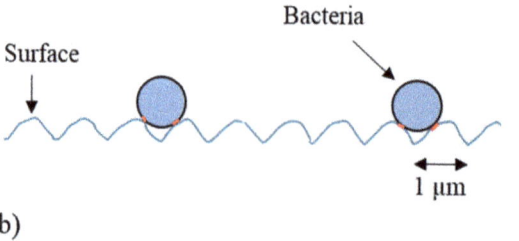

Figure 6. The bacteria retained on the surfaces were bound in the highest amounts on the surfaces with (a) irregular topographies rather than on (b) topographically regular surfaces.

4. Discussion

Product contact surfaces may contaminate meat products directly with microbial or organic material contaminants [23]. The properties of a surface play a pivotal role in bacterial and organic material retention, but nevertheless, the way in which the substrata can mediate such binding remains unclear [28,52,53].

The surfaces with regular surface topographies demonstrated clearly defined features or regular size, shape, depth, and periodicity. However, surfaces with irregular topographies, such at the fine polished stainless steel (FPSS) and the titanium coated fine polished stainless steel (TiFP), contained features of different sizes with irregular frequencies, which dependent on their size may contribute to increased or decreased bacterial binding. In this study, more cells were retained initially on the topographically irregular surfaces, which suggests that these irregular features enhanced the bacterial cell: surface interaction. The amount of bacteria retained on the irregular surface features was higher following the initial inoculation and cleans. In agreement with these findings, micropatterned topography films were utilised to determine the attachment and survival of *Escherichia coli* and *Listeria innocua* and it was demonstrated that initial bacteria attachment to the micro-pattern topography films were significantly lower in the short term [41]. In addition, after incubation with a methicillin-resistant *Staphylococcus pseudintermedius*, it was determined that bacterial biofilms tended to form in crevices [54]. However, such findings were carried out using retention and biofilm assays and were not subject to cleaning or physical forces.

Throughout this study, bacterial retention and meat exudate (e.g., the conditioning film) was quantified via differential staining and epifluorescence microscopy. The samples were prepared by adding DAPI and Rhodamine B directly to the surface and spread across the surface and dried. Although it may be considered that the methodology used in the staining method may affect the distribution of the retained material, previous studies in our laboratories have demonstrated that this is not the case since the material retained is dried onto the surface and is extremely well retained [51]. In addition, all the samples in this study were prepared using the same method; any effect which may be due to the staining process is negligible. In order for epifluorescence microscopy to be utilised effectively, samples must be prepared in a consistent manner, as was the case in this study [55].

Surfaces with features of microbial dimensions similar to those of microbial cells have been shown to promote bacterial binding, whilst the morphology of the bacterial cell can also influence such mechanisms [37,38]. All the surfaces used in this study contained surface topographies with microbial dimensions. The findings in this research demonstrated that surfaces with periodically regular dimensions decreased bacterial retention regardless of the direction of clean and removed the greatest amount of meat exudate following cleaning along the linear surface features. Although features of microbial decisions may readily retain bacteria, when a physical force is applied, it may be that the shape of the topographical feature is of importance, with the periodic regularity of the surface combined with the cell size enabling the bacteria to be easily rolled across the surface. Thus, in the context of cleaning, surface with regular topographies may enhance surface hygiene following cleaning procedures.

In addition to the surface topography, the surface chemistry may affect bacterial retention. The results demonstrated that the bacteria and meat exudate were retained in lower amounts and coverage on the titanium surfaces. In agreement with our findings, Jeyachandran et al. (2007) demonstrated that a titanium oxide film retained fewer bacteria than other materials [56]. Furthermore, Ma et al. (2008) demonstrated that the heterogeneous chemistry of a surface may provide specific contact points for bacterial retention; such points may be found on stainless steel surfaces [43]. Hence, the more homogeneous surface chemistry of the titanium coating may have resulted in a reduced number of chemically different sites, resulting in lowered bacterial and meat exudate retention. Surface wettability can interact with other surface parameters, resulting in preferential or disadvantageous bacterial retention [57,58]. In the current study, the FPSS and the TiFP surfaces were more wettable than the RG surfaces. However, the bacteria and meat extract were deposited directly onto the surfaces and hence the physicochemical effects may have been negated.

The processing of meat products results in high level of organic material remaining on food contact surfaces which conditions the underlying substrata, and it is onto the proteinaceous conditioning film to which the bacteria become retained [9,27]. It has been demonstrated that the attachment of *Pseudomonas fragi* to beef resulted in the bacteria becoming entrapped within the collagen fibres of the raw meat [59]. It has been suggested that contamination of the meat product by bacteria could be transferred to a surface, therefore thorough cleaning of surfaces and meat residues during meat production is critical to reduce the bacterial load [60]. The results from this study demonstrated that all the surfaces retained similar levels of meat extract initially, but following cleaning, the meat exudate was more difficult to remove from the surfaces with the irregular topographies. When the surfaces were cleaned in the direction along the surface features, the meat exudate was also easier to remove from the titanium coated regular surface (RG) than the titanium coated irregular surface (TiFP) or the stainless steel (FPSS). However, a clear trend on the effect of the surface properties, on the amount of meat exudate removal was not demonstrated when the surfaces were cleaned perpendicular to the linear features. Although only small amounts of organic material were retained, the difference in the trends in the effects of the surfaces properties on meat exudate retention may be due to the composition of the meat exudate, which will consist of much smaller molecules than the bacterial cells. It may be that although the bacteria can be removed by the physical force due to their larger size, the smaller organic molecules can only be pushed out of the linear features when cleaned in the direction along the linear features, as this will offer little resistance. In contrast, when the cleaning action is perpendicular to the surface features, the organic material is pushed against the wall of the surface feature where it becomes retained. This may explain the differences observed in the results.

By ten cleans, the surfaces demonstrated similar amounts of bacteria and meat exudate retained on the surfaces. One of the reasons for this is that a key component of the meat exudate is protein [50]. Protein adsorption on surfaces is a major issue in the food industry and the adsorption of proteins onto surfaces is a complex phenomenon influenced by many factors [61,62]. Protein adsorption to a surface occurs due to a range of forces and will continue until a state of equilibrium occurs [63]. It may be that as the number of cleans increased a state of equilibrium of the protein binding that occurred on the surfaces, masking the original surface properties, albeit at levels of concentrations below the detection limits of the analyses used in this study. This would effectively make the surfaces similar in terms of their characteristics.

The fouling of surfaces with proteins derived from organic foulants such as meat exudates can change the properties of a surface. A recent study conducted by Slate et al. (2019) demonstrated that the surface properties of Ti-ZrN/Ag became more hydrophilic with greater anti-adhesive properties following the introduction of a conditioning film [15]. Furthermore, the presence of a conditioning film may alter the properties of the bacterial cells themselves. When *Staphylococcus* spp. was exposed to a 10% solution of bovine serum albumin (BSA), the bacteria were demonstrated to have a reduction in their hydrophobicity and their propensity to donate electrons [64]. A linear correlation between the negative charge on the bacterial cell surface and the initial attachment to beef lean muscle and fat tissue has also been reported [65]. Such differences in the surface and bacterial properties will influence the interactions between the cell:organic material and the interface.

Standard operating procedures, which include regular cleaning, are used in the food industry to eliminate foodborne pathogens and to reduce contamination, yet despite such measures, surface contamination in food processing facilities still occurs [65]. A fundamental understanding of bacterial attachment to meat surfaces should be the basis for the development of procedures for physical removal of microorganisms that contaminate meat surfaces [11]. The determination of the removal of bacteria in the presence of meat exudate is important since although pathogens have been demonstrated to be easily destroyed by commercial sanitizers in water, the presence of organic matter may significantly affect the function of sanitizers [27,66]. A key aspect of this work is the uneven distribution of fouling across the surface. When surfaces are tested in pristine condition, this allows for easily comparative data between laboratories. However, such methodology although comparable, does not reflect a true environmental situation. The uneven distribution of the conditioning film across the surface demonstrates that the surface in a real environment will be subjected to very different material-biological interface interactions than occur when a pristine surface is used in such studies. Hence, the use of such organic material in surface-biological interactions is imperative to understand such systems.

The results from our work demonstrated that repeated cleaning of the surfaces resulted in residual organic fouling. When meat processing plants were sampled for biofilms by placing stainless steel and cast iron chips in or on floor drains and food contact areas, it was found that biofilms were formed on the drain samples but were not formed on chips placed on food contact surfaces [67]. Gibson et al. (1999) found that bacterial attachment to surfaces in the food processing environment readily occurred; however, extensive surface colonization and biofilm formation only occurred on environmental surfaces that were not regularly cleaned [23]. In addition, surfaces that were not cleaned daily, resulted in the occurrence of biofilm formation; the bacteria established in a biofilm could not be eradicated by using one single treatment or one single detergent or disinfectant, and the most effective cleaning methods were shown to require scrubbing of the surfaces [68]. With specific regards to a wipe clean, Lopez et al. (2015) showed that using a disinfectant-wipe intervention to clean a contaminated work area that was used in the preparation of chicken fillets decreased the exposure to *Campylobacter jejuni* by 2 to 3 orders of magnitude [69]. Hence, understanding the physical actions of cleaning systems is an important factor in the maintenance of hygienic systems. The cleaning process throughout the food industry is in debate over the best methods, equipment, monitoring, frequency, benchmarks, and standards to be used [70]. Thus, it is important to understand the effects that surface properties have on the cleaning efficacy of the substrata.

5. Conclusions

This work demonstrated that more bacteria were retained in higher amounts, initially on the stainless steel (FPSS) and titanium coated surfaces with the irregular topographies (TiFP). With subsequent cleaning, the amount of bacteria decreased and was most easily removed from the surfaces that had regular surface features and/or were titanium coated. The direction of cleaning (along or perpendicular to the linear features of the surface) did not have an effect on the amount of bacteria but did affect the amount of meat exudate retained whereby surfaces cleaned along the linear features removed more organic material. After ten cleans, the bacteria and meat exudate retained on the surfaces was not significantly different and suggested that a steady state of the surface properties had been reached. This study highlights the importance of surface properties and cleaning method selection to be utilised within the meat production industry to reduce microbial contamination and surface biofouling.

Author Contributions: J.V. devised the project and the main conceptual ideas presented in this study; J.V., I.D.A. and A.J.S. contributed to the manuscript preparation; K.A.W. drafted the final manuscript; A.E. was involved in data generation and analysis; and P.J.K. led the surface design. All authors have read and agreed to the published version of the manuscript.

Funding: This research received no external funding.

Institutional Review Board Statement: Not applicable.

Informed Consent Statement: Not applicable.

Data Availability Statement: The datasets generated during the current study are available from the corresponding author on reasonable request.

Acknowledgments: The authors would like to thank Brigitte Carpentier for her kind gift of the *E. coli*. This research was part of the project FOOD-CT-2005-007081 (PathogenCombat) supported by the European Commission through the Sixth Framework Programme for Research and Development.

Conflicts of Interest: The authors declare no conflict of interest.

References

1. Lindsay, D.; von Holy, A. What food safety professionals should know about bacterial biofilms. *Br. Food J.* **2006**, *108*, 27–37. [CrossRef]
2. Yuan, L.; Hansen, M.F.; Røder, H.L.; Wang, N.; Burmølle, M.; He, G. Mixed-species biofilms in the food industry: Current knowledge and novel control strategies. *Crit. Rev. Food Sci. Nutr.* **2020**, *60*, 2277–2293. [CrossRef] [PubMed]
3. Whitehead, K.A.; Benson, P.; Verran, J. Developing application and detection methods for *Listeria monocytogenes* and fish extract on open surfaces in order; to optimize cleaning protocols. *Food Bioprod. Process.* **2015**, *93*, 224–233. [CrossRef]
4. Bintsis, T. Foodborne pathogens. *AIMS Microbiol.* **2017**, *3*, 529–563. [CrossRef]
5. Van Houdt, R.; Michiels, C.W. Biofilm formation and the food industry, a focus on the bacterial outer surface. *J. Appl. Microbiol.* **2010**, *109*, 1117–1131. [CrossRef] [PubMed]
6. Chlebicz, A.; Śliżewska, K. Campylobacteriosis, salmonellosis, yersiniosis, and listeriosis as zoonotic foodborne diseases: A review. *Int. J. Environ. Res. Public Health* **2018**, *15*, 863. [CrossRef] [PubMed]
7. Food Standard Agency. *Foodborne Disease Strategy 2010–2015: An FSA Programme for the Reduction of Foodborne Disease in the UK*; Food Standard Agency: London, UK, 2011.
8. Yemmireddy, V.K.; Hung, Y.C. Using photocatalyst metal oxides as antimicrobial surface coatings to ensure food safety—Opportunities and challenges. *Compr. Rev. Food Sci. Food Saf.* **2017**, *16*, 617–631. [CrossRef]
9. Genigeorgis, C. Biofilms: Their Significance to Cleaning in the Meat Sector. In *New Challenges in Meat Hygiene: Specific Problems in Cleaning and Disinfection*; Bart, S.A., Bauer, F., Eds.; ECCEAMST: Utrecht, The Netherlands, 1995; pp. 29–49.
10. CDC. *Multistate Out Break of Shiga Toxin-Producing Escherichia coli O157:H7 Infections Linked to Ground Beef*; CDC: Atlanta, GA, USA, 2014.
11. Pordesimo, L.O.; Wilkerson, G.; Womac, R.; Cutter, N. Process Engineering Variables in the Spray Washing of Meat. *J. Food Prot.* **2002**, *65*, 222–237. [CrossRef]
12. Gristina, A.G. Biomaterial-centered infection: Microbial adhesion versus tissue integration. *Science* **1987**, *237*, 1588–1595. [CrossRef]
13. Bos, R.; Van der Mei, H.C.; Busscher, H.J. Physico-chemistry of initial microbial adhesive interactions—its mechanisms and methods for study. *FEMS Microbiol. Rev.* **1999**, *23*, 179–230. [CrossRef]
14. Hori, K.; Matsumoto, S. Bacterial adhesion: From mechanism to control. *Biochem. Eng. J.* **2010**, *48*, 424–434. [CrossRef]
15. Slate, A.J.; Wickens, D.; Wilson-Nieuwenhuis, J.; Dempsey-Hibbert, N.; West, G.; Kelly, P.; Verran, J.; Banks, C.E.; Whitehead, K.A. The effects of blood conditioning films on the antimicrobial and retention properties of zirconium-nitride silver surfaces. *Colloids Surf. B* **2019**, *173*, 303–311. [CrossRef] [PubMed]
16. Lorite, G.S.; Rodrigues, C.M.; De Souza, A.A.; Kranz, C.; Mizaikoff, B.; Cotta, M.A. The role of conditioning film formation and surface chemical changes on *Xylella fastidiosa* adhesion and biofilm evolution. *J. Colloid Interface Sci.* **2011**, *359*, 289–295. [CrossRef] [PubMed]
17. Kokare, C.; Chakraborty, S.; Khopade, A.; Mahadik, K.R. Biofilm: Importance and Applications. *Indian J. Biotechnol.* **2009**, *8*, 159–168.
18. Moreira, J.; Gomes, L.; Whitehead, K.; Lynch, S.; Tetlow, L.; Mergulhão, F. Effect of surface conditioning with cellular extracts on *Escherichia coli* adhesion and initial biofilm formation. *Food Bioprod. Process.* **2017**, *104*, 1–12. [CrossRef]
19. Guyard-Nicodème, M.; Tresse, O.; Houard, E.; Jugiau, F.; Courtillon, C.; El Manaa, K.; Laisney, M.J.; Chemaly, M. Characterization of *Campylobacter* spp. transferred from naturally contaminated chicken legs to cooked chicken slices via a cutting board. *Int. J. Food Microbiol.* **2013**, *164*, 7–14. [CrossRef] [PubMed]
20. Birk, T.; Ingmer, H.; Andersen, M.T.; Jørgensen, K.; Brøndsted, L. Chicken juice a food-based model system suitable to study survival of *Campylobacter jejuni*. *Lett. Appl. Microbiol.* **2004**, *38*, 66–71. [CrossRef]
21. Brown, H.L.; Reuter, M.; Salt, L.J.; Cross, K.L.; Betts, R.P.; van Vliet, A.H.M. Chicken juice enhances surface attachment and biofilm formation of *Campylobacter Jejuni*. *Appl. Environ. Microbiol.* **2014**, *80*, 7053–7060. [CrossRef]
22. Otto, C.; Zahn, S.; Rost, F.; Zahn, P.; Jaros, D.; Rohm, H. Physical Methods for Cleaning and Disinfection of Surfaces. *Food Eng. Rev.* **2011**, *3*, 171–188. [CrossRef]
23. Gibson, H.; Taylor, J.H.; Hall, K.E.; Holah, J.T. Effectiveness of cleaning techniques used in the food industry in terms of the removal of bacterial biofilms. *J. Appl. Microbiol.* **1999**, *87*, 41–48. [CrossRef]
24. Yang, X.; Wang, H.; He, A.; Tran, F. Microbial efficacy and impact on the population of *Escherichia coli* of a routine sanitation process for the fabrication facility of a beef packing. *Plant Food Control* **2017**, *71*, 353–357. [CrossRef]
25. Yang, X.; Badoni, M.; Youssef, M.K.; Gill, C.O. Enhanced control of microbiological contamination of product at a large beef packing plant. *J. Food Prot.* **2012**, *75*, 144–149. [CrossRef] [PubMed]
26. Youssef, M.K.; Badoni, M.; Yang, X.; Gill, C.O. Sources of *Escherichia coli* deposited on beef during breaking of carcasses carrying few *E. coli* at two packing plants. *Food Control* **2013**, *31*, 166–171. [CrossRef]
27. Genigeorgis, C.; Rosales, J.; Verder-Elepano, M. Affect of selected sanitizer cleaners and soaps on *Listeria* spp., *S. typhimurium*, *E. coli*, and *P. aeruginosa* in the presence or absence of organic matter. In Proceedings of the International Conference Listeria and Food Safety—ASEPT, Laval, France, 13–14 June 1991; p. 186.
28. Whitehead, K.A.; Verran, J. The effect of surface topography on the retention of microorganisms. *Food Bioprod. Process.* **2006**, *84*, 253–259. [CrossRef]
29. Jullien, C.; Bénézech, T.; Carpentier, B.; Lebret, V.; Faille, C. Identification of surface characteristics relevant to the hygienic status of stainless steel for the food industry. *J. Food Eng.* **2003**, *56*, 77–87. [CrossRef]

30. Mettler, E.; Carpentier, B. Hygienic quality of floors in relation to surface texture. *Food Bioprod. Process.* **1999**, *77*, 90–96. [CrossRef]
31. Whitehead, K.A.; Verran, J. The effect of application method on the retention of *Pseudomonas aeruginosa* on stainless steel, and titanium coated stainless steel of differing topographies. *Inter. Biodeter. Biodeg.* **2007**, *60*, 74–80. [CrossRef]
32. Whitehead, K.; Benson, P.; Smith, L.; Verran, J. The use of physicochemical methods to detect organic food soils on stainless steel surfaces. *Biofouling* **2009**, *25*, 749–756. [CrossRef]
33. Jullien, C.; Benezech, T.; Le Gentil, C.; Boulange-Petermann, L.; Dubois, P.; Tissier, J.P.; Traisnel, M.; Faille, C. Physico-chemical and hygienic property modifications of stainless steel surfaces induced by conditioning with food and detergent. *Biofouling* **2008**, *24*, 163–172. [CrossRef]
34. Tuson, H.H.; Weibel, D.B. Bacteria-surface interactions. *Soft Matter.* **2013**, *9*, 4368–4380. [CrossRef]
35. Song, F.; Koo, H.; Ren, D. Effects of material properties on bacterial adhesion and biofilm formation. *J. Dent. Res.* **2015**, *94*, 1027–1034. [CrossRef]
36. Wu, S.; Zhang, B.; Liu, Y.; Suo, X.; Li, H. Influence of surface topography on bacterial adhesion: A review. *Biointerphases* **2018**, *13*, 060801. [CrossRef]
37. Whitehead, K.A.; Colligon, J.; Verran, J. Retention of microbial cells in substratum surface features of micrometer and sub-micrometer dimensions. *Colloids Surf. B* **2005**, *41*, 129–138. [CrossRef]
38. Hsu, L.C.; Fang, J.; Borca-Tasciuc, D.A.; Worobo, R.W.; Moraru, C.I. Effect of micro- and nanoscale topography on the adhesion of bacterial cells to solid surfaces. *Appl. Environ. Microbiol.* **2013**, *79*, 2703–2712. [CrossRef] [PubMed]
39. Verran, J. Testing surface cleanability in food processing. In *Handbook of Hygiene Control in the Food Industry*; Lelieveld, A.H.L.M., Holah Mostert, J.T., Eds.; CRC Press: New York, NY, USA, 2005; pp. 556–571.
40. Cheng, Y.; Feng, G.; Moraru, C.I. Micro and Nanotopography Sensitive Bacterial Attachment Mechanisms: A Review. *Front. Microbiol.* **2019**, *10*, 191. [CrossRef] [PubMed]
41. Lee, J.; Pascal, M.A. Effect of micro-pattern topography on the attachment and survival of foodborne microorganisms on food contact surfaces. *Food Saf.* **2018**, *38*, e12379. [CrossRef]
42. Kamerud, K.L.; Hobbie, K.A.; Anderson, K.A. Stainless steel leaches nickel and chromium into foods during cooking. *J. Agric. Food Chem.* **2013**, *61*, 9495–9501. [CrossRef]
43. Ma, H.; Winslow, C.J.; Logan, B.E. Spectral force analysis using atomic force microscopy reveals the importance of surface heterogeneity in bacterial; and colloid adhesion to engineered surfaces. *Colloids Surf. B* **2008**, *62*, 232–237. [CrossRef]
44. Ribeiro, C.F.; Cogo-Müller, K.; Franco, G.C.; Silva-Concílio, L.R.; Campos, M.S.; de Mello Rode, S.; Neves, A.C.C. Initial oral biofilm formation on titan;ium implants with different surface treatments: An in vivo study. *Arch. Oral. Biol.* **2016**, *69*, 33–39. [CrossRef] [PubMed]
45. Akhidime, I.D.; Saubade, F.; Benson, P.S.; Butler, J.A.; Olivier, S.; Kelly, P.; Verran, J.; Whitehead, K.A. The antimicrobial effect of metal substrates on food pathogens. *Food Bioprod. Process.* **2019**, *113*, 68–76. [CrossRef]
46. Lausmaa, J. Surface spectroscopic characterization of titanium implant materials. *J. Electron. Spectros. Relat. Phenom.* **1996**, *81*, 343–361. [CrossRef]
47. Verran, J.; Packer, A.; Kelly, P.; Whitehead, K.A. The retention of bacteria on hygienic surfaces presenting scratches of microbial dimensions. *Lett. Appl. Microbiol.* **2010**, *50*, 258–263. [CrossRef] [PubMed]
48. Whitehead, K.A.; Olivier, S.; Benson, P.S.; Arneborg, N.; Verran, J.; Kelly, P. The effect of surface properties of polycrystalline, single phase metal coatin;gs on bacterial retention. *Int. J. Food Microbiol.* **2015**, *197*, 92–97. [CrossRef] [PubMed]
49. Caballero, L.; Whitehead, K.; Allen, N.; Verran, J. Inactivation of *Escherichia coli* on immobilized TiO_2 using fluorescent light. *J. Photochem. Photobiol. A* **2009**, *202*, 92–98. [CrossRef]
50. Whitehead, K.; Benson, P.; Verran, J. The detection of food soils on stainless steel using energy dispersive X-ray and Fourier transform infrared spectroscopy. *Biofouling* **2011**, *27*, 907–917. [CrossRef]
51. Whitehead, K.A.; Benson, P.; Verran, J. Differential fluorescent staining of *Listeria monocytogenes* and a whey food soil for quantitative analysis of surfac;e hygiene. *Int. J. Food Microbiol.* **2009**, *135*, 75–80. [CrossRef]
52. Boyd, R.D.; Verran, J.; Jones, M.; Bhakoo, M. Use of the atomic force microscope to determine the effect of substratum surface topography on bacterial adhesion. *Langmuir* **2002**, *18*, 2343–2346. [CrossRef]
53. Slate, A.J.; Wickens, D.J.; El Mohtadi, M.; Dempsey-Hibbert, N.; West, G.; Banks, C.E.; Whitehead, K.A. Antimicrobial activity of Ti-ZrN/Ag coatings for use in biomaterial applications. *Sci. Rep.* **2018**, *8*, 1497. [CrossRef]
54. McGaffey, M.; zur Linden, A.; Bachynski, N.; Oblak, M.; James, F.; Weese, J.S. Manual polishing of 3D printed metals produced by laser powder bed fusion reduces biofilm formation. *PLoS ONE* **2019**, *14*, e0212995. [CrossRef]
55. Wilson, C.; Lukowicz, R.; Merchant, S.; Valquier-Flynn, H.; Caballero, J.; Sandoval, J.; Okuom, M.; Huber, C.; Brooks, T.D.; Wilson, E.; et al. Quantitative and qualitative assessment methods for biofilm growth: A mini-review. *Res. Rev. J. Eng. Technol.* **2017**, *6*, 30214915.
56. Jeyachandran, Y.; Venkatachalam, S.; Karunagaran, B.; Narayandass, S.K.; Mangalaraj, D.; Bao, C.; Zhang, C. Bacterial adhesion studies on titanium, titanium nitride and modified hydroxyapatite thin films. *Mater. Sci. Eng. C* **2007**, *27*, 35–41. [CrossRef]
57. Spriano, S.; Chandra, V.S.; Cochis, A.; Uberti, F.; Rimondini, L.; Bertone, E.; Vitale, A.; Scolaro, C.; Ferrari, M.; Cirisano, F. How do wettability, zeta potential and hydroxylation degree affect the biological response of biomaterials? *Mater. Sci. Eng. C* **2017**, *74*, 542–555. [CrossRef]

58. Wassmann, T.; Kreis, S.; Behr, M.; Buergers, R. The influence of surface texture and wettability on initial bacterial adhesion on titanium and zirconium oxide dental implants. *Int. J. Implant. Dent.* **2017**, *3*, 1–11. [CrossRef]
59. Scwach, T.S.; Zottola, E.A. Scanning electron microscopic study on some effects of sodium hypochloride on attachment of bacteria to stainless steel. *J. Food. Prot.* **1984**, *47*, 656–759.
60. Li, J.; Feng, J.; Ma, L.; de la Fuente Núñez, C.; Gölz, G.; Lu, X. Effects of meat juice on biofilm formation of Campylobacter and Salmonella. *Int. J. Food Microbiol.* **2017**, *253*, 20–28. [CrossRef] [PubMed]
61. Nakanishi, K.; Sakiyama, T.; Imamura, K. On the adsorption of proteins on solid surfaces, a common but very complicated phenomenon. *J. Biosci. Bioeng.* **2001**, *91*, 233–244. [CrossRef]
62. Rechendorff, K.; Hovgaard, M.B.; Foss, M.; Zhdanov, V.; Besenbacher, F. Enhancement of protein adsorption induced by surface roughness. *Langmuir* **2006**, *22*, 10885–10888. [CrossRef] [PubMed]
63. Thyparambil, A.A.; Wei, Y.; Latour, R.A. Experimental characterization of adsorbed protein orientation, conformation, and bioactivity. *Biointerphases* **2015**, *10*, 019002. [CrossRef] [PubMed]
64. Saubade, F.J.; Hughes, S.; Wickens, D.J.; Wilson-Nieuwenhuis, J.; Dempsey-Hibbert, N.; Crowther, G.S.; West, G.; Kelly, P.; Banks, C.E.; Whitehead, K.A. Effectiveness of titanium nitride silver coatings against Staphylococcus spp. in the presence of BSA and whole blood conditioning agents. *Int. Biodeterior. Biodegrad.* **2019**, *141*, 44–51. [CrossRef]
65. Dickson, J.S.; Koohmaraie, M. Cell surface charge characteristics and their relationship to bacterial attachment to meat surfaces. *Appl. Environ. Microbiol.* **1989**, *55*, 832–836. [CrossRef]
66. van de Weyer, A.; Devleeschouwer, M.J.; Dony, J. Bactericidal activity of disinfectants on Listeria. *J. Appl. Bacteriol.* **1993**, *74*, 480–483. [CrossRef]
67. Spurlock, A.T.; Zottola, E.A. Growth and attachment of *Listeria monocytogenes* to cast iron. *J. Food Prot.* **1991**, *54*, 925–929. [CrossRef] [PubMed]
68. Jessen, B.; Lammert, L. Biofilm and disinfection in meat processing plants. *Int. Biodeter. Biodeg.* **2003**, *51*, 265–269. [CrossRef]
69. Lopez, G.U.; Kitajima, M.; Sherchan, S.P.; Sexton, J.D.; Sifuentes, L.Y.; Gerba, C.P.; Reynolds, K.A. Impact of disinfectant wipes on the risk of *Campylobacter jejuni* infection during raw chicken preparation in domestic kitchens. *J. Appl. Microbiol.* **2015**, *119*, 245–252. [CrossRef] [PubMed]
70. Bloomfield, S.F.; Carling, P.C.; Exner, M. A unified framework for developing effective hygiene procedures for hands, environmental surfaces and laundry in healthcare, domestic, food handling and other settings. *GMS Hyg. Infect. Control* **2017**, *12*, 1–16. [CrossRef]

Article

Toxic Metals in Cereals in Cape Verde: Risk Assessment Evaluation

Carmen Rubio-Armendáriz [1,*], Soraya Paz [1], Ángel J. Gutiérrez [1], Verena Gomes Furtado [2], Dailos González-Weller [1,3], Consuelo Revert [4] and Arturo Hardisson [1]

1. Department of Toxicology, Universidad de La Laguna, 38071 La Laguna (Canary Islands), Spain; spazmont@ull.edu.es (S.P.); ajguti@ull.edu.es (Á.J.G.); dgonwel@gmail.com (D.G.-W.); atorre@ull.edu.es (A.H.)
2. Entidade Regulatora Independiente da Saúde, Avenida Cidade de Lisboa, 296-A Praia, Cape Verde; Verena.Furtado@eris.cv
3. Health Inspection and Laboratory Service, Servicio Canario de Salud, 38004 S/C de Tenerife (Canary Islands), Spain
4. Departament of Physical Medicine and Pharmacology, Universidad de La Laguna, 38071 La Laguna (Canary Islands), Spain; mgirones@ull.edu.es
* Correspondence: crubio@ull.es; Tel.: +34-615422540

Abstract: Consumption of cereals and cereal-based products represents 47% of the total food energy intake in Cape Verde. However, cereals also contribute to dietary exposure to metals that may pose a risk. Strengthening food security and providing nutritional information is a high-priority challenge for the Cape Verde government. In this study, toxic metal content (Cr, Ni, Sr, Al, Cd, and Pb) is determined in 126 samples of cereals and derivatives (rice, corn, wheat, corn flour, wheat flour, corn gofio) consumed in Cape Verde. Wheat flour samples stand out, with the highest Sr (1.60 mg/kg), Ni (0.25 mg/kg) and Cr (0.13 mg/kg) levels. While the consumption of 100 g/day of wheat would contribute to 13.2% of the tolerable daily intake (TDI) of Ni, a consumption of 100 g/day of wheat flour would contribute to 8.18% of the tolerable weekly intake (TWI) of Cd. Results show relevant Al levels (1.17–13.4 mg/kg), with the highest level observed in corn gofio. The mean Pb average content in cereals is 0.03–0.08 mg/kg, with the highest level observed in corn gofio. Al and Pb levels are lower in cereals without husks. Without being a health risk, the consumption of 100 g/day of wheat contributes to 17.5% of the European benchmark doses lower confidence limit (BMDL) of Pb for nephrotoxic effects; the consumption of 100 g/day of corn gofio provides an intake of 1.34 mg Al/day (13.7% of the TWI) and 8 μg Pb/day (20% of the BMDL for nephrotoxic effects). A strategy to minimize the dietary exposure of the Cape Verdean population to toxic metals from cereals should consider the continuous monitoring of imported cereals on arrival in Cape Verde, the assessment of the population's total diet exposure to toxic metals and educational campaigns.

Keywords: Cape Verde; cereals; metals; dietary intake; risk assessment

1. Introduction

The Macaronesian region consists of a collection of four volcanic archipelagos in the North Atlantic Ocean (Cape Verde, Azores and Madeira in Portugal and the Canaries in Spain). The four archipelagos share features such as a volcanic origin, a contrasting landscape, a gentle climate and a particularly rich biodiversity. The archipelago of Cape Verde is located on the West African coast, 500 km from Senegal, and comprises ten islands, nine of which are inhabited and one of which is uninhabited. The population of the island of Santiago is approximately 260,000 inhabitants, while that of São Vicente is 76,000. The Cape Verdean diet is characterized by the consumption of significant amounts of cereals and cereal-based products. According to the preliminary results of the 2015 Ínquérito Ás Despesase e Receitas Familiares (IDRF), the ingestion of cereals occupies the highest annual per capita consumption expenditure (about 11,611$) compared to other food products consumed. However, internal cereal production satisfies only 6.9% of the population's consumption needs, contributing to the highly vulnerable state of the country regarding food security. Food security in Cape Verde is also affected by agroclimatic variations and external market fluctuations. National cereal production in 2019 was estimated at about 1000 tons, almost 70% below the mean average of the previous five years [1]. Therefore, about 85% of the domestic cereal demand (mostly rice and wheat for human consumption) was covered by imports. The cereal import requirements in the 2019/2020 marketing year (November to October) were forecasted at an above-average level of 87,000 tons [1]. From 2016 to 2020, the cereal imports reached a total of 419,749.30 tons, with an emphasis on corn (159,979.30 tons), rice (144,799.33 tons) and wheat grain (91,623.39 tons). The market supply of cereals stems both from food aid through cooperative relations with development partners and through commercial imports [2]. Current domestic corn production does not meet the internal demand, and so the cereal must be imported for food and fodder [3]. Moreover, the main drivers of food insecurity in Cape Verde are the effects of dry weather events (such as drought) and pest attacks on cereal and fodder production [1]. As mentioned above, food insecurity in Cape Verde has a structural and multifactorial nature: It demonstrates a structural deficit in national food production, strong dependence on the international market and economic accessibility weaknesses. Strengthening the Food Security and Nutrition Information System (FSNIS) is an important challenge for the Cape Verde government [4].

According to the Food and Agriculture Organization (FAO), in 2017, about 13% of the population was undernourished. The data available indicate that 20% of rural families lived in a situation of food insecurity, with 13% in a moderate position and 7% in a severe position [2]. Cape Verde is in a nutritional transition period characterized both by the high consumption of fat, refined carbohydrates, cholesterol and sugar, and by the low consumption of fruit and vegetables, causing a rapid and significant increase in the prevalence of being overweight and obese [5]. However, the consumption of cereals and cereal-based products is still relevant, representing 47% of the total food energy intake. In Cape Verde, the cereal balance for 2002/2003 estimated a cereal consumption of 242 kg/year per person, comprising 123 kg of corn (337 g/day), 67 kg of rice (184 g/day) and 52 kg of wheat (142 g/day).

Although the nutritional value of cereals is noteworthy, cereals may also contain elements that are harmful to health [6,7], as is the case with elements such as Al, Cd, Cr, Ni, Pb and Sr. Each of these elements has standards of tolerable daily/weekly intake (TDI/TWI) and/or benchmark dose (lower confidence limit) (BMDL) levels set by reference bodies in food safety, such as the European Food Safety Authority (EFSA) and the World Health Organization (WHO) (Table 1).

Table 1. Reference intakes of the analyzed elements.

Element	Parameter	Guideline Value	References
Cr (III)		0.3 mg/kg bw/day	[8]
Ni	TDI	13 µg/kg bw/day	[9]
Sr		0.13 mg/kg bw/day	[10]
Al	TWI	1 mg/kg bw/week	[11]
Cd		2.5 µg/kg bw/week	[12]
Pb	BMDL	0.63 [1] µg/kg bw/day 1.50 [2] µg/kg bw/day	[13]

TDI, tolerable daily intake; TWI, tolerable weekly intake; BMDL, benchmark dose level; bw, body weight; Nephrotoxicity [1] and Cardiovascular effects [2].

Al is a neurotoxic metal with no function in the human body [14]. Prolonged exposure to Al is related to neurodegenerative diseases such as Alzheimer's, and the estimation of its dietary exposure is the subject of previous studies [15–17]. In 2008, the EFSA estimated the dietary intake of Al in the European population to be 0.2–1.5 mg/kg of body weight per week for an adult weighing 60 kg, and concluded that cereals and cereal derivatives are among the main foods that contribute to Al dietary intake [18]. In 2010, González-Weller estimated the total intake of Al in the Canary Islands to be 10.171 mg/day [15].

Cd is a toxic element with a long half-life and a tendency to bioaccumulate [19]. Its presence in cultivation soils favors its transfer to and accumulation in cereals [20]. Known to compete in the body with other essential divalent cations, it affects the renal system, causing irreversible damage to the renal tubules [21,22]. In 2006, Rubio et al. [23] assessed dietary exposure to Cd in the Macaronesian archipelago of the Canary Islands, estimating the intake of Cd from cereals at 1.065 µg/day, and identifying cereals as one of the food categories contributing the most to the dietary intake of Cd. In 2012, the EFSA also identified cereals as one of the food categories that contributes most to the dietary intake of Cd in the European population [24].

Cr is mainly found in the trivalent ion form in food. Although oral Cr (III) is not particularly toxic [25], high intakes of Cr can trigger chronic kidney failure, dermatitis, bronchitis and asthma [26,27]. While cereals were found to contribute most to the dietary intake of Cr (0.087 mg/day) in the Canary Islands archipelago [28] compared to other food categories, a study by Filippini et al. [29] concluded that beverages, cereals and meat provided the highest dietary contributions of Cr in a northern Italian population.

Ni is essential for plants [30], and grains and grain-based products are considered the most important contributors to Ni exposure in the European diet, even though Ni is only regulated in drinking water and not in other food groups [9]. Individuals with hypersensitivity to Ni or with kidney disease are susceptible to damage from a high dietary intake of Ni [26].

Sr is an element that is found in food; however, there are no reported cases of food poisoning from Sr to date. Nevertheless, Sr competes with essential elements such as phosphorus [31], and recent studies in experimental animals reported hepatotoxic effects associated with Sr [32]. The total intake of Sr in the Canary Islands archipelago was estimated at 1.923 mg/day, and cereal intake was estimated at 1.276 ± 0.711 mg/kg w.w. [28].

Pb is a neurotoxic metal that accumulates in the body, causing serious damage to the central nervous system (CNS) as well as contributing to kidney disease, gastrointestinal tract disorders and Alzheimer's [13]. Pb traces can be found in large quantities in food and drinking water [33,34], especially in fruits, vegetables and cereals due to the deposit of Pb particles from the atmosphere. Bread and rolls (8.5%), tea (6.2%) and tap water (6.1%) are among the food categories found to contribute to high Pb exposure in Europe [35]. While Pb intake of the Canarian population was estimated at 72.8 µg/day in 2005 [33], in 2012, mean lifetime dietary exposure in the European population was estimated at 0.68 µg/kg b.w. per day based on middle bound mean lead occurrence [35].

Food risk surveillance and food safety strategies encourage the monitoring of metal in each of the food groups consumed by different populations. The aims of the present study are to determine the levels of Al, Cd, Cr, Ni, Pb or Sr in commonly consumed cereals and cereal-based products in the Cape Verde islands, and to assess their subsequent risk.

2. Material and Methods

2.1. Samples

A total of 126 samples of cereals (rice, corn and wheat) and cereal-based products (corn flour, wheat flour and corn gofio) (Table 2) that are marketed and consumed in Cape Verde were acquired from two different islands of the Cape Verde archipelago, specifically, Santiago and São Vicente (Figure 1). Gofio is a traditional artisan food derived from cereals, mainly corn, that is made by first roasting the cereal in its husk and then grinding it until a powder similar to flour is obtained [36–38].

Table 2. Analyzed cereal and derived product samples.

Type	No. Samples	Sampling Location	Origin
Rice	56	Santiago	Brazil, Vietnam, Thailand, Japan, USA (California),
	5	São Vicente	Cape Verde (Mindelo), Pakistan
Corn gofio	6	Santiago	
	1	São Vicente	Unknown
Corn flour	10	Santiago	
	1	São Vicente	Portugal, The Netherlands
Wheat flour	17	Santiago	
	2	São Vicente	Portugal, France
Corn	13	Santiago	
	2	São Vicente	Argentina, France, Russia, South America
Wheat	2	Santiago	
	11	São Vicente	Russia, France, Cape Verde (Mindelo), Spain

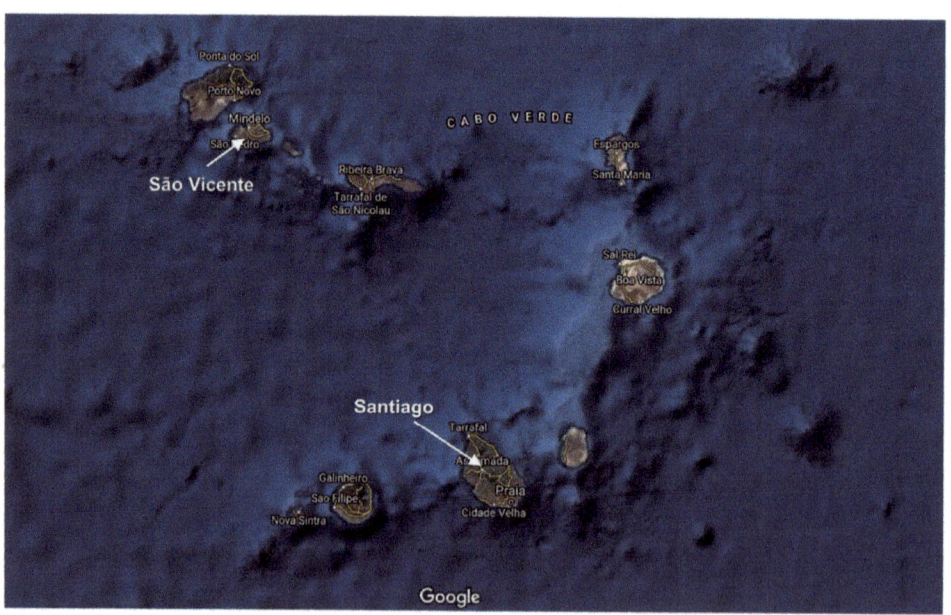

Figure 1. Map of the Cape Verde islands showing the sampling areas (São Vicente and Santiago) (Source: Google Maps).

Sampling took place from 2017 to 2019 at establishments that import and sell cereal on the Santiago and São Vicente islands. Because most of the samples were not commercialized in packages, but instead, were mainly sold by weight in local markets, it was not possible to obtain the origin of each individual sample. Nevertheless, according to Entidade Regulatora Independiente da Saúde (ERIS) from Cape Verde, the origins of the cereal samples distributed in Cape Verde are diverse (Table 2).

2.2. Sample Treatment

One gram of each sample was added to pressure vessels (HVT50, Anton Paar, Graz, Austria) previously washed with laboratory detergent and Milli-Q quality distilled water. Then, 4 mL 65% nitric acid (Sigma Aldrich, Darmstadt, Germany) and 2 mL hydrogen peroxide (Sigma Aldrich, Darmstadt, Germany) were added to the samples. The pressure vessels were closed and placed in a microwave oven (Multiwave Go Plus, Anton Paar, Graz, Austria) for subsequent digestion according to the conditions described in Table 3. After the samples were digested, they were transferred to 10 mL volumetric flasks and made up with Milli-Q quality distilled water. Finally, they were transferred to airtight jars with a lid for later measurement.

Table 3. Microwave digestion process instrumental conditions.

No.	Ramp (min)	Temperature (°C)	Time (min)
1	15	50	5
2	5	60	4
3	5	70	3
4	3	90	2
5	20	180	10

Microwave processing power: 850 W; Limit temperature: 200 °C; Cooling temperature: 50 °C.

2.3. Analytical Method

The determination of metal content was conducted by Inductively Coupled Plasma Atomic Emission Spectrometry (ICP-OES) model ICAP 6300 Duo Thermo Scientific (Waltham, MA, USA), with an Auto Sampler automatic sampler (CETAX model ASX-520).

The instrumental conditions of the method comprised the following: RF power of 1150 W; gas flow (nebulizer gas flow, make up gas flow) of 0.5 L/min; injection of the sample to the 50-rpm flow pump; stabilization time of zero s [39,40]. Instrumental wavelengths (nm) of the analyzed elements were Al (167.0), Cd (226.5), Cr (267.7), Ni (231.6), Pb (220.3) and Sr (407.7).

The quantification limits of the toxic metals, calculated as ten times the standard deviation (SD) resulting from the analysis of 15 targets under reproducibility conditions [41], were: 0.012 mg/L (Al), 0.001 mg/L (Cd), 0.008 mg/L (Co), 0.003 mg/L (Ni), 0.001 mg/L (Pb) and 0.003 mg/L (Sr).

The quality control of the method (Table 4) was based on the recovery percentage obtained with reference material (SRM 1515 Apple Leaves, SRM 1548a Typical Diet, SRM 1567a Wheat Flour) under reproducible conditions. The recovery percentages obtained with the reference material were above 94% in all cases. The statistical analysis did not detect significant differences ($p < 0.05$) between the certified concentrations and the concentrations obtained.

Table 4. Recovery study results and reference materials used.

Metal	Material	Concentration Found (mg/kg)	Certified Concentration (mg/kg)	R (%)
Al	SRM 1515 Apple Leaves	286 ± 9	285.1 ± 26	99.7
Sr		25.0 ± 2.0	24.6 ± 4.0	98.3
Cr		0.29 ± 0.03	0.30 ± 0.00	97.8
Ni	SRM 1548a Typical Diet	0.37 ± 0.02	0.38 ± 0.04	102.3
Pb		0.044 ± 0.000	0.044 ± 0.013	98.9
Cd	SRM 1567a Wheat Flour	0.026 ± 0.002	0.026 ± 0.008	98.4

2.4. Statistical Analysis

The IBM Statistics SPSS 24.0 computer software for Windows was used for statistical analysis. Two studies were conducted in order to check the significance of the differences ($p < 0.05$) in the metal contents both between cereals and derived product types and between locations. Kolmogorov-Smirnov and Shapiro-Wilk tests were used to check normality, and Levene's test was applied to check the homogeneity of the variances based on the mean, median and trimmed mean. Data followed a non-normal distribution, and consequently, the Kruskal-Wallis nonparametric test was applied [42]. A one-way study was conducted with the fixed factor "Cereal type" and six levels of variation: *rice, corn gofio, corn flour, wheat flour, corn, wheat*. The Mann-Whitney test was also conducted (95% confidence interval) to determine significant differences in the concentrations of elements according to the cereal type or product. Another one-way study was conducted with the fixed factor "Location" and two levels of variation: *Santiago, São Vicente*. Finally, another Mann-Whitney test was used, and 166 data were analyzed with a 95% confidence interval.

2.5. Calculation of Dietary Intake

The assessment of dietary exposure was based on the calculation of the estimated daily intake (EDI) and the subsequent obtained percentage contribution to the reference value (TDI for Cr, Ni and Sr; TWI for Al and Cd; BMDL for Pb) of each of the metals under study (Table 1).

EDI (mg/day) = Mean consumption (kg/day) × Element concentration (mg/kg fresh weight)

Contribution (%) = [EDI/Reference value] × 100

3. Results and Discussion

Figure 2 shows box plots with the mean concentrations (mg/kg fresh weight), standard deviations (SD) and comparisons of the concentrations between the different cereals and the derived products.

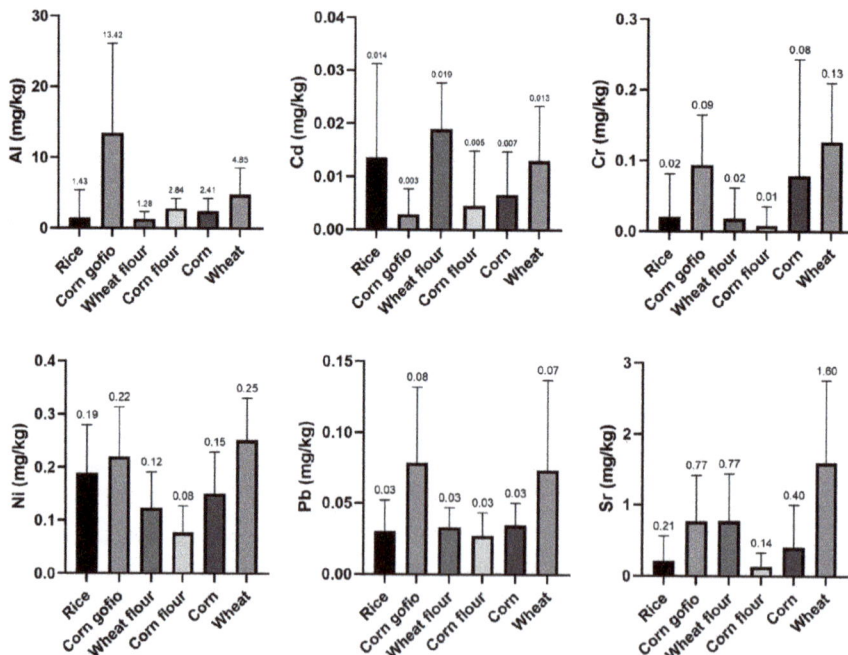

Figure 2. Box plot of mean trace element concentrations (mg/kg) by cereals and derived products.

Al was found in the highest concentrations in all analyzed cereal samples, most clearly in corn gofio, where it reached a mean average concentration of 13.4 ± 12.7 mg/kg fresh weight. This concentration differs significantly from the rest of the cereals ($p < 0.05$). Liu et al. [43] concluded that cereal husks contain higher concentrations of metals than the grain. Accordingly, the differences in the Al content recorded here in corn gofio may be due to the use of the whole cereal, including the husk, in the manufacture of this corn-derived product [35], which may explain the higher Al content. However, despite the toxicological considerations of this neurotoxic element, current European legislation does not include maximum levels of Al in food.

The wheat flour samples are worth mentioning, as they presented the highest levels of Sr (1.60 mg/kg fresh weight), Ni (0.25 mg/kg fresh weight) and Cr (0.13 mg/kg fresh weight). The Second French Total Diet Study (TDS) had a mean level of Sr in breakfast cereals of 0.842 mg/kg fresh weight [44]; this value was lower than the level obtained in the wheat samples of the present study. In addition, Cubadda et al. [45] reported lower Ni levels in flour and wheat (0.035 mg/kg) than those observed in this study. However, Mathebula et al. [46] observed a mean Cr level in wheat of 2.629 mg/kg fresh weight, higher than the mean level recorded in this study.

As observed for Sr, Ni and Cr, the wheat flour samples also presented the highest mean concentration of Cd (0.02 ± 0.01 mg/kg fresh weight). Tejera et al. [47] recorded mean Cd concentrations of 0.027 mg/kg fresh weight in wheat flour, values similar to those recorded in the present study. However, regarding wheat grain, Škrbić et al. [48] observed Cd levels in Serbian wheat of 2.4–252 µg/kg fresh weight, higher than those registered in the wheat analyzed here (0.01 ± 0.01 mg/kg fresh weight).

As for Pb, the highest mean level was observed in the corn gofio samples, with a mean concentration of 0.08 ± 0.05 mg/kg fresh weight. Furthermore, this concentration may indicate that Pb tends to accumulate in the husk of cereals, since in cereal-based products manufactured without the husk, the Pb levels were lower. A study conducted by Bilo et al. [49] on rice and rice husks concluded that rice husks accumulated higher concentrations of toxic metals than rice. This suggests that gofio, being a derivative produced from whole-grain cereal, including the husk, may have higher Pb levels than flours produced from dehusked cereal.

The statistical analysis showed significant differences ($p < 0.05$) in the Pb content between wheat and the rest of the samples, in the Al content between the rice and wheat samples and in the Sr and Ni content of the rice and corn samples when compared to the wheat samples.

Figure 3 presents box plots with the mean concentrations (mg/kg fresh weight), standard deviations (SD) and the comparisons of the concentrations between the sampling locations. The samples from São Vicente presented the highest mean concentrations of Al, Cd, Cr, Ni, Sr and Pb. Considering that these differences may be due to multiple factors [48,50], it is suggested that in future risk-assessment studies, correlations between metal levels and the origin of the imports are calculated. Minimizing the dietary exposure of the Cape Verdean population to metals of toxicological relevance involves risk management actions, including continuous monitoring of these metals in the different food commodities upon arrival in Cape Verde, as well as importing higher-quality cereals that also have lower concentrations of Al, Cd, Cr, Ni, Sr and Pb. In addition, cereals with higher levels of metals, such as Pb and Al, should not be used for the manufacture of cereal-based products containing the husk, but rather, should be used in the manufacture of flours after being dehusked.

In Cape Verde, the cereal balance for 2002/2003 estimated a cereal consumption of 242 kg/year per person, made up of 123 kg maize (337 g/day), 67 kg rice (184 g/day) and 52 kg wheat (142 g/day). However, since there are no additional current data on the consumption habits of cereals and cereal-based products, the estimations here of the dietary exposure (Estimated Daily Intake, EDI) of the Cape Verdean population to the metals under study were performed using a mean ration of 100 g/day of each cereal and its derivatives (Table 5). The European reference limits (Table 1) were used for the evaluation of the EDI of the Cape Verde population. The TDI, TWI, and BMDL were used, along with an estimated mean average weight of an adult individual of 68.48 kg (similar to that of the Spanish population) [51].

Table 5. Metal dietary intake assessment and evaluation.

Element	Rice EDI (mg/day)	Rice Contribution	Corn EDI (mg/day)	Corn Contribution	Corn Flour EDI (mg/day)	Corn Flour Contribution	Wheat Flour EDI (mg/day)	Wheat Flour Contribution	Corn Gofio EDI (mg/day)	Corn Gofio Contribution	Wheat EDI (mg/day)	Wheat Contribution
Cr	0.002	0.01% TDI	0.008	0.04%TDI	0.001	0.005%TDI	0.002	0.01%TDI	0.009	0.04%TDI	0.01	0.05%TDI
Ni	0.02	10.00% TDI	0.02	7.89%TDI	0.008	4.21%TDI	0.01	6.32%TDI	0.02	11.6%TDI	0.03	13.2%TDI
Sr	0.02	0.24% TDI	0.04	0.45%TDI	0.01	0.16%TDI	0.08	0.87%TDI	0.08	0.87%TDI	0.16	1.80%TDI
Al	0.14	1.46%TWI	0.24	2.46%TWI	0.12	1.20% TWI	0.27	2.80% TWI	1.34	13.7% TWI	0.49	4.96% TWI
Cd	0.001	4.09% TWI	0.0007	2.86%TWI	0.0005	2.04% TWI	0.002	8.18% TWI	0.0003	1.23% TWI	0.001	4.09% TWI
Pb	0.003	7.50% BMDL for Nephrotoxicity 3.00% BMDL for Cardiovascular Effects	0.003	7.50% BMDL for Nephrotoxicity 3.00% BMDL for Cardiovascular Effects	0.003	7.50% BMDL for Nephrotoxicity 3.00% BMDL for Cardiovascular Effects	0.003	7.50% BMDL for Nephrotoxicity 3.00% BMDL for Cardiovascular Effects	0.008	20.0% BMDL for Nephrotoxicity 8% BMDL for Cardiovascular Effects	0.007	17.5%BMDL for Nephrotoxicity 7% BMDL for Cardiovascular Effects

Estimated daily intake (mg/day) when consuming 100 g/day; Percentage of contribution (%) to the Reference Intake (Table 1) when consuming 100 g/day. Considering a mean average weight of an adult of 68.48 kg [50].

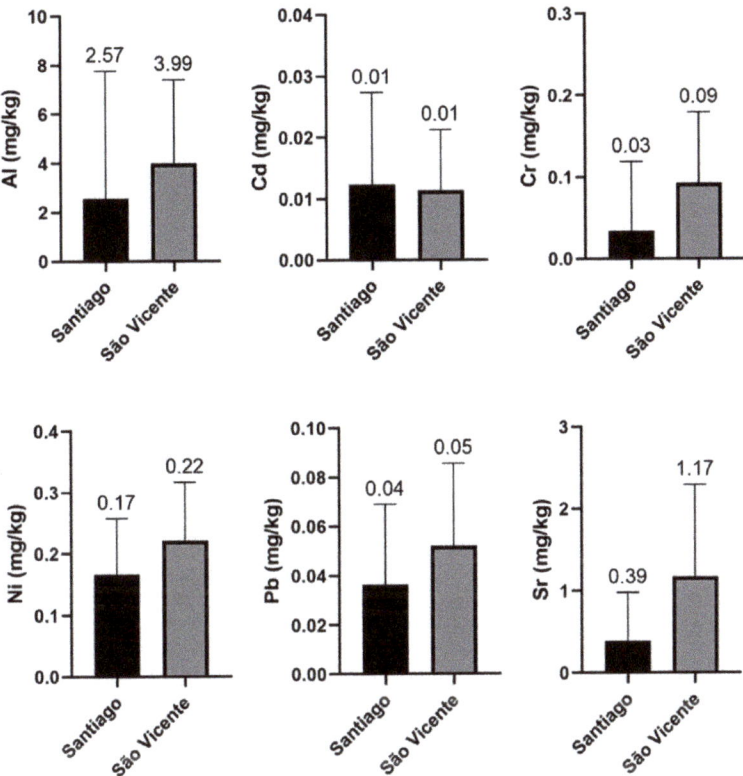

Figure 3. Box plot of mean trace element concentrations (mg/kg) by sampling location.

Thus, the consumption of 100 g/day of wheat represents a contribution percentage of 13.2% to the TDI (tolerable daily intake) of Ni, i.e., 13 µg/kg bw/day. In the case of sensitive individuals or people with kidney problems, a high intake of Ni may be a dietary hazard and health risk [9]. The consumption of 100 g/day of wheat was found to provide a contribution percentage of 17.5% of the European BMDL of Pb set at 0.63 µg/kg bw/day for nephrotoxic effects [13]. This percentage may represent a relevant contribution to the total intake of Pb with the consequent risk to health. Similarly, the consumption of 100 g/day (700 g/week) of corn gofio contributes 13.7% of the TWI (tolerable weekly intake) of Al set in Europe at 1 mg/kg bw/week [11].

The Al levels detected in the corn gofio differed between the Santiago and Sào Vicente islands; in the case of Sào Vicente (39 mg Al/kg fresh weight), the consumption of 100 g/day with an Al content of 39 mg/kg fresh weight would mean an intake of 3.9 mg Al/day from this food alone, i.e., almost 39.9% of the TWI for Al.

Assuming that food risk management needs to be accompanied by a communication plan, the authors believe that the nutritional re-education campaigns and actions provided in the PERVEMAC2 Project could contribute to communicating and disseminating this knowledge to the Cape Verdean population, risk managers and policy regulators. Previous studies carried out in Cape Verde [52] have pointed to the success of involving women in health promotion because of their decision-making power; their multidimensional role in purchasing, processing and preparing food as the pillar of familial food security; and their contribution via nonformal economic activities for their families. Focus group discussions and intensive fieldwork reinforced the higher participation of residents in the informal unit and women in all stages, suggesting the practicability of health-promotion campaigns; this work also showcases the potential of the social capital of the informal settlements and the role of the woman in the family and society in Cape Verde [52].

4. Conclusions

In this study, the existence of significant differences in the content of elements analyzed between different cereals is confirmed, which reaffirms the need for continuous monitoring of both locally produced and imported cereals upon arrival in Cape Verde as risk management and minimization strategies, while also continuing to monitor the population's total dietary exposure to toxic metals. Furthermore, cereals with higher levels of metals such as Pb and Al should not be used with the husk for the manufacture of cereal-based products, but rather, should be used in the manufacture of flours only after removing the husk. In the case of Al, it would be advisable for the food safety authorities to set a maximum limit for this element in cereals and cereal-based products, thus allowing quality control and minimizing the population's exposure to this neurotoxic element. The evaluation of dietary exposure to the toxic metals studied here in cereals and their cereal-based products should undoubtedly be complemented with future studies targeting other groups of basic foods in the diet of the Cape Verde population.

Author Contributions: Conceptualization, C.R.-A. and Á.J.G.; Data curation, V.G.F.; Formal analysis, C.R.-A., Á.J.G. and D.G.-W.; Funding acquisition, C.R.-A. and A.H.; Investigation, C.R.-A., S.P., Á.J.G. and A.H.; Methodology, C.R.-A., S.P., Á.J.G., V.G.F. and A.H.; Project administration, C.R.-A., Á.J.G. and A.H.; Resources, A.H.; Software, Á.J.G.; Supervision, C.R.-A., S.P., Á.J.G., C.R. and A.H.; Writing—original draft, C.R.-A., S.P. and C.R.; Writing—review & editing, C.R.-A., Á.J.G., V.G.F. and A.H. All authors have read and agreed to the published version of the manuscript.

Funding: This research was funded by PERVEMAC II: Programa de Cooperación INTERREG V-A España-Portugal MAC (Madeira-Azores-Canarias) 2014–2020 grant number MAC/1.1a/049. Project "Sustainable Agriculture and Food Security in Macaronesia: Investigation of the benefits and risks of the intake of plant products for the health of consumers and development of minimization strategies"

Institutional Review Board Statement: Not applicable.

Informed Consent Statement: Not applicable.

Data Availability Statement: The datasets generated during the current study are not publicly available but are available from the corresponding author on reasonable request.

Conflicts of Interest: The authors declare no conflict of interest.

References

1. FAO (Food and Agriculture Organization of the United Nations). GIEWS Country Brief Cabo Verde. Available online: http://www.fao.org/giews/countrybrief/country.jsp?code=CPV (accessed on 29 January 2021).
2. Governo de Cabo Verde. Informe Económico y Comercial. Cabo Verde. Available online: https://www.google.com/url?sa=t&rct=j&q=&esrc=s&source=web&cd=&ved=2ahUKEwji7eXpsOXuAhXKTcAKHfgUD5wQFjADegQIBRAC&url=https%3A%2F%2Fwww.icex.es%2Ficex%2FGetDocumento%3FdDocName%3DDOC2018793032%26urlNoAcceso%3D%2Ficex%2Fes%2Fregistro%2Finiciar-sesion%2Findex.html%3FurlDestino%3Dhttps%3A%2F%2Fwww.icex.es%3A443%2Ficex%2Fes%2Fnavegacion-principal%2Ftodos-nuestros-servicios%2Finformacion-de-mercados%2Festudios-de-mercados-y-otros-documentos-de-comercio-exterior%2Findex.html%26site%3DicexES&usg=AOvVaw3NgJEPVkUw8wwZvuF-iJz1 (accessed on 29 January 2021).
3. Monteiro, F.; Fortes, A.; Ferreira, V.; Pereira Essoh, A.; Gomes, I.; Correia, A.M.; Romeiras, M.M. Current Status and Trends in Cabo Verde Agriculture. *Agronomy* **2020**, *10*, 74. [CrossRef]
4. SDG (Sustainable Development Goals). Cabo Verde. Voluntary National Report on the Implementation of the 2030 Agenda for Sustainable Development. Governo de Cabo Verde. June 2018. Available online: https://sustainabledevelopment.un.org/content/documents/19580Cabo_Verde_VNR_SDG_Cabo_Verde_2018_ING_final_NU_280618.pdf (accessed on 29 January 2021).
5. Craveiro, I.; Alves, D.; Amado, M.; Santos, Z.; Fortes, A.T.; Delgado, A.P.; Correia, A.; Gonçalves, L. Determinants, health problems, and food insecurity in urban areas of the largest city in Cape Verde. *Int. J. Environ. Res. Pub. Health* **2016**, *13*, 1155. [CrossRef]

6. Brizio, P.; Benedetto, A.; Squadrone, S.; Curcio, A.; Pellegrino, M.; Ferrero, M.; Abete, M.C. Heavy metals and essential elements in Italian cereals. *Food Addit. Contam. PB* **2016**, *9*, 261–267. [CrossRef] [PubMed]
7. Wei, J.; Cen, K. Contamination and health risk assessment of heavy metals in cereals, legumes, and their products: A case study based on the dietary structure of the residents of Beijing, China. *J. Clean. Prod.* **2020**, *260*, 121001. [CrossRef]
8. EFSA (European Food Safety Authority). Scientific Opinion on the risks to public health related to the presence of chromium in food and drinking water. *EFSA J.* **2014**, *12*, 3595. [CrossRef]
9. EFSA. Update of the risk assessment of nickel in food and drinking water. *EFSA J.* **2020**, *18*, 6268. [CrossRef]
10. WHO (World Health Organization). Strontium and strontium compounds. *Concise Int. Chem. Assess. Doc.* **2010**, *77*, 1–63.
11. EFSA. Statement on the evaluation on a new study related to thee bioavailability of aluminum in food. *EFSA J.* **2011**, *9*, 2157. [CrossRef]
12. EFSA. Panel on Contaminants in the Food Chain (CONTAM). Statement on tolerable weekly intake for cadmium. *EFSA J.* **2010**, *9*, 1975.
13. EFSA. Scientific Opinion on Lead in Food. *EFSA J.* **2010**, *8*, 1570.
14. Exley, C. The toxicity of aluminum in humans. *Morphologie* **2016**, *100*, 51–55. [CrossRef]
15. González-Weller, D.; Gutiérrez, A.J.; Rubio, C.; Revert, C.; Hardisson, A. Dietary Intake of Aluminum in a Spanish Population (Canary Islands). *J. Agric. Food Chem.* **2010**, *58*, 10452–10457. [CrossRef]
16. Hardisson, A.; Revert, C.; Gonzales-Weler, D.; Rubio, C. Aluminium exposure through the diet. *Food Sci. Nutr.* **2017**, *3*, 19.
17. Zhao, Y.; Dang, M.; Zhang, W.; Lei, Y.; Ramesh, T.; Veeraraghavan, V.P.; Hou, X. Neuroprotective effects of Syringic acid against aluminium chloride induced oxidative stress mediated neuroinflammation in rat model of Alzheimer's disease. *J. Func. Foods* **2020**, *71*, 104009. [CrossRef]
18. EFSA (European Food Safety Authority). Safety of aluminium from dietary intake-Scientific Opinion of the Panel on Food Additives, Flavourings, Processing Aids and Food Contact Materials (AFC). *EFSA J.* **2008**, *6*, 754.
19. Barbier, O.; Jacquillet, G.; Tauc, M.; Cougnon, M.; Poujeol, P. Effect of Heavy Metals on, and Handling by, the Kidney. *Nephron Physiol.* **2005**, *99*, 105–110. [CrossRef]
20. Azhar, M.; Rehman, M.Z.; Ali, S.; Qayyum, M.F.; Naeem, A.; Ayub, M.A.; Haq, M.A.; Iqbal, A.; Rizwan, M. Comparative effectiveness of different biochars and conventional organic materials on growth, photosynthesis and cadmium accumulation in cereals. *Chemosphere* **2020**, *227*, 72–81. [CrossRef] [PubMed]
21. Rubio, C.; Napoleone, G.; Luis-González, G.; Gutiérrez, A.J.; González-Weller, D.; Hardisson, A.; Revert, C. Metals in edible seaweed. *Chemosphere* **2017**, *173*, 572–579. [CrossRef] [PubMed]
22. Huang, Y.; He, C.; Shen, C.; Guo, J.; Mubeen, S.; Yuan, J.; Yang, Z. Toxicity of cadmium and its health risks from leafy vegetable consumption. *Food Funct.* **2017**, *8*, 1373–1401. [CrossRef] [PubMed]
23. Rubio, C.; Hardisson, A.; Reguera, J.I.; Revert, C.; Lafuente, M.A.; Gonzalez-Iglesias, T. Cadmium dietary intake in the Canary Islands, Spain. *Environ. Res.* **2006**, *100*, 123–129. [CrossRef]
24. EFSA. Cadmium dietary exposure in the European population. *EFSA J.* **2012**, *10*, 2551. [CrossRef]
25. Løvik, M.; Frøyland, L.; Haugen, M.; Henjum, S.; Stea, T.; Strand, T.A.; Parr, C.; Holvik, K. Assessment of Dietary Intake of Chromium (III) in Relation to Tolerable Upper Intake Level. *Euro. J. Nutr. Food Saf.* **2018**, *8*, 195–197. [CrossRef]
26. IOM (Institute of Medicine). Food and Nutrition Board of the Institute of Medicine of the National Academies. *Dietary Reference Intakes for Vitamin A, Vitamin K, Arsenic, Boron, Chromium, Copper, Iodine, Iron, Manganese, Molybdenum, Nickel, Silicon, Vanadium, and Zinc*; National Academy Press: Washington, DC, USA, 2001.
27. Krejpcio, Z. Essentiality of Chromium for Human Nutrition and Health. *Polish J. Environ. Stud.* **2001**, *10*, 399–404.
28. González-Weller, D.; Rubio, C.; Gutiérrez, A.J.; Luis González, G.; Caballero Mesa, J.M.; Revert Gironés, C.; Burgos Ojeda, A.; Hardisson, A. Dietary intake of barium, bismuth, chromium, lithium, and strontium in a Spanish population (Canary Islands, Spain). *Food Chem. Toxicol.* **2013**, *62*, 856–868. [CrossRef]
29. Filippini, T.; Cilloni, S.; Malavolti, M.; Violi, F.; Malagoli, C.; Tesauro, M.; Bottecchi, I.; Ferrari, A.; Vescovi, L.; Vinceti, M. Dietary intake of cadmium, chromium, copper, manganese, selenium and zinc in a Northern Italy community. *J. Trace Elem. Med. Biol.* **2018**, *50*, 508–517. [CrossRef] [PubMed]
30. Carver, P.L. *Essential Metals in Medicine: Therapeutic Use and Toxicity of Metal Ions in the Clinic*; Walter de Gruyter GmbH&Co KG: Berlin, Germany, 2019.
31. Nielsen, S.P. The biological role of strontium. *Bone* **2004**, *35*, 583–588. [CrossRef] [PubMed]
32. Liu, Z.; Chen, B.; Li, X.; Wang, L.; Xiao, H.; Liu, D. Toxicity assessment of artificially added zinc, selenium, and strontium in water. *Sci. Total Environ.* **2019**, *670*, 433–438. [CrossRef] [PubMed]
33. Rubio, C.; González-Iglesias, T.; Revert, C.; Reguera, J.I.; Gutiérrez, A.J.; Hardisson, A. Lead dietary intake in a Spanish population (Canary Islands). *J. Agric. Food Chem.* **2005**, *53*, 6543–6549. [CrossRef]
34. Tinggi, U.; Schoendorfer, N. Analysis of lead and cadmium in cereal products and duplicate diets of a small group of selected Brisbane children for estimation of daily metal exposure. *J. Trace Elem. Med. Biol.* **2018**, *50*, 671–675. [CrossRef]
35. EFSA. Scientific Report of EFSA. Lead dietary exposure in the European population. *EFSA J.* **2012**, *10*, 2831.
36. Caballero-Mesa, J.M.; Alonso Marrero, S.; González Weller, D.M.; Afonso Gutiérrez, V.L.; Rubio Armendáriz, C.; Hardisson de la Torre, A. Implementation and evaluation of critical hazards and checkpoints analysis (CHCPA) in gofio-producing industries from Tenerife. *Nutr. Hosp.* **2006**, *21*, 189–198. [PubMed]

37. Caballero, J.M.; Tejera, R.L.; Caballero, A.; Rubio, C.; González-Weller, D.; Gutiérrez, A.J.; Hardisson, A. Mineral composition of different types of Canarian gofio; Factors affecting the presence of Na, Mg, Ca, Mn, Fe, Cu y Zn. *Nutr. Hosp.* **2014**, *29*, 687–694. [CrossRef]
38. Luzardo, O.P.; Bernal-Suárez, M.M.; Camacho, M.; Henríquez-Hernández, L.A.; Boada, L.D.; Rial-Berriel, C.; Almeida-González, M.; Zumbado, M.; Díaz-Díaz, R. Estimated exposure to EU regulated mycotoxins and risk characterization of aflatoxin-induced hepatic toxicity through the consumption of the toasted cereal flour called "gofio", a traditional food of the Canary Islands (Spain). *Food Chem. Toxicol.* **2016**, *93*, 73–81. [CrossRef]
39. Rubio, C.; Paz, S.; Tius, E.; Hardisson, A.; Gutierrez, A.J.; Gonzalez-Weller, D.; Caballero, J.M.; Revert, C. Metal contents in the most widely consumed commercial preparations of four different medicinal plants (aloe, senna, ginseng, and ginkgo) from Europe. *Biol. Trace Elem. Res.* **2018**, *186*, 562–567. [CrossRef] [PubMed]
40. Padrón, P.; Paz, S.; Rubio, C.; Gutiérrez, Á.J.; González-Weller, D.; Hardisson, A. Trace element levels in vegetable sausages and burgers determined by ICP-OES. Biol. *Trace Elem. Res.* **2020**, *194*, 616–626. [CrossRef] [PubMed]
41. IUPAC (International Union of Pure and Applied Chemistry). Nomenclature in Evaluation of Analytical Methods including Detection and Quantification Capabilities. *Pure Appl. Chem.* **1995**, *67*, 1699–1723. [CrossRef]
42. Razali, N.M.; Wah, Y.B. Power comparisons of Shapiro-Wilk, Kolmogorov-Smirnov, Lilliefors and Anderson-Darling tests. *J. Stat. Model. Anal.* **2011**, *2*, 21–33.
43. Liu, H.; Probst, A.; Liao, B. Metal contamination of soils and crops affected by the Chenzhou lead/zinc mine spill (Hunan, China). *Sci. Total Environ.* **2005**, *339*, 153–166. [CrossRef]
44. Millour, S.; Noël, L.; Kadar, A.; Chekri, R.; Vastel, C.; Sirot, V.; Guérin, T. Pb, Hg, Cd, As, Sb and Al levels in foodstuffs from the 2nd French total diet study. *Food Chem.* **2011**, *126*, 1787–1799. [CrossRef]
45. Cubadda, F.; Iacoponi, F.; Ferraris, F.; D'Amato, M.; Aureli, F.; Raggi, A.; Sette, S.; Turrini, A.; Mantovnai, A. Dietary exposure of the Italian population to nickel: The national Total Diet Study. *Food Chem. Toxicol.* **2020**, *146*, 111813. [CrossRef]
46. Mathebula, M.W.; Mandiwana, K.; Panichev, N. Speciation of chromium in bread and breakfast cereals. *Food Chem.* **2017**, *217*, 655–659. [CrossRef] [PubMed]
47. Tejera, R.L.; Luis, G.; González-Weller, D.; Caballero, J.M.; Gutiérrez, A.J.; Rubio, C.; Hardisson, A. Metals in wheat flour; comparative study and safety control. *Nutr. Hosp.* **2013**, *28*, 506–513. [PubMed]
48. Škrbić, B.; Durišić-Mladenović, N.; Cvejanov, J. Principal Component Analysis of Trace Elements in Serbian Wheat. *J. Agric. Food Chem.* **2005**, *53*, 2171–2175. [CrossRef] [PubMed]
49. Bilo, F.; Lodolo, M.; Borgese, L.; Bosio, A.; Benassi, L.; Depero, L.E.; Bontempi, E. Evaluation of Heavy Metals Contamination from Environment to Food Matrix by TXRF: The Case of Rice and Rice Husk. *J. Chem.* **2015**, *2015*, 274340. [CrossRef]
50. Bakirciouglu, D.; Bakircioglu Kurtulus, Y.; Ibar, H. Investigation of trace elements in agricultural soil by BCR sequential extraction method and its transfer to wheat plants. *Environ. Monit. Assess.* **2011**, *175*, 303–314. [CrossRef] [PubMed]
51. AESAN (Agencia Española de Seguridad Alimentaria y Nutrición). *Modelo de Dieta Española para la Determinación de la Exposición del Consumidor a Sustancias Químicas*; Ministerio de Sanidad y Consumo: Madrid, Spain, 2006.
52. Gonçalves, L.; Santos, Z.; Amado, M.; Alves, D.; Simões, R.; Delgado, A.P.; Correia, A.; Cabral, J.; Lapão, L.V.; Craveiro, I. Urban Planning and Health Inequities: Looking in a Small-Scale in a City of Cape Verde. *PLoS ONE* **2015**, *23*, e0142955. [CrossRef] [PubMed]

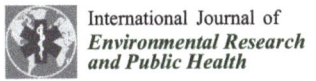

Article

Indigenous Community Perspectives of Food Security, Sustainable Food Systems and Strategies to Enhance Access to Local and Traditional Healthy Food for Partnering Williams Treaties First Nations (Ontario, Canada)

Ashleigh Domingo [1,*], Kerry-Ann Charles [2], Michael Jacobs [2], Deborah Brooker [3] and Rhona M. Hanning [1]

1 School of Public Health and Health Systems, Faculty of Health, University of Waterloo, Waterloo, ON N2L 3G1, Canada; rhanning@uwaterloo.ca
2 Cambium Indigenous Professional Services, Curve Lake, ON K0L 1R0, Canada; ka.charles@indigenousaware.com (K.-A.C.); m.jacobs@indigenousaware.com (M.J.)
3 Ontario Ministry of Food, Agriculture and Rural Affairs, Guelph, ON N1G 4Y2, Canada; deborah_brooker@hotmail.com
* Correspondence: ashleigh.domingo@uwaterloo.ca

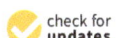

Citation: Domingo, A.; Charles, K.-A.; Jacobs, M.; Brooker, D.; Hanning, R.M. Indigenous Community Perspectives of Food Security, Sustainable Food Systems and Strategies to Enhance Access to Local and Traditional Healthy Food for Partnering Williams Treaties First Nations (Ontario, Canada). *Int. J. Environ. Res. Public Health* **2021**, *18*, 4404. https://doi.org/10.3390/ijerph18094404

Academic Editors: António Raposo, Fernando Ramos, Dele Raheem, Conrado Javier Carrascosa Iruzubieta and Ariana Saraiva

Received: 19 March 2021
Accepted: 18 April 2021
Published: 21 April 2021

Publisher's Note: MDPI stays neutral with regard to jurisdictional claims in published maps and institutional affiliations.

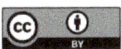

Copyright: © 2021 by the authors. Licensee MDPI, Basel, Switzerland. This article is an open access article distributed under the terms and conditions of the Creative Commons Attribution (CC BY) license (https:// creativecommons.org/licenses/by/ 4.0/).

Abstract: In partnership with communities of the Williams Treaties First Nations in southern Ontario (Canada), we describe an approach to work with communities, and highlight perspectives of food security and sustainability, including priorities and opportunities to revitalize local food systems as a pathway to food security and food sovereignty. The objectives of our project were: (1) to build a shared understanding of food security and sustainability; and (2) to document community priorities, challenges and opportunities to enhance local food access. Utilizing an Indigenous methodology, the conversational method, within the framework of community-based participatory research, formative work undertaken helped to conceptualize food security and sustainability from a community perspective and solidify interests within the four participating communities to inform community-led action planning. Knowledge generated from our project will inform development of initiatives, programs or projects that promote sustainable food systems. The community-based actions identified support a path towards holistic wellbeing and, ultimately, Indigenous peoples' right to food security and food sovereignty.

Keywords: Indigenous health; food security; food sovereignty; food systems; sustainability; colonialism; community-based; participatory

1. Introduction

Indigenous communities are increasingly driving the reclamation of traditional food systems (the term, *traditional food systems*, has been described as all foods identified within a particular culture that derive from local natural resources and includes sociocultural meanings associated with acquisition and use of such foods) as a means to enhance food security, food sovereignty and to sustain traditional food practices [1–4]. Indigenous holistic wellness has been supported by deep relations with the environment, including the natural resources it provides such as food and water for generations [3,4]. In Canada, however, the inequities faced by Indigenous peoples, tied to the loss of land, forced displacement from traditional territories and the history of colonization, have threatened the resilience of Indigenous food systems and impacted the right to food security and food sovereignty [1–6]. (Food sovereignty is the *"right of peoples to healthy and culturally appropriate food produced through ecologically sound and sustainable methods. It entails peoples' right to participate in decision making and define their own food, agriculture, livestock and fisheries systems"* ([6]). The traditions and cultural practices to acquire, grow or prepare food have consequently been affected [1,4,7]. Challenges to ensuring food security have been further amplified by global climate change and environmental contamination of food systems, which have impacted access to, and quality of, land, water, plants and animal resources [8–11]. In addition to such processes that have threatened Indigenous food systems, rising costs of traditional food acquisition activities and local food production, along with the introduction of westernized food, has driven greater use of store-bought less nutritious food [12–14]. This nutrition transition has been tied to obesity and diet-related chronic diseases: a nutritional burden impacting Indigenous peoples worldwide [15–18].

In Canada, food insecurity has been felt most strongly by Indigenous peoples, recognized as First Nations, Inuit and Métis [12–21]. Food insecurity, an outcome and determinant of health, can range from worry about having enough food to limited access to, or reduced intake of, sufficient, safe, personally accepted, healthy food and even to hunger [21–24]. First Nations households on-reserve (Crown land designated by Canadian government for primary use of First Nations with registered Indian status [3]) in Ontario, have experienced a rate of food insecurity (41.7%) far greater than reported provincial household levels for the general population (11.6%) [24,25]. The extreme injustices exposed by the disproportionate rates of food insecurity impacting First Nations households highlight the need for community identified approaches to enhance food security in culturally safe and relevant ways. Sustainable food systems are central to long-term food and nutrition security [26] and extend beyond usual considerations for supportive economic, social and environmental conditions [27] to encompass cultural integrity.

In partnership with communities of the Williams Treaties First Nations in southern Ontario, Canada, we describe an approach to work with communities, and highlight perspectives of food security and sustainability, including priorities and opportunities to revitalize local food systems as a pathway to food security. Given the diverse challenges to food security described, momentum for the current work stemmed from broad considerations for the ecological health of the Lake Simcoe watershed under the Lake Simcoe Protection Plan and encompassed environment, climate change, agriculture and human health (the Lake Simcoe Protection Plan is part of the Lake Simcoe Protection Act, 2008, an Ontario government strategy to protect and restore the health of the Lake Simcoe watershed). Importantly, protecting and honouring harvesting rights for food, social and ceremonial purposes have long been recognized as essential to wellness by the Williams Treaties First Nations communities. Hence, creating opportunities to enhance and sustain local and traditional food access and knowledge has been identified as necessary to improve food security. As such, this participatory formative work was initiated and driven by communities to address food insecurity and enhance sustainability of food systems.

The objectives of our project were to: (1) build a shared understanding of food security and sustainability; and (2) document community priorities, challenges and opportunities to enhance local food access. The Williams Treaties First Nations, Cambium Indigenous Professional Services, the Ontario Ministry of Food, Agriculture and Rural Affairs, and the University of Waterloo coordinated and documented the process of data collection. Through the participatory process, we hope the formative work will initiate community capacity building and set the stage for further community-led action. The overall goal of this participatory formative work, is to inform a pathway of community driven solutions to strengthen food security and sustainable food systems, thereby promoting Indigenous people's right to food and holistic wellness.

2. Materials and Methods

2.1. Project Team and Guiding Principles: Indigenous Communities and Academic Partnership

A project advisory committee with liaisons within each of the four partnering communities was established to guide project activities. Respectful and reciprocal relationships, approached through a decolonizing and participatory process, represents the foundational core of how this formative project was undertaken in ways that are culturally safe and ethical. The project team consisted of both Indigenous and non-Indigenous partners who engaged directly with participating Williams Treaties First Nations communities to identify culturally-relevant capacity building approaches to increase access to affordable, nutritious foods.

The project teams' skills and knowledge positioned this participatory project to advance community-identified priorities and enhance access to sustainable local food systems. Project co-investigators from Cambium Indigenous Professional Services provided First Nations led expertise in environmental consulting and engineering services as members of Georgina Island First Nation and Curve Lake First Nation. Pre-existing relationships established with each of the partnering communities provided the opportunity to engage directly with community-identified expert advisors to continue ongoing food security and sustainability dialogues. Academic partners from the University of Waterloo supported by co-facilitating conversations with community advisors, evaluating and synthesizing findings and preparing project reports for funder and communities. Community members, identified through Cambium Indigenous Professional Services contacts and snowball approaches, were critical to the integrity of the process and relevance and utility of the findings.

Guided by the First Nations principles of Ownership, Control, Access and Possession (OCAP) [28], the project partners ensured engagement with communities was respectful, appropriate, beneficial and relevant to the communities involved. Information was only collected when informed assent was provided by participants, whose personal identification information remained anonymous. The OCAP principles applied helped to ensure integrity and meaningful engagement with communities to inform and control the direction of priorities identified throughout. Funding support was provided by the Ontario Ministry of Agriculture, Food and Rural Affairs as part of a broader commitment to the Lake Simcoe Protection Plan. Canada's Tri-Council Policy Statement: Ethical Conduct for Research Involving Humans ([29], article 6.11, p. 77), indicates the *"initial exploratory phase, which is intended to establish research partnerships or to inform the design of a research proposal, and may involve contact with individuals or communities"* does not require full REB review (U Waterloo, Office of Research Ethics).

2.2. Partnering Communities of the Williams Treaties First Nations

The Williams Treaties First Nations are located in the province of Ontario, Canada within the Georgian Bay, Lake Simcoe and Lake Ontario watersheds of Treaty 20. The First Nations of the Williams Treaties comprise of the Chippewas of Georgina Island First Nations, Beausoleil First Nation, and Rama First Nation; and the Mississaugas of Curve Lake First Nation, Alderville First Nations, Hiawatha First Nation and Scugog Island First Nation. These communities, which include First Nations with non-registered and registered Indian status (Registered Indian status refers to an individual registered under the Canadian Indian Act [30]), are a diverse and growing population that strongly embrace a holistic relationship with the land, water and its local food systems. Communities of Georgina Island First Nation, Beausoleil First Nation, Curve Lake First Nation and Rama First Nation expressed interest in participating in this project as community partners.

The Beausoleil First Nation is situated at the Southern tip of Georgian Bay on Christian Island, Ontario. It is a small remote community, home to approximately 800 year-round residents, and has a membership of approximately 2214 people. The Island's main access is by ferry transportation except, during the winter months, when access to the island is made over ice roads or hovercraft. As such, community members need to travel by vehicle and ferry to access the nearest store for groceries. The Island is also referred to as Chimnissing, which means "Big Island" in the Ojibway language. The First Nation consists of three Islands known as Christian, Hope and Beckwith, as well as 25 acres on the mainland at Cedar Point. Members predominately reside on Christian Island, however, several families live year-round on Cedar Point.

Curve Lake First Nation is also an Ojibway community, located 25 km northwest of Peterborough, Ontario. It has a diverse population of 2500, which includes First Nation members and non-First Nation members alike residing on territorial lands. There are 1918 registered status Indian members (1161 off reserve and 764 on reserve). The territory has a communal land base of 900 hectares, which consists of a mainland peninsula, a large island (Fox Island) and several other smaller islands located throughout the Trent Severn Waterway system. Curve Lake First Nation is a proud community known for its leadership and promoting Anishinabe culture. The health centre in Curve Lake, offers a range of programs and services including a healthy eating programming and a food bank. While there is access to convenience stores and a coffee shop, many must travel to Peterborough to shop at the nearest grocery store.

The Chippewas of Georgina Island First Nation is located both on and off the east shore of Lake Simcoe in the Region of York and is approximately 100 km north of the Greater Toronto Area. Georgina Island First Nation Reserve No. 33 consists of three separate islands and two mainland access points. The three islands (Georgina Island, Snake Island and Fox Island) are approximately 3 km off the southern shore of Lake Simcoe. The main population of the reserve resides on the largest island, Georgina Island, with approximately 90 households. The island's land mass is approximately 15 km, which is 4.5 km long and 3.2 km wide with an area of 1415 hectors. Snake Island is approximately 135 hectors; and Fox Island is approximately 20 hectors, both of which are comprised of seasonal cottage residence and non-First Nation member residence. Travel by vehicle and ferry is needed to access the nearest store for groceries.

The Chippewas of Rama First Nation has been known as 'the gathering place', where travelers journeyed to trade, to seek counsel or medicines, and attend great meetings. Rama is now home to Casino Rama, a tourism attraction that brings many visitors to the area for gaming, shows, conventions, shopping and fine dining. Rama First Nation is approximately 1.5 h north of Toronto, Ontario. The community has over 2500 acres of interspersed land, nestled in "Ontario's Lake Country" on the eastern side of Lake Couchiching. The community has over 1800 members including over 700 living off-reserve. Rama has a food bank and some local food and restaurant access but most travel to nearby Orillia (14 km) for groceries.

2.3. Project Design and Process

Applying a decolonizing theoretical perspective [31–35], we employed a community-based participatory research (CBPR) [33] methodological approach to advance the following formative project objectives: (1) to conceptualize food security and food sustainability from a First Nations perspective; and (2) to identify community-based approaches to enhance, protect and sustain local food systems in support of food security and sustainable food systems (Figure 1).

A participatory orientation emphasizes strong collaboration, non-hierarchical relations, and sharing of perspectives throughout the research process [36–38]. Given the partner centred and collaborative approach underpinning CBPR, it has increasingly been accepted as an appropriate methodology to engage with Indigenous communities as its relational component aligns with an Indigenous paradigm [35,39–41]. Applying CBPR within Indigenous contexts can facilitate space for Indigenous knowledge systems by shifting a focus on community values, perspectives and priorities [33,34,38,39,41].

To support communities with enhancing local food security and sustainability, the principles of CBPR were applied to facilitate the identification of community-led action and enablers for project planning. Further, CBPR in conjunction with Indigenous approaches to inquiry, akin to *two-eyed seeing* [41,42], was used to decolonize the research process and draw on the strengths and wisdom of Indigenous knowledge and ways of knowing. Formative work helped conceptualize food security and sustainability from a local community perspective and solidify interest within the four participating communities to inform and support community-led action planning in moving forward with their identified priorities.

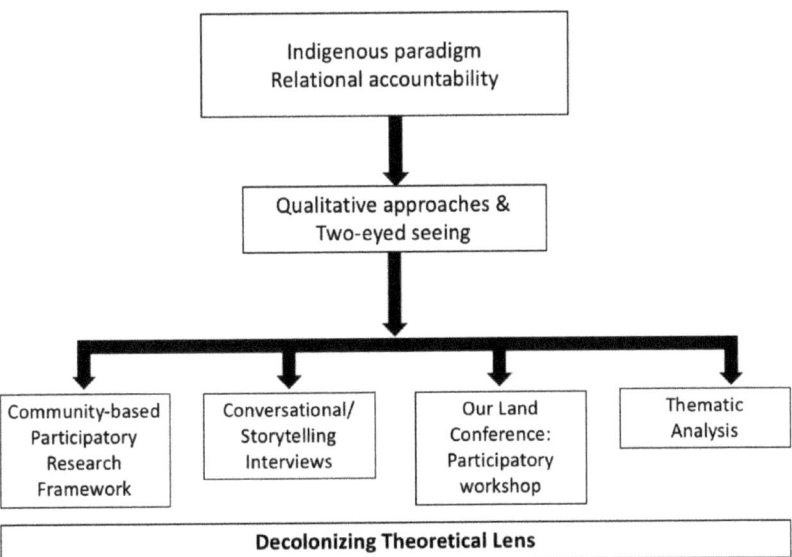

Figure 1. Overview of project design and Indigenous approach to inquiry.

2.4. Indigenous Approach to Inquiry

Recognizing the importance of telling stories in Indigenous culture, we used the conversational method to facilitate the sharing of reflections and experiences [33,34]. The conversational method is a dialogic approach to generating and gathering knowledge through oral storytelling and is congruent with Indigenous methodologies [33,34]. This was applied to facilitate community-based conversational/storytelling interviews involving semi-structured open-ended questions guided by the literature. This approach was undertaken with the aim of decolonizing the proposed work by enabling the creation of a safe space for partnering Williams Treaties First Nations community voices to be heard (Figure 1) [33]. As such, conversations were co-facilitated by an experienced community member to enable a safe environment for dialogue.

Using the conversational method, a series of community engagement meetings were held between December 2017 and March 2018 with four First Nation communities. Community liaisons in each partnering community, employed by the First Nation on climate change adaptation in their community, helped to identity advisors to engage in community dialogue sessions. Advisors with extensive knowledge of and expertise in environmental sustainability, food systems, traditional food practices, health, education and community development were invited to be engaged in the project. Academic partners, co-facilitated conversations with community expert advisors. Engagement sessions provided the opportunity to build relationships with respective community members and solicit input from the communities on perspectives of food security and food sustainability. In conversations with communities, informants identified priorities, challenges and opportunities for community-driven food-related projects to enhance food security and support sustainable local food systems.

Our Land, Building Capacity in Ontario First Nation Communities (Our Land) was a First Nations led and informed conference that was held on January 2018 at Rama, Ontario. This annual conference, organized by the project partners from Cambium Indigenous Professional Services, convened over 30 First Nations community representatives across Ontario.

The conference featured keynote presentations, panel presentations, participatory workshops, as well as an interactive digital survey to engage with conference delegates. On day one of the conference, we planned and facilitated a participatory workshop to explore ways to increase access to healthy food through the development of local food initiatives. The workshop featured a short video on food sustainability and food security, preliminary digital information gathering, an ice-breaker activity (trivia game and card game), facilitated break-out group discussions, and a dot-voting method to identify shared priorities. Conference attendees visiting the project booth were also invited to complete an optional survey to provide input on priorities and challenges to food security in their community. On day two of the conference, a digital survey of all delegates took place, based in part, on the findings of day one information gathering. All notes, flip charts and votes were collected.

The workshop guiding questions and both the paper-based and digital surveys were informed by knowledge gained from a review of the literature and community engagement sessions with partnering communities as a way to fill any knowledge gaps. In addition, early findings from the workshop helped to refine questions included in the digital survey on day two of the conference. The purpose of the workshop, the paper-based survey, and digital survey was to solicit input from Our Land Conference delegates on understandings of food security and food sustainability, and perspectives on community-level initiatives and capacity needed to achieve food security.

2.5. Data Analyses

Information gathered from the community-based conversational/storytelling interviews was transcribed and thematically analyzed [43,44]. Data used in this project are owned by communities as per First Nations Ownership, Control, Access and Possession guidelines (OCAP^{TM}). In addition, notes from the participatory workshop at the conference and surveys were also analyzed to inform cross-cutting themes across all four partnering communities. Thematic analysis was used to systematically identify and organize patterns of meaning and experiences as described by Braun, Clarke and colleagues [43] and Cresswell and Cresswell [44]. The approach identified insights and patterns of meaning as they related to perspectives of food security and strategies to enhance local access to food. The code book and emergent themes were reviewed by the project team for refinement and to ensure inclusiveness and appropriate representation of community voices.

3. Results

3.1. Project Participants

Community key informants ($n = 15$) who were engaged in conversational/storytelling interviews (2–6 participants per community) included leaders in food security, environmental and energy sustainability, local food producers, and educators. Attendees of the conference included key partners and stakeholders working in the areas of climate change, environmental sustainability, energy, agriculture, public health, food security, and government. Conference delegates shared their perspectives through a participatory workshop ($n = 65$), and survey ($n = 22$ delegates), and large group feedback ($n = 85$). In addition to partnering communities of the project, the experiences and voices shared by First Nations community representatives across Ontario who attended the conference contributed to knowledge generation of priorities and opportunities for food security. The perspectives of key informants from each community on food security, food sustainability and associated challenges had common themes, though preliminary ideas for initiatives to strengthen local food systems were sometimes context specific. Given the small numbers, perspectives are not distinguished by respondent position or community.

3.2. Food Security

Food security was broadly understood from a holistic wellness perspective by all partnering communities. It was viewed as both an outcome and determinant of wellbeing. Participants highlighted the importance of access to food, knowledge of how to grow your own food, and the skills and resources to prepare food. Also emphasized was the importance that food procurement from the land, whether through hunting, fishing or gardening, should honour traditional practices and be carried out in ways that protect the environment.

Perspectives of individual and community food security were shared. Food security was commonly described as a way of life: promoting and maintaining overall wellness from a holistic perspective. Perspectives shared largely centred around access and use of traditional foods and store-bought food (non-traditional food sources). The ability to grow and produce food all year round and the opportunity to share food with others within the community was widely appreciated by community members.

> Community advisor 1: *"I'll give you my whole idea on it, on what would be the dream for me, which would essentially be people growing their own food. Maybe having greenhouses to supply the things you're not getting from the summer. Having root cellars for storage. Having community freezers for those who hunt, fish, trap, but then also using the hide using the furs and putting that towards either making clothing or whatever it ends up being. But also knowing your medicines around, being able to identify trees, what parts of the plant are edible what parts are medicine."*

> Community advisor 2: *"I mean to me food security is everyone having access to healthy foods."*

In addition, the value of having the knowledge and skills to undertake traditional food activities was expressed. This was inclusive of community reflections on the importance of practicing ceremony associated with traditional food acquisition activities, as well as being able to partner with other communities to acquire local foods within a community established trading system. These were recognized as essential to supporting community's ability to provide its own food (e.g., grow, hunt, harvest, self-produce) for multiple generations.

> Community advisor 4: *"Food is medicine. If you're sick and have a cold, you don't take vitamin C capsules, you boil a light batch of cedar tea."*

3.3. Sustainable Food Systems

While food security was the primary topic of community engagement dialogues, the connection between sustainable food systems and food security was recognized by each community. Communities often discussed the importance of engaging in environmentally responsible food production as a way to protect the environment, while also growing and sustaining food within the community. In addition, communities expressed the importance of not relying on external food sources and also having the ability to control what goes into your food as a way to control the health of the community.

> Community advisor 7: *"The ability to produce all year round would be nice. Trying to get the younger generations interested in fishing again, if we could tap into that a little."*

3.4. Challenges to Food Security

Community identified challenges to food security centred around the impacts of climate change and environmental degradation, income, food knowledge and skills, and limited availability of healthy food options (Table 1).

Table 1. Community perspectives of challenges and priorities to enhance food security and strengthen local food systems.

Challenges	Priorities
Climate change and environmental degradation	Access to food
Income	Availability and use of fresh, nutritious food
Traditional food knowledge and skills	Restoring community connections to the land and traditions
	Support for locally grown food in the community

3.4.1. Climate Change and Environmental Degradation

Community members shared observations about changes in the abundance, distribution, and health of species (e.g., fish are smaller and have sores). Drivers of these changes identified include climate-related differences observed over time, from more drought in the summer (necessitating frequent fire bans) to longer growing seasons. Also shared was the observation of a growing number of invasive species that have altered plants and local food, including the presence of wildlife in the area. Some shared that environmental contaminants have also been responsible for impacting water and soil quality (road spraying oil and salts), including chemical waste dumped in waterways from a factory (reports of agent orange). As a result of these changes to local sources of food, communities have expressed having to travel further distances to hunt and fish because there's not the same accessibility as there used to be.

> Community advisor 6: " ... under our environmental assessment that we just had completed, one of the major issues on there that kind of held up the whole process for us would be the stuff that they spray on the road the dust control. And so that gives people a lot of concerns because you know we are so close, like a lot of the houses are so close to the road, our water sources [is] there and you know what's running off into the water.
>
> So [this] makes you think about, you know, if you were to have a garden, if each family had a garden, what's running off into the gardens?"

> Community advisor 8: "People travel further to hunt and fish to trap because it's not the same like it used to be. So if they're hunting muskrat there's no muskrat left here really. There might be a few beavers."

3.4.2. Income

Concerns were shared related to the high cost of food within the community, including high costs associated with travelling to grocery stores outside of the community. In addition, the costs to engage in traditional food activities related to travel to hunting areas, and access to tools or equipment to hunt was a concern. Amplifying these challenges is the dependency on social assistance due to low employment opportunities and rates in the community.

> Community advisor 2: "Food insecurity is huge for us. What is the root problem? It's income basically."

> Community advisor 6: "I think also because we live in the cottage country that really determines the price especially meat and produce. I think sometimes we end up as during summer months like we are paying more for stuff that you know if you lived in the city you wouldn't be paying that price. I think costs is the biggest factor."

3.4.3. Traditional Food Knowledge and Skills

The loss of traditional knowledge, language and skills to engage in traditional food acquisition practices was emphasized as a barrier to food security. In particular, reflections were made on how the loss of traditional knowledge is tied to colonization and the Indian Act which have contributed to a lack of sovereignty and control over access to land to hunt, fish and gather (The Constitution Act (1876), Canada has the responsibility for 'Indians and Lands Reserved for Indians' under the Indian Act [3]. The Indian Act, which formally recognizes First Nations ancestry, is recognized as legislative authority that remains a source of internal colonization [3,30]). Shared was that such circumstances have not only led to less traditional food available to be consumed, but has also changed the perception and taste for traditional food.

> Community advisor 6: "I think we need to start with the younger generations because I think with the older generation we're slowly losing that link to the past especially the ones that remember what it's like way back when times were simpler, when people helped themselves, help each other, they didn't have to rely with a lot of programs."

Emphasized, was the implication of limited traditional knowledge, in particular the lack of opportunities for traditional knowledge of food and culture to be passed down to younger generations on how to engage in community food gathering and harvesting practices, including knowing the location of hunting grounds and how to use tools or equipment to hunt.

> Community advisor 9: *"I think there's a gap that needs to be bridged somehow because we are losing our traditions and cultures within our own community. Because of that we are having to bring other people in that are teaching the same skills, but they are not our community's skills."*

3.5. Priorities to Enhance Food Security and Strengthen Local Food Systems

Priorities and actions were identified within each community to enhance food security (Table 1). These ranged from specific interests in food production, types of food, sustainability practices and developing food knowledge and skills, to community-based projects to implement in the short-term to support community interests and priorities.

3.5.1. Access to Food

Access to grocery stores outside of the community was emphasized. Within each community, the importance of having access to means of transportation (either by bus, car or boat) was commonly expressed, as this was recognized as essential to accessing food, and especially healthy food of good quality.

Having a community-based travel system in place with appropriate storage was identified as an opportunity to support access to grocery stores outside of the community. For example, having a community-based bus that could accommodate large grocery portions and preserve freshness of vegetables in the summer was discussed.

> Community advisor 5: *" ... my one Aunt she won't even buy bananas in the winter because they are brown by the time they get on the boat across the bay, but I think too, a lot of people like having to transport and so many people are on the boat. So if the ice starts building up then we use our passenger ferry only, so if you have 70 people riding a ferry then all their food and stuff like you kinda have to watch yourself."*

> Community advisor 6: *"But again it's just our access has always been an issue because you know you have to bring stuff over. We do have farmers market in the summer, sometimes they are well received and sometimes they are not. It depends who's bringing stuff over; sometimes it's fresh, sometimes it's not."*

Also highlighted as key to supporting access to food, was ensuring sufficient income and employment opportunities within the community. Creating jobs within the community to support economic growth and security was emphasized.

> Community advisor 2: *"And we know about [how] income and accessing affordable fresh produce in general, changes their body. Chronic disease goes down, you feel good. You're not losing limbs because you're eating sugary bread all the time."*

3.5.2. Availability and Use of Fresh, Nutritious Food

The importance of making fresh produce available and affordable for communities to access at wholesale costs was emphasized. Having food markets in the community with a variety of vendors of locally produced food and other essential products was identified as an action that could support greater access to fresh food. Having stable and reliable access to enough healthy and affordable food year-round without worry was broadly understood by communities as having secure access to food.

Support for health promoting activities to increase food literacy and knowledge of healthy foods and recipes was also identified as a priority that can support community in healthy eating practices. Developing incentives to have community members engaged at local markets and community-based food initiatives was also discussed.

Community advisor 7: *"I think with our community, I've heard from [a] few people that the issue too is education and equipment right. So, I mean, just finding out from people like, Ellen, you know getting that knowledge in order [to know] 'where do I start?'. Some areas in our community are so sandy that you probably couldn't get a garden, 'so what do you have to do, okay fine you need to build up, so you have to build a crib right.' 'Who do I talk to?' 'Who has the skills to build this crib right?'*

Community advisor 3: *"I think it's trying to find ways to provide fresh foods and vegetables. Cause like I said, they have this program called, the good food box, but that's only catered towards certain people right; it's not available to everybody."*

An existing initiative within one of the partnering communities, Nourish, provides affordable access to local produce and market foods, was identified as an opportunity to support local food production and enhance community food security.

Community advisor 2: *"Nourish is a collaboration from Peterborough and public health from the YMCA which we are housed out of. We are a small group. We try to bring people into the system to help with system change ... It's all about food. We have people entering into our programs so we do cooking, we do growing, we have community meals, and we do advocacy work. Basically, the bottom line is to empower people to make decisions for themselves in order to make system changes."*

Accelerating the uptake of existing projects within the community to support scale-up efforts, including support for local business to enhance traditional food supply (e.g., Nourish Project JustFood Boxes, restoration of wild rice beds, fish habitat improvements) [45,46] is an approach that can be taken and led by community to improve access to and availability of local, fresh and nutritious food.

3.5.3. Restoring Community Connections to the Land and Traditions

Restoring and maintaining access to traditional food sources and distribution systems, such as wild rice production within the community, was emphasized. Communities shared the importance of promoting traditional food acquisition activities such as fishing, hunting and cultivating (e.g., wild rice production). This was discussed as an opportunity to re-establish connections to traditions, culture and the environment (e.g., water ceremony teachings, traditional medicines). This included promoting greater engagement with youth in traditional food teachings and encouraging younger generations to be advocates for local food projects and traditional food activities. In addition, utilizing social media platforms to engage youth and generate interest in learning more about traditional food and ways to contribute to food security in their community through gardening, gathering of traditional medicines, fishing, hunting, and harvesting and production (e.g., wild rice, maple syrup, net making), was emphasized. An approach identified to support this was having hunters and trappers from the community share their knowledge and skills to other members of the community (i.e., community-specific, not just northern FN community coming down to teach), including teachings of food as medicine. In addition, having a communal resource for members of the community to access tools and equipment for hunting was also identified as an opportunity to enable greater engagement in traditional food acquisition practices.

Community advisor 8: *"I think if we are able somehow to find a way to get the kids excited about farming, gardening, and fishing that we might see a difference, you know? Them bringing that home to their own parents and then getting them interested as well, but I think we need to offer some, I don't know some ways to get them involved."*

3.5.4. Support for Locally Grown Food in the Community

Creating a sustainable food system, that can support healthy eating in the community and opportunities to achieve food security through approaches that enable local food production (e.g., community gardening), was discussed. Communities highlighted the importance of having policies that enable better management, protection and preservation of the land from pesticides/herbicides, and industry related activities. This was identified as an important process to ensure food safety and minimize food system exposure to environmental contaminants.

Regulations in place, with community input to support ongoing environmental assessment of water and soil quality, was identified as a priority to support local food production and a way to build legislative trust within the community. As invasive species can pose a potential threat to traditional food systems, programs and services in place that can remove invasive species were identified as an opportunity to support long-term environmental health in the community. Holding workshops that can enhance community members' skills and knowledge to engage in local food production and activities that promote energy sustainability was also emphasized.

> Community advisor 7: " ... well I think there is movement already to tell you the truth. From what I see from the people who have access to programs and their wants and their needs. I think even the younger are more [willing] now to try things. We've done canning workshops here. The only thing that I think of is if people were to grow their own food and they have all this extra produce. They get overwhelmed by okay, what do I do with all this kale? So, there's education in that and how to do that or maybe have a barter system set up or whatever trading and things."

4. Discussion

The formative work undertaken in this participatory project aimed to facilitate the building of shared understandings of food security and food sustainability, including opportunities to strengthen access to nutritious and sustainable food systems. The Indigenous approaches utilized for knowledge generation and sharing helped to ensure appropriate engagement that centred the priorities of First Nations communities at the core. In addition, the findings will support community-led action planning and will be used to inform next steps for implementation. Knowledge generated from our project is intended to help develop initiatives, programs or projects that promote sustainable food systems. Such community-based action supports a path towards holistic wellbeing and, ultimately, Indigenous peoples' right to food security and food sovereignty.

4.1. Strengthening Indigenous Food Security, Food Sustainability and Food Sovereignty

Food security was broadly understood from a holistic wellness perspective by all partnering communities. It was viewed as both an outcome and determinant of wellbeing. Participants highlighted the importance of access to food, knowledge of how to grow your own food, and the skills and resources to prepare food. Also emphasized was the importance of food procurement from the land, whether through hunting, fishing or gardening, should honour traditional practices and be carried out in ways that protect the environment.

Conceptualizations of food security underscored the importance of considering unique dimensions as related to access, availability and use of market and traditional food systems in efforts aimed at enhancing food security in Indigenous communities [21]. For Indigenous communities, this means a consideration of factors such as income and transportation that impact access to and use of market and traditional food; climate change and environmental degradation impacts on availability, use and access to traditional food and locally produced food; and how traditional food knowledge and skills, and connections to the land influence preparation and use of traditional and local food. In addition to such unique considerations of food security, an underlying theme was food sovereignty [5,6,47–51].

Food sovereignty is closely aligned with how partnering communities described food security, food sustainability and opportunities to improve access to food [47–51]. Underpinning community interests and priorities are actions that can support reclamation of access to land, revitalization of local food systems, reconnection with culture, traditional food and ways of knowing, and having greater control over ways to obtain healthy food within local food environments of the community. Such priorities align closely with what has been described as Indigenous food sovereignty.

Dawn Morison, for example, describes Indigenous food sovereignty as *"present day strategies that enable and support the ability of Indigenous communities to sustain traditional hunting, fishing, gathering, farming and distribution practices, the way we have done for thousands of years prior to contact with the first European settlers"* ([51], p. 98). Promoting food security and nutrition in a sustainable, culturally relevant and just way, as described by community members, is a window to enhancing Indigenous food sovereignty. Activities identified by communities that can improve greater access to food, restore connections and cultural ties to the environment, and support local food production, highlight their need to protect and restore the right to food and food sovereignty. As such, efforts to support revitalization of local food systems as a way to restore, protect and sustain community food practices is a community identified priority and opportunity to strengthen food security and food sovereignty.

4.2. Moving from Priorities to Community-Led Action

While partnering communities recognize the need to mobilize interests towards creating more sustainable and accessible food systems, moving from priorities to actions requires a level of readiness and capacity to plan, develop and implement initiatives. In addition, it requires working within the specific context of each community's traditional and market food systems. Building on the momentum to better understand their local context as it relates to challenges and opportunities to strengthen access and availability of food, communities can begin thinking about how to create an environment for transformation and meaningful change. Existing implementation and change frameworks have highlighted the importance of understanding local context to build shared knowledge, assumptions and practices to define the change pursuits of interest as an initial step before effective implementation can take place [51–53].

The community-identified priorities from this formative work therefore present opportunities for change, whereby communities mobilize their interest for sustainable food systems, food sovereignty and food security by identifying and building on existing strengths within the community to enhance readiness and capacity for action. This may include identification of key system actors and champions, along with existing projects, initiatives and programs that can be scaled-up within the community. In addition, successes and lessons identified from existing or previous projects can also be leveraged. For example, an existing initiative, Nourish, was identified by community members as an opportunity for scale-up; extending its reach to nearby First Nations communities and incorporating traditional food could support their access to nutritious, culturally-relevant food. Strengthening relational capacities with key system actors has been identified as a critical process to support successful change pursuits [52,53]. Within the context of Indigenous communities, this is especially critical to align change efforts with community identified priorities and interests [54]. Indigenous scholars have continuously emphasized the importance of appropriate and respectful approaches to engage with communities to build shared understandings of knowledge and practices as required to support the implementation of programs or policies intended to improve Indigenous health and wellbeing [31,35,54].

Ongoing engagement with key community members from this preliminary work will be essential to identifying key system actors and champions that can lead and sustain implementation efforts and ensure success is achieved in the community. Furthermore, such engagement, driven by the community, will be fundamental to ensuring that actions, including partner-support of implementation strategies, are taken in a culturally safe way that best serves the interests of communities.

4.3. Limitations

Community-based participatory work, though well respected and recognized as an appropriate approach to working with Indigenous communities, is not without challenges or shortcomings. Short-term funding cycles may not support additional efforts to plan and implement community-identified projects of interest. While time and resource constraints limited the immediate uptake of the current project, partners continue to identify opportunities to utilize and leverage the findings from this project to inform other areas of existing or future funded projects.

5. Conclusions

We use Indigenous methodologies and western approaches to partner with communities and engage with community advisors to solicit input on priorities and opportunities to enhance food security, strengthen sustainability of food systems, and in doing so support the promotion of food sovereignty. The shared understanding of community perspectives, priorities, challenges and opportunities to strengthen food security will benefit participating Williams Treaties First Nations communities directly. Moreover, the approach taken in this formative initiative will help to inform other work to integrate robust Indigenous practices and approaches to community engagement critical to building shared knowledge and understanding as an initial step and requirement of implementation of programs intended to improve Indigenous health. Hence, the contributions made to understanding ways to support the wellbeing of partnering Williams Treaties First Nations by taking a community driven and participatory approach to identifying priorities and opportunities to revive local food systems, will promote greater food security, sustainability and food sovereignty that may resonate with other Indigenous communities.

The current research can serve as an important foundation for planning Indigenous community-based projects and initiatives to strengthen food security, create more sustainable food systems and work towards food sovereignty.

Author Contributions: Conceptualization, design and methodology were conducted by K.-A.C., M.J., A.D. and R.M.H.; validation, K.-A.C., M.J., A.D. and R.M.H.; formal analysis, A.D. and R.M.H.; investigation, K.-A.C., M.J., A.D. and R.M.H.; resources, K.-A.C., M.J., A.D., R.M.H. and D.B.; writing—original draft preparation, A.D.; writing—review and editing, A.D., K.-A.C., M.J., R.M.H. and D.B.; supervision, R.M.H. and K.-A.C.; project administration, K.-A.C., M.J., A.D. and R.M.H.; funding acquisition K.-A.C., M.J., R.M.H., D.B. and A.D. All authors have read and agreed to the published version of the manuscript.

Funding: This work was funded by Ontario Ministry of Agriculture, Food and Rural Affairs.

Institutional Review Board Statement: Canada's Tri-Council Policy Statement: Ethical Conduct for Research Involving Humans (TCPS2, article 6.11, p. 77), indicates the *"initial exploratory phase, which is intended to establish research partnerships or to inform the design of a research proposal, and may involve contact with individuals or communities"* does not require full REB review (U Waterloo, Office of Research Ethics).

Informed Consent Statement: Not applicable.

Data Availability Statement: Data used are owned by communities as per First Nations Ownership, Control, Access and Possession guidelines (OCAP[TM]). Availability is dependent on reasonable request to the corresponding author and permission from the partnering communities.

Acknowledgments: The authors would like to acknowledge all partnering communities for their time, commitment and leadership in shaping this work. The authors also appreciate the financial support provided by the Ontario Ministry of Agriculture, Food and Rural Affairs and coordinative and technical support provided.

Conflicts of Interest: The authors declare no conflict of interest. A representative of the funder, OMAFRA, participated in managing the grant but the organization had no role in the design of the study; in the collection, analyses, or interpretation of data, the writing of the manuscript or in the decision to publish the results.

References

1. Kuhnlein, H.; Erasmus, B.; Creed-Kanashiro, H.; Englberger, L.; Okeke, C.; Turner, N.; Bhattacharjee, L. Indigenous peoples' food systems for health: Finding interventions that work. *Public Health Nutr.* **2006**, *9*, 1013–1019. [CrossRef]
2. Lemke, S.; Delormier, T. Indigenous Peoples' Food Systems, Nutrition, and Gender: Conceptual and Methodological Considerations. *Matern. Child Nutr.* **2017**, *13* (Suppl. 3), e12499. [CrossRef]
3. Richmond, C.A.M.; Ross, N.A. The Determinants of First Nation and Inuit Health: A Critical Population Health Approach. *Health Place* **2009**, *15*, 403–411. [CrossRef]
4. Kuhnlein, H.V. Dietary Change and Traditional Food Systems of Indigenous Peoples. *Annu. Rev. Nutr.* **1996**, *16*, 417–442. [CrossRef]
5. Desmarais, A.A.; Wittman, H. Farmers, Foodies and First Nations: Getting to Food Sovereignty in Canada. *J. Peasant Stud.* **2014**, *41*, 1153–1173. [CrossRef]
6. International Steering Committee. Nyéléni: Forum for Food Sovereignty; Sélingué, Mali; 23–27 February 2007. Synthesis Report. Available online: https://nyeleni.org/spip.php?article334 (accessed on 9 April 2021).
7. Socha, T.; Chambers, L.; Zahaf, M.; Abraham, R.; Fiddler, T. Food availability, food store management, and food pricing in a northern community First Nation community. *Int. J. Humanit. Soc. Sci.* **2011**, *1*, 49–61.
8. Spring, A.; Carter, B.; Blay-Palmer, A. Climate Change, Community Capitals, and Food Security: Building a More Sustainable Food System in a Northern Canadian Boreal Community. *Can. Food Stud.* **2018**, *5*, 111–141. [CrossRef]
9. Burnett, K.; Skinner, K.; LeBlanc, J. From Food Mail to Nutrition North Canada: Reconsidering Federal Food Subsidy Programs for Northern Ontario. *Can. Food Stud.* **2015**, *2*, 141. [CrossRef]
10. Ford, J.D.; Beaumier, M. Feeding the Family during Times of Stress: Experience and Determinants of Food Insecurity in an Inuit Community: Feeding the Family during Times of Stress. *Geogr. J.* **2011**, *177*, 44–61. [CrossRef]
11. Zavaleta-Cortijo, C.; Ford, J.D.; Arotoma-Rojas, I.; Lwasa, S.; Lancha-Rucoba, G.; García, P.J.; Miranda, J.J.; Namanya, D.B.; New, M.; Wright, C.J.; et al. Climate Change and COVID-19: Reinforcing Indigenous Food Systems. *Lancet Planet. Health* **2020**. [CrossRef]
12. Egeland, G.M. IPY Inuit Health Survey Speaks to Need to Address Inadequate Housing, Food Insecurity and Nutrition Transition. *Int. J. Circumpolar Health* **2011**, *70*, 444–446. [CrossRef]
13. Kuhnlein, H.V.; Receveur, O.; Soueida, R.; Egeland, G.M. Arctic Indigenous Peoples Experience the Nutrition Transition with Changing Dietary Patterns and Obesity. *J. Nutr.* **2004**, *134*, 1447–1453. [CrossRef] [PubMed]
14. Gracey, M.; King, M. Indigenous Health Part 1: Determinants and Disease Patterns. *Lancet* **2009**, *374*, 65–75. [CrossRef]
15. Pal, S.; Haman, F.; Robidoux, M.A. The Costs of Local Food Procurement in Two Northern Indigenous Communities in Canada. *Food Foodways* **2013**, *21*, 132–152. [CrossRef]
16. Bhawra, J.; Cooke, M.J.; Hanning, R.; Wilk, P.; Gonneville, S.L.H. Community Perspectives on Food Insecurity and Obesity: Focus Groups with Caregivers of Métis and Off-Reserve First Nations Children. *Int. J. Equity Health* **2015**, *14*, 96. [CrossRef]
17. Sharma, S.; Cao, X.; Roache, C.; Buchan, A.; Reid, R.; Gittelsohn, J. Assessing Dietary Intake in a Population Undergoing a Rapid Transition in Diet and Lifestyle: The Arctic Inuit in Nunavut, Canada. *Br. J. Nutr.* **2010**, *103*, 749–759. [CrossRef]
18. Hanley, A.J.G.; Harris, S.B.; Mamakeesick, M.; Goodwin, K.; Fiddler, E.; Hegele, R.A.; Spence, J.D.; House, A.A.; Brown, E.; Schoales, B.; et al. Complications of Type 2 Diabetes Among Aboriginal Canadians: Prevalence and Associated Risk Factors. *Diabetes Care* **2005**, *28*, 2054–2057. [CrossRef]
19. Skinner, K.; Hanning, R.M.; Desjardins, E.; Tsuji, L.J.S. Giving Voice to Food Insecurity in a Remote Indigenous Community in Subarctic Ontario, Canada: Traditional Ways, Ways to Cope, Ways Forward. *BMC Public Health* **2013**, *13*, 427. [CrossRef]
20. Skinner, K.; Hanning, R.M.; Tsuji, L.J.S. Prevalence and Severity of Household Food Insecurity of First Nations People Living in an On-Reserve, Sub-Arctic Community within the Mushkegowuk Territory. *Public Health Nutr.* **2014**, *17*, 31–39. [CrossRef]
21. Power, E.M. Conceptualizing Food Security for Aboriginal People in Canada. *Can. J. Public Health* **2008**, *99*, 95–97. [CrossRef]
22. Tarasuk, V. Household Food Insecurity in Canada. *Top. Clin. Nutr.* **2005**, *20*, 299–312. [CrossRef]
23. McIntyre, L. Food security: More than a determinant of health. *Policy Options Montr.* **2003**, *24*, 46–51.
24. Tarasuk, V.; Mitchell, A.; Dachner, N. *Household Food Insecurity in Canada: 2011*; Research to Identify Policy Options to Reduce Food Insecurity (PROOF): Toronto, ON, Canada, 2014; Volume 15.
25. Domingo, A.; Spiegel, J.; Guhn, M.; Wittman, H.; Ing, A.; Sadik, T.; Fediuk, K.; Tikhonov, C.; Schwartz, H.; Chan, H.M.; et al. Predictors of Household Food Insecurity and Relationship with Obesity in First Nations Communities in British Columbia, Manitoba, Alberta and Ontario. *Public Health Nutr.* **2021**, *24*, 1021–1033. [CrossRef] [PubMed]
26. Slater, J.; Yeudall, F. Sustainable Livelihoods for Food and Nutrition Security in Canada: A Conceptual Framework for Public Health Research, Policy, and Practice. *J. Hunger Environ. Nutr.* **2015**, *10*, 1–21. [CrossRef]
27. Nguyen, H. Sustainable Food Systems Concepts and Framework, 2018. Food and Agriculture Organization of the United Nations. Available online: http://www.fao.org/3/ca2079en/CA2079EN.pdf (accessed on 20 April 2021).
28. The First Nations Information Governance Centre. *Ownership, Control, Access and Possession (OCAP™): The Path to First Nations Information Governance*; The First Nations Information Governance Centre: Ottawa, ON, Canada, May 2014. Available online: https://achh.ca/wp-content/uploads/2018/07/OCAP_FNIGC.pdf (accessed on 20 April 2021).

29. Government of Canada, Interagency Advisory Panel on Research Ethics. Tri-Council Policy Statement: Ethical Conduct for Research Involving Humans—TCPS 2 (2018). Available online: https://ethics.gc.ca/eng/policy-politique_tcps2-eptc2_2018.html (accessed on 20 April 2021).
30. Adelson, N. The Embodiment of Inequity: Health Disparities in Aboriginal Canada. *Can. J. Public Health* **2005**, *96*, S45–S61. [CrossRef] [PubMed]
31. Smylie, J.; Kaplan-Myrth, N.; McShane, K. Métis Nation of Ontario-Ottawa Council Pikwakanagan First Nation; Tungasuvvingat Inuit Family Resource Centre. Indigenous Knowledge Translation: Baseline Findings in a Qualitative Study of the Pathways of Health Knowledge in Three Indigenous Communities in Canada. *Health Promot. Pr.* **2009**, *10*, 436–446.
32. Smith, L.T. *Decolonizing Methodologies: Research and Indigenous Peoples*, 2nd ed.; Zed Books: London, UK, 2012.
33. Kovach, M.E. *Indigenous Methodologies: Characteristics, Conversations, and Contexts*; University of Toronto Press: Toronto, ON, Canada, 2010.
34. Kovach, M. Conversational Method in Indigenous Research. *First Peoples Child Fam. Rev.* **2010**, *14*, 123–136.
35. Evans, M.; Miller, A.; Hutchinson, P.; Dingwall, C. Decolonizing Research Practice: Indigenous Methodologies, Aboriginal Methods, and Knowledge/Knowing. In *The Oxford Handbook of Qualitative Research*; Oxford University Press: Oxford, UK, 2014; pp. 179–191.
36. Israel, B.A.; Schulz, A.J.; Parker, E.A.; Becker, A.B. Review of Community-Based Research: Assessing Partnership Approaches to Improve Public Health. *Annu. Rev. Public Health* **1998**, *19*, 173–202. [CrossRef] [PubMed]
37. Minkler, M.; Wallerstein, N. Part One: Introduction to Community-Based Participatory Research. *Community-Based Participatory Research for Health*; Jossey-Bass: San Francisco, CA, USA, 2003.
38. Tobias, J.K.; Richmond, C.A.M.; Luginaah, I. Community-Based Participatory Research (CBPR) with Indigenous Communities: Producing Respectful and Reciprocal Research. *J. Empir. Res. Hum. Res. Ethics* **2013**, *8*, 129–140. [CrossRef]
39. Wilson, S. What is an Indigenous research methodology? *Can. J. Nativ. Educ.* **2001**, *25*, 175–179.
40. Drawson, A.S.; Toombs, E.; Mushquash, C.J. Indigenous Research Methods: A Systematic Review. *Int. Indig. Policy J.* **2017**, *8*. [CrossRef]
41. Hyett, S.; Marjerrison, S.; Gabel, C. Improving Health Research among Indigenous Peoples in Canada. *CMAJ* **2018**, *190*, E616–E621. [CrossRef]
42. Marshall, M.; Marshall, A.; Bartlet, C. *Determinants of Indigenous Peoples' Health in Canada: Beyond the Social*; Greenwood, M., de Leeuw, S., Lindsay, N.M., Reading, C., Eds.; Canadian Scholars' Press Inc.: Toronto, ON, Canada, 2015; pp. 16–24.
43. Braun, V.; Clarke, V.; Hayfield, N.; Terry, G. Thematic Analysis. In *Handbook of Research Methods in Health Social Sciences*; Springer: Singapore, 2018; pp. 1–18.
44. Creswell, J.W.; Creswell, J.D. *Research Design: Qualitative, Quantitative, and Mixed Methods Approaches*; Sage Publications: Thousand Oaks, CA, USA, 2008.
45. Sustainable Local Food Systems Research Group. Nourishing Communities. Inspiring Reconcile-Action through Dialogue. Available online: http://nourishingontario.ca/blog/tag/james-whetung/ (accessed on 27 October 2020).
46. Just Food. Available online: https://nourishproject.ca/justfood (accessed on 27 October 2020).
47. Grey, S.; Patel, R. Food sovereignty as decolonization: Some contributions from Indigenous movements to food system and development politics. *Agric. Hum. Values* **2015**, *32*, 431–444. [CrossRef]
48. Wittman, H. Food sovereignty: A new rights framework for food and nature? *Environ. Soc. Adv. Res.* **2011**, *2*, 87–105.
49. Wittman, H.; Desmarais, A.A.; Wiebe, N. (Eds.) *Food Sovereignty in Canada: Creating Just and Sustainable food Systems*; Fernwood Publishing: Halifax, NS, Canada, 2011.
50. Menezes, F. Food Sovereignty: A Vital Requirement for Food Security in the Context of Globalization. *Development* **2001**, *44*, 29–33. [CrossRef]
51. Morrison, D. *Indigenous Food Sovereignty—A Model for Social Learning*; Wittman, H., Desmarais, A.A., Wiebe, N., Eds.; Fernwood Publishing: Halifax, NS, Canada, 2011.
52. Foster-Fishman, P.G.; Watson, E.R. The ABLe Change Framework: A Conceptual and Methodological Tool for Promoting Systems Change. *Am. J. Community Psychol.* **2012**, *49*, 503–516. [CrossRef]
53. Meyers, D.C.; Durlak, J.A.; Wandersman, A. The Quality Implementation Framework: A Synthesis of Critical Steps in the Implementation Process. *Am. J. Community Psychol.* **2012**, *50*, 462–480. [CrossRef]
54. Morton Ninomiya, M.E.; Atkinson, D.; Brascoupé, S.; Firestone, M.; Robinson, N.; Reading, J.; Ziegler, C.P.; Maddox, R.; Smylie, J.K. Effective Knowledge Translation Approaches and Practices in Indigenous Health Research: A Systematic Review Protocol. *Syst. Rev.* **2017**, *6*. [CrossRef]

Article

How Capital Endowment and Ecological Cognition Affect Environment-Friendly Technology Adoption: A Case of Apple Farmers of Shandong Province, China

Hongyu Wang [1,2,†], Xiaolei Wang [3,†], Apurbo Sarkar [1] and Fuhong Zhang [4,*]

1. Department of Economics & Management, College of Economics & Management, Northwest A&F University, Yangling 712100, China; wanghongyu@nwafu.edu.cn (H.W.); apurbo@nwafu.edu.cn (A.S.)
2. The Sixth Industry Research Institute, Northwest A&F University, Yangling 712100, China
3. Department of Information Science and Engineering, College of Information Science and Engineering, Shandong Agricultural University, Tai'an 271018, China; 2018110568@sdau.edu.cn
4. Department of Economics & Management, College of Economics & Management, Shandong Agricultural University, Tai'an 271018, China
* Correspondence: sdzhangfuhong@sdau.edu.cn
† These authors contributed equally to the study.

Abstract: Ever-increasing global environmental issues, land degradation, and groundwater contamination may significantly impact the agricultural sector of any country. The situation worsens while the global agricultural sectors are going through the unsustainable intensification of agricultural production powered by chemical fertilizers and pesticides. This trend leads the sector to exercise environmentally friendly technology (EFT). Capital endowment and ecological cognition may significantly impact fostering farmers' adoption of environmentally friendly technology. The government also tends to change the existing policies to cope with ever-increasing challenges like pollution control, maintaining ecological balance, and supporting agricultural sectors substantially by employing ecological compensation policy. The study's main objective is to explore the impacts of farmer's ecological compensation, capital endowment, and ecological cognition for the adoption of EFT. The empirical setup of the study quantifies with survey data of 471 apple farmers from nine counties of Shandong province. The study used Heckman's two-stage model to craft the findings. The results showed that 52.02% of fruit farmers adopted two environmentally friendly technologies, and 23.99% of fruit farmers adopted three forms of environmentally friendly technologies. At the same time, we have traced that the capital endowment, planting scale, family income, and technical specialization of fruit farmers significantly impact adopting EFT. The study also revealed that understanding ecological compensation policy has a significant positive effect on adopting environmentally friendly technology. Seemingly, ecological compensation policy has a specific regulatory effect on fruit farmers' capital endowment and ecological cognition. Therefore, it is necessary to extend the demonstration facilities, training, and frequently arrange awareness-building campaigns regarding rural non-point source pollution hazards and improve the cognition level of farmers. The agriculture extension department should strengthen the agricultural value chain facilities to make farmers fully realize the importance of EFT. Government should promote and extend the supports for availing new and innovative EFT at a reasonable price. Moreover, cooperative, financial, and credit organizations need to lead for the smooth transition of EFT. The agricultural cooperatives and formal risk-taking networks should act responsibly for shaping the behavioral factors of farmers.

Keywords: capital endowment; ecological cognition; environment-friendly technology; adoption level; Hackman model

1. Introduction

China has gained relatively swift development in agricultural sectors by employing intense inputs within the last decade. It has a long history of given priorities for intensifying agriculture production to support the massive population with limited arable land [1]. For mitigating these challenges, widespread and overuse of chemical fertilizers and pesticides has been adopted by Chinese agriculture sectors [2]. However, China is achieving the challenges of food security by employing intensive agro-productivity powered by intensive interactions of chemical components, but those activities have drawn exacerbated controversies for maintaining the sustainable development goals set by the united nations (UN) [3]. The impermissible utilization of chemical components and overuse of natural resources resulted in extra production costs and staggering ecological issues from the soil, water, and air contaminations by greenhouse gas emissions [4–6]. These concerns are not only slowing down sustainable development goals achievement but also threatened human wellbeing and existence. Therefore, China is confronting significant sustainability issues as a densely populated and agriculture-based nation [7]. Intensive and chemical input-based agricultural production methods have been updated, and innovative eco-friendly technology is rigorously studied, introduced, and reviewed to reduce farm emissions from non-point sources and enhance its influence. As a result, Chinese farmers are trying to improve their environmental stand while sustaining or increasing crop production [8]. Global studies have shown that the usage of environmentally friendly technologies could be crucial to reduce the rural non-point source of pollution and improve the quality of products [6,9]. Seemingly, several eco-friendly technologies have been applied in horticultural production, such as soil testing and formula fertilization, organic fertilizer instead of chemical fertilizer, green prevention and control technology, soil improvement technology, and so on [10]. Moreover, it revealed a smooth progression from emphasizing scientific research facilities to participative field trials [11].

Interestingly, research has shown that by adopting environment-friendly technology, farmers can improve product quality, protect the ecological environment, and effectively integrate into the high-value industrial chain [12,13]. The continuous adjustment of the agricultural and industrial structure has forced more farmers to turn their limited land resources to planting high-yield and high-value products [14]. From the effect, the application of the technologies reduces the rural non-point source pollution. It also improves the quality of products conducive to obtaining the food quality and safety certification to lay a foundation for products to enter the high-end and dynamic consumption market [15,16]. The strategies of reducing the non-point cause of agricultural emissions are entirely satisfactory within demonstration zones and experimental stages, whether the effectiveness of those innovative tactics and the promotions and adoption intentions are not sufficiently explored yet [17]. Thus, the areas where small farms can practically use this advanced technology would have to be assessed appropriately. According to Grzelak et al. [18], resource endowments such as human and materials resources of capital approach to farming may impact fostering EFT. It is apparent that if a farmer has certain freedom and resource supports, it provides confidence for farmers to try many forms of potential technology [4]. Several pieces of research also indicate that farmers' cognition level largely influences the farmers to adopt environmentally friendly technologies [19,20]. If farmers possess a positive attitude towards a certain EFT, it is easier for them to make decisions for adopting EFT in the future [21]. In terms of emerging countries, the ecological compensation policies may significantly impact the impacts of EFT [22]. Especially among the smallholder farmers, the impacts of such policies may have crucial impacts to build up a positive attitude and eventually improve their cognition level. Therefore, based on apple farmers' actual situation in Shandong and from the capital endowment and ecological cognition prospects, this paper analyzes the impact mechanism of environment-friendly technology adoption. It further explores the mediating impacts of ecological compensation for shaping cognition and improving farmer's capital endowment capabilities.

Related literature mainly focuses on influencing factors and adopting decision-making by using environment-friendly technologies [23]. Due to the difference in endowment, the heterogeneity of their technology adoption behavior is apparent, and the age factor is usually included in the estimation model first. For example, Wang et al. [20] provided a brief assessment on the adoption behavior of soil testing, and formula fertilization technology for grain crop farmers shows that the older the age, the lower the possibility of technology adoption, which is in line with the previous studies on Integrated Pest Management of vegetable farmers. However, Zhou et al. [24] also argued that experienced farmers might have a greater willingness to adopt water-saving and labor-saving technologies. Seemingly, Ma et al. [25] addressed that farmers with higher education tend to have a deeper understanding of using chemical products scientifically and rationally to reduce the impacts of excessive use and have a higher adoption rate of environment-friendly technologies.

Moreover, the promotions and guidance from suppliers also have a significant impact on practical usage of chemical products and technology adoption behavior of farmers [26], while the planting years, scale, number of laborers, and whether to join cooperatives also have an impact on the adoption behavior of environment-friendly technologies [27]. Interestingly, farmers' new technology adoption decision-making is different from the adoption intention [19], which is a rational choice after comparing the expected cost and benefit [28]. Farmers show a low awareness of green prevention and control technologies such as biological pesticides, have uncertainty about the effect [25], and demand a profound paradox in the application, willingness, and behavioral changes [29]. Whether farmers adopt environment-friendly technologies depends on the potential performance that can be improved after technology adoption, such as market share, yield level, and cost–benefit comparison [30]. However, the government's subsidies, for example, price concession for innovative machinery utilization, price and procurement subsidies on organic fertilizers (cash grant and interest-free loans), and pest control, facilitating low-interest loans, accelerated depreciation, and rent rebates (indirect subsidies) to farmers who adopt environment-friendly technologies could have a good effect on improving the adoption of environment-friendly technologies and controlling rural non-point source pollution [9].

The existing studies mainly focus on single technology adoption, centered within the crop farmers' context. In contrast, a minimal number of publications have been traced that can quantify adoption behavior towards environmental-friendly technologies among apple or other orchard-based products [31]. Moreover, the research on the adoption behavior and degree of farmer's environment-friendly technology around capital endowment, ecological cognition, and ecological compensation policy is relatively rare, quantifying the article's strength and prime novelty. Therefore, for fulfilling the research mentioned above the gap, these articles used the survey of 471 apple farmers from nine counties (cities, districts) of Shandong Province, and adopted the Heckman sampling model to provide an in-depth assessment of the adoption behavior and measured the degree of adoption of environmentally friendly technologies by orchard farmers from the perspective of capital endowment and ecological cognition.

The article is designed as follows: Section 1 comprised the introduction and theoretical baseline. Section 2 described a brief overview of the data sources and theoretical outline. Section 3 outlined the variables and research approaches, whereas Section 4 denotes the results and analytical framework. Section 5 comprised the discussion and Section 6 explored the conclusions of the study and policy recommendations.

2. Methodology

2.1. Data Sources

The empirical data were collected through the field survey among the apple orchard farmers listed in the "National Research Center for Apple Engineering and Technology (NRCAET), Shandong Agricultural University," situated in the most specialized apple production counties of Shandong province from December 2018 to January 2019. The surveyed regions were covered by nine major apple production counties (Penglai, Laiyang, Qixia, Haiyang, Longkou, Zhaoyuan, Zibo, and Linyi). Whereas we randomly selected 5-6 apple-growing townships from each county, each township selects a core apple-growing village. Finally, we randomly selected 10–15 apple growers from each selected village with sufficient communication skills to answer the questionnaire. A total of 500 questionnaires were distributed, and 471 valid questionnaires were collected, with an effective rate of 94.20%. Shandong is one of China's largest apple-growing areas, and it is one of the largest exporter provinces in China, having strong market competitiveness within South Asia and Europe. However, due to the excessive application of fertilizers and pesticides, the local agricultural and environmental pollution problems are very prominent, so it is pertinent to study environmentally friendly technologies by apple growers. The nine counties surveyed in this article are also the core clusters of apple growers in Shandong. Thus, the data of the growers in these nine counties are representative in terms of the high demand of chemical usage, production rate, market values, and trends of synthetic pesticide usage of the selected area. Before the survey, a pilot test was conducted within the targeted areas to grasp the basic characteristics of the targeted area and respondents. Moreover, before the formal interviews were taken, the investigator briefly explained the content of the questionnaire, which might have influenced the high response rate. Figure 1 represents the theoretical framework adopted by the study.

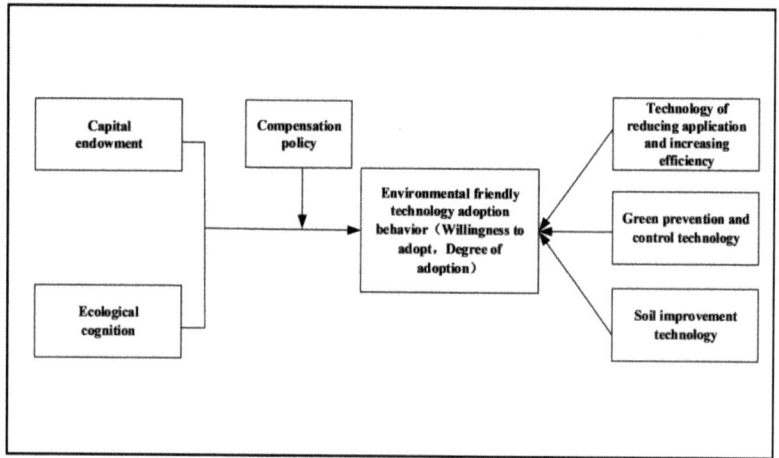

Figure 1. Theoretical model for the adoption of environment-friendly technology by farmers. Here, capital endowment and ecological cognition have been set as independent variables and "willingness to adopt" and "adoption" as dependent variables. In addition, compensation policy is composed of moderating variables.

2.2. Demographic Profile of the Respondent

The respondents are primarily middle-aged farmers, whereas 57.96% are over 50 years old, and 79.9% had junior high school education. Moreover, the planting scale is smaller than the average planting scale in these scales; 74.31% of them are less than 1.4 acres. On the other hand, the degree of specialization is high, 87.69% of apple production income accounts for more than 60% of the total income, and 80.3% joined the agricultural cooperatives. On the whole, the sample farmers are representative. The results show that the adoption rate of soil improvement technology is relatively high, reaching 87.26%. Among those, Penglai City, Qixia City, Yiyuan County, and Mengyin County are covered around 90% because they are situated within the pilot areas to replace chemical fertilizer with organic fertilizer. Simultaneously, reducing application and efficiency increasing technology has been found moderate, about 54.26%. It could have happed due to the favorable subsidy policy introduced by China. The results showed that the adoption level of reducing application and efficiency increasing technology in the above four pilot counties is higher than average.

In contrast, the adoption level of green prevention and control technology (biological control, physical trapping) is relatively low, only 18.47%, which may have happened for relatively high cost and slow effect of this technology, and the low recognition of the effect of this technology. Besides, 52.02% of the fruit farmers adopted two environmentally friendly technologies (soil improvement technology, reduction, and efficiency technology, green prevention, and control technology), 23.99% of the fruit farmers adopted three environmentally friendly technologies (soil improvement technology, reduced application efficiency technology, green prevention, and control technology). Therefore, it can be seen that fruit farmers' subjective willingness to adopt environmentally friendly technology is more optimistic. However, the willingness and acceptance rate of green prevention and control technology in environmentally friendly technology is relatively low.

2.3. Theoretical Basis and Research Hypothesis

2.3.1. The Direct Impact of Capital Endowment and Ecological Cognition on Farmer's Adoption of Environment-Friendly Technology

The environment-friendly technologies in this paper mainly refer to the technologies of reducing and increasing efficiency of chemical fertilizer (soil testing and formula fertilization, water, and fertilizer integration technology), green prevention and control technology (artificial release of natural enemies, physical trapping), soil improvement technology (using organic fertilizer to replace chemical fertilizer, garden grass). Farmers need to invest in improving the human and material resources in adopting environment-friendly technology. EFT can be termed as applying knowledge that leads the sectors to enjoy not harming or less harming farming practices in agriculture. In the context of the study, we chose the three types of technologies as EFT, (i) technologies regarding reducing application and increasing efficiencies, (ii) green preventions and control technology, and (iii) soil improvement technology. Low-input technologies could act as a crucial EFT as the technology allows farmers to practice lower resource usage by increasing firm utility management while not compromising productivity [32]. Seemingly, green prevention and control technology directly allows farmers not to use or reduce the chemical intersection by employing bio-based organic components or integrated pest management practices to control the pests and diseases of the farm [33]. Finally, eco-friendly soil-management practices positively address serious environmental issues and maintain productivity [34,35].

When farmers make decisions, they are usually constrained by their capital endowment. The capital endowment has a significant impact on the farmer's behavior choice and decision-making [36]. Due to the limitation of capital endowment, farmers may show lower adoption behavior when making adoption decisions [37]. On the contrary, if farmers possessed a sound capital endowment, it would be beneficial to them to take more risks and implement their innovativeness [38]. Thus, the study put forward Hypothesis 1 as (H1) capital endowment positively impacts the farmer's adoption of environment-friendly technology. Seemingly, according to the planned behavior theory, farmers' decisions will also be affected by subjective cognition [39]. In production, farmers will get an idea about the surrounding ecological environment, which will encourage farmers to make different decisions to adapt to the ecological environment changes [40,41]. Moreover, farmers' cognition of changes positively impacts their living environment and eventually shaped the adoption behavior of environment-friendly technologies [42,43]. Additionally, farmers' awareness of environmental risk positively impacts their adoption of environment-friendly behavior [44]. Therefore, capital endowment and ecological cognition will affect farmers' adoption of environment-friendly technologies. Based on the above analysis, the author puts forward Hypothesis 2 as (H2) ecological cognition has a positive impact on the farmer's adoption of environment-friendly technologies.

2.3.2. Impact of Ecological Compensation Policy on Farmer's Adoption of Environment-Friendly Technology

As a rational decision-maker, whether farmers finally decide to adopt new technologies is usually rational after comparing the expected costs and benefits. Therefore, if the government can provide certain policy subsidies to farmers (for example, price concession for innovative machinery utilization, subsidies on organic fertilizers, and pest control), it will help them eliminate their endowments' restrictions and urge farmers to adopt environment-friendly technologies [38–40] actively. Additionally, ecological compensation (see above and references [22,45]) policy improves farmers' awareness of environmental protection policies, thus promoting their enthusiasm to adopt environment-friendly technologies because farmers will adjust their production behavior according to agricultural subsidy policies [46]. Thus, the study put forward Hypothesis 3 as (H3) ecological compensation policy has a regulatory effect on farmers' capital endowment and ecological cognition.

3. Variables and Research Approaches

3.1. Variables

3.1.1. Dependent Variable

The dependent variables are "willingness to adopt" and "adoption" of environment-friendly technologies. The measurement of "willingness to adopt" uses the binary valuation method. To measure the "adoption" of environment-friendly technology, the values are 1–3 according to the number of types adopted by farmers to reduce application efficiency technology, green prevention and control technology, and soil improvement technology. If the farmers adopt any two or more of the above three technologies, the willingness to adopt environment-friendly technologies is relatively positive, and the value is 1. On the contrary, it is not active enough to adopt environment-friendly technology if the value is 0. Thus, the farmers' willingness to adopt environment-friendly technologies indicates their views for the ecological management of orchards, and the degree of adoption of environment-friendly technologies indicates the efficiency of technology adoption.

3.1.2. Independent Variables

This paper selects age, education, labor force, and duration of farming as the human aspects of capital endowment, which comprises exploring the local and international scholars within similar approaches (for more details, please see references [47–49]). In addition, the study selects planting scale, quality of agricultural pieces of machinery, income, and specialization as a material aspect of the capital endowment. Meanwhile, the respondents' cognition on the harm of excessive fertilization, the cognition of soil environmental protection policy, and the cognition of environment-friendly technology to improve the ecological environment was selected to represent the ecological cognition.

3.1.3. Moderating Variables

This paper selects the impact of ecological compensation policy as the moderating variable. The attitude and willingness of farmers to adopt environment-friendly technology will affect the ecological compensation policy and its implementation after technology adoption. We can learn from the relevant research results of Zhang Yu et al. [50] and Huang Xiaohui et al. [51]. The influence of compensation policy is represented by the degree of understanding, the satisfaction with ecological compensation policy, and the benefit to ecological compensation policy. The definition and descriptive statistics of variables are shown in Table 1.

3.1.4. Research Approaches

Theoretically, in terms of adopting environment-friendly technology, in most cases, farmers will face a dilemmatic situation of whether they are willing to adopt it or not [52–54]. Previous studies mainly involved the issue of willingness to adapt [55–57], but not enough attention was paid to the degree of the farmer's adoption intentions. From the perspective of subjective adoption intention, the first issue is whether the farmers are willing to adopt environment-friendly technologies, and if the farmers' subjective willingness is not favorable, they will not fully adopt the three environment-friendly technologies. While the Heckman two-stage model can control the selectivity deviation caused by unobservable factors [58,59], it can deal with effect evaluation based on binary selection [60,61]. Therefore, this paper uses Heckman sampling to solve effect evaluation based on binary selection, as suggested by Lambrecht et al. [62].

Table 1. Variable definition and descriptive statistics.

Variables	Meaning and Assignment	AVG	Standard Deviation	Minimum	Maximum
Dependent variable					
Y1: The willingness	Adopting (two or more) positive = 1; otherwise = 0	0.51	0.49	0	1
Y2: Adaptation	Adoption	2.06	0.78	0	3
Capital endowment					
X1: Sex	F = 0; M = 1	0.37	0.48	0	1
X2: Age	By 2017	51.03	9.48	25	85
X3: Education	Years of education	7.64	5.22	0	11
X4: Duration of farming	Duration of farming	27.63	5.07	4	58
X5: Scale	AVG of the area in 2017	4.13	0.48	1	12
X6: Labor	Labors in family	3	1.49	0	12
X7: Machinery	Machinery	0.48	0.65	0	4
X8: Family income	income in 2017	10.52	0.95	7.60	13.30
X9: Specialization	Proportion to total income in 2017	68.47	7.89	60	86
Ecological cognition					
X10: Awareness of the hazards of over chemicals use	Do not know = 1; have heard of = 2; know something = 3; know very well = 4	1.83	1.02	1	3
X11: Awareness of soil environmental protection policy	Do not know = 1; have heard of = 2; know something = 3; know very well = 4	2.53	0.70	1	3
X12: Awareness on effect of environment-friendly technology	No = 1; little effect = 2; large action = 3; great effect = 4	2.28	0.50	1	4
The Impact of Environmental Policy					
X13: Understanding of ecological policy	1 = totally do not understand, 2 = do not understand, 3 = general, 4 = understand, 5 = fully understand	3.38	0.87	2	5
X14: Satisfaction with ecological policy	1 = very dissatisfied, 2 = not very satisfied, 3 = general, 4 = satisfied, 5 = very satisfied	3.18	2.04	1	5
X15: Benefit	1 = significant decrease, 2 = slight decrease, 3 = constant, 4 = slight increase, 5 = obvious increase	3.42	0.98	1	5

Moreover, Heckman's two-stage model can effectively solve the two-stage characteristics [63,64] of environmentally friendly technology adoption and is conducive to unbiased estimation [65]. The specific steps of the study are as follows: in the first stage, a probit selection model is established. The probit selection model is used to estimate the possibility of selection bias and calculate the inverse mills ratio (IMR). The function of IMR is to calculate a value for each sample to correct the sample selection bias. If the IMR is greater than 0, it indicates a selective bias in the sample. In the second stage, the estimated IMR of the first stage is put into the regression model of the second stage together with other variables by using the selective sample observations. Thus, the selection model's self-selection problem was modified in the first stage and reflected by IMR in the second stage. After that, with the help of the Heckman sample selection model, the article estimates the farmers' subjective willingness to adopt environmentally friendly technology y_{1i} and the degree of farmers' adoption of environmentally friendly technology y_{2i} and verifies the hypothesis. On this basis, the study constitutes the interaction among the degree of ecological compensation, capital endowment, and ecological cognition to verify whether they significantly impact EFT adoption. Finally, the degree of farmers' understanding, satisfaction, and benefits of ecological compensation policy were calculated and averaged. Then, the average value was used as the grouping standard, and those below and above the average value were divided into a group to examine the regulatory role of ecological compensation policy and test its robustness.

Although Heckman's two-step selection model can effectively solve the endogenous problem caused by sample selection, it is very consistent with the two-stage technology adoption process [66]. However, there may still be data quality problems in data collection due to farmers' lack of cooperation, and the model itself cannot solve these problems [67]. In addition, another major limitation of this methodology is that it is unable to carry out extensive statistical inference, the research sample is based on a specific region, and the research object is relatively single [68]. Finally, Heckman's two-step selection model can only solve the endogenous problem caused by sample selection but cannot solve missing variables and reverse causality caused by other possible factors [69].

The sample selection model is used to deal with the above problems, which is as follows:

$$y_{1i} = X_{1i}\alpha + \mu_{1i}; y_{1i} = \begin{cases} 1 & y_{1i}^* > 0 \\ 0 & y_{1i}^* \leq 0 \end{cases} \quad (1)$$

$$y_{2i} = X_{2i}\beta + \mu_{2i}; y_{2i} = \begin{cases} b & y_{1i} > 0 \\ 0 & y_{1i} \leq 0 \end{cases} \quad (2)$$

$$\begin{aligned} E(y_{2i}|y_{2i}=c) &= E(y_{2i}|y_{1i}^* > 0) = E(X_{2i}\beta + \mu_{2i}|X_{1j}\alpha + \mu_{1i} > 0) \\ &= E(X_{2i}\beta + \mu_{2i}|\mu_{1i} > -X_{1i}\alpha) = X_{2i}\beta + E(\mu_{2i}|\mu_{1i} > -X_{1i}\alpha) \\ &= X_{2i}\beta + \rho\sigma\mu_2\lambda(-X_{1i}\alpha) \end{aligned} \quad (3)$$

Equation (1) represents the selection equation, and Equation (2) represents the resulting equation. Where i represents the number of the grower; y_{1i} represents the willingness to adopt environmentally friendly technologies; y_{2i} represents the degree of adoption of technologies, which are the dependent variable; X_{1i} and X_{2i} are the independent variables of the two equations; y_{1i}^* is latent variables that cannot be observed; b indicates that several technologies were adopted. The selection mechanism is as follows: only when $y_{1i}^* > 0$, y_{2i} can be observed. Meanwhile, α and β are the parameters to be estimated μ_{1i} and μ_{2i} are residual, consistent with the normal distribution.

The conditional expectation of farmers' adoption of environment-friendly technology is as follows:

In (3), where λ is the inverse mills ratio function. While ρ is the coefficient of correlation of y_{1i} and y_{2i}, when $\rho = 0$, it means that y_{2i} it will not be affected by y_{1i}, and when $\neq 0$, y_{2i} will be affected by y_{1i}. Therefore, there is an ample selection bias, σ denotes the standard deviation.

4. Results and Analysis

4.1. Impact Analysis of Farmer's Willingness to Adopt Environment-Friendly Technologies

The estimated results in Table 2 show that the ownership of agricultural machinery, the cognition of environment-friendly technology to improve the ecological environment, and the understanding of farmers' ecological compensation policy have passed the positive significance test of 10%. It shows that the more agricultural machinery owned by farmers in the capital endowment, the higher the intensity of adopting environment-friendly technology. In ecological cognition, the higher the awareness of environment-friendly technology to improve the ecological conditions, the easier it is to adopt environment-friendly technology, which further leads farmers to improve the ecological environment of the orchard. As for the impact of ecological compensation policy, farmers are more likely to adopt environment-friendly technology to improve the ecological environment. Farmers' understanding of ecological compensation policies positively affects their willingness to adopt environment-friendly technologies. Farmers need to pay a specific cost to adopt environmentally friendly technologies. If they cannot get the compensation, farmers' views to adopt environment-friendly technologies will be affected. Therefore, understanding and mastering the ecological compensation policies can promote them to adopt environment-friendly technologies.

Table 2. Model regression results.

Variable	Willingness to Adopt		Degree of Adoption	
	Coefficient	Standard Error	Coefficient	Standard Error
x1 Sex	−0.214	0.150	−0.082	0.075
x2 Age	−0.006	0.008	−0.002	0.004
x3 Education	0.036	0.021	0.003	0.009
x4 Duration of farming	0.005	0.012	0.034	0.005
x5 Scale	−0.012	0.046	0.002 *	0.020
x6 Labor	−0.076	0.047	0.011	0.026
x7 Machinery	0.138 *	0.080	0.019	0.040
x8 Family income	0.011	0.078	0.059 *	0.035
x9 Specialization	−0.005	0.010	0.011 ***	0.004
x10: Awareness of excessive use	−0.011	0.072	−0.036	0.031
x11: Awareness of soil protection policy	0.140	0.103	0.215	0.052
x12: Awareness on improving effect	0.113 *	0.146	0.019	0.069
x13: Awareness of ecological compensation	0.111 *	0.082	0.053 *	0.040
x14: Satisfaction with ecological compensation	−0.072	0.080	−0.057	0.038
x15: Satisfaction with ecological compensation	0.083	0.076	0.015	0.037
x13: Awareness of ecological compensation * x5 Scale	—	—	0.029 *	0.020
x13: Awareness of ecological compensation * x8 Family income	—	—	0.042 *	0.155
x13: Awareness of ecological compensation * x9 Specialization	—	—	0.011 *	0.017
x13: Awareness of ecological compensation * Awareness of soil protection policy	—	—	0.277 *	0.151
x13: Awareness of ecological compensation * x12: Awareness on improving effect	—	—	0.302 *	0.166
The constant	1.295	1.306	1.694 ***	0.575
Log-likelihood	−440.6671			
Wald chi2(15)		22.41		

Note: *, **, and *** represent significant at 10%, 5% and 1% confidence levels, respectively.

4.2. Analysis of the Impact of the Adoption of Environment-Friendly Technologies

From the adoption degree perspective, the planting scale, family income level, and a specialization degree in capital endowment have significant positive effects on farmers' adoption of environment-friendly technologies. The larger the planting scale is for adopters, the higher the utilization efficiency of adopting environment-friendly technologies will be, and the adoption cost will be relatively reduced. In contrast, the high family income level has been found crucial for farmers to adopt environment-friendly technologies. If the farmer possessed higher income and specialized farming, the more likely they could be willing to adopt the environment-friendly technology [21,70,71]. Thus, Hypothesis 1 holds, but Hypothesis 2 has not been quantified. Besides, the understanding degree of ecological compensation policy significantly positively affects the adoption degree of farmers' environment-friendly technology [22,72]. It indicates that an acceptable ecological compensation policy can enhance farmers' willingness to adopt environment-friendly technology and help to improve the degree of farmers' adoption of environment-friendly technology. From the perspective of the interaction between ecological compensation policy and farmers' capital endowment and ecological cognition, the interaction coefficient of farmers understanding of ecological compensation and planting scale, family income level and specialization degree, soil environmental protection policy cognition, and environmental improvement effect cognition all have a positive impact on the adoption of environment-friendly technology at the level of 10%. The results show that the ecological compensation policy has a specific moderating effect on farmers' capital endowment and ecological cognition.

5. Discussion

To further verify the robustness of the estimation results, this paper measures the ecological compensation policy variables and calculates the average value of the impact of ecological compensation policy on farmers by calculating the degree of understanding, satisfaction, and benefits of ecological compensation policy, which are parallel with Zhang Yu et al. [50] and Huang Xiaohui et al. [51]. Then, the average values are used as the grouping standard, and the groups below the average value and higher than the average value are divided into a group. The Heckman model was then used to quantify the influence of capital endowment and ecological cognition on the willingness and degree of adoption of environment-friendly technology in the two groups. Finally, the ecological compensation policy's regulatory effect was investigated by examining the significant changes of different variable coefficients in the two groups [45,46,73]. The specific analysis results are shown in Table 3.

Table 3. Regression results of the robustness test.

Variable	High Group on Ecological Compensation		Low Group on Ecological Compensation	
	Willingness to Adopt	Degree	Willingness to Adopt	Degree
	Coefficient	Coefficient	Coefficient	Coefficient
X5: Scale	0.008 *	0.035 **	−0.002	0.032 *
	(0.016)	(0.208)	(0.074)	(0.020)
X7: Machinery	0.137 **	0.012	0.116	0.052
	(0.210)	(0.056)	(0.144)	(0.056)
lnX8: Family income	0.028	0.042 **	−0.160	−0.013
	(0.100)	(0.247)	(0.133)	(0.055)
X9: Specialization	0.009	0.008 **	−0.016	0.004 **
	(0.013)	(0.206)	(0.017)	(0.007)
X12: Cognition of improving environmental effect	0.078 **	0.087 *	−0.030	0. 017
	(0.019)	(0.012)	(0.252)	(0. 016)
The constant	−0.361	2.124 **	6.272 **	0.236
	(1.767)	(0.876)	(2.518)	(1.082)
Log likelihood	−266.0604		−177.2996	
Wald chi2(15)		24.46		27.46

Note: *, **, and *** represent significant at 10%, 5% and 1% confidence levels.

From the perspective of capital endowment, the group estimation results show that the influence coefficient of planting scale, family income level, and specialization degree on farmer's adoption of environment-friendly technology has passed the significance test of 5%, and the regression results are consistent with the estimation results as shown in Table 2. Further, the coefficients of the ecological compensation policy are affected by the more extensive the scale of planting area, the higher the level of family income and the degree of specialization of farmers, the higher the enthusiasm of farmers to adopt environment-friendly technology, and the more comfortable to benefit from the ecological compensation policy, which is supported by Zhang et al. [74], Liu et al. [75] and Ke-Guo [76].

Seemingly, from the perspective of ecological cognition, the improved cognition effect of environment-friendly technology has a significant impact on farmers' adoption of environment-friendly technology at the level of 10%, and the coefficient level of the high group is affected by the ecological compensation policy greater than that of the low group. It further verifies that the ecological compensation policy has a certain regulatory effect on farmers' ecological cognition. Thus, the findings are verified by the study of Cai and Zhang [77], Home et al. [78], and Xuehai et al. [79]. However, it is worth noting that farmers' ecological cognition has no significant impact on adopting environment-friendly technologies. This shows that the ecological compensation policy is conducive to help the majority of farmers to improve their awareness regarding improving the ecological environment [80–82]. Only if most farmers can acquire benefit from the process of technology adoption will they be attracted more towards the positive impact on the improvement of environment-friendly technology adoption in the future [78,83]. The assumption is also supported by Yuanquan and Wangsheng [84] and Dezdar [85]. Therefore, the government should continue to strengthen the ecological compensation policy and provide full support to enhance the awareness-building activities such as training facilities, boost the demonstration process, and massive circulation of the advantages of new and improved eco-friendly technologies.

6. Conclusions

The environmentally friendly technology adoption may crucial for fostering sustainable development goals set by the United Nations (UN). The adoption decision is a complex and dynamic phenomenon that could be affected by several factors. As per the core economic thought, farmers could adopt the EFT if they possessed enough capital endowment and the possibilities of economic benefit. Moreover, the proactive policy supports may also have significant impacts to improve the adoption tendencies. Within these circumstances, the article has been quantified by three pillars—capital endowment, ecological cognition, and ecological compensation policy and evaluated the impacts of those to foster environmentally friendly technology under the premise of maximizing profit. More specifically, the article explored the impacts of capital endowment and ecological cognition for facilitating EFT employing green preventions and control, efficient soil improvement, and low input production technologies. It also evaluated the underlying factors of human and material aspects of capital endowments for EFT adoption. Further, it also covered the factors associated with adoption willingness and degree of adoption to understand better the willingness and the actual adoption intensity of EFT.

The article utilized a dataset of 471 apple farmers extracted from a survey from nine counties of Shandong province to craft its findings. Overall, farmers positively responded to adopting environment-friendly technologies. However, there were significant differences in adopting the three kinds of environment-friendly technologies. The soil improvement technology was triggered the highest by comprising the adoption level of 87.26%, the middle rate of application was found for reduction and efficiency enhancement technology (54.26%). However, the lowest was found at 18.47% in terms of green pest control and management technologies. Whereas 52.02% of farmers adopted two kinds of environment-friendly technologies, 23.99% of farmers adopted three environment-friendly technologies. The study traces a positive connection between capital endowment and ecological cognition and reveals significant moderating effects of ecological compensation policy for facilitating EFT. From the perspective of capital endowment, the planting scale, family income level, and specialization degree have significant positive effects on adopting environment-friendly technology. The understanding of ecological compensation policy has a significant positive impact on farmers' adoption of environment-friendly technology. Hence, the article's findings will help formulate and implement relevant agricultural policies as it provided a theoretical basis for adopting environment-friendly technologies for orchards, especially apple farmers. Furthermore, this article is helpful to further research to understand the mechanism of the adoption of environmentally friendly technologies.

This paper draws the following policy recommendations: (i) as human capital is an integrated part of the capital endowment, the human capital empowering tactics such as training and demonstration facilities should be extended. Furthermore, to improve the farmer's materials aspects of capital endowment, modern machinery and improved technologies should be introduced to harness the potentialities of modern science and technology. (ii) It is necessary to strengthen the information circulating facilities and education regarding rural non-point source pollution and the hazards of those within rural communities, to improve the cognitive level of the majority of farmers to participate in green development. Awareness-building campaigns should also be implemented to make farmers fully realize the importance of adopting environment-friendly technology in improving the ecological environment of the orchard, improving land fertility, and improving fruit quality. In addition, the potentialities of EFT should be highlighted among rural farmers, which will eventually improve the cognition level of farmers. (iii) Ecological compensation should be utilized by extending the existing agricultural subsidy policy for green development. Especially, instead of providing chemical fertilizer subsidies, the government should implement rewards programs for those who intend to or already utilize organic-based fertilizers and pesticides. (iv) The financial institutions and farmer's organizations such as agricultural cooperatives should provide more financial support introducing new and innovative technologies, which could play a significant role in shaping cognition and improving access towards material aspects of capital endowments. Productivity may be increased by using environmentally friendly technology, which is also viable towards the farm's profitability. Not essentially all the profitable technologies must be adopted by the farmers since barriers to practice innovative technologies and market uncertainty for environmental attributes interlinked with green technologies limit their effectiveness. The adoption and diffusion of alternative practices are also influenced by the factors such as the size of the farm, economic risk, and geographical location. It should be one of the crucial issues for policy consideration.

Apart from the monetary tools (direct subsidies), the government should emphasize indirect subsidies (insurance, low-interest loans, accelerated depreciation, rent rebates). The direct and indirect benefits of environmentally friendly technology, such as enhancing the ecological environment and biodiversity of the orchard, improving soil fertility and fruit quality, should also be highlighted and demonstrated among the farmers. Moreover, a sound interaction of e-commerce and value chain network facilities should also be implemented to make farmers fully utilize the betterment of modern science and technology. The social supports and obligations should also be prioritized, aligned with the other monetary incentives. The formal and informal risk-sharing organizations should also prioritize their scheme regarding risk minimizations and diffusions. This might be helpful to improve the cognition level and willingness of farmers to adopt environment-friendly technology.

Although the study revealed that the ecological compensation policy is helpful to trigger the majority of fruit growers to improve their understanding regarding EFT, how and to what extent the compensation policy triggers the adoption of EFT should be explored more distinctively. For example, if potential researchers could have traced whether there are any specific effects of several subsidies (subsidies per hectors or subsidies regarding modern equipment) for adopting EFT. Furthermore, the study focuses only on a single region with specific types of farmers; if more depth studies with several regions are combined, it would be more interesting. In addition, the social network will have a certain impact on the adoption of environment-friendly technology by influencing farmers' information acquisition; the potential researchers should include this crucial factor into the core variable. Finally, as there are differences in the suitable orchard planting environment and planting scale of various environment-friendly technologies, further studies should trigger the specific planting environment and planting scale of various environment-friendly technologies combined with the social network in the future.

Author Contributions: Conceptualization H.W. and X.W.; data curation H.W. and X.W.; formal analysis H.W. and F.Z.; investigation H.W. and X.W.; resources A.S. and F.Z.; software H.W. and A.S.; validation H.W., X.W. and A.S.; writing—original draft H.W., X.W. and A.S.; writing—reviewing and editing A.S., X.W. and F.Z.; funding acquisition F.Z. and H.W.; resources and supervision F.Z. All authors have read and agreed to the published version of the manuscript.

Funding: This research was funded by (i) "Research on Multidimensional Control Mechanism of Quality and Safety of Fruits and Vegetables Agricultural Products in the Context of the Internet (No.: ZR2018MG013), the program of Shandong 434 provincial natural fund" (ii) Research on the Realization Path of Enabling High-quality Development of Agriculture in 436 Shandong Province, (No.: 20CSDJ44), the project of social science planning and research of Shandong Province. (iii) Research on demand induction mechanism of Conservation Tillage Technology: organizational support, inter-temporal selection, and incentive effect (No.: 7197030867), The program of National Natural Science Foundation of China.

Institutional Review Board Statement: As the study does not involve any personal data and the respondent was well aware that they can opt-out anytime during the data collection phase, any written institutional review board statement is not required.

Informed Consent Statement: As the study does not involve any personal data and the respondent was well aware that they can opt-out anytime during the data collection phase, any written Informed Consent Statement is not required.

Data Availability Statement: The associated dataset of the study is available upon request to the corresponding author.

Acknowledgments: The author(s), are grateful to Asfikur Rahman, faculty member, School of Social Science, Khulna University, and Saleh Mohammad Shariar, College of Economics and Management, Northwest A&F University, for critically reviewing the study and valuable inputs for improving the quality of the study. We extend our gratitude to Rob Gilles, Queens Management School, Queens University Belfast, for the help with the study's presentation improvement.

Conflicts of Interest: The authors declare no conflict of interest.

References

1. Zuo, L.; Zhang, Z.; Carlson, K.M.; MacDonald, G.K.; Brauman, K.A.; Liu, Y.; Zhang, W.; Zhang, H.; Wu, W.; Zhao, X.; et al. Progress towards Sustainable Intensification in China Challenged by Land-Use Change. *Nat. Sustain.* **2018**, *1*, 304–313. [CrossRef]
2. Wang, X.; Dou, Z.; Shi, X.; Zou, C.; Liu, D.; Wang, Z.; Guan, X.; Sun, Y.; Wu, G.; Zhang, B.; et al. Innovative Management Programme Reduces Environmental Impacts in Chinese Vegetable Production. *Nat. Food* **2021**, *2*, 47–53. [CrossRef]
3. Veeck, G.; Veeck, A.; Yu, H. Challenges of Agriculture and Food Systems Issues in China and the United States. *Geogr. Sustain.* **2020**, *1*, 109–117. [CrossRef]
4. Smith, E.; Klein, K.K. Development and Adoption of Dryland Cropping Technologies in Hebei Province of Northern China. *Can. J. Agric. Econ. Rev. Can. Dagroecon.* **2000**, *48*, 573–583. [CrossRef]
5. Huang, W.; Jiang, L. Efficiency Performance of Fertilizer Use in Arable Agricultural Production in China. *China Agric. Econ. Rev.* **2019**, *11*, 52–69. [CrossRef]
6. Hu, Y.; Su, M.; Wang, Y.; Cui, S.; Meng, F.; Yue, W.; Liu, Y.; Xu, C.; Yang, Z. Food Production in China Requires Intensified Measures to Be Consistent with National and Provincial Environmental Boundaries. *Nat. Food* **2020**, *1*, 572–582. [CrossRef]
7. Bryan, B.A.; Gao, L.; Ye, Y.; Sun, X.; Connor, J.D.; Crossman, N.D.; Stafford-Smith, M.; Wu, J.; He, C.; Yu, D.; et al. China's Response to a National Land-System Sustainability Emergency. *Nature* **2018**, *559*, 193–204. [CrossRef]
8. El Bilali, H.; Allahyari, M.S. Transition towards Sustainability in Agriculture and Food Systems: Role of Information and Communication Technologies. *Inf. Process. Agric.* **2018**, *5*, 456–464. [CrossRef]
9. Selvi, S.; Karthikeyan, R.; Vanitha, U. Organic Farming: Technology for Environment-Friendly Agriculture. In Proceedings of the IEEE-International Conference On Advances In Engineering, Science And Management (ICAESM-2012), Nagapattinam, India, 30–31 March 2012; pp. 132–136.
10. Pretty, J.; Benton, T.G.; Bharucha, Z.P.; Dicks, L.V.; Flora, C.B.; Godfray, H.C.J.; Goulson, D.; Hartley, S.; Lampkin, N.; Morris, C.; et al. Global Assessment of Agricultural System Redesign for Sustainable Intensification. *Nat. Sustain.* **2018**, *1*, 441–446. [CrossRef]
11. Frank, S.; Havlík, P.; Stehfest, E.; van Meijl, H.; Witzke, P.; Pérez-Domínguez, I.; van Dijk, M.; Doelman, J.C.; Fellmann, T.; Koopman, J.F.L.; et al. Agricultural Non-CO_2 Emission Reduction Potential in the Context of the 1.5 °C Target. *Nat. Clim. Chang.* **2019**, *9*, 66–72. [CrossRef]
12. Eisenstein, M. Natural Solutions for Agricultural Productivity. *Nature* **2020**, *588*, S58–S59. [CrossRef]

13. Hofmann, T.; Lowry, G.V.; Ghoshal, S.; Tufenkji, N.; Brambilla, D.; Dutcher, J.R.; Gilbertson, L.M.; Giraldo, J.P.; Kinsella, J.M.; Landry, M.P.; et al. Technology Readiness and Overcoming Barriers to Sustainably Implement Nanotechnology-Enabled Plant Agriculture. *Nat. Food* **2020**, *1*, 416–425. [CrossRef]
14. Horton, P.; Long, S.P.; Smith, P.; Banwart, S.A.; Beerling, D.J. Technologies to Deliver Food and Climate Security through Agriculture. *Nat. Plants* **2021**, *7*, 250–255. [CrossRef] [PubMed]
15. Scialabba, N.E.-H. *Greening the Economy with Agriculture*; FAO: Rome, Italy, 2012.
16. Kliestik, T.; Valaskova, K.; Nica, E.; Kovacova, M.; Lazaroiu, G. Advanced Methods of Earnings Management: Monotonic Trends and Change-Points under Spotlight in the Visegrad Countries. *Oeconomia Copernic.* **2020**, *11*, 371–400. [CrossRef]
17. Bukchin, S.; Kerret, D. Character Strengths and Sustainable Technology Adoption by Smallholder Farmers. *Heliyon* **2020**, *6*, e04694. [CrossRef]
18. Grzelak, A.; Guth, M.; Matuszczak, A.; Czyżewski, B.; Brelik, A. Approaching the Environmental Sustainable Value in Agriculture: How Factor Endowments Foster the Eco-Efficiency. *J. Clean. Prod.* **2019**, *241*, 118304. [CrossRef]
19. Wang, H.; Sarkar, A.; Qian, L. Evaluations of the Roles of Organizational Support, Organizational Norms and Organizational Learning for Adopting Environmentally Friendly Technologies: A Case of Kiwifruit Farmers' Cooperatives of Meixian, China. *Land* **2021**, *10*, 284. [CrossRef]
20. Wang, N.; Gao, Y.; Wang, Y.; Li, X. Adoption of Eco-Friendly Soil-Management Practices by Smallholder Farmers in Shandong Province of China. *Soil Sci. Plant Nutr.* **2016**, *62*, 185–193. [CrossRef]
21. Srivara Buddhi Bhuvaneswari, S. Eco-Friendly Technologies in Vegetable Cultivation-Farmers' Awareness, Knowledge, Adoption and Attitude. *Madras Agric. J.* **2005**, *92*, 132–137.
22. Liu, M.; Xiong, Y.; Yuan, Z.; Min, Q.; Sun, Y.; Fuller, A.M. Standards of Ecological Compensation for Traditional Eco-Agriculture: Taking Rice-Fish System in Hani Terrace as an Example. *J. Mt. Sci.* **2014**, *11*, 1049–1059. [CrossRef]
23. Barnes, A.P.; Soto, I.; Eory, V.; Beck, B.; Balafoutis, A.T.; Sanchez, B.; Vangeyte, J.; Fountas, S.; van der Wal, T.; Gomez-Barbero, M. Influencing Factors and Incentives on the Intention to Adopt Precision Agricultural Technologies within Arable Farming Systems. *Environ. Sci. Policy* **2018**, *93*, 66–74. [CrossRef]
24. Zhou, S.; Herzfeld, T.; Glauben, T.; Zhang, Y.; Hu, B. Factors Affecting Chinese Farmers' Decisions to Adopt a Water-Saving Technology. *Can. J. Agric. Econ. Rev. Can. Dagroecon.* **2008**, *56*, 51–61. [CrossRef]
25. Ma, J.; Li, X.; Wen, H.; Fu, Z.; Zhang, L. A Key Frame Extraction Method for Processing Greenhouse Vegetables Production Monitoring Video. *Comput. Electron. Agric.* **2015**, *111*, 92–102. [CrossRef]
26. Suri, T. Selection and Comparative Advantage in Technology Adoption. *Econometrica* **2011**, *79*, 159–209. [CrossRef]
27. Kaine, G.; Bewsell, D. Adoption of Integrated Pest Management by Apple Growers: The Role of Context. *Int. J. Pest Manag.* **2008**, *54*, 255–265. [CrossRef]
28. Bukchin, S.; Kerret, D. Food for Hope: The Role of Personal Resources in Farmers' Adoption of Green Technology. *Sustainability* **2018**, *10*, 1615. [CrossRef]
29. Zeng, Y.; Zhang, J.; He, K.; Cheng, L. Who Cares What Parents Think or Do? Observational Learning and Experience-Based Learning through Communication in Rice Farmers' Willingness to Adopt Sustainable Agricultural Technologies in Hubei Province, China. *Environ. Sci. Pollut. Res.* **2019**, *26*, 12522–12536. [CrossRef] [PubMed]
30. Lordan, J.; Gomez, M.; Francescatto, P.; Robinson, T.L. Long-Term Effects of Tree Density and Tree Shape on Apple Orchard Performance, a 20 Year Study—Part 2, Economic Analysis. *Sci. Hortic.* **2019**, *244*, 435–444. [CrossRef]
31. Adnan, N.; Nordin, S.M.; Bahruddin, M.A.; Tareq, A.H. A State-of-the-Art Review on Facilitating Sustainable Agriculture through Green Fertilizer Technology Adoption: Assessing Farmers Behavior. *Trends Food Sci. Technol.* **2019**, *86*, 439–452. [CrossRef]
32. Tal, A. Making Conventional Agriculture Environmentally Friendly: Moving beyond the Glorification of Organic Agriculture and the Demonization of Conventional Agriculture. *Sustainability* **2018**, *10*, 1078. [CrossRef]
33. Zhao, Z.; Yin, Z.; Yang, P. Advances in the applications of green crop pest control techniques. *Plant Prot.* **2011**, *37*, 29–32.
34. Kim, D.; Park, K. An Environmentally Friendly Soil Improvement Technology with Microorganism. *Int. J. Railw.* **2013**, *6*, 90–94. [CrossRef]
35. Rajabi Agereh, S.; Kiani, F.; Khavazi, K.; Rouhipour, H.; Khormali, F. An Environmentally Friendly Soil Improvement Technology for Sand and Dust Storms Control. *Environ. Health Eng. Manag. J.* **2019**, *6*, 63–71. [CrossRef]
36. Jian, C. The Effect Analysis of Fund Loan on Adoption of Agricultural Technology under the Condition of Different Capital Endowment. *Forum Sci. Technol. China* **2013**, *10*, 93–98.
37. Eor, M.K. Analysis of the Factor Endowments and Agricultural Trade for Economic Cooperation in Northeast Asia. *East Asian Econ. Rev.* **2004**, *8*, 143–167. [CrossRef]
38. Anik, A.R.; Rahman, S.; Sarker, J.R. Agricultural Productivity Growth and the Role of Capital in South Asia (1980–2013). *Sustainability* **2017**, *9*, 470. [CrossRef]
39. Alavion, S.J.; Allahyari, M.S.; Al-Rimawi, A.S.; Surujlal, J. Adoption of Agricultural E-Marketing: Application of the Theory of Planned Behavior. *J. Int. Food Agribus. Mark.* **2017**, *29*, 1–15. [CrossRef]
40. Gustafson, C.R.; Nganje, W.E. Value of Social Capital to Mid-Sized Northern Plains Farms. *Can. J. Agric. Econ. Rev. Can. Dagroeconomie* **2006**, *54*, 421–438. [CrossRef]
41. Deng, Z.; Zhang, J.; Xu, Z. Research on Farmers' Cognition and Behavior Response in Rural Living Environment Improvement—Taking the Main Rice Production Area of Dongting Lake Wetland Reserve As An Example. *J. Agric. Econ.* **2013**, 72–79.

42. Liu, Z.; Zhou, J. Information Capability, Environmental Risk Perception and Farmers' Adoption of Pro-Environmental Behavior: An Empirical Test Based on Broiler Farmers in Liaoning Province. *J. Agric. Econ.* **2018**, 135–144.
43. Atinkut, H.B.; Yan, T.; Zhang, F.; Qin, S.; Gai, H.; Liu, Q. Cognition of Agriculture Waste and Payments for a Circular Agriculture Model in Central China. *Sci. Rep.* **2020**, *10*, 10826. [CrossRef]
44. Rude, J.; Weersink, A. The Potential for Cross-Compliance in Canadian Agricultural Policy: Linking Environmental Goals with Business Risk Management Programs. *Can. J. Agric. Econ. Rev. Can. Dagroecon.* **2018**, *66*, 359–377. [CrossRef]
45. Hu, Y.; Huang, J.; Hou, L. Impacts of the Grassland Ecological Compensation Policy on Household Livestock Production in China: An Empirical Study in Inner Mongolia. *Ecol. Econ.* **2019**, *161*, 248–256. [CrossRef]
46. Huang, X.; Lu, Q.; Wang, L.; Cui, M.; Yang, F. Does Aging and Off-Farm Employment Hinder Farmers' Adoption Behavior of Soil and Water Conservation Technology in the Loess Plateau? *Int. J. Clim. Chang. Strateg. Manag.* **2020**, *12*, 92–107. [CrossRef]
47. Bhaumik, S.K.; Dimova, R. Does Human Capital Endowment of Foreign Direct Investment Recipient Countries Really Matter? Evidence from Cross-Country Firm Level Data. *Rev. Dev. Econ.* **2013**, *17*, 559–570. [CrossRef]
48. Ju, J.; Lin, J.Y.; Wang, Y. Endowment Structures, Industrial Dynamics, and Economic Growth. *J. Monet. Econ.* **2015**, *76*, 244–263. [CrossRef]
49. Rosochatecká, E.; Tomšík, K.; Žídková, D. Selected Problems of Capital Endowment of Czech Agriculture. *Agric. Econ.* **2008**, *54*, 108–116. [CrossRef]
50. Zhang, Y.; Qi, Z.; Meng, X.; Zhang, D.; Wu, L. Study on the Influence of Family Endowments on the Environmental Behavior of Massive Pig Farmers Under the Situation of Ecological Compensation Policy: Based on the Survey of 248 Massive Pig Farmers in Hubei Province. *Issues Agric. Econ.* **2015**, *6*, 82–91.
51. Huang, X.; Wang, L.; Lu, Q. Farmers' cognition, government Support and Farmers' soil and Water Conservation Technology Adoption in Loess Plateau. *J. Arid. Land Resour. Environ.* **2019**, *12*, 21–25.
52. Razzaghi Borkhani, F.; Mohammadi, Y. Perceived Outcomes of Good Agricultural Practices (GAPs) Technologies Adoption in Citrus Farms of Iran (Reflection of Environment-Friendly Technologies). *Environ. Sci. Pollut. Res.* **2019**, *26*, 6829–6838. [CrossRef]
53. Hall, T.J.; Dennis, J.H.; Lopez, R.G.; Marshall, M.I. Factors Affecting Growers' Willingness to Adopt Sustainable Floriculture Practices. *HortScience* **2009**, *44*, 1346–1351. [CrossRef]
54. Abbas, T.; Ali, G.; Adil, S.A.; Bashir, M.K.; Kamran, M.A. Economic Analysis of Biogas Adoption Technology by Rural Farmers: The Case of Faisalabad District in Pakistan. *Renew. Energy* **2017**, *107*, 431–439. [CrossRef]
55. Feng, L.; Xu, J. Farmers' Willingness to Participate in the Next-Stage Grain-for-Green Project in the Three Gorges Reservoir Area, China. *Environ. Manag.* **2015**, *56*, 505–518. [CrossRef]
56. Channa, H.; Chen, A.Z.; Pina, P.; Ricker-Gilbert, J.; Stein, D. What Drives Smallholder Farmers' Willingness to Pay for a New Farm Technology? Evidence from an Experimental Auction in Kenya. *Food Policy* **2019**, *85*, 64–71. [CrossRef] [PubMed]
57. Memon, J.A.; Alizai, M.Q.; Hussain, A. Who Will Think Outside the Sink? Farmers' Willingness to Invest in Technologies for Groundwater Sustainability in Pakistan. *Environ. Dev. Sustain.* **2020**, *22*, 4425–4445. [CrossRef]
58. Wang, H.; Yu, F.; Reardon, T.; Huang, J.; Rozelle, S. Social Learning and Parameter Uncertainty in Irreversible Investments: Evidence from Greenhouse Adoption in Northern China. *China Econ. Rev.* **2013**, *27*, 104–120. [CrossRef]
59. Tilahun, U.; Bedemo, A. Farmers' Perception and Adaptation to Climate Change: Heckman's Two Stage Sample Selection Model. *Ethiop. J. Environ. Stud. Manag.* **2014**, *7*, 832–839. [CrossRef]
60. Esfandiari, M.; Mirzaei Khalilabad, H.R.; Boshrabadi, H.M.; Mehrjerdi, M.R.Z. Factors Influencing the Use of Adaptation Strategies to Climate Change in Paddy Lands of Kamfiruz, Iran. *Land Use Policy* **2020**, *95*, 104628. [CrossRef]
61. Amfo, B.; Ali, E.B. Climate Change Coping and Adaptation Strategies: How Do Cocoa Farmers in Ghana Diversify Farm Income? *For. Policy Econ.* **2020**, *119*, 102265. [CrossRef]
62. Lambrecht, I.; Vanlauwe, B.; Merckx, R.; Maertens, M. Understanding the Process of Agricultural Technology Adoption: Mineral Fertilizer in Eastern DR Congo. *World Dev.* **2014**, *59*, 132–146. [CrossRef]
63. Rabbi, F.; Ahamad, R.; Ali, S.; Chandio, A.A.; Ahmad, W.; Ilyas, A.; Din, I.U. Determinants of Commercialization and Its Impact on the Welfare of Smallholder Rice Farmers by Using Heckman's Two-Stage Approach. *J. Saudi Soc. Agric. Sci.* **2019**, *18*, 224–233. [CrossRef]
64. Geniaux, G.; Martinetti, D. Heckman Two-Stage Spatial Models for Agricultural Land Use Change. In Proceedings of the AgroMed International Conference 2016, Avignon, France, 1–2 December 2016; p. 1.
65. Certo, S.T.; Busenbark, J.R.; Woo, H.; Semadeni, M. Sample Selection Bias and Heckman Models in Strategic Management Research. *Strateg. Manag. J.* **2016**, *37*, 2639–2657. [CrossRef]
66. Goldberger, A.S. Abnormal selection bias. In *Studies in Econometrics, Time Series, and Multivariate Statistics*; Karlin, S., Amemiya, T., Goodman, L.A., Eds.; Academic Press: Stanford, CA, USA, 1983; pp. 67–84. ISBN 978-0-12-398750-1.
67. Newey, W.; Powell, J.L.; Walker, J. Semiparametric Estimation of Selection Models: Some Empirical Results. *Am. Econ. Rev.* **1990**, *80*, 324–328.
68. Nawata, K. Estimation of Sample Selection Bias Models by the Maximum Likelihood Estimator and Heckman's Two-Step Estimator. *Econ. Lett.* **1994**, *45*, 33–40. [CrossRef]
69. Puhani, P. The Heckman Correction for Sample Selection and Its Critique. *J. Econ. Surv.* **2000**, *14*, 53–68. [CrossRef]
70. Luthra, S.; Kumar, S.; Kharb, R.; Ansari, M.D.F.; Shimmi, S.L. Adoption of Smart Grid Technologies: An Analysis of Interactions among Barriers. *Renew. Sustain. Energy Rev.* **2014**, *33*, 554–565. [CrossRef]

71. Ali, E. Farm Households' Adoption of Climate-Smart Practices in Subsistence Agriculture: Evidence from Northern Togo. *Environ. Manag.* **2021**, *67*, 949–962. [CrossRef] [PubMed]
72. Gabel, V.M.; Home, R.; Stolze, M.; Birrer, S.; Steinemann, B.; Köpke, U. The Influence of On-Farm Advice on Beliefs and Motivations for Swiss Lowland Farmers to Implement Ecological Compensation Areas on Their Farms. *J. Agric. Educ. Ext.* **2018**, *24*, 233–248. [CrossRef]
73. Zhang, Y.; Qi, Z.; Meng, X. Impact of Family Resource Endowment on Environmental Behavior of Pig Farmers in the Context of Ecological Compensation Policy: Based on the Investigation of 248 Professional Farmers (Farms) in Hubei Province. *Issues Agric. Econ.* **2015**, *36*, 82–91.
74. Zhang, Q.; Hong, J.; Wu, F.; Yang, Y.; Dong, C. Gains or Losses? A Quantitative Estimation of Environmental and Economic Effects of an Ecological Compensation Policy. *Ecol. Appl.* **2021**, *31*, e2341. [CrossRef]
75. Liu, J.; Li, S.; Ouyang, Z.; Tam, C.; Chen, X. Ecological and Socioeconomic Effects of China's Policies for Ecosystem Services. *Proc. Natl. Acad. Sci. USA* **2008**, *105*, 9477–9482. [CrossRef]
76. Ke-guo, L.I. Reflections on Ecological Compensation Policy. *J. Environ. Manag. Coll. China* **2007**, *1*, 19–22.
77. Cai, Y.Y.; Zhang, A.L. Researching Progress and Trends of Agricultural Land's Ecological Compensation under Land Use Planning Control. *J. Nat. Resour.* **2010**, *5*, 868–880.
78. Home, R.; Balmer, O.; Jahrl, I.; Stolze, M.; Pfiffner, L. Motivations for Implementation of Ecological Compensation Areas on Swiss Lowland Farms. *J. Rural. Stud.* **2014**, *34*, 26–36. [CrossRef]
79. Ju, X.; Xue, Y.; Xi, B.; Jin, T.; Xu, Z.; Gao, S. Establishing an Agro-Ecological Compensation Mechanism to Promote Agricultural Green Development in China. *Jore* **2018**, *9*, 426–433. [CrossRef]
80. Zhang, Y.; Ji, Y.; Zhou, Y.; Sun, H. *Ecological Compensation Standard for Non-Point Pollution from Farmland*; Social Science Research Network: Rochester, NY, USA, 2017.
81. Ge, Y.; Wu, F.; Wang, B.; Liang, L. Valley Ecological Compensation: The Comparison and Selection between the Government Compensation and the Market Compensation. *J. Shandong Agric. Univ. (Soc. Sci. Ed.)* **2007**, *4*, 48–53.
82. Gebru, B.M.; Wang, S.W.; Kim, S.J.; Lee, W.-K. Socio-Ecological Niche and Factors Affecting Agroforestry Practice Adoption in Different Agroecologies of Southern Tigray, Ethiopia. *Sustainability* **2019**, *11*, 3729. [CrossRef]
83. He, K.; Zhang, J.; Wang, X.; Zeng, Y.; Zhang, L. A Scientometric Review of Emerging Trends and New Developments in Agricultural Ecological Compensation. *Environ. Sci. Pollut. Res.* **2018**, *25*, 16522–16532. [CrossRef] [PubMed]
84. Yuanquan, C.; Wangsheng, G. On the Principles and Decision-Making Model of Ecological Compensation for Agriculture. *Chin. Agric. Sci. Bull.* **2007**, *23*, 163–166.
85. Dezdar, S. Green Information Technology Adoption: Influencing Factors and Extension of Theory of Planned Behavior. *Soc. Responsib. J.* **2017**, *13*, 292–306. [CrossRef]

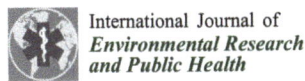

Article

Updating the Mediterranean Diet Pyramid towards Sustainability: Focus on Environmental Concerns

Lluís Serra-Majem [1,2,3,*], Laura Tomaino [1,4], Sandro Dernini [2,5], Elliot M. Berry [2,6], Denis Lairon [7], Joy Ngo de la Cruz [2], Anna Bach-Faig [8,9], Lorenzo M. Donini [10], Francesc-Xavier Medina [8], Rekia Belahsen [11], Suzanne Piscopo [12], Roberto Capone [13], Javier Aranceta-Bartrina [1,3,14], Carlo La Vecchia [4] and Antonia Trichopoulou [15]

1. Research Institute of Biomedical and Health Sciences, University of Las Palmas de Gran Canaria, and Complejo Hospitalario Universitario Insular—Materno Infantil (CHUIMI), Canarian Health Service, 35016 Las Palmas de Gran Canaria, Spain; laura.tomaino@unimi.it (L.T.); javieraranceta@gmail.com (J.A.-B.)
2. International Foundation of Mediterranean Diet, Nutrition Research Foundation, Barcelona Science Park, 08028 Barcelona, Spain; s.dernini@tiscali.it (S.D.); elliotb@ekmd.huji.ac.il (E.M.B.); alegria.ngo@gmail.com (J.N.d.l.C.)
3. CIBEROBN, Biomedical Research Networking Center for Physiopathology of Obesity and Nutrition, Instituto de Salud Carlos III, 28029 Madrid, Spain
4. Department of Clinical Medicine and Community Health (DISCCO), Università degli Studi di Milano, 20122 Milan, Italy; carlo.lavecchia@unimi.it
5. Forum on Mediterranean Food Cultures, 00148 Rome, Italy
6. Braun School of Public Health, Hebrew University Hadassah Medical School, 91120 Jerusalem, Israel
7. Human Nutrition, Aix Marseille University, INSERM, INRA, C2VN, 13005 Marseille, France; denis.lairon@orange.fr
8. FoodLab Research Group (2017SGR 83), Faculty of Health Sciences, Universitat Oberta de Catalunya (Open University of Catalonia, UOC), 08018 Barcelona, Spain; anbachf@gmail.com (A.B.-F.); fxmedina@uoc.edu (F.-X.M.)
9. Food and Nutrition Area, Barcelona Official College of Pharmacists, 08009 Barcelona, Spain
10. Department of Experimental Medicine, Sapienza University, 00136 Rome, Italy; lorenzomaria.donini@uniroma1.it
11. Training and Research Unit on Nutrition & Food Sciences, Biotechnology, Biochemistry & Nutrition Laboratory, Chouaib Doukkali University, El Jadida 24000, Morocco; belrekia@hotmail.com
12. Department of Health, Physical Education and Consumer Studies, Faculty of Education, University of Malta, MSD2080 Msida, Malta; suzanne.piscopo@um.edu.mt
13. International Center for Advanced Mediterranean Agronomic Studies (CIHEAM), 70010 Valenzano (Bari), Italy; capone@iamb.it
14. Department of Food Sciences and Physiology, University of Navarra, 31008 Pamplona, Spain
15. Hellenic Health Foundation, 11527 Athens, Greece; atrichopoulou@hhf-greece.gr
* Correspondence: lluis.serra@ulpgc.es

Received: 9 October 2020; Accepted: 23 November 2020; Published: 25 November 2020

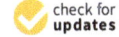

Abstract: Background: Nowadays the food production, supply and consumption chain represent a major cause of ecological pressure on the natural environment, and diet links worldwide human health with environmental sustainability. Food policy, dietary guidelines and food security strategies need to evolve from the limited historical approach, mainly focused on nutrients and health, to a new one considering the environmental, socio-economic and cultural impact—and thus the sustainability—of diets. Objective: To present an updated version of the Mediterranean Diet Pyramid (MDP) to reflect multiple environmental concerns. Methods: We performed a revision and restructuring of the MDP to incorporate more recent findings on the sustainability and environmental impact of the Mediterranean Diet pattern, as well as its associations with nutrition and health. For each level of the MDP we provided a third dimension featuring the corresponding environmental aspects related to it. Conclusions: The new environmental dimension of the MDP enhances food intake recommendations addressing both health and environmental issues. Compared to the previous 2011 version, it emphasizes more strongly a lower consumption of red meat and bovine dairy products, and a higher consumption of legumes and locally grown eco-friendly plant foods as much as possible.

Keywords: Mediterranean diet; Mediterranean diet pyramid; sustainable diets; sustainability; environmental concerns; nutrition; food-based dietary guidelines

1. Introduction

The global population is constantly increasing and, according to estimates, from 7.7 billion people worldwide in 2019 it could rise to around 8.5 billion by 2030 and up to 9.7 billion by 2050 [1]. Feeding this global population with healthy food will be a growing concern for governments. Adequate nutrition is not only a survival issue, but is also highly related to the environment and its fragile balance. Food production is the major cause of global environmental change: agriculture occupies about 40% of global land [2], and food production is responsible for up to 30% of global greenhouse gas (GHG) emissions [3] and 70% of freshwater use [4,5]. In other words, diets link worldwide human health with environmental sustainability [6]. Thus, providing an increasing world population with a healthy and sustainable diet represents a major challenge [6]. Food policy, dietary guidelines and food security measures need to move from the traditional approach focused primarily on nutrients and health, to one that takes into consideration sustainability, and its environmental, economic and social dimensions [7]. This also needs to reflect food system factors influencing dietary choices, with their various implications for policy interventions and actions in education, agriculture and the food industry, among others [8,9]. The Mediterranean Diet (MD) has been presented as part of the solution [9,10].

Over the past 50 years, the notion of the MD has undergone a progressive evolution. The limited perception of the MD solely as a healthy dietary pattern [11] has been extended to portray a sustainable dietary pattern embracing the important socio-cultural, economic and environmental benefits of the diet [3,12]. This was done primarily by linking food consumption with production and distribution [13,14], three aspects which are among the main causes of ecological pressure on the natural environment [10]. The MD as a traditional dietary pattern is rich in plant-based foods (cereals, legumes, nuts, fruits, vegetables and herbs) and low in red and processed meat. It includes a moderate intake of fish, seafood, eggs, white meat and dairy products, a moderate intake of alcohol (mainly wine during meals, where culturally acceptable) and olive oil as the main source of added fat [11,14]. Since the 1960s, increasing evidence has shown the protective effect of the MD for cardiovascular diseases, metabolic syndrome, diabetes mellitus, and certain neurodegenerative disorders and cancers [15–22]. However, it has also recently been observed that dietary patterns such as the MD, rich in plant-based foods and low in animal foods are healthier and exert a lower impact on the environment [23–26].

Indeed, the Mediterranean Diet Pattern (MD-P) has been shown to have a better ecological footprint than current dietary habits in industrialized countries, particularly when compared to the Western dietary pattern [25,27–30]. This is mainly due to the higher consumption of local and in-season plant-derived foods and lower consumption of animal products. Yet, unfortunately, the current dietary pattern in many Mediterranean countries has shifted from the traditional MD-P. A return to the latter would be beneficial for human health and the natural environment. This can be explained by the fact that the MD is not only a model of cultural food choices, cooking methods, meal patterns and, more broadly, a lifestyle [31–34]; it is also a sustainable framework that attenuates the environmental pressure of food production and consumption [35–40]. A broader adherence to this dietary model would make a significant contribution to greater sustainability of the food system (from producer to consumer), with a myriad of benefits for human and planetary well-being [41].

The transition from the currently consumed diet in most European Mediterranean countries towards a traditional MD-P requires substantial changes in consumers' values, education and choices.

Improvements would also be required in the training of primary care and nutrition professionals [42], as well as changes in agri-food and fishing industry practices, public catering supply, trade policies and areas of research to inform policy and practice. Thus, many stakeholders need to be involved in this change process in order to reach a convergence of the health sector, food production systems and consumer demands. Using a common practical, flexible and science-based graphical guide to illuminate the process would be both efficient and acceptable to all involved.

The aim of the present work is to refine the Mediterranean Diet Pyramid (MDP) with particular attention to the environmental impact of food and based on a consensus between experts in the field. While non-prescriptive from a nutritional (as in specific food) point of view, this update aims to foster the debate about food chain sustainability and to promote the necessary changes for a healthier life, both for humankind and for the planet.

2. Materials and Methods

2.1. A Historical Overview

The first graphical representation of the (traditional) MDP was developed in 1993 in collaboration with Oldways, Harvard University and the World Health Organization (WHO) [11]. The 1993 MDP was updated in 2009 and 2010 by a group of experts, including one author of the 1993 MDP (AT), as part of this long-standing collaboration. This update was coordinated by the Mediterranean Diet Foundation in collaboration with the Forum on Mediterranean Food Cultures, the Hellenic Health Foundation, the Hebrew University, the International Commission on the Anthropology of Food and Nutrition (ICAF), the Centre International de Hautes Etudes Agronomiques Méditerranéennes (CIHEAM), the Centro Interuniversitario Internazionale di Studi sulle Culture Alimentari Mediterranee (CIISCAM), the Federation of European Nutrition Societies (FENS), the Federation of African Nutrition Societies (FANUS) and the International Union of Nutritional Sciences (IUNS). This review gathered and updated recommendations considering the lifestyle, dietary, socio-cultural, environmental and health challenges that the current Mediterranean populations were facing [14]. The traditional MDP being used at that time was significant as it was intended not only to provide dietary guidance to meet nutritional needs, but also to describe a healthy and sustainable lifestyle using a simple, practical framework which could be adapted to the different cultural and socio-economic contexts of the countries in the Mediterranean region [14]. In 2010, the international symposium "Biodiversity and sustainable diets: united against hunger", was held in Rome at the Food and Agriculture Organization (FAO), during which a consensus position on a definition of "sustainable diets" was reached, with an entire program session devoted to the MD as an example of a sustainable diet (FAO/Biodiversity, 2012). Subsequently, at the end of 2010, the MD was recognized as an Intangible Cultural Heritage of Humanity by the United Nations Educational, Scientific and Cultural Organization (UNESCO) [31].

After this watershed and historical moment, the MDP continued to be developed as has been outlined in Figure 1. In 2011, an international FAO/CIHEAM workshop was organized to assess the sustainability of the MD model in the Mediterranean region, considering its four dimensions and impacts: health and nutrition, environment including biodiversity, economy, and socio–cultural factors. Initially, a comprehensive list of 74 potential indicators was compiled (FAO/CIHEAM, 2012); this was later reduced to 24 indicators, which was deemed more feasible considering the availability of data sources and the methodological approaches developed. Then from 2013–2015 an international working group from different institutions collaborated to identify 13 nutritional indicators with which to assess the sustainability of a healthy diet, using the MD as a case study and the 2011 MD pyramid model as a reference [43]. In November 2014, the International Mediterranean Diet Foundation (IFMeD) was founded by a group of previous MDP co-authors. The goal was to establish an international center of multi-disciplinary knowledge and expertise, with the objective to revalorize and enhance the MD as a healthy and sustainable lifestyle model, adapting it to current socio-economic and cultural changes, as well as preserving and enhancing it as an intangible cultural heritage of humankind.

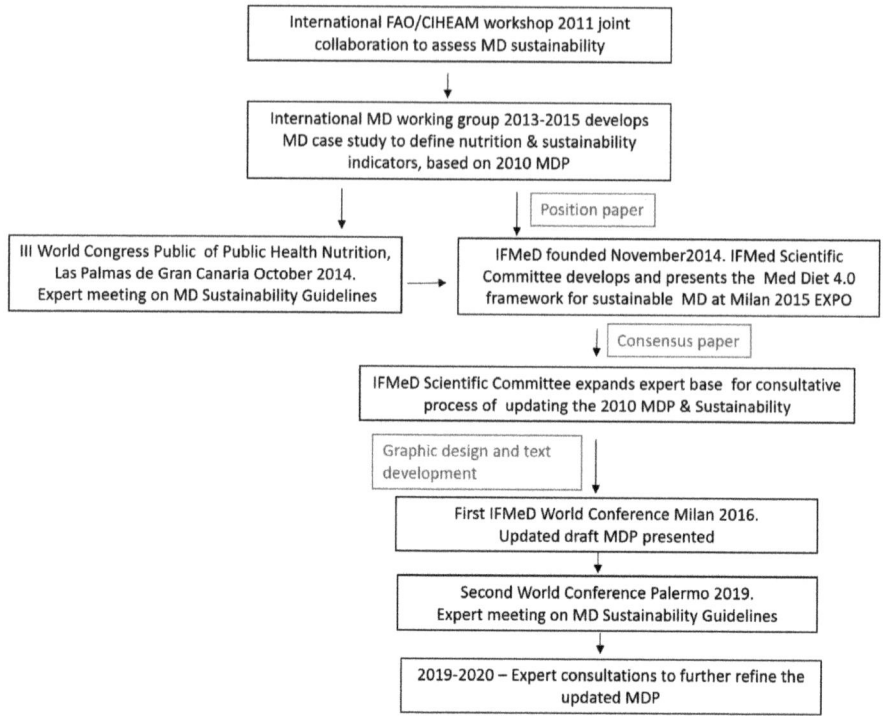

Figure 1. Consensus process for an updated graphical representation of the Mediterranean Diet Pyramid.

As a follow up of these collaborative efforts, the Med Diet 4.0 framework was presented at the Milan 2015 EXPO to valorize the MD as a dietary pattern with multiple sustainability benefits and country-specific variations, embodying the following characteristics: (1) recognized and well-documented major health and nutrition benefits, in the prevention of chronic diseases and in reducing public health costs as well as in the overall improvement of well-being; (2) low environmental impacts and richness in biodiversity, appreciation of biodiversity value, reduction of pressure on natural resources and mitigation of climate change; (3) high positive local economic returns, sustainable territorial development, reduction of rural poverty, and high performance in reduction of food waste and loss; (4) high social and cultural value of food, growth of mutual respect, identity recovery, social inclusion and consumer empowerment. The Med Diet 4.0 framework was released as a joint contribution of the IFMeD scientific committee [13].

IFMeD then continued this consultation process with the goal of establishing an updated consensus position on a newly revised representation of the MD pyramid that incorporated recent scientific evidence highlighting the benefits of the MD as a sustainable and healthy diet. In this exercise IFMeD sought to involve those nutrition, health and socio- culture experts who had been involved in the previous revision of the MDP, as well as new authorities on the subject and a broader expert view. Greater attention was given to environmental issues such as climate change, use of land, use of water, protection of seas and waterways, sourcing and distribution of food, respect for food producers and communication of the value of the MD as a diet in line with scientific environmental recommendations. With this in mind, the first MD world conference "Revitalizing the Mediterranean Diet: from a healthy dietary pattern to a healthy Mediterranean sustainable lifestyle" was organized by IFMeD in Milan on July 2016, and provided a major opportunity to continue this consensus process supporting sustainability and 'respect' for the planet. Sustainability and the MD were then addressed more comprehensively in the second MD world conference "Strategies toward more sustainable food systems in the Mediterranean region: the Mediterranean Diet as a lever for bridging consumption and production in a sustainable and healthy way", organized by CIHEAM-Bari and the Forum on Mediterranean Food Cultures in Palermo, in May 2019.

During the latter half of 2019 and early 2020, further online consultations were held in order to reach consensus regarding an updated MDP. At the same time, the current scientific literature was also examined. The proposed new graphical representation of the MDP responds to the need for a common framework among Mediterranean countries in the form of food-based dietary guidelines [44] which are in line with the 2010 definition of sustainable diets elaborated by FAO [45]. Moreover, it embodies the result of a continuous and rigorous process of consensus building between all relevant stakeholders.

2.2. Consensus on an Updated Graphical Representation of the Mediterranean Diet Pyramid

This revision fostered an interdisciplinary dialogue among scientists and experts in public health nutrition, food science, dietetics, social anthropology, sociology, cultural heritage, family and consumer sciences, agriculture, resource management and environmental sciences in order to provide a unified representation of the MD as a sustainable dietary pattern encompassing the entirety of the Mediterranean area. This new revision of the MD Pyramid is created by scientific consensus among experts and is grounded in evidence from research in the fields of nutrition, health and environmental issues. However, it should be emphasized that the MDP described here is not prescriptive. Rather, we suggest that each country uses the basic updated MDP and the recommendations aligned with it as an aid to developing their own guidelines suited to their food systems and culture-rooted cuisines.

3. Results

3.1. The Updated Mediterranean Diet Pyramid

This new graphical representation was conceived as a simplified pyramid framework, to be adapted by different countries in the Mediterranean region to their geographical, socio-economic and cultural contexts, dietary needs and meal patterns. The recommendations target the healthy adult population (18–65 years old) and should be modified to meet the special nutritional needs and diets of children, pregnant women, elderly, and individuals with health problems such as cardiovascular diseases. In this updated pyramid, food items at the base of the pyramid continue to contribute the highest intake levels in terms of grams/day. Animal protein sources are positioned to suggest a lower frequency of consumption and contribution to total intake, having been shifted from daily to weekly consumption. The top of the pyramid presents both animal and sugar-rich foods that should only be consumed occasionally (e.g. red and processed meat, pastries and sweets). Preference for local, seasonal, fresh and minimally processed food is emphasized, supporting biodiversity and eco-friendly and traditional foods. The novelty of the updated MDP lies in its third dimension as shown in Figure 2. This represents the environmental impact of the food items included, as well as aspects of food production sustainability.

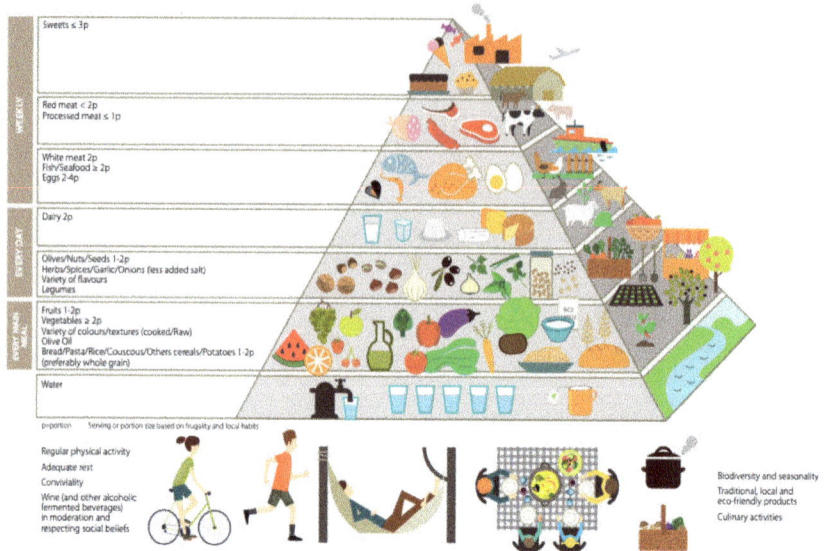

Figure 2. New Pyramid for a Sustainable Mediterranean Diet.

3.2. Meal Composition

Main meals consumed daily should be a combination of three elements: cereals, vegetables and fruits, and a small quantity of legumes, beans or other (though not in every meal). Cereals in the form of bread, pasta, rice, couscous or bulgur (cracked wheat) should be consumed as one–two servings per meal, preferably using whole or partly refined grains. Vegetable consumption should amount to two or more servings per day, in raw form for at least one of the two main meals (lunch and dinner). Fruit should be considered as the primary form of dessert, with one–two servings per meal. Consuming a variety of colors of both vegetables and fruit is strongly recommended to help ensure intake of a broad range of micronutrients and phytochemicals. The less these foods are cooked, the higher the retention of vitamins and the lower use of fuel, thus minimizing environmental impact.

The highlighted triad of elements for the main meals constitutes the core of the MDP, is based on plant foods, and is responsible for the prevention of numerous chronic diseases and for healthy weight management, as well as for reduced use of natural resources and GHG emissions [22]. Plant foods produced by agro-ecological methods (free from chemical pesticides) can markedly minimize human and nature's exposure to pesticides [46]. The preference should always be for fresh, seasonal and minimally processed vegetables and fruits. Similarly, choosing local cereal-based products (i.e., bread, couscous, polenta, pasta, rice etc.) when possible and available will support the local economy and reduce the ecologic impact of the production chain.

Agriculture has historically shaped the rich biodiversity heritage of European Union (EU) countries, including those of the South, but over the last decades this synergistic relationship has been undermined [47]. This is why the sustainable management of natural resources is now part of the objectives of the EU's Common Agricultural Policy agenda, focused on protecting biodiversity and the environment within agriculture [48–50]. Food consumption and production have implications for both land use and GHG emissions [51]. In 2017 the total GHG emissions in the EU's 28 member states (EU-28) were 4483 million tons of CO_2 equivalents, of which agricultural practices represented around 10% [52]. At the same time, the quantity and type of food consumed directly influences land use. Overall, scientific evidence now supports the general concept that a plant-based diet, compared to the current widely consumed animal food-based diet (especially rich in ruminant foodstuffs), markedly minimizes land, water and resources use for production, along with reducing GHG emissions. Such a diet appears to have significant potential for ensuring food security for all, reducing impacts on climate change and facilitating the realization of the 2030 UN Sustainable Development Goals, as discussed below [53].

However, the nature of this land-food/diet relationship depends on other factors, such as population growth, agricultural productivity, land ownership and investment patterns, as well as land use efficiency [54]. A major limitation to addressing these issues consists of the difficulty in obtaining such estimates for each country.

Olive Oil

Olive oil should be the principal source of dietary lipids. Due to its composition and resistance to high temperatures, Extra Virgin Olive Oil (EVOO) is recommended both for cooking and dressing food. Traditionally, in the Mediterranean region, vegetables, other plant foods and staple starchy foods served at principal meals, including pasta, potatoes or rice, are cooked with olive oil, thus amplifying their nutritional value. EVOO has been reported to have a key role in the primary prevention of cardiovascular diseases [18,55] and is inversely associated with certain cancers [56–59].

Olive production (for use as oil or as olives) represents a significant utilization of land in the southern regions of the EU, particularly Spain (2.4 million ha), Italy (1.4 million ha), Greece (1 million ha) and Portugal (0.5 million ha) [60]. According to the International Olive Council (IOC), the production of table olives in the EU during 2019–2020 was 808.4 (×1000) tons, of which 500 were in Spain, 207 in Greece, 74.1 in Italy and 22.5 in Portugal. Of note, among the other countries of the IOC, Egypt produced 690, Turkey 414, Algeria 300 and Morocco 130 (×1000) tons of table olives [61]. In the olive sector, the negative environmental effects of intensification could be reduced considerably by means of sustainable farming practices. Moreover, with appropriate support, traditional low-input plantations could continue to maintain important natural and social values in marginal areas [60]. On the other hand, several studies [62,63] have shown that olive oil production is associated with adverse effects on the environment during the fruit growth and olive oil production phases. For this reason, it is crucial to identify those phases with greater environmental impacts in order to minimize their effects [62,63]. On a positive note, olive trees are a barrier to desertification and erosion and olive orchards are a CO_2 sink, removing CO_2 from the atmosphere and fixing it in the soil. In the production of 1 L of olive oil, olive trees remove 10 kg of CO_2 from the atmosphere [64].

It is relevant here to discuss palm oil, an industrial alternative to olive oil in the Mediterranean countries. Due to its properties, it is used in many commercial products (e.g., processed foods, cosmetics, biofuels). Globally, palm oil cultivation has increased in the past years, resulting in deforestation (particularly in Indonesia and Malaysia), biodiversity loss, and net GHG emissions. However, Europe remains the leading market for sustainably sourced palm oil, although progress on the number of voluntary initiatives and commitments by industry has been slow [65].

3.3. Daily Intake

3.3.1. Olives, Nuts and Seeds

Olives (apart from olive oil), nuts and seeds should be present on a daily basis since they are good sources of unsaturated healthy fats, minerals, vitamins and fiber as well as other compounds with antioxidant potential that contribute to general well-being [66]. Nuts have an important role in the primary prevention of cardiovascular and other diseases [18]. Nuts and olives are high in monounsaturated fatty acids contributing to a desirable monounsaturated/saturated fats ratio. A reasonable consumption (i.e., a handful) of nuts and seeds (minimally salted or unsalted) represent a healthy snack choice, offering plant protein and having good satiety value, amongst others. If possible, locally produced nuts, seeds and olives should be opted for.

3.3.2. Herbs, Spices, Garlic and Onions

Herbs, spices, garlic and onions give dishes flavor, increasing palatability while allowing for a reduction in salt use. They constitute, to different degrees, a source of multiple micronutrients and antioxidant compounds helping to enrich the dishes they are used in. These foodstuffs are staples in many countries in and around the Mediterranean basin and contribute to the regional cultural identities and culinary specialties (e.g., "sofrito" in Italy and Spain and "ladera" in Greece).

3.3.3. Legumes

As indicated earlier, in this updated MDP, preference is given to plant protein sources such as legumes, though animal protein sources low in saturated fats, such as fish, poultry, rabbit and certain lean meats, as well as eggs, are allowed in reasonable amounts. Thus, a daily amount of plant protein sources should be prioritized (at least one small serving per day). Indeed, in this update, legumes have been incorporated into the category of daily consumption. There is no health reason to limit legumes consumption, but there are a number of environmental reasons to increase it. Legumes may substitute animal protein foods in the diet, decreasing the environmental impact of the current MD. Legumes also help to fix atmospheric nitrogen in the soil, improving soil fertility and reducing dependence on energy-intensive or artificial fertilizers. Legumes share some of the health attributes of vegetables with respect to micronutrients and also provide large amounts of protein and soluble fibers. Although of moderate quality, their protein content can be improved if combined with cereals. Legumes are highly satiating with a low glycemic index and glycemic load and the soluble fibers help in controlling blood glucose and cholesterol levels. The versatility of legumes enhances their culinary value. They may be bought dried and then cooked or bought fresh or frozen. Fresh legumes are seasonally available, while frozen and dried versions are available all year round.

3.3.4. Dairy Products

Milk and dairy products should be consumed on a daily basis in a moderate amount (maximum of two servings per day). Traditionally, in the Mediterranean region, the most consumed dairy products were in the form of yogurt and cheese (particularly from sheep's milk) and these should continue to be consumed in moderation. Dairy products like milk, cheese and yogurt have numerous benefits for bone and muscle health, as they are a source of proteins, calcium and micronutrients. Moreover, due to their probiotic content, they boost digestive tract health and positively affect the microbiome [67,68].

However, dairy products together with meat represent a major concern because of their environmental impact. Dairy farming in the EU is becoming more intensive and more specialized, with imported grains and soybeans being used as feed. There is a move towards fewer and larger farms, except where national authorities actively intervene to help maintain small producers or promote organic production [69]. These trends lead to problems regarding atmospheric, land and water pollution (e.g., from transportation and animal waste) and put pressure on marginal habitats and landscape features, biodiversity and soil integrity. Thus, eating a variety of dairy products and, as much as possible, milk and dairy products from small producers and local farmers should be preferred, as well as consuming organic products. This will help to reduce the environmental impact of these products (i.e., harm to soil quality, or impacts from packaging and transport), sustain the local economy, and yield better quality products, as grazing leads to better lipid profiles in milk.

3.4. Weekly Intake

Fish and seafood are integral to the MD and a varied consumption (oily fish, lean fish and shellfish) is recommended based on local availability and culinary traditions. Not only are they important sources of proteins, but Mediterranean Sea fish, such as sardines and others, are rich in omega-3 fatty acids—eicosapentaenoic acid (EPA) and docosahexaenoic (DHA)—reported to reduce the risk of coronary heart disease and to have anti-inflammatory properties [70]. Yet fish and shellfish are largely a wild resource that is at risk of being depleted; therefore, adequate management is needed in order to maintain fish stocks [71]. Apart from seeking sustainably sourced and captured wild fish, aquaculture can be considered as an alternative. Aquaculture fish have equally valid nutritional characteristics, though the lipid profile may be altered due to the feed [72]. Moreover, aquaculture production is now often being redesigned to take on a circular economy approach where waste is reused for other functions, such as feeding plants in aquaponics, or creating energy [73].

Poultry and eggs are also included in the MDP. Poultry provides high quality protein and does not contain the high levels of saturated fat found in red meat. Whole eggs, including those used for cooking or baking, should not exceed four per week. Poultry meat and eggs have moderate impacts on natural resources and environment. Organically produced varieties should be sought, as animal welfare is safeguarded, and this also helps to enrich the soil where these animals roam and deposit waste.

A key recommendation concerns red and processed meats. Red meats should be eaten less frequently ($\leq$2 servings/week), preferably as lean cuts. Similarly, processed meat consumption should also be limited ($\leq$1 serving/week). Both red and processed meats should be seen as a condiment to add palatability to dishes and recipes, and not as the main item in a dish- a common characteristic in the Western dietary pattern. Intake of meat, particularly red and processed meats, has been consistently associated with certain chronic diseases (i.e., increased risk of type 2 diabetes, cardiovascular disease, cancer) and all-cause mortality [74,75]. Thus, a decrease in consumption is beneficial for multiple health reasons. Moreover, this decrease also has high environmental value. In fact, most of the estimated global GHG emissions deriving from agriculture and land use come from livestock production. The process of raising ruminants produces significant amounts of methane, a GHG with detrimental global warming potential. Moreover, livestock production affects land use and GHG emission in different ways: deforestation for grazing land and cropland for soy-feed production, soil carbon loss in pastures, energy required for growing feed-grains and processing and transporting grains and meat, NO releases from the use of nitrogenous fertilizers, and gases from animal manure (especially methane) and enteric fermentation [54,76]. In the future, if acceptability is tackled, alternative protein sources could potentially be in the form of sustainable novel foods such as insects and jellyfish.

Finally, at the top of the MDP, one finds that high fat and/or high sugar sweets, pastries and beverages are represented. Sweets and ultra-processed high sugar, high fat, foods and drinks should be consumed in small amounts and only occasionally. They should be limited to maximum one–two servings per week or reserved for special occasions and celebrations. Sweetness in the diet should preferably be added with fresh and, to a lesser extent, dried fruits, honey or carob syrup. Of note, a lower consumption of highly processed long shelf life sweets, pastries and snacks may contribute to less use by the food industry of palm fats, which are typical ingredients in such foods, and which as described earlier are harmful to the environment unless sustainably produced.

3.5. Drinks and Fluid Balance

3.5.1. Water

Water and non-sweetened beverages (1.5–2 L per day, corresponding to an average amount of six–eight servings per day), in addition to water from food are essential to preserve body water balance and maintain an active lifestyle. According to the European Food Safety Authority (EFSA), the reference values for adequate water intake are 2.0 and 2.5 L per day for adult females and males, respectively [77]. These values include drinking water, water from other beverages and water present in food, and apply to individuals engaging in moderate physical activity levels and are at moderate ambient temperature. Water requirements may vary according to age, personal clinical/health status, physical activity intensity, weather and other environmental conditions. Water should be consumed freely, preferably from the tap, according to hygienic safety. Tap water is preferred in order to reduce the environmental footprint of commercial drinking water (mainly packaging and transport).

In general, local tap or bottled water should be the order of choice [78] and always prioritizing glass over plastic containers.

3.5.2. Other Beverages

Coffee, tea and herbal infusions (rich in flavonoids) are also included, but consumption should be with a minimal use of sugar or honey, or preferably without any sweetener. Each of these beverages, in varying degrees, offers another source of beneficial flavonoids and can potentially decrease consumption of highly sweetened beverages. Certified fair trade and sustainably produced coffee and tea should be opted for as much as possible, and recipes for local, traditional herbal brews should be recorded for posterity.

3.6. Portion Size

Portion sizes (formerly called servings) should be based on frugality and moderation and aligned with the energy needs of urban and modern lifestyles where applicable. In general, the portion sizes of the foods represented at the base of the pyramid should be larger and the foods from this section consumed more frequently (while avoiding food waste). In contrast, those foods at the upper levels should be consumed in much smaller amounts and less frequently.

It is worth noting that in countries adopting the Western diet pattern, most individuals have protein intakes largely exceeding their needs, with red meat being one of the main contributors. Thus, limiting portion sizes of protein-rich foods, particularly red meat, will better fit with a healthy, sustainable diet, and has the added benefit of reducing monetary costs.

3.7. The Base of the Pyramid

Situated outside, but at the base of the pyramid, the new concepts of sustainability and affordability are highlighted, adding on to aspects already present in the previous version [14]. Physical activity, adequate rest and socialization during meals are also represented, being practices integral to the definition of the Mediterranean lifestyle.

3.7.1. Physical Activity

The importance of the regular practice of moderate-intensity physical activity (150 min throughout the week, or at least 30 min a day for 5 days per week) and muscle-strengthening activities at least twice a week, are emphasized as a basic complement to the MD for balancing energy intake, maintaining a healthy body weight and for many other health benefits.

3.7.2. Sleep and Rest

A restorative nightly sleep, as well as resting during the day (usually after the mid-day meal) are part of a balanced lifestyle, contributing to health maintenance. A slower lifestyle with reduced stress levels should also be sought. Being active or relaxing in a natural setting (e.g., swimming, walking and hiking, or responsible picnicking) is in keeping with the MD whilst not being detrimental to the natural environment.

3.7.3. Culinary Activities and Conviviality

Mealtimes have a social and cultural value which transcends their nutritional and nourishing functions [79]. Cooking from scratch is typical of the MD, whereas shared culinary activities and shared dining allow for trans-generational transmission of culinary knowledge and recipes in an enjoyable atmosphere. These are key elements for the revitalization of the MD, at least in the Mediterranean region itself.

3.7.4. Wine

As shown by the available scientific literature, there is no safe level for alcohol consumption [80]. Nevertheless, while fully respecting religious principles, cultural beliefs and social norms, an optional moderate consumption of wine (one glass per day for women and two glasses per day for men), preferably during meals, as well as other fermented beverages, might be indicated. In Muslim Mediterranean countries where alcoholic drinks are not consumed, there is a high intake of tea infusions, rich in polyphenols similar to wine, and sometimes accompanied with herbs such as mint. The habit of tea and infusion drinking is commendable from both a health and environmental perspective.

3.7.5. Biodiversity and Seasonal and Local Foods

The value of eating a variety of local and seasonal foods is emphasized. Consuming a range of locally available foods—animal, fish and shellfish and plants—will aid in maintaining biodiversity in the region. As far as possible, fresh, seasonal and minimally processed foods should be preferred. This will maximize their nutritional properties and markedly reduce the environmental footprints of food production and processing, as well as long-distance transport of imported foods. Moreover, local production chains will be sustained, with beneficial effects on the local economy and employment.

3.7.6. Traditional

The selection and preference of traditional and local foods will sustain the local culinary heritage, promote the use of indigenous ingredients, and thus support the (sustainable) production (plants and animal) and capture (e.g., fish, wild rabbit, fowl) of foods which are familiar, and also those less known. Many traditional MD dishes are plant-based and high in vegetables, legumes, nuts and cereals making them more environment-friendly.

3.7.7. Eco-Friendly Products

Consuming eco-friendly products will help the preservation of Mediterranean landscapes and sea. Eco-friendly production methods, such as agro-ecology or organic agriculture, result in biodiversity promotion and reduction or elimination of harmful chemical use [80]. Thus, health for consumers as well as nature (land, rivers, sea, etc.) will be promoted. Indeed, recent large epidemiological studies have shown that consumers whose diet comprises a high share of organic foods adopt a healthier plant-based dietary pattern with lower pesticide exposure, lower body mass, lower impact on natural resources and lower GHG emissions [26,81,82]. Combining the MD with regular organic food consumption appears to be the optimal option [30].

3.7.8. Affordability

Adherence to a MD does not necessarily increase the expense of one's diet significantly [83,84]. Basing meals on legumes, cereals and local and seasonal vegetables, fruit and fish can help to offset the cost of other potentially more expensive foods such as meat or less healthy processed foods. Following the guidance of the updated MDP can assist those who are financially insecure in consuming a healthier diet.

4. Discussion

The seminal EAT LANCET study established a global food system modelling framework to evaluate which combinations of feasible measures (dietary shift, standard and high levels of improved production practices, reduced food waste and loss) were needed to stay within sustainable food production limits (GHG emissions, nitrogen cycling, phosphorus cycling, freshwater use, biodiversity loss and land system change) while still supplying nutritious and healthful diets by 2050. Their findings suggest that a shift towards a dietary pattern comprising more plant-based foods than animal foods (obviating the need to become a strict vegan, and emphasizing fish and poultry, legumes, whole grains, vegetables, fruits and nuts) would provide environmental benefits, nutrient adequacy and improved health [6]. The nutritional adequacy of the traditional MD has been demonstrated, despite being lower in animal products and less caloric, as it contains smaller amounts of proteins and fats and is richer in fiber and micronutrients [11,14,34,43,81].

The proposed new graphical representation of the MDP has considered various aspects outlined by the recent EAT LANCET study and fulfills an expressed need for a common framework among countries in the Mediterranean regions to develop sustainability-promoting Food-Based Dietary Guidelines [38]. It represents a concerted effort at consensus-building among experts from different disciplines, reflective of the complexity of food systems, as well as the need to adhere to the latest scientific evidence.

Assessing the sustainability and especially the environmental impact of the MD has been perceived as a complex task, but one which is urgently required. With this objective, during 2012–2016 an informal international working group from different institutions collaborated to identify nutritional indicators for assessing the sustainability of a healthy diet [43,85]. The group identified thirteen indicators belonging to five areas (biochemical characteristics, food quality, and environmental, lifestyle and clinical aspects). Such indicators were proposed as a useful methodological framework to address health, education and agricultural policies [43]. The significance of the diet for environmental protection or degradation was integral to the choice of indicators, and the role of agriculture and fisheries in facilitating a sustainable diet was considered from different angles.

The role of agriculture has been crucial in historically shaping the biodiversity of EU countries, but over the last decades this synergistic relationship has been undermined. Intensification and specialization of agricultural production has been established increasing production potential, but also causing the marginalization and abandonment of many areas of land and consequently losses of species and habitats associated with farmland [47]. For these reasons, the sustainable management of natural resources is part of the objectives of the EU's Common Agricultural Policy agenda [48–50].

Moreover, changes in food consumption and production could have important implications for land use and GHG emissions [51]. The nature of this land-food relationship depends on the type of food consumed and also on other factors, such as population growth, agricultural productivity, land ownership and investment patterns, and land use efficiency [54].

With the identification of the food production chain as one of the main contributors towards a negative environmental impact in the last decades, the study of such effects has often involved using the Life Cycle Assessment (LCA) method. This method comprises a tool for appraising the environmental impacts and resources used throughout a product's life cycle. For example, in the case of food production, the LCA investigates the environmental impact of each phase, from agricultural production to final consumption, examining industrial processing, packaging, distribution and retail, cooking and finally waste management [86,87]. Muñoz et al.'s 2010 study analyzed the average Spanish diet (consisting of water 75%, protein 3.6%, fat 5.8%, carbohydrate 13% and fiber 0.78% of ingested food weight) with the LCA method [88]. Results showed that the net Global Warming Potential (GWP) related to feeding a Spanish citizen for one year amounted to 2.1 tons of CO_2 equivalent. Considering the whole food production chain from production to wastewater treatment, this figure was dominated by the production stage. Moreover, the contribution of meat and dairy production represented around 54% of total GWP for food production. Similarly, eutrophication potential and primary energy use were dominated by the food production stage [88].

The sustainability of the updated MD versus present-day Spanish and Western dietary patterns in the context of the Spanish population was analyzed in 2012–2013 comparing the reference pattern of the MD pyramid [14] with an estimation of the current Spanish and Western dietary patterns derived from FAO data [27]. The MD emerged as having the lowest environmental impact compared to current Spanish and Western dietary patterns, having an agricultural land use of 8365×10^3 Ha/year (Spanish and Western dietary patterns $12,342 \times 10^3$ Ha/year and $33,162 \times 10^3$ Ha/year, respectively), energy consumption of 239,042 TJ/year (Spanish and Western dietary patterns 285,968 TJ/year and

611,314 TJ/year, respectively), water consumption of 13.2 Km^3/year (Spanish and Western dietary patterns 13.4 Km^3/year and 22.0 Km^3/year respectively) and GHG emissions amounting to 35,510 Gg CO$_2$ eq/year (Spanish and Western dietary patterns 72,758 Gg CO$_2$ eq/year and 217,128 Gg CO$_2$ eq/year, respectively). The food groups mainly responsible for environmental pressure were meat and dairy products [27].

The environmental burden of the MD applied in the Italian context was also analyzed [89]. The authors recognize that the LCA method inevitably suffers from omissions (which are required to make the method applicable) that could lead to underestimation of the total impact when applied to household consumption. For this reason, they chose to assess the environmental footprint of the MD using a hybrid method. This method addresses stages of food production and consumption through the LCA and other methodologies (in this case input-output analysis). It was observed that the national average diet led to 402.91 kg CO$_2$ eq/month of GHG emissions, while the MD presented a 6.81% lower CO$_2$ eq/month [89]. These results are in agreement with the findings of the study of Muñoz et al. [87], recording slightly higher values of GWP. This is probably due to the authors taking into account the actual consumption of a Spanish citizen, as well as solid waste management, which were not considered in the Italian study.

Two recent studies (2013 and 2018) dealt with sustainability of the MD and dietary patterns in Spain. In the first study, based on the SUN cohort (20,363 adults), it was observed that better adherence to the MD was significantly associated with lower land use, water and energy consumption and GHG emissions, making it an eco-friendly option [28]. In the second study evaluating a cohort of 18,929 adults, the MD was compared to a partly vegetarian diet or Western diet, after ten years of follow-up. Overall, the MD was healthier, whereas the partly vegetarian diet was slightly better than the MD for environmental impacts, whilst the Western diet was better only because of its lower monetary cost. Thus, according to the findings of this study, the MD seemed to be the more sustainable option, closely followed by the partly vegetarian diet [29].

It is important to note (as briefly mentioned earlier) that the environmental impact of food production also involves water use. Water availability is an important issue in some countries of the Mediterranean basin (e.g., in Spain and Malta), linked to the increasing water demand for agriculture plus the desertification process. For these reasons, the concept of a water footprint is gaining importance when analyzing the link between water resources and the food production chain. In the last decades, methodologies such as the Water Footprint Assessment (WFA) and the LCA have been implemented to study such relationships.

The concept of a water footprint (WF) represents an indicator of freshwater use, including both direct water use of a consumer or producer and the indirect water use. In other words, the WF of a product is the volume of freshwater used to produce a food, measured over the whole supply chain. WFA refers to the quantification and location of the WF of a food production chain, and to the assessment of the environmental, social and economic sustainability of this WF. This is carried out with the objective of informing policies and formulating response strategies [90,91].

A study conducted in 2019 [92] investigated the nutritional and water usage implications of the current Spanish diet compared with the MD. The findings showed that the current Spanish dietary habits presented higher WF than the recommended MD: the former consumed 2554 L/capita per day and the latter 1835 L/capita per day. This difference was mainly due to the higher consumption of red and processed meat, sugars, pastries, beverages and dairy products [92]. The authors observed that, in addition to its beneficial effects on health, the adoption of the MD by the Spanish population (approx. 46.6 million) would save 474 million m^3 of blue water, a valuable resource that could be allocated to other uses. Thus, the MD emerged as a healthy, more sustainable and more water-efficient model than the average Spanish diet. This finding is of major relevance, considering that some of the areas in the Mediterranean region are semi-arid zones.

Widespread international scientific consensus and a large body of evidence support the assertion that plant-based diets are healthier and more protective of natural resources and the general environment, including GHG emissions [11,24,25,93,94]. It is also worth noting that more and more countries are integrating sustainability into their Food-Based Dietary Guidelines (FBDG). For instance, in France the FBDG were extensively updated in 2019 by the Ministry of Health [95]. They now include the concept of environmental preservation and the reduction of pesticide exposure. In brief, they recommend adopting a plant-based diet with increased consumption of all plant foods (vegetables, fruits, whole grains, legumes and nuts) and preferably of organic origin, a reduction in dairy products and limitation of red and processed meats. In an article based on the NutriNet-Santé cohort (28,240 participants), the authors showed that better adherence to the 2019 FBDG was related to higher plant-based food consumption, lower energy intake, lower exposure to chemical pesticides, lower expected population mortality and lower overall environmental impacts (land use, energy demand, GHGs), albeit at a somewhat higher cost [46]. These results suggest that overall, the French 2019 FBDG are generally in line with the multiple dimensions of diet sustainability, including health, although adherence is associated with a slight increase in cost. If adopted by a large part of the population, these dietary guidelines may help to prevent chronic diseases while reducing environmental impacts related to food consumption. The small increase in monetary cost would be balanced by lower externalized costs for the society. This implies that governments should take appropriate measures to help citizens and farmers to adopt sustainable attitudes and practices.

Nevertheless, the evidence supporting the environmental sustainability of the MD has some limitations that should be considered. First of all, there is limited information about each step of the food production chain, and assumptions are sometimes made in environmental impact analyses. Secondly, the food production system is a complex one which requires that many aspects should be controlled and kept in mind. Unfortunately, this remains a challenge as the food production system, transport, distribution and retail are extremely globalized and also diverse. The evaluation of the sustainability of a certain dietary pattern should be context-specific and involve different professionals from the health, medical, sociological and educational fields, as well as from systems engineering, and from agronomic, veterinary and environmental sciences. Moreover, extreme caution must be exerted when discussing the sustainability of food system issues in order to avoid the risk of trivializing problems characterized by extreme complexity, as well as their consequences and/or possible solutions.

Finally, evidence shows that to stay within the guidelines that foster sustainable food systems, a combination of dietary changes and production and management-related measures are required [11,14]. Although putting some of the measures into practice may be sufficient to stay within particular environmental limits, no single intervention is enough to simultaneously meet all the recommended environmental guidelines. This can be seen in the negative effect of climate change on food production, thus emphasizing the need to concurrently address reducing food waste and loss, apart from shifting to more sustainable dietary patterns.

5. Conclusions

Past versions of the MDP aimed to describe and summarize the MD patterns of different countries in the Mediterranean area whilst highlighting health benefits or recommendations. The various MD-Ps have all evolved as a result of modern technology, food processing and globalization (e.g., many developments and innovations have changed the range of foods currently available throughout the year). The MD-P is a shared cultural heritage that is widely recognized for its contribution to health and well-being and which should be preserved among the Mediterranean populations. Moreover, according to the United Nations Sustainable Development Goals (SDGs), the MD complies with at least 11 out of 17 goals: SDG2 Zero Hunger: End hunger, achieve food security and improved nutrition and promote sustainable agriculture; SDG3 Good Health and Well-Being: Ensure healthy lives and promote well-being for all at all ages; SDG4 Quality Education: Ensure inclusive and equitable quality education and promote lifelong learning opportunities for all; SDG5 Gender Equality: Achieve gender equality and empower all women and girls; SDG6 Clean Water and Sanitation: Ensure availability and sustainable management of water and sanitation for all; SDG7 Affordable and Clean Energy:

Ensure access to affordable, reliable, sustainable and modern energy for all; SDG8 Decent Work and Economic Growth: Promote sustained, inclusive and sustainable economic growth, full and productive employment and decent work for all; SDG11 Sustainable Cities and Communities: Make cities and human settlements inclusive, safe, resilient and sustainable; SDG12 Responsible Consumption and Production: Ensure sustainable consumption and production patterns; SDG13 Climate Action: Take urgent action to combat climate change and its impacts; SDG14 Life Below Water: Conserve and sustainably use the oceans, seas and marine resources for sustainable development; SDG15 Life on Land: Protect, restore and promote sustainable use of terrestrial ecosystems, sustainably manage forests, combat desertification, and halt and reverse land degradation and halt biodiversity loss [53].

The updated edition of the MDP presented here stresses the need to increase the sustainability of the MDP, decreasing the contribution of meat, high fat dairy products and highly processed foods, and increasing the consumption of legumes and as many locally grown vegetables, fruits, nuts and their products, preferably as eco-friendly products, as feasible. The final point to remember is that there should be a comprehensive approach to the MD, promoting it not just as a healthy diet, but also as a culturally coherent way of life to be enjoyed in a sustainable manner. Even if other food models may have a better performance on given points (e.g., certain environmental impacts of plant-based diets) the overall value of the MD on four dimensions, that is environmental, social, cultural, economic and nutritional/health levels, makes it a sustainable diet model that has been also recognized as an intangible heritage of humanity [3], but with added environmental value. The virtues of the MD and particularly its significance for environmental preservation and protection as presented in this new version of the MD pyramid need to be efficiently communicated and applied in an integrated manner at multiple levels. This implies starting from the level of policymakers, and expanding to mass media and social media influencers, to community development NGOs, to educators, to food innovators in production and processing, to restaurateurs and finally to the individuals and families in households.

This revision was fostered by an interdisciplinary dialogue amongst a multidisciplinary team of scientists and experts in order to provide a unified representation of the MD as a sustainable dietary pattern relevant to the entire Mediterranean region. This new revision of the MD Pyramid is grounded in scientific consensus among experts, as well as in evidence from research in the areas of nutrition, health and the natural and socio-economic environments; but it does not intend to be prescriptive. The idea is that each country uses the basic updated MDP and related recommendations as a guide, adapting the contents to their own country-specific contexts and cuisines.

This updated representation of the MD pyramid is released in order to marry the worldwide interest in the MD with increasing attention to sustainability, and especially to environmental concerns. Such representation aims to contribute towards a significantly greater adherence to this dietary pattern and lifestyle in the Mediterranean basin, as well as in other similar countries. The main goal is to shift the perception of the MD benefits from a person-centered, individual focus, to a broader focus embracing the benefits of the MD pattern for the planet and its populations.

Author Contributions: L.S.-M. and L.T. are joint first authors of this manuscript. L.S.-M. and L.T. conceptualization, methodology, writing—original draft preparation, review and editing. S.D., E.M.B., D.L., L.M.D., F.-X.M., R.B., S.P., R.C., A.B.-F., J.A.-B., C.L.V. and A.T. contributed substantially to the paper within their field of research as well as in reviewing drafts. L.T., L.S.-M., S.P., A.B.-F. and J.N.d.l.C. reviewed the final version of the manuscript. All authors have read and agreed to the published version of the manuscript.

Funding: This research received no external funding.

Acknowledgments: This consensus paper represents many rounds of discussions among the authors. They all agreed on the major issues presented herein; however, there remain some outstanding points where some authors dissented. It is hoped that these will be resolved through in-depth academic debate following publication. We realize that the Mediterranean Diet is in constant evolution and therefore subject to constant updates and clarifications such as regarding the environmental, economic and socio-cultural aspects.

Conflicts of Interest: The authors declare no conflict of interest.

References

1. World Population Prospects 2019. Available online: http://www.ncbi.nlm.nih.gov/pubmed/12283219 (accessed on 6 October 2020).
2. Foley, J.A.; DeFries, R.; Asner, G.P.; Barford, C.; Bonan, G.; Carpenter, S.R.; Chapin, F.S.; Coe, M.T.; Daily, G.C.; Gibbs, H.K.; et al. Global Consequences of Land Use. *Science* **2005**, *309*, 570–574. [CrossRef] [PubMed]
3. Vermeulen, S.J.; Campbell, B.M.; Ingram, J. Climate Change and Food Systems. *Annu. Rev. Environ. Resour.* **2012**, *37*, 195–222. [CrossRef]
4. Molden, D. *Water for Food Water for Life*; Routledge: London, UK, 2013.
5. Steffen, W.; Richardson, K.; Rockström, J.; Cornell, S.E.; Fetzer, I.; Bennett, E.; Biggs, R.; Carpenter, S.R.; De Vries, W.; De Wit, C.A.; et al. Planetary boundaries: Guiding human development on a changing planet. *Science* **2015**, *347*, 1259855. [CrossRef] [PubMed]
6. Willett, W.; Rockström, J.; Loken, B.; Springmann, M.; Lang, T.; Vermeulen, S.; Garnett, T.; Tilman, D.; Declerck, F.; Wood, A.; et al. Food in the Anthropocene: The EAT–Lancet Commission on healthy diets from sustainable food systems. *Lancet* **2019**, *393*, 447–492. [CrossRef]
7. Berry, E.M.; Dernini, S.; Burlingame, B.; Meybeck, A.; Conforti, P. Food security and sustainability: Can one exist without the other? *Public Health Nutr.* **2015**, *18*, 2293–2302. [CrossRef] [PubMed]
8. Food Security and Nutrition—Building a Global Narrative towards 2030. Available online: http://www.fao.org/3/ca9731en/ca9731en.pdf (accessed on 6 October 2020).
9. Food and Agriculture Organization of the United Nations. World Health Organization. Sustainable Healthy diets—Guiding Principles. Available online: http://www.fao.org/documents/card/en/c/ca6640en/ (accessed on 6 October 2020).
10. Dernini, S.; Berry, E.M. Mediterranean Diet: From a Healthy Diet to a Sustainable Dietary Pattern. *Front. Nutr.* **2015**, *2*, 15. [CrossRef] [PubMed]
11. Willett, W.C.; Sacks, F.; Trichopoulou, A.; Drescher, G.; Ferro-Luzzi, A.; Helsing, E.; Trichopoulos, D. Mediterranean diet pyramid: A cultural model for healthy eating. *Am. J. Clin. Nutr.* **1995**, *61* (Suppl. 6), 1402S–1406S. [CrossRef]
12. Trichopoulou, A. Diversity v. globalization: Traditional foods at the epicentre. *Public Health Nutr.* **2012**, *15*, 951–954. [CrossRef]
13. Dernini, S.; Berry, E.; Serra-Majem, L.; La Vecchia, C.; Capone, R.; Medina, F.; Aranceta-Bartrina, J.; Belahsen, R.; Burlingame, B.; Calabrese, G.; et al. Med Diet 4.0: The Mediterranean diet with four sustainable benefits. *Public Health Nutr.* **2017**, *20*, 1322–1330. [CrossRef]
14. Bach-Faig, A.; Berry, E.M.; Lairon, D.; Reguant, J.; Trichopoulou, A.; Dernini, S.; Medina, F.X.; Battino, M.; Belahsen, R.; Miranda, G.; et al. Mediterranean diet pyramid today. Science and cultural updates. *Public Health Nutr.* **2011**, *14*, 2274–2284. [CrossRef]
15. Serra-Majem, L.; Roman, B.; Estruch, R. Scientific evidence of interventions using the Mediterranean Diet: A systematic review. *Nutr. Rev.* **2006**, *64* (Suppl. 1), S21–S47. [CrossRef]
16. Sofi, F.; Cesari, F.; Abbate, R.; Gensini, G.F.; Casini, A. Adherence to Mediterranean diet and health status: Meta-analysis. *BMJ* **2008**, *337*, a1344. [CrossRef] [PubMed]
17. Benetou, V.; Trichopoulou, A.; Orfanos, P.; Naska, A.; Lagiou, P.; Boffetta, P.; Trichopoulos, D. Conformity to traditional Mediterranean diet and cancer incidence: The Greek EPIC cohort. *Br. J. Cancer* **2008**, *99*, 191–195. [CrossRef] [PubMed]
18. Estruch, R.; Ros, E.; Salas-Salvadó, J.; Covas, M.-I.; Corella, D.; Arós, F.; Gómez-Gracia, E.; Ruiz-Gutiérrez, V.; Fiol, M.; Lapetra, J.; et al. Primary Prevention of Cardiovascular Disease with a Mediterranean Diet Supplemented with Extra-Virgin Olive Oil or Nuts. *N. Engl. J. Med.* **2018**, *378*, e34. [CrossRef] [PubMed]
19. Kargın, D.; Tomaino, L.; Serra-Majem, L. Experimental Outcomes of the Mediterranean Diet: Lessons Learned from the Predimed Randomized Controlled Trial. *Nutrients* **2019**, *11*, 2991. [CrossRef]
20. Martínez-González, M.A.; Salas-Salvadó, J.; Estruch, R.; Corella, D.; Fitó, M.; Ros, E. Benefits of the Mediterranean Diet: Insights from the PREDIMED Study. *Prog. Cardiovasc. Dis.* **2015**, *58*, 50–60. [CrossRef]
21. Martínez-González, M.Á.; Bes-Rastrollo, M.; Serra-Majem, L.; Lairon, D.; Estruch, R.; Trichopoulou, A. Mediterranean food pattern and the primary prevention of chronic disease: Recent developments. *Nutr. Rev.* **2009**, *67*, S111–S116. [CrossRef]

22. Serra-Majem, L.; Román-Viñas, B.; Sanchez-Villegas, A.; Guasch-Ferré, M.; Corella, D.; La Vecchia, C. Benefits of the Mediterranean diet: Epidemiological and molecular aspects. *Mol. Asp. Med.* **2019**, *67*, 1–55. [CrossRef]
23. E Nelson, M.; Hamm, M.W.; Hu, F.B.; Abrams, S.A.; Griffin, T.S. Alignment of Healthy Dietary Patterns and Environmental Sustainability: A Systematic Review. *Adv. Nutr.* **2016**, *7*, 1005–1025. [CrossRef]
24. Aleksandrowicz, L.; Green, R.; Joy, E.J.M.; Smith, P.; Haines, A. The Impacts of Dietary Change on Greenhouse Gas Emissions, Land Use, Water Use, and Health: A Systematic Review. *PLoS ONE* **2016**, *11*, e0165797. [CrossRef]
25. Tilman, D.; Clark, M. Global diets link environmental sustainability and human health. *Nat. Cell Biol.* **2014**, *515*, 518–522. [CrossRef] [PubMed]
26. Baudry, J.; Pointereau, P.; Seconda, L.; Vidal, R.; Taupier-Letage, B.; Langevin, B.; Allès, B.; Galan, P.; Hercberg, S.; Amiot, M.-J.; et al. Improvement of diet sustainability with increased level of organic food in the diet: Findings from the BioNutriNet cohort. *Am. J. Clin. Nutr.* **2019**, *109*, 1173–1188. [CrossRef] [PubMed]
27. Sáez-Almendros, S.; Obrador, B.; Bach-Faig, A.; Serra-Majem, L. Environmental footprints of Mediterranean versus Western dietary patterns: Beyond the health benefits of the Mediterranean diet. *Environ. Health* **2013**, *12*, 118. [CrossRef] [PubMed]
28. Fresán, U.; Martínez-González, M.-A.; Sabaté, J.; Bes-Rastrollo, M. The Mediterranean diet, an environmentally friendly option: Evidence from the Seguimiento Universidad de Navarra (SUN) cohort. *Public Health Nutr.* **2018**, *21*, 1573–1582. [CrossRef] [PubMed]
29. Fresán, U.; Martínez-González, M.A.; Sabaté, J.; Bes-Rastrollo, M. Global sustainability (health, environment and monetary costs) of three dietary patterns: Results from a Spanish cohort (the SUN project). *BMJ Open* **2019**, *9*, e021541. [CrossRef] [PubMed]
30. Seconda, L.; Baudry, J.; Allès, B.; Hamza, O.; Boizot-Szantai, C.; Soler, L.-G.; Galan, P.; Hercberg, S.; Lairon, D.; Kesse-Guyot, E. Assessment of the Sustainability of the Mediterranean Diet Combined with Organic Food Consumption: An Individual Behaviour Approach. *Nutrients* **2017**, *9*, 61. [CrossRef] [PubMed]
31. Serra Majem, L.; Medina, F.X. The Mediterranean Diet as an Intangible and Sustainable Food Culture. In *The Mediterranean Diet: An Evidence-Based Approach*; Academic Press: London, UK, 2015; pp. 37–46.
32. Medina, F.X. Mediterranean diet, culture and heritage: Challenges for a new conception. *Public Health Nutr.* **2009**, *12*, 1618–1620. [CrossRef]
33. Medina, F.X. Food consumption and civil society: Mediterranean diet as a sustainable resource for the Mediterranean area. *Public Health Nutr.* **2011**, *14*, 2346–2349. [CrossRef]
34. CIHEAM/FAO. Mediterranean food consumption patterns: Diet, environment, society, economy and health. In *A White Paper Priority 5 of Feeding Knowledge Programme Expo Milan 2015*; CIHEAM-Bari/FAO: Rome, Italy, 2015.
35. Burlingame, B.; Dernini, S. Sustainable diets: The Mediterranean diet as an example. *Public Health Nutr.* **2011**, *14*, 2285–2287. [CrossRef]
36. Donini, L.M.; Serra-Majem, L.; Bulló, M.; Gil, Á.; Salas-Salvadó, J. The Mediterranean diet: Culture, health and science. *Br. J. Nutr.* **2015**, *113*, S1–S3. [CrossRef]
37. Gussow, J.D. Mediterranean diets: Are they environmentally responsible? *Am. J. Clin. Nutr.* **1995**, *61*, 1383S–1389S. [CrossRef] [PubMed]
38. Galli, A.; Iha, K.; Halle, M.; El Bilali, H.; Grunewald, N.; Eaton, D.; Capone, R.; Debs, P.; Bottalico, F. Mediterranean countries' food consumption and sourcing patterns: An Ecological Footprint viewpoint. *Sci. Total Environ.* **2017**, *578*, 383–391. [CrossRef] [PubMed]
39. Grosso, G.; Fresán, U.; Bes-Rastrollo, M.; Marventano, S.; Galvano, F. Environmental Impact of Dietary Choices: Role of the Mediterranean and other Dietary Patterns in an Italian Cohort. *Int. J. Environ. Res. Public Health* **2020**, *17*, 1468. [CrossRef] [PubMed]
40. De Boer, J.; Helms, M.; Aiking, H. Protein consumption and sustainability: Diet diversity in EU-15. *Ecol. Econ.* **2006**, *59*, 267–274. [CrossRef]
41. Berry, E.M. Sustainable Food Systems and the Mediterranean Diet. *Nutrients* **2019**, *11*, 2229. [CrossRef] [PubMed]
42. Medina, F.X.; De Moura, A.P.; Vázquez-Medina, J.A.; Frías, J.; Aguilar-Martínez, A. Feeding the online: Perspectives on food, nutrition and the online higher education. *Int. J. Educ. Technol. High. Educ.* **2019**, *16*, 1–8. [CrossRef]

43. Donini, L.M.; Dernini, S.; Lairon, D.; Serra-Majem, L.; Amiot, M.-J.; Del Balzo, V.; Giusti, A.-M.; Burlingame, B.; Belahsen, R.; Maiani, G.; et al. A Consensus Proposal for Nutritional Indicators to Assess the Sustainability of a Healthy Diet: The Mediterranean Diet as a Case Study. *Front. Nutr.* **2016**, *3*. [CrossRef]
44. World Health Organization. Dietary Recommendations/Nutritional Requirements List of Publications. 2020. Available online: https://www.who.int/nutrition/publications/nutrientrequirements/en/ (accessed on 23 June 2020).
45. Sustainable Diets and Biodiversity. Available online: https://www.bioversityinternational.org/e-library/publications/detail/sustainable-diets-and-biodiversity/ (accessed on 23 June 2020).
46. Kesse-Guyot, E.; Chaltiel, D.; Wang, J.; Pointereau, P.; Langevin, B.; Allès, B.; Rebouillat, P.; Lairon, D.; Vidal, R.; Mariotti, F.; et al. Sustainability analysis of French dietary guidelines using multiple criteria. *Nat. Sustain.* **2020**, *3*, 377–385. [CrossRef]
47. Elbersen, B.; Beaufoy, G.; Jones, G.; Noij, I.; Van Doorn, A.; Breman, B. Aspects of Data on Diverse Relationships between Agriculture and the Environment. Rep DG-Environment Contract no 07-0307/2012/633993/ETU/B1 Alterra Wageningen, April 2014 [Internet]. 2012. Available online: http://library.wur.nl/WebQuery/wurpubs/456846 (accessed on 6 October 2020).
48. European Commission DG Environment. *Integrated Crop Managementsystems in the EU*; DG Environ: Brussels, Belgium, 2002.
49. Hart, K.; Allen, B.; Lindner, M.; Keenleyside, C.; Burgess, P.; Eggers, J.; Buckwell, A. Land as an Environmental Resource. February 2013, p. 262. Available online: http://ec.europa.eu/environment/agriculture/pdf/LER-FinalReport.pdf (accessed on 6 October 2020).
50. High Nature Value Farming throughout EU-27 and Its Financial Support under the CAP Executive Summary. Available online: https://ec.europa.eu/environment/agriculture/pdf/High%20Nature%20Value%20farming.pdf (accessed on 6 October 2020).
51. Springmann, M.; Mason-D'Croz, D.; Robinson, S.; Garnett, T.; Godfray, H.C.J.; Gollin, D.; Rayner, M.; Ballon, P.; Scarborough, P. Global and regional health effects of future food production under climate change: A modelling study. *Lancet* **2016**, *387*, 1937–1946. [CrossRef]
52. Greenhouse Gas Emission Statistics-Emission Inventories (Redirected from Greenhouse Gas Emission Statistics). Available online: https://ec.europa.eu/eurostat/statistics-explained/index.php?title=Greenhouse_gas_emission_statistics&redirect=no#Trends_in_greenhouse_gas_emissions (accessed on 9 March 2020).
53. United Nations. Sustainable Development Goals. 2020. Available online: https://www.un.org/sustainabledevelopment/sustainable-development-goals/ (accessed on 23 June 2020).
54. Strapasson, A.; Woods, J.; Mbuk, K. Land Use Futures in Europe. *Grantham Inst. Brief. Pap.* **2016**, *17*, 16.
55. Estruch, R.; Ros, E.; Salas-Salvadó, J.; Covas, M.-I.; Corella, D.; Arós, F.; Gómez-Gracia, E.; Ruiz-Gutiérrez, V.; Fiol, M.; Lapetra, J.; et al. Mediterranean diet for primary prevention of cardiovascular disease. *N. Engl. J. Med.* **2013**, *368*, 1279–1290. [CrossRef]
56. Bosetti, C.; Pelucchi, C.; La Vecchia, C. Diet and cancer in Mediterranean countries: Carbohydrates and fats. *Public Health Nutr.* **2009**, *12*, 1595–1600. [CrossRef] [PubMed]
57. Perezjimenez, F.; Lista, J.D.; Pérez-Jiménez, F.; Lopez-Segura, F.; Fuentes, F.; Cortes, B.; Lozano, A.; Miranda, J.L. Olive oil and haemostasis: A review on its healthy effects. *Public Health Nutr.* **2006**, *9*, 1083–1088. Available online: https://www.cambridge.org/core/product/identifier/S1368980007668566/type/journal_article (accessed on 6 March 2020). [CrossRef]
58. Pelucchi, C.; Bosetti, C.; Negri, E.; Lipworth, L.; La Vecchia, C. Olive oil and cancer risk: An update of epidemiological findings through 2010. *Curr. Pharm. Des.* **2011**, *17*, 805–812. [CrossRef]
59. La Vecchia, C. Association between Mediterranean dietary patterns and cancer risk. *Nutr. Rev.* **2009**, *67*, S126–S129. [CrossRef] [PubMed]
60. Beaufoy, G. The Environmental Impact of Olive Oil Production in the European Union. *Eur. Com.* **2000**, *52100–521073*. Available online: http://ec.europa.eu/environment/agriculture/pdf/oliveoil.pdf (accessed on 6 October 2020).
61. International Olive Oil Council. Newsletter: INTERNATIONAL OLIVE COUNCIL. 2019. Available online: https://www.internationaloliveoil.org/wp-content/uploads/2019/12/NEWSLETTER_144_ENGLISH.pdf (accessed on 6 October 2020).
62. Salomone, R.; Ioppolo, G. Environmental impacts of olive oil production: A Life Cycle Assessment case study in the province of Messina (Sicily). *J. Clean. Prod.* **2012**, *28*, 88–100. [CrossRef]

63. Tsarouhas, P.; Achillas, C.; Aidonis, D.; Folinas, D.; Maslis, V. Life Cycle Assessment of olive oil production in Greece. *J. Clean. Prod.* **2015**, *93*, 75–83. [CrossRef]
64. Granitto, Y. Sustainable Olive Oil Production Helps Mitigate Climate Change. 2016. Available online: https://www.oliveoiltimes.com/production/sustainable-olive-oil-production-can-help-mitigate-climate-change/53615 (accessed on 6 October 2020).
65. Barthel, M.; Jennings, S.; Schreiber, W.; Sheane, R.; Royston, S.; Fry, J.; Khor, Y.L.; McGill, J. *Study on the Environmental Impact of Palm Oil Consumption and on Existing Sustainability Standards*; DG Environment: Brussels, Belgium, 2018.
66. De Souza, R.G.M.; Schincaglia, R.M.; Pimentel, G.D.; Mota, J.F. Nuts and Human Health Outcomes: A Systematic Review. *Nutrients* **2017**, *9*, 1311. [CrossRef]
67. National Health and Medical Research Council (2013) Australian Dietary Guidelines. Canberra: National Health and Medical Research Council. Available online: https://www.eatforhealth.gov.au/sites/default/files/files/the_guidelines/n55_australian_dietary_guidelines.pdf (accessed on 6 October 2020).
68. Eu Science Hub. Summary of FBDG Recommendations for Milk and Dairy Products for the the EU, Iceland, Norway, Switzerland and the United Kingdom. Available online: https://ec.europa.eu/jrc/en/health-knowledge-gateway/promotion-prevention/nutrition/food-based-dietary-guidelines (accessed on 22 June 2020).
69. The Environmental Impact of Dairy Production in the Eu: Practical Options for the Improvement of the Environmental Impact. Available online: https://ec.europa.eu/environment/agriculture/pdf/dairy.pdf (accessed on 6 October 2020).
70. Office of Dietary Supplements. Omega-3 Fatty Acids-Fact Sheet for Health Professionals. 2019. Available online: https://ods.od.nih.gov/factsheets/Omega3FattyAcids-HealthProfessional/ (accessed on 22 June 2020).
71. FAO. *The State of World Fisheries and Aquaculture 2020*; FAO: Rome, Italy, 2020; Available online: http://www.fao.org/documents/card/en/c/ca9229en (accessed on 6 October 2020).
72. Huntington, T.; Hasan, M.R. Fish as feed inputs for aquaculture–practices, sustainability and implications: A global synthesis. In *Fish as Feed inputs for Aquaculture: Practices, Sustainability and Implications FAO Fisheries and Aquaculture Technical Paper No 518*; Hasan, M., Halwart, M., Eds.; FAO: Rome, Italy, 2009; pp. 1–61.
73. Veronesi Burch, M.; Rigaud, A.; Binet, T.; Barthélemy, C.; Vertigo, L. *Circular Economy in Fisheries and Aquaculture Areas-Guide #17*; European Commission, Directorate-General for Maritime Affairs and Fisheries, Director-General: Luxembourg, 2019.
74. Abete, I.; Romaguera, D.; Vieira, A.R.; De Munain, A.L.; Norat, T. Association between total, processed, red and white meat consumption and all-cause, CVD and IHD mortality: A meta-analysis of cohort studies. *Br. J. Nutr.* **2014**, *112*, 762–775. [CrossRef]
75. Qian, F.; Riddle, M.C.; Wylie-Rosett, J.; Hu, F.B. Red and Processed Meats and Health Risks: How Strong Is the Evidence? *Diabetes Care* **2020**, *43*, 265–271. [CrossRef] [PubMed]
76. McMichael, A.J.; Powles, J.W.; Butler, C.D.; Uauy, R. Food, livestock production, energy, climate change, and health. *Lancet* **2007**, *370*, 1253–1263. [CrossRef]
77. EFSA. Scientific Opinion on Dietary Reference Values for water. *EFSA J.* **2010**, *8*, 1–48.
78. Botto, S. Tap Water vs. Bottled Water in a Footprint Integrated Approach. *Nat. Précéd.* **2009**. [CrossRef]
79. Medina, F.X. Food Culture: Anthropology of Food and Nutrition. In *Encyclopedia of Food Security and Sustainability*; Ferranti, P., Berry, E.M., Anderson, J.R., Eds.; Elsevier: Amsterdam, The Netherlands, 2019; pp. 307–310.
80. Barański, M.; Średnicka-Tober, D.; Volakakis, N.; Seal, C.; Sanderson, R.; Stewart, G.B.; Benbrook, C.; Biavati, B.; Markellou, E.; Giotis, C.; et al. Higher antioxidant and lower cadmium concentrations and lower incidence of pesticide residues in organically grown crops: A systematic literature review and meta-analyses. *Br. J. Nutr.* **2014**, *112*, 794–811. [CrossRef] [PubMed]
81. Kesse-Guyot, E.; Baudry, J.; Assmann, K.E.; Galan, P.; Hercberg, M.D.P.G.; Lairon, D. Prospective association between consumption frequency of organic food and body weight change, risk of overweight or obesity: Results from the NutriNet-Santé Study. *Br. J. Nutr.* **2017**, *117*, 325–334. Available online: https://www.cambridge.org/core/article/prospective-association-between-consumption-frequency-of-organic-food-and-body-weight-change-risk-of-overweight-or-obesity-results-from-the-nutrinetsante-study/1B800116CA8AFD21D26B6DF877EF7AC1 (accessed on 2 July 2017). [CrossRef]

82. Baudry, J.; Assmann, K.E.; Touvier, M.; Allès, B.; Seconda, L.; Latino-Martel, P.; Ezzedine, K.; Galan, P.; Hercberg, S.; Lairon, D.; et al. Association of Frequency of Organic Food Consumption with Cancer Risk. *JAMA Intern. Med.* **2018**, *178*, 1597–1606. [CrossRef]
83. Tong, T.Y.N.; Imamura, F.; Monsivais, P.; Brage, S.; Griffin, S.J.; Wareham, N.J.; Forouhi, N.G. Dietary cost associated with adherence to the Mediterranean diet, and its variation by socio-economic factors in the UK Fenland Study. *Br. J. Nutr.* **2018**, *119*, 685–694. [CrossRef]
84. Saulle, R.; Semyonov, L.; La Torre, G. Cost and Cost-Effectiveness of the Mediterranean Diet: Results of a Systematic Review. *Eur. J. Public Health* **2014**, *24*, 166–171. [CrossRef]
85. Food and Agriculture Organization of the United Nations. Proceedings of a Technical Workshop. Development of Voluntary Guidelines for the Sustainability of the Mediterranean Diet in the Mediterranean Region. 2017, p. 144. Available online: www.ciheam.org/en/publications (accessed on 6 October 2020).
86. Finnveden, G.; Hauschild, M.; Ekvall, T.; Guinée, J.; Heijungs, R.; Hellweg, S.; Koehler, A.; Pennington, D.W.; Suh, S. Recent developments in Life Cycle Assessment. *J. Environ. Manag.* **2009**, *91*, 1–21. [CrossRef]
87. Heller, M.C.; Keoleian, G.A.; Willett, W.C. Toward a Life Cycle-Based, Diet-level Framework for Food Environmental Impact and Nutritional Quality Assessment: A Critical Review. *Environ. Sci. Technol.* **2013**, *47*, 12632–12647. [CrossRef] [PubMed]
88. Muñoz, I.; I Canals, L.M.; Fernández-Alba, A.R. Life cycle assessment of the average Spanish diet including human excretion. *Int. J. Life Cycle Assess.* **2010**, *15*, 794–805. [CrossRef]
89. Pairotti, M.B.; Cerutti, A.K.; Martini, F.; Vesce, E.; Padovan, D.; Beltramo, R. Energy consumption and GHG emission of the Mediterranean diet: A systemic assessment using a hybrid LCA-IO method. *J. Clean. Prod.* **2015**, *103*, 507–516. [CrossRef]
90. Hoekstra, A.; Chapagain, A.; Aldaya, M.; Mekonnen, M. *The Water Footprint Assessment Manual*; Routledge: London, UK, 2011.
91. Vanham, D.; Del Pozo, S.; Pekcan, A.; Keinan-Boker, L.; Trichopoulou, A.; Gawlik, B. Water consumption related to different diets in Mediterranean cities. *Sci. Total Environ.* **2016**, *573*, 96–105. [CrossRef]
92. Blas, A.; Garrido, A.; Unver, O.; Willaarts, B. A comparison of the Mediterranean diet and current food consumption patterns in Spain from a nutritional and water perspective. *Sci. Total Environ.* **2019**, *664*, 1020–1029. [CrossRef]
93. Scarborough, P.; Appleby, P.N.; Mizdrak, A.; Briggs, A.D.M.; Travis, R.C.; Bradbury, K.E.; Key, T.J. Dietary greenhouse gas emissions of meat-eaters, fish-eaters, vegetarians and vegans in the UK. *Clim. Chang.* **2014**, *125*, 179–192. [CrossRef]
94. Seconda, L.; Baudry, J.; Allès, B.; Boizot-Szantai, C.; Soler, L.-G.; Galan, P.; Hercberg, S.; Langevin, B.; Lairon, D.; Pointereau, P.; et al. Comparing nutritional, economic, and environmental performances of diets according to their levels of greenhouse gas emissions. *Clim. Chang.* **2018**, *148*, 155–172. [CrossRef]
95. Lemoine, V.; Humez, M.; Bessarion, C. Santé Publique France. Recommandations sur L'alimentation, L'activité Physique e la Sédentarité Pour les Adultes. 2019. Available online: https://www.santepubliquefrance.fr (accessed on 6 October 2020).

Publisher's Note: MDPI stays neutral with regard to jurisdictional claims in published maps and institutional affiliations.

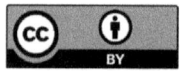

© 2020 by the authors. Licensee MDPI, Basel, Switzerland. This article is an open access article distributed under the terms and conditions of the Creative Commons Attribution (CC BY) license (http://creativecommons.org/licenses/by/4.0/).

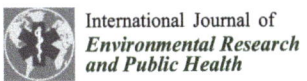

Commentary

Mediterranean Dietary Pyramid

Walter Willett

Departments of Nutrition and Epidemiology, Harvard T.H. Chan School of Public Health, Boston, MA 02115, USA; wwillett@hsph.harvard.edu

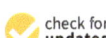

Citation: Willett, W. Mediterranean Dietary Pyramid. *Int. J. Environ. Res. Public Health* **2021**, *18*, 4568. https://doi.org/10.3390/ijerph18094568

Academic Editor: Paul B. Tchounwou

Received: 13 April 2021
Accepted: 23 April 2021
Published: 26 April 2021

Publisher's Note: MDPI stays neutral with regard to jurisdictional claims in published maps and institutional affiliations.

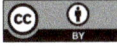

Copyright: © 2021 by the author. Licensee MDPI, Basel, Switzerland. This article is an open access article distributed under the terms and conditions of the Creative Commons Attribution (CC BY) license (https://creativecommons.org/licenses/by/4.0/).

The updated Mediterranean Dietary Pyramid (MDP) described by Serra-Majem et al. [1] is a highly welcome addition to the nutritional landscape, built on the solid foundations of earlier versions. As its construction over the last decade was a collective effort by an expanded circle of experts representing additional countries around the Mediterranean region, this update incorporates additional insights on regional dietary traditions and engages a broader network in the transformation of our food systems to be healthier and more sustainable. Although many new scientists have contributed to this effort, I am pleased to note the input of Antonia Trichopoulou, who has been a consistent, knowledgeable thread connecting the first MDP with this update.

The description of the foods comprising this updated pyramid has been fine tuned to be more specific and emphasize the central role of healthy plant foods and the modest role of meat, especially red meat, and dairy. This is consistent with Mediterranean dietary traditions, and the evidence linking this pattern with better health has strengthened with time. Notably, the EAT-Lancet commission, charged with identifying a pathway to healthy and sustainable diets for the expected world population by 2050, reviewed the available evidence on diet and health to develop global targets for specific food groups. When these targets were combined into an overall dietary pattern, they aligned tightly with the traditional Mediterranean diet as described in the updated MDP. This was invaluable proof that these targets were not just a conceptual goal but were consistent with a way of eating that had been tested over millennia and were found to be associated with well-documented longevity and wellbeing.

The fundamental innovation in the updated MDP is a dimension representing environmental sustainability. When my colleagues and I designed the first Traditional MDP in 1993, health effects were our focus. This was impactful because the emphasis of dietary guidelines had been to reduce dietary fat as much as possible and encourage high carbohydrate intake. This was not consistent with scientific evidence emerging at that time, and the MDP made a transformative statement that the type of fat, not total fat, was important for long-term health. At that time, we appreciated the importance of the environmental impacts of food systems, but most of us thought that the impact of climate change would be felt centuries into the future. Since then, global warming has accelerated, and we are already experiencing adverse effects in many ways. At present, we are far off track to achieve the United Nations goal of limiting temperature increases by 2100 to less than 2 degrees C; instead, we are on course for disastrous and irreversible environmental changes. Thus, environmental sustainability has become an urgent issue and the addition of this new dimension in the updated MDP is important and timely. Notably, work cited in this report suggests that the adoption of the traditional Mediterranean dietary pattern could reduce greenhouse gas emissions from the food system by half or more compared to current Western diets. This, combined with transition to green energy sources, could enable us to pass on a sustainable world to future generations. All countries can benefit by considering this updated MDP when developing their dietary guidelines and food systems.

Funding: This research received no external funding.

Institutional Review Board Statement: Not applicable.

Informed Consent Statement: Not applicable.

Data Availability Statement: No new data were created or analyzed in this study. Data sharing is not applicable to this article.

Conflicts of Interest: The author declares no conflict of interest.

Reference

1. Serra-Majem, L.; Tomaino, L.; Dernini, S.; Berry, E.M.; Lairon, D.; Ngo de la Cruz, J.; Bach-Faig, A.; Donini, L.M.; Medina, F.X.; Belahsen, R.; et al. Updating the Mediterranean Diet Pyramid towards Sustainability: Focus on Environmental Concerns. *Int. J. Environ. Res. Public Health* **2020**, *17*, 8758. [CrossRef] [PubMed]

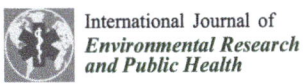

Commentary

Highlights of Current Dietary Guidelines in Five Continents

Maria Luz Fernandez [1,*], Dele Raheem [2], Fernando Ramos [3,4], Conrado Carrascosa [5], Ariana Saraiva [5] and António Raposo [6,*]

1. Department of Nutritional Sciences, University of Connecticut, Storrs, CT 06269, USA
2. Northern Institute for Environmental and Minority Law (NIEM), Arctic Centre, University of Lapland, 96101 Rovaniemi, Finland; braheem@ulapland.fi
3. Pharmacy Faculty, University of Coimbra, Azinhaga de Santa Comba, 3000-548 Coimbra, Portugal; framos@ff.uc.pt
4. REQUIMTE/LAQV, Rua Dom Manuel II, Apartado 55142, 4051-401 Oporto, Portugal
5. Department of Animal Pathology and Production, Bromatology and Food Technology, Faculty of Veterinary, Universidad de Las Palmas de Gran Canaria, Trasmontaña s/n, 35413 Arucas, Spain; conrado.carrascosa@ulpgc.es (C.C.); ariana_23@outlook.pt (A.S.)
6. CBIOS (Research Center for Biosciences and Health Technologies), Universidade Lusófona de Humanidades e Tecnologias, Campo Grande 376, 1749-024 Lisboa, Portugal
* Correspondence: maria-luz.fernandez@uconn.edu (M.L.F.); antonio.raposo@ulusofona.pt (A.R.)

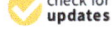

Abstract: The dietary guidelines as well as the organizations that establish the recommendations are not homogeneous across regions of the world. Each country utilizes specific icons to better describe to the public easy ways to follow specific recommendations, including the use of pyramids, plates, and other forms of presenting key information. All dietary guidelines are updated within certain periods to ensure that new findings or specific changes are communicated to the public. The purpose of this commentary is to describe the most updated information as well as some history on how these symbols are utilized in different countries or areas of the world. The updated Mediterranean pyramid as well as MyPlate and the Pyramids utilized in South Africa, Japan, and Argentina are discussed in this commentary.

Keywords: dietary guidelines; Mediterranean; the USA; Japan; Argentina; South Africa

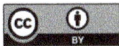

1. Introduction

The importance of communicating the dietary guidelines to the public in a comprehensive yet easy to follow approach is well-recognized [1]. Therefore, the need to identify the means to exemplify these guidelines led to the creation of dietary pyramids and MyPlate to better illustrate these recommendations. The first dietary pyramid was published in Sweden in 1974 followed by the United States (US) pyramid in 1992 [2]. The idea was to illustrate that foods that should be consumed in greater amounts should be located in the base of the pyramid, while those that should be eaten sparingly should be at the top [2]. Later, a number of countries decided to convey a similar message regarding specific guidelines, which followed cultural and regional food recommendations. An example is the Mediterranean Diet Pyramid, created in 1993, which illustrates the healthy food choices followed by the Mediterranean region.

Other dietary pyramids that were created early on and that have been recently updated are those from Argentina created in 2000, South Africa created in 2003, and Japan created in 2014. Recently, in June of 2011, The US Department of Agriculture (USDA) created MyPlate to have a better visualization of the recommended portions of different food groups including grains, vegetables, fruits, dairy, and high-protein foods [2].

The Food and Agriculture Organization (FAO) emphasized food-based dietary guidelines with key messages for many countries including USA, South Africa, Argentina, and Japan [3]. In this commentary, we have chosen to briefly discuss different representations of the updated dietary guidelines in five countries/regions. We highlight the way these recommendations are conveyed and briefly discuss their strengths and weaknesses.

2. Dietary Pyramid and My Plate

MyPlate (Figure 1) was created to substitute the US Dietary Pyramid in 2011 resulting in the ending of 19 Dietary Pyramids since 1992 [4]. MyPlate is the representation of a plate setting with a glass that includes five groups: grains, vegetables, fruits, protein foods, and dairy. Several strengths have been identified in how MyPlate is represented: (1) MyPlate has been adapted to cover the needs of pregnancy and breastfeeding, toddlers, children, adults, and older adults and thus is more precise in its recommendations across the life cycle [4]; (2) the web site created by USDA also provides a list of recipes and innovative ways to follow MyPlate; (3) MyPlate also recommends moderate to vigorous physical activity 150 min per week [5]. Further, studies have shown that following MyPlate contributes to the maintenance of a healthy body weight plus a lower risk of hypertension in adults over 50 years of age [6]. MyPlate also recommends more satiating foods to treat obesity rather than caloric counting. The key messages from MyPlate are to follow a healthy eating pattern that supports adequate nutrient intake to prevent the risk of chronic disease; to focus on a variety of nutrient dense foods; to limit calories from added sugars, saturated fat, and sodium; and to shift to healthier beverage choices.

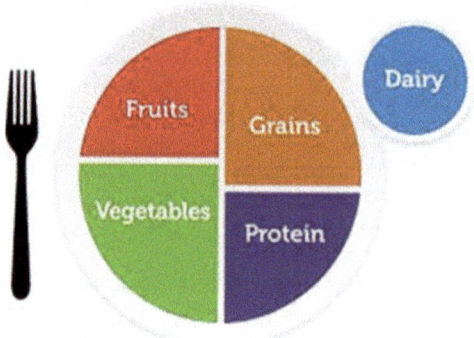

Figure 1. MyPlate [4].

Although MyPlate is the newest way by which USDA depicts dietary recommendations, the Pyramid is still used. There is a Harvard Dietary Pyramid (Figure 2), which in addition to including the type of foods that should be consumed most at the base of the pyramid also provides additional information regarding exercise and lifestyle practices [7]. This pyramid has several strengths that are worth mentioning: (1) the bottom of the pyramid, instead of including food groups, states the importance of both exercise and maintenance of a healthy body weight. (2) The food groups are arranged differently than in the original pyramid, since whole grains, healthy oils, fruits, and vegetables are recognized as the foods that should be consumed the most, followed by fish, poultry and eggs, nuts, seeds, and beans, of which equal intake is recommended; the next portion of the pyramid recommends dairy as well as Vitamin D and calcium supplements, and the tip of the pyramid includes red meat, butter, refined grains, sugar, and salt to consume in moderation. (3) Other recommendations include optional alcohol intake in moderation (not meant for all populations) and intake of daily multivitamin plus Vitamin D for most people.

THE HEALTHY EATING PYRAMID

Department of Nutrition, Harvard School of Public Health

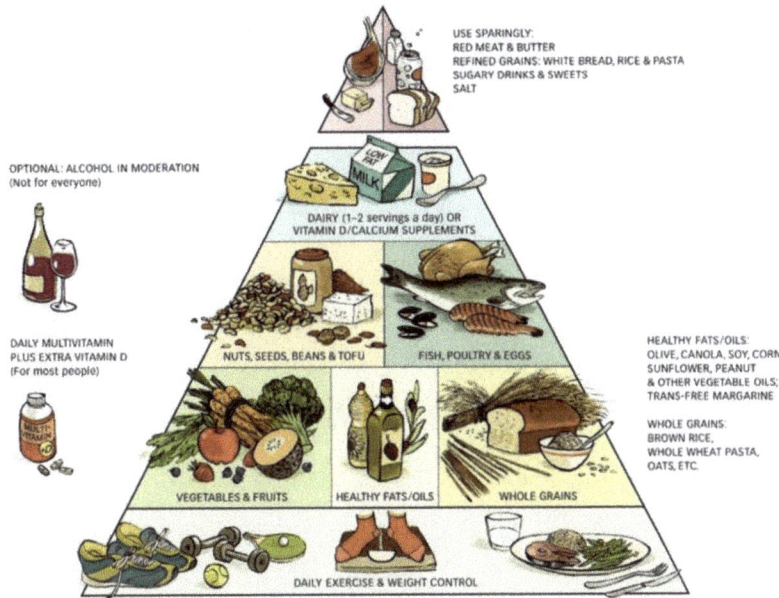

Figure 2. Harvard Dietary Pyramid [7]. Copyright © 2008. For more information about The Healthy Eating Pyramid, please see The Nutrition Source, Department of Nutrition, Harvard T.H. Chan School of Public Health, www.thenutritionsource.org (accessed on 1 February 2021), and Eat, Drink, and Be Healthy, by Walter C. Willett, M.D. and Patrick J. Skerrett (2005), Free Press/Simon & Schuster Inc.

These two approaches for dietary recommendations in US have a number of strengths in that they do not only focus on foods but also on maintenance of healthy body weight and exercise. However, they do not address sustainability or environmental concerns associated with food production.

3. Mediterranean Diet Pyramid

Serra-Majem et al. recently reported the updated Mediterranean Diet Pyramid (MDP) (Figure 3) [8], a sequel of the previous study by Bach-Faig et al. [9], which summarized and updated the traditional Mediterranean Diet (MD) of those basin areas that have developed with modernization. This region includes all the countries that surround the Mediterranean Sea: France, Portugal, Italy Spain, Greece, Malta, and Cyprus, which is characterized by specific climate and by a biodiversity of species [10].

The MDP was a shared and dynamic cultural heritage recognized in 2010 by UNESCO [8]. This updated MDP highlights the fact that it takes into consideration not only nutrition but also sustainability and the environment as well as economic implications and sociocultural factors and comprises the combined effort of a number of expert individuals who updated the pyramid based on current challenges that Mediterranean populations are confronting [8]. This updated MDP constitutes a logical follow-up to the original MDP that was created in 1993 and updated in 2010 by a group of professionals and organizations who have dedicated many years to the evaluation and promotion of the MD [11]. Such collaborative efforts on the Med Diet 4.0 framework in the years 2015 and 2016 and the early part of 2020 led to a continuous update of the MDP.

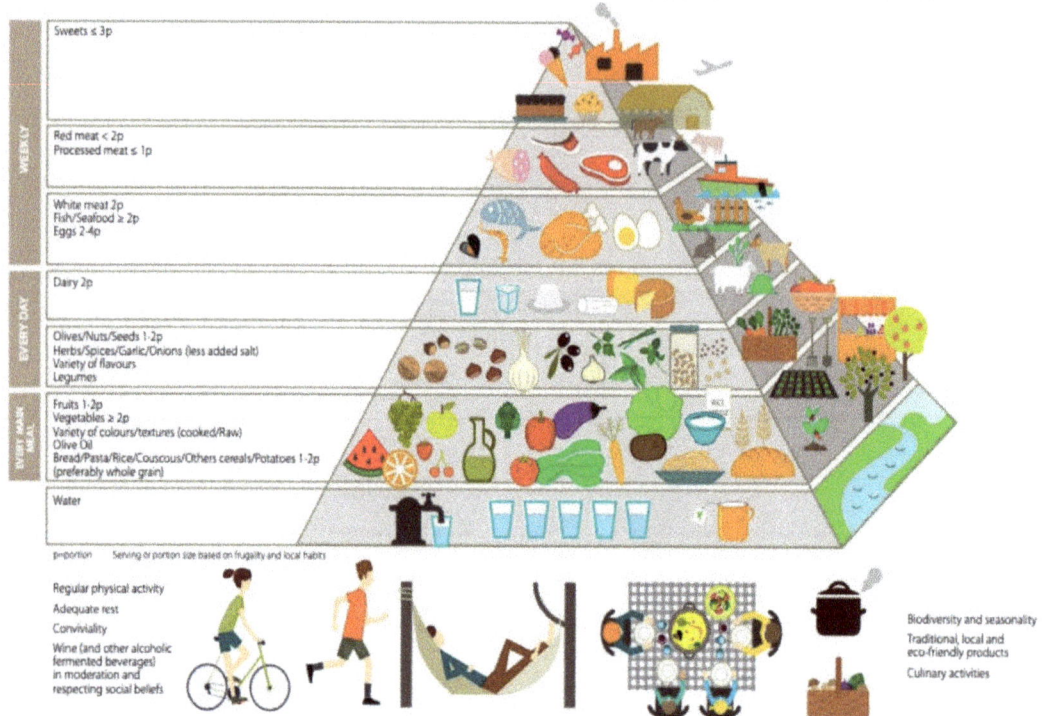

Figure 3. Updated Mediterranean Diet Pyramid [8].

It is well established that the MD has been recognized as a healthy diet that not only protects against chronic disease including heart disease, Type-2 diabetes, and cancer, but also provides numerous healthy dietary components that promote health and well-being [12,13]. The updated pyramid provides very detailed information on the main food items that constitute the MD as well as a clear description of the different nutrients and antioxidants present in foods and their precise role in promoting health. A clear description of the portions that should be consumed either daily or weekly is also included, which are easy to follow and comprehend. In addition, authors rationalize that different countries adapt the components of the MD according to their own traditions, an example being the consumption of wine that is replaced by herbal teas in Muslim societies. Since a healthy dietary pattern needs to be linked to food production and sustainability [14,15], the updated MDP, in addition to the well-described nutritional components of the diet, also emphasizes exercise, conviviality, biodiversity, and culinary activities associated with the consumption of eco-friendly local seasonal products.

A summary of the salient points of this MDP are presented in Figure 4, which exemplifies the benefits of the Mediterranean diet for (1) nutrition and health, (2) the environment, (3) the economy, and (4) sociocultural factors.

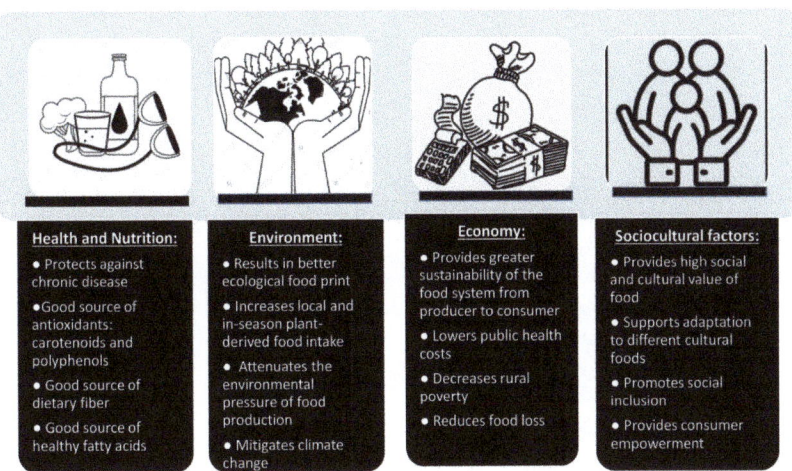

Figure 4. The updated Mediterranean Diet Pyramid is characterized for its contribution to Health and Nutrition, the Environment, the Economy and the incorporation of Sociocultural Factors. Some of the elements supporting these claims are depicted in this figure.

The Mediterranean Diet (MD) is unique as it complies with at least 11 out of 17 goals of the United Nations Sustainable Development Goals (SDGs), mainly SDG2–SDG8 and SDG11–SDG15 [8], which are related to Zero Hunger, Good Health, Quality Education, Gender Equity, Clean Water, Affordable and Clean Energy, Economic Growth, Sustainable Cities and Communities, Responsible Consumption and Production, Climate Action, and Life Below Water [8].

4. South African Dietary Pyramid

South Africa first published food-based dietary guidelines (FBDG) in 2003. A revised version was launched in 2012 (Figure 5). Seven differently sized circles are used by the Circles of South Africa to "symbolically reflect the proportional volume that the group should contribute to the total daily diet" [16]. Each circle reflects a food group and healthy eating recommendations that are associated. In order to preserve good health, the South African model reflects what should be consumed, as opposed to what should be avoided. The key messages are related to specific foods consumed in that region, including starchy foods, dry beans, split peas, lentils, and soy, and it also emphasizes the consumption of fruit and vegetables. The South African Pyramid also recommends to drink milk every day as well as to consume fish, lean meat, and eggs daily while emphasizing that sugars, saturated fat, and salt should be eaten sparingly.

Food groups are not written on the FBDG image itself; however, they are otherwise indicated in the accompanying FBDG [16]. As exemplified by ethnically varied staples such as corn meal, rice, potatoes, and bread, the main group includes distinct grains and starches. These starchy foods make up the largest of the seven circles, a relatively large part of the proposed South African diet. In the next larger circle, fresh fruits and vegetables are pictured; the overall amount ingested should be somewhat equal to that of starches, since the circle is somewhat narrower. By analogy, legumes, animal proteins, and dairy products, as indicated by their smaller circle sizes, are to be eaten in comparatively smaller volumes. The South African model illustrates socio-economic facts and accessibility problems, as numerous items are sold in boxes, bags, cans, plastic jugs, and cartons, since not everybody can afford fresh ingredients. Fats and oils make up the smallest group, while water and tea are placed at the top. Compared to other dietary guidelines, the FBDG shows the relevance of daily water consumption by placing the image at the top of the graph.

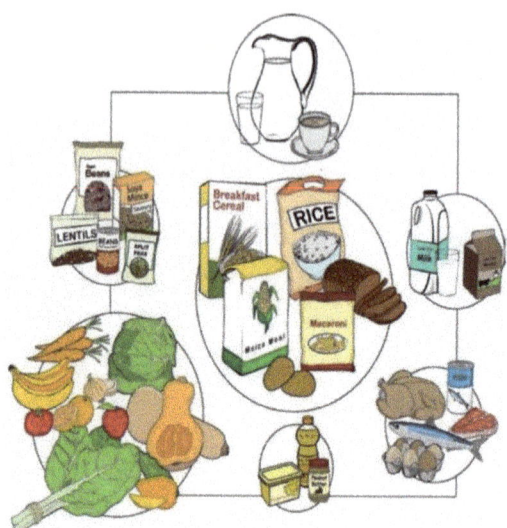

Figure 5. Food-based dietary guidelines (South Africa) [3].

5. Argentinian Dietary Pyramid

Argentina first launched its food-based dietary guidelines and food guide in 2000. They were revised in 2015 (Figure 6). The Dietary Guidelines for the Argentinian Population (DGAP) constitute a fundamental tool to promote the dissemination of knowledge. The DGAP are an educational instrument whose main aim is to promote more equitable intake of healthy food as well as improved dietary behaviors in the whole country. They translate the nutritional goals established for Argentina into practical messages, written in simple and understandable language. This pyramid, in addition to the recommendations of consuming five portions of fruits and vegetables, milk, yogurt, and cheese daily, has specific recommendations, including drinking eight glasses of water per day and 30 minutes of physical activity daily, plus it emphasizes that alcohol should not be consumed while driving and pregnant women and children should not drink alcohol.

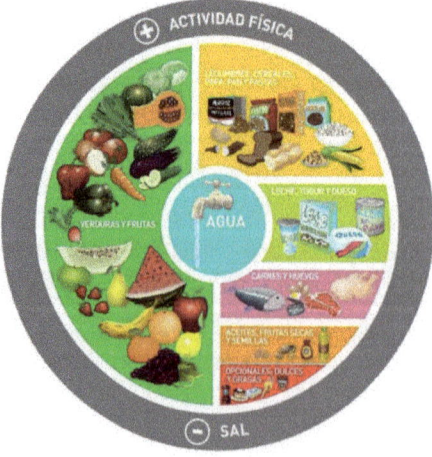

Figure 6. Food-based dietary guidelines—Argentina [3].

The DGAP are also a planning tool for the sectors of health, education, production, industry, commerce, and all those who work in the food area [17]. The highlighted recommendations include the consumption of safe water, the practice of physical activity, the lower consumption of salt and a higher consumption of fibers, polyunsaturated fatty acids with a decrease in the consumption of saturated fats and sugars [17,18]. However, the Argentinian pyramid does not address sustainability or the environment.

6. Japanese Dietary Pyramid

In 2005, the Japanese government launched the Japanese Food Guide Spinning Top (JFG) to help Japanese citizens adopt nutritional recommendations to encourage healthier eating [19]. The JFG was revised in 2010 (Figure 7), and it is distinctive in that the quantity of food eaten in a daily diet is represented in amounts of the "dish" rather than in the "food" format and it uses the analogy of the shape of a spinning top, which reflects an element of Japanese culture [19].

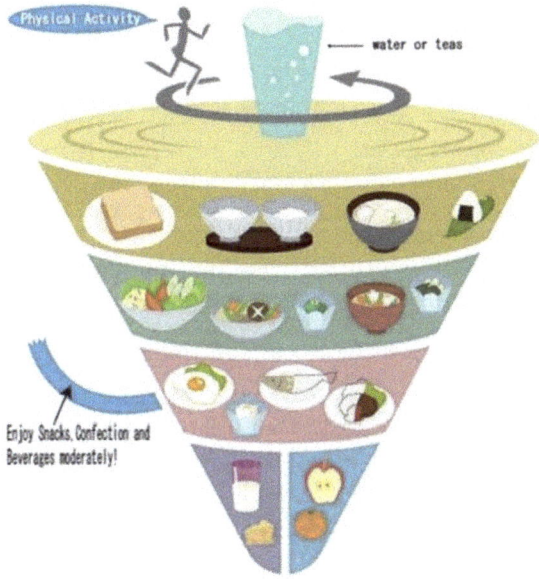

Figure 7. Japanese Food Guide Spinning Top [3].

The following categories of food are included in the JFG: grain dishes (rice, bread, noodles, etc.), vegetable dishes (vegetables, mushrooms, potatoes, and seaweed), fish and meat dishes (meat, fish, eggs, soybeans, etc.), milk (milk and milk products), fruit, confectionaries, sugar-sweetened drinks, and alcoholic drinks. The order of the food groups is determined by the size of the specified daily servings. It is advised to eat a combination of the food groups daily. There are special messages emphasized by this pyramid, including keeping regular hours for meals, enjoying the meals, maintaining a healthy body weight by physical activity, using proper cooking and storage methods, and tracking your food to monitor your diet.

The JFG is a valuable instrument for the assessment of Japanese people's dietary consistency [20]. Previous investigations assessing the degree of compliance to the JFG (Food Guide score) have identified correlations between the Food Guide score and the risk of total mortality [21], depressive symptoms [22], and metabolic risk factors [23]. However, the JFG does not address environmental issues or take into consideration the economy.

7. Conclusions

In summary, all the updated pyramids and MyPlate provide more detailed information on nutrient consumption and food groups and include exercise as an important component, [3,4,8,16,17,19]. Further, they all cater to the specific socio-cultural factors of each country or region. However, most of the updated pyramids with the exception of the MDP do not address the environment or the sustainability of local production. The South African Pyramid does address the economy. The MDP addresses all these important points, resulting in a stronger message to consumers. It would be important that the US, Japan, Argentina, and South Africa update their recommendations, taking into consideration the environment and the economy. The major points addressed by of each of these pyramids is depicted in Table 1.

Table 1. Points addressed by the Updated Pyramids from MyPlate and the Harvard Pyramid in the US, the Updated Mediterranean Pyramid (UMP), and the Argentinian and Japanese Pyramids.

Dietary Pyramids	Clear Dietary Recommendations	Physical Activity	Socio-Cultural Factors	Environment	Economy
MyPlate	Yes	Yes	Yes	No	No
Harvard Pyramid	Yes	Yes	Yes	No	No
UMP	Yes	Yes	Yes	Yes	Yes
South African Pyramid	Yes	Yes	Yes	No	Yes
Argentinian Pyramid	Yes	Yes	Yes	No	No
Japanese Pyramid	Yes	Yes	Yes	No	No

Author Contributions: M.L.F. developed the layout of the manuscript, edited the content, and designed the figure. D.R., F.R., C.C., A.S., and A.R. critically evaluated the draft and edited the content. All authors have read and agreed to the published version of the manuscript.

Funding: This article received no external funding.

Conflicts of Interest: The authors declare no conflict of interest.

References

1. Pencina, M.J.; Millen, B.E.; Hayes, L.J.; D'Agostino, J.B. Performance of a Method for identifying the Unique Dietary Patterns of Adult Women and Men: The Framingham Nutrition Studies. *J. Am. Diet. Assoc.* **2008**, *108*, 1453–1460. [CrossRef] [PubMed]
2. U.S. Department of Agriculture; U.S. Department of Health and Human Services. *Nutrition and Your Health: Dietary Guidelines for Americans 1995*, 4th ed.; US Department of Agriculture and US Department of Health and Humans Services: Washington, DC, USA, 1995.
3. FAO. Food-based Dietary Guidelines for Countries and Regions. 2021. Available online: http://www.fao.org/nutrition/education/food-dietary-guidelines/home/en/ (accessed on 1 February 2021).
4. U.S Department of Agriculture. Available online: https://www.myplate.gov/ (accessed on 1 February 2021).
5. Gelberg, L.; Rico, M.W.; Herman, D.R.; Belin, T.R.; Chandler, M.; Ramirez, E.; Love, S.; McCarthy, W.J. Comparative effectiveness trial comparing MyPlate to calorie counting for mostly low-income Latino primary care patients of a federally quali-fied community health center: Study design, baseline characteristics. *BMC Public Health* **2019**, *19*, 990. [CrossRef] [PubMed]
6. Vernarelli, J.; Di Sarrro, R. Forget the Fad Diets: Use of the Usda's Myplate Plan Is Associated with Better Dietary Intake in Adults Over Age 50 (Or14-06-19). *Curr. Dev. Nutr.* **2019**, *3*. [CrossRef]
7. Harvard School of Public Health. Available online: https://www.hsph.harvard.edu/nutritionsource/healthy-eating-pyramid/ (accessed on 1 February 2021).
8. Serra-Majem, L.; Tomaino, L.; Dernini, S.; Berry, E.M.; Lairon, D.; Ngo de la Cruz, J.; Bach-Faig, A.; Donini, L.M.; Medina, F.-X.; Belahsen, R.; et al. Updating the Mediterranean diet Pyramid towards sustainability: Focus on environmental concerns. *Int. J. Environ. Res. Public Health* **2020**, *17*, 8758. [CrossRef] [PubMed]

9. Bach-Faig, A.; Berry, E.M.; Lairon, D.; Reguant, J.; Trichopoulou, A.; Dernini, S.; Xavier Medina, F.; Battino, M.; Belahsen, R.; Miranda, G.; et al. Mediterranean diet pyramid today. Science and cultural updates. *Public Health Nutr.* **2011**, *14*, 2274–2284. [CrossRef] [PubMed]
10. The Mediterranean Region. Available online: https://ec.europa.eu/environment/nature/natura2000/biogeog_regions/mediterranean/index_en.htm (accessed on 1 February 2021).
11. Willett, W.C.; Sacks, F.; Trichopoulou, A.; Drescher, G.; Ferro-Luzzi, A.; Helsing, E.; Trichopoulou, D. Mediterranean diet pyramid: A cultural model for healthy eating. *Am. J. Clin. Nutr.* **1995**, *61*, 1402S–1406S. [CrossRef] [PubMed]
12. Martinez-Gonzalez, M.A.; Salas-Salvado, J.; Estruch, R.; Corella, D.; Fito, M.; Ros, E. Mediterranean Diet: Insights from the PREDIMED Study. *Prog. Cardiovasc. Dis.* **2015**, *58*, 50–60. [CrossRef] [PubMed]
13. Sofi, F.; Abbate, R.; Gensini, G.F.; Casini, A. Adherence to the Mediterranean diet and health status: Meta-analysis. *BMJ* **2008**, *337*, a1344. [CrossRef] [PubMed]
14. Burlingame, B.; Dernini, S. Sustainable diets: The Mediterranean diet as an example. *Public Health Nutr.* **2011**, *14*, 2285–2287. [CrossRef] [PubMed]
15. Nelson, M.E.; Hamm, M.W.; Hu, F.B.; Abrams, S.A.; Griffin, T.S. Alignment of Healthy Dietary Patterns and Environmental Sustainability: A Systematic Review. *Adv. Nutr.* **2016**, *7*, 1005–1025. [CrossRef] [PubMed]
16. Vorster, H.H.; Badham, J.B.; Venter, C.S. An introduction to the revised food-based dietary guidelines for South Africa. *South Afr. J. Clin. Nutr.* **2013**, *26*, S5–S12.
17. Fortino, A.; Vargas, M.; Berta, E.; Cuneo, F.; Ávila, O. Valoración de los patrones de consumo alimentario y actividad física en universitarios de tres carreras respecto a las guías alimentarias para la población argentina. *Rev. Chil. Nutr.* **2020**, *47*, 906–915. [CrossRef]
18. Arrieta, E.M.; González, A.D. Impact of current, National Dietary Guidelines and alternative diets on greenhouse gas emissions in Argentina. *Food Policy* **2018**, *79*, 58–66. [CrossRef]
19. Yoshiike, N.; Hayashi, F.; Takemi, Y.; Mizoguchi, K.; Seino, F. A new food guide in Japan: The Japanese food guide Spinning Top. *Nutr. Rev.* **2007**, *65*, 149–154. [CrossRef] [PubMed]
20. Yamamoto, K.; Ota, M.; Minematsu, A.; Motokawa, K.; Yokoyama, Y.; Yano, T.; Watanabe, Y.; Yoshizaki, T. Association between adherence to the Japanese food guide spinning top and sleep quality in college students. *Nutrients* **2018**, *10*, 1996. [CrossRef] [PubMed]
21. Kurotani, K.; Akter, S.; Kashino, I.; Goto, A.; Mizoue, T.; Noda, M.; Sasazuki, S.; Sawada, N.; Tsugane, S.; Japan Public Health Center based Prospective Study Group. Quality of diet and mortality among Japanese men and women: Japan Public Health Center based prospective study. *BMJ* **2016**, *352*, i1209. [CrossRef] [PubMed]
22. Sakai, H.; Murakami, K.; Kobayashi, S.; Suga, H.; Sasaki, S. Food-based diet quality score in relation to depressive symptoms in young and middle-aged Japanese women. *Br. J. Nutr.* **2017**, *117*, 1674–1681. [CrossRef] [PubMed]
23. Nishimura, T.; Murakami, K.; Livingstone, M.B.E.; Sasaki, S.; Uenishi, K. Adherence to the food-based Japanese dietary guidelines in relation to metabolic risk factors in young Japanese women. *Br. J. Nutr.* **2015**, *114*, 645–653. [CrossRef] [PubMed]

MDPI
St. Alban-Anlage 66
4052 Basel
Switzerland
Tel. +41 61 683 77 34
Fax +41 61 302 89 18
www.mdpi.com

International Journal of Environmental Research and Public Health Editorial Office
E-mail: ijerph@mdpi.com
www.mdpi.com/journal/ijerph

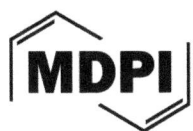

www.ingramcontent.com/pod-product-compliance
Lightning Source LLC
LaVergne TN
LVHW070249100526
838202LV00015B/2196